OXFORD MEDICAL PUBLICATIONS

Brain Systems, Disorders, and Psychotropic Drugs

Brain Systems, Disorders, and Psychotropic Drugs

HEATHER ASHTON

University of Newcastle upon Tyne

OXFORD   NEW YORK   TOKYO

OXFORD UNIVERSITY PRESS

1987

Oxford University Press, Walton Street, Oxford OX2 6DP
Oxford New York Toronto
Delhi Bombay Calcutta Madras Karachi
Petaling Jaya Singapore Hong Kong Tokyo
Nairobi Dar es Salaam Cape Town
Melbourne Auckland
and associated companies in
Beirut Berlin Ibadan Nicosia

Oxford is a trade mark of Oxford University Press

Published in the United States
by Oxford University Press, New York

British Library Cataloguing in Publication Data
Ashton, Heather
Brain systems, disorders and psychotropic
drugs.—(Oxford medical publications)
1. Nervous system—Diseases—Chemotherapy
I. Title
616.8'0461   RC350.C54
ISBN 0–19–261436–3

Library of Congress Cataloging-in-Publication Data
Ashton, Heather,
Brain systems, disorders, and psychotropic drugs.
(Oxford medical publications)
Bibliography: p.
Includes index
1. Psychotropic drugs—Physiological effect.
2. Brain.   3. Brain—Effect of drugs on.   4. Mental
illness—Chemotherapy.   5. Neuropsychopharmacology.
I. Title. II. Series.   [DNLM: 1. Brain—drug effects.
2. Brain—physiology.   3. Mental Disorders—
physiopathology.   4. Psychotropic Drugs—
pharmacodynamics.   WL 300 A828b]
RM315.A75   1986   615'.788   86-17971
ISBN 0–19–261436–3

Processed by the Oxford Text System
Printed in Great Britain
at The Alden Press, Oxford

Preface

My growing awareness of a need for a book of this kind stemmed from the requirement of teaching the principles of psychopharmacology to second year medical students. It was clear that the actions of psychotropic drugs could not be discussed without first giving some idea of the mechanisms of the disorders for which they are used. In turn, disorders of mood, thought, and behaviour are not comprehensible without a basic knowledge of the brain systems which normally control these variables. And so one is led full circle, for it is also necessary to know how psychotropic drugs affect normal brain function in order to interpret their effects on malfunctioning systems. How is it that many psychotropic drugs produce dysphoria in normal subjects yet improve symptoms in disturbed subjects, while others have euphoric effects in normal subjects but aggravate some mental disorders? A single book describing the brain systems which govern the behaviour of man, suggesting how these systems may malfunction to produce various types of mental disorder, and discussing how drugs might affect these systems, was not, to my knowledge, available.

From the viewpoint of research, a similar lack seemed to exist. In this case, a somewhat different order applies: Knowledge of pharmacodynamics can shed light on the mechanisms of brain disorders, and also on normal brain function. The partial illumination of anxiety disorders and of the GABA-receptor complex by benzodiazepines, of pain mechanisms and opioid receptors by opiate analgesics, and of schizophrenia and dopaminergic systems by antipsychotic drugs are examples of this 'reverse' process. However, workers in different aspects of these problems sometimes appear limited by their specialities. 'Rat pharmacologists' (a term used disparagingly by the late Dr. Henry Miller) occasionally have little conception of clinical problems; the same may be true of 'rat psychologists' and other laboratory-based researchers in neuropharmacology. Yet a broad understanding is needed to answer important questions raised by laboratory studies. What relation, for instance, does the behaviour of an infant monkey separated from its mother bear to human depression, or that of an electrically punished rat to human anxiety neurosis?

There also seemed to be a gap in the literature for those concerned with the treatment of clinical problems. Psychiatrists, clinical psychologists, physicians, and general practitioners do not always display an understanding of

normal brain systems, and have often appeared ignorant of the pharmacodynamics of the drugs they use with such profligacy. For example,
the enormous prescribing of benzodiazepines and the ensuing problem of
benzodiazepine dependence need not have occurred if more attention had
been paid to basic knowledge of the reward systems of the brain and the
part they play in drug dependence (especially after previous experience with
barbiturates and amphetamines). Similarly, deaths from some food and drug
interactions with monoamine oxidase inhibitors could have been prevented
if contemporary knowledge about their mode of action had been applied.

All those concerned with the workings of the brain, whether for teaching,
research, clinical practice, or for pure interest, might thus find a use for a
book which draws together three aspects of brain function: normal systems,
dysfunction in neuropsychiatric disorders, and responses to psychotropic
drugs. Not finding such a book, I have undertaken—with feelings both of
humility and temerity—to fill this need. Inevitably my conception is limited
by my experience and training, and the book is written from a neuropharmacological point of view. I realise that specialists may be irritated by
lack of depth in certain aspects, while generalists may wish for wider cover-
age. It is of course impossible to include the full range of human brain
function in any one book and I am conscious of omissions in many areas,
including the clinically important subjects of aggression, sexual disorders,
and disorders of appetite. A further difficulty is that, in spite of recent major
advances in many fields, we are still only beginning dimly to see how the
brain achieves feeling, thinking, and behaving. Nevertheless, I hope I have
succeeded in my main aim which is to attempt to show how various brain
systems function together to produce integrated behavioural responses, and
to stress that these normal systems must be considered in interpreting disorders of behaviour and responses to drugs.

I am deeply grateful to Professor J. Z. Young, Dr. P. J. Cowen, Professor
J. W. Thompson, and Dr. J. F. Golding who read parts or all of the
manuscript and provided encouragement and valuable advice. The book
could not have been completed without the assistance of Mrs. Valerie Wright,
both in the library and in the preparation of the manuscript, and I remain
forever in her debt. Finally, I thankfully acknowledge the forebearance of
my family who put up with years of preoccupation and neglect while I
pondered on the brain.

Newcastle upon Tyne   H. A.
April 1986

Contents

1
Overview

Functional systems of the brain

The behaviour of man is governed by three main functional systems in the brain: the systems for arousal, for reward, and for learning and memory. Each of these systems encompasses a spectrum of active states. Mechanisms for waking interact with those for sleeping; reward mechanisms interact with those for punishment; learning and memory include forgetting and unlearning. The three major systems operate together throughout life. Their combined state of activity determines an individual's responsiveness at any moment, his state of consciousness, his motivation, and the effect of previous experiences. Together they define his perception and interpretation of environmental stimuli, and together they shape the degree and direction of his behavioural reactions. Interplay between the systems allows for an almost infinite variety of responses and subjective mental states.

In determining behaviour, these systems are inextricably interconnected and operationally indivisible. They are simultaneously active, utilize the same neurotransmitters and neuromodulators, and share overlapping anatomical pathways. Yet, paradoxically, it is necessary to separate the systems in order to describe them, and in the following chapters arousal and sleep, reward and punishment, and learning and memory are considered sequentially. This forced distinction is artificial, since activity in each system is influenced by, and itself influences, activity in the others. Inevitably, the sequential arrangement leads to a certain amount of repetition since the mode of operation of the different systems is fundamentally similar. Some constantly recurring themes which apply to all the systems are mentioned in general terms at this stage; more detailed examples are given later in relation to particular topics.

Patterns of neural activity

Stimulation of each system can be envisaged to generate a complex three-dimensional pattern of neural activity extending through many levels of the nervous system. The shape of the pattern is characteristic of the system or subsystem activated and is initially constrained by the anatomy of its neural connections. However, the pattern of one system may merge and intermingle

1

with patterns simultaneously generated by other systems. As the neural pathways cross and recross, the resultant activity is modulated, facilitated or inhibited here and there, with the formation of further intricate patterns coalescing at some points, separating at others, to produce continuously shifting complexes, ebbing, flowing, and reforming moment by moment. An emotion, a memory, a thought exists as a transitory shape; it has a form and structure composed of the temporal and spatial firing patterns of multisynaptic neuronal complexes, but it is evanescent. When not actually occurring, it is represented only by a network of potential pathways. The pathways are constitutionally 'hardwired' as a result of evolution, but are functionally adaptable and changeable through the process of learning and memory. The pathways themselves and the intensity of neural traffic within them differ subtly between individuals, and influence personality characteristics, vulnerability to psychiatric disease, and response to psychotropic drugs.

A feature of the patterns generated by different types of neural activity appears to be a considerable degree of hemispheric asymmetry both at cortical and subcortical levels. Such asymmetry may reflect an evolution towards the more efficient use of neural space by specialization of functions in each hemisphere. Thus, in most individuals the processes of language, logical analysis, and symbolic reasoning occur largely in the left hemisphere while those of selective attention, visuospatial discrimination, and certain sensory experiences occur mainly in the right hemisphere. It is possible that the symptoms of certain psychiatric disorders, such as depression and schizophrenia, result from asymmetric disturbances of hemispheric functions, or from defective interhemispheric transfer of information.

Multiple neurotransmitter systems

Combinations of the same neurotransmitters and neuromodulators are utilized by all the main functional systems in complex multisynaptic circuits connected in series and in parallel, and containing many regulatory feedback loops. The behavioural effect produced by a transmitter released at a synapse depends on the system in which it is operating. For example, serotonergic activity may promote sleep in one system, but generate anxiety, activate punishment mechanisms, inhibit reward mechanisms, or suppress pain in other systems. The effect of a neurotransmitter may also depend on the degree of activity in a particular circuit. Thus, certain levels of noradrenergic and dopaminergic activity can be rewarding in some brain areas, but excessive activity in the same areas becomes aversive. Different receptors for the same transmitter may mediate different (excitatory or inhibitory) actions, as described below, so that the effect of the same transmitter also depends on the population of its receptors activated at any site. The effect of a transmitter, which may in isolation initiate a relatively rapid, phasic, synaptic response, is in integrated systems further influenced by the action of other neurotransmitters and neuromodulators, which can produce long-lasting changes in neuronal excitability, thus tonically altering the background on which the transmitter acts (Bloom 1985).

Redundant back-up systems

Many systems employ a redundancy of multiple back-up circuits, each performing similar functions via different anatomical and chemical pathways. For example, feeding behaviour in animals can be increased through specific dopaminergic, alpha-noradrenergic, or opioid pathways in the hypothalamus. The same behaviour can be decreased through serotonergic or beta-noradrenergic pathways and by the polypeptide calcitonin. Activity in separate, but connected GABA-ergic pathways can produce either effect by inhibition of the dopaminergic neurones that promote feeding or of the serotonergic neurones which suppress feeding. Similarly, pain sensation can be suppressed through discrete noradrenergic, serotonergic, or opioid and perhaps cholinergic pathways. The particular pain suppression system activated may depend partly on the type of stress to which the animal is exposed. This elaborate organization of redundant back-up systems appears to be a feature of many, if not all, vital, life-sustaining processes.

Diversity of neuronal receptors

Neurotransmitters and neuromodulators exert their various effects in the central nervous system by interacting with specific neuronal receptors. This interaction initiates a cascade of biochemical and biophysical events within the neurone which lead to modification of its activity. The modification may consist of an initiation, an inhibition, or an alteration in the rate of firing of the neurone. The type of cascade triggered by the transmitter/receptor interaction and the direction and degree of the final effect on the firing of the neurone depend on the properties and distribution of the receptors (as well as on the 'conditioning' effects of other transmitters and modulators acting upon the receptor at the same time).

Of great importance in the operation of the functional systems which determine behaviour is the fact that receptors for transmitters are diverse. There are several subtypes of receptor for each neurotransmitter, and the different subtypes mediate different effects. For example, one type of post-synpatic receptor for noradrenaline (alpha-1-adrenoreceptor) probably mediates excitatory effects in some brain systems. Another post-synpatic receptor subtype (beta-adrenoreceptor) may mediate inhibitory effects. Both these post-synpatic receptors interact with noradrenaline, so that release of this transmitter may produce either stimulant or depressant effects depending on the distribution of receptor subtypes in particular neural circuits. Receptor subtypes mediating excitatory or inhibitory effects exist for many of the other known neurotransmitters. In addition, pre-synaptic autoreceptors appear to control transmitter release and to be sensitive to different concentrations of transmitter. Details of the biochemistry of individual neurotransmitters, the molecular conformation of the various receptors, or the biochemical cascade produced by their interactions are beyond the scope of this book, but various receptor subtypes are described where relevant in the ensuing chapters.

Plasticity of neuronal receptors

In addition to their diversity, receptors for neurotransmitters exhibit plasticity. They are dynamic structures whose density and sensitivity undergo adaptive changes in response to alterations in agonist supply. A chronic decrease in the supply of a neurotransmitter to its receptors, for example by a drug which inhibits its release, leads to the emergence of new or previously inactive receptors so that the functional activity of the synapse is restored. Conversely, a chronic increase in receptor activation is followed by a reduction in receptor density. In some cases receptors appear to be actually engulfed into the cell membrane. By this and other mechanisms the balance of synaptic activity is reinstated.

The phenomenon of receptor plasticity is of particular importance in relation to the chronic administration of drugs, since many drugs affect the synaptic release of neurotransmitters, or act as agonists and antagonists at specific neurotransmitter receptors. For example, amphetamine exerts central stimulant effects by releasing dopamine and noradrenaline in catecholaminergic pathways involved in arousal systems. After chronic administration, arousing effects of the drug decline, partly because of a compensatory decrease in dopaminergic and adrenergic receptor density in these pathways. Similarly, the narcotic analgesics, such as heroin, produce hedonic effects by stimulating opioid receptors in reward pathways. Due to receptor adaptations, this effect declines with repeated use, so that heroin addicts may find it necessary to escalate their dosage. On the other hand, receptor adaptations may possibly be necessary for the therapeutic efficacy of some chronically administered drugs, such as antidepressant and antipsychotic agents. Whether an individual can become tolerant to his own endogenous neurotransmitters or neuromodulators, without the intervention of drugs, is a debatable point which is discussed later in relation to chronic pain syndromes and depressive disorders.

Other forms of neural plasticity in the brain include axonal growth and regeneration, the establishment of new synaptic connections after lesioning, and modification of synaptic efficiency by learning and memory.

Disorders of functional systems

In such an intricate and dynamic organization, it is not surprising that occasional dysfunction or maladaptation occurs. It is emphasized here that certain behavioural and psychiatric disorders can be viewed as dysfunctions of the brain systems controlling behaviours. Thus, in later chapters, anxiety neurosis and sleep disorders are considered as dysfunctions of arousal systems; drug dependence and chronic pain syndromes are discussed as dysfunctions of reward and punishment systems; the various amnesic syndromes clearly constitute disorders of learning and memory systems. Depression and mania appear to involve primarily reward and punishment systems, while some forms of schizophrenia may reflect abnormalities of integration between the various systems.

This classification may seem obvious, but in medical practice such disorders are usually described and classified in terms of their symptoms, with little consideration of the underlying systems or processes producing the symptoms. Depressive disorders, for example, are defined in clinical psychiatry as consisting of a cluster of symptoms (a syndrome) in which depression of mood is a central feature. The clinical syndrome is carefully separated from the symptom of depression which may occur in various organic disorders, or as a result of certain infections, drugs, or environmental events in normal subjects. Similarly, the psychiatric diagnosis of schizophrenia depends on the presence of certain alterations of thought and affect, after the exclusion of known organic causes (such as drugs, brain tumours, and epilepsy) which can cause the same psychotic symptoms.

Consideration of psychological symptoms in terms of functional systems of the brain may give a greater insight into the mechanisms of the syndromes, and provide a more rational basis for pharmacological and other treatments. This view takes into account the extensive overlap between different psychiatric states, as exemplified by the clinical terms anxiety/depression and schizoaffective psychosis, since the functional systems themselves overlap. It accommodates the fact that the same symptoms may be found in a variety of disorders and can be experienced by normal subjects. The patterns of neuronal firing described above could be similarly perturbed or distorted by an endogenous biochemical abnormality, a physical lesion, a virus, a drug, an outside event, and many other agents, to produce the same mental state. In fact, it is becoming clear that many psychiatric disorders, including schizophrenia and depression, are not clinical entities, but heterogeneous illnesses. Thirdly, the systems view draws no sharp distinction between normality, and psychiatric or behavioural disease. Instead, it allows for a continuum of individuals who, depending on the details of their structural and functional brain organization, are more or less likely to develop insomnia, anxiety, depression, schizophrenia, drug dependence, or chronic pain (or any combination of these) when exposed to greater or lesser 'doses' of precipitating or aggravating agents. The particular symptoms developed would depend on the site and degree of the perturbation, and the neurological background on which it was acting. Borderline states between normality and various forms of behavioural disease are indeed recognized.

Psychotropic drugs

Psychotropic drugs exert their effects on mental state and behaviour by interacting directly or indirectly with neurotransmitter and neuromodulator systems in the brain. Many of them act as agonists or antagonists at specific receptor sites; others affect the synthesis, storage, release, reuptake, or metabolism of one or more neurotransmitter, while some disrupt neurotransmission by altering the properties of neuronal membranes. Particular attention is paid in following chapters to pharmacodynamics, the mechanisms of drug action. This aspect is relatively neglected in textbooks of medicine, psychiatry, and clinical pharmacology, which are more orientated towards the practical aspects of pharmacokinetics and toxicology. However, the dynamics of drug action are of greater importance for providing a rational basis of drug treatment of psychiatric disorders and for understanding the factors which produce them.

For several reasons the effects of psychotropic drugs on the functional systems of the brain are relatively unspecific. First as, already mentioned, the same neurotransmitters and neuromodulators are utilized by all systems. Thus, even drugs which affect only one transmitter can alter the function of several systems. Secondly, because of the integration between and within the systems, alteration of function of one neurotransmitter affects the balance of activity in antagonistic or synergistic transmitter systems.

Thirdly, drug actions are rarely confined to one transmitter system, to one receptor type or subtype, or to one part of the brain. In the case of the antipsychotic drugs, a stereospecific interaction with one dopamine receptor subtype (dopamine-2 receptor) in particular limbic structures may be responsible for the therapeutic effects in some types of schizophrenia. However, the simultaneous action of the drugs on the same receptor subtype and possibly other dopamine receptors in a different part of the brain (basal ganglia) can give rise to serious adverse effects, while interactions with adrenergic, cholinergic, and histaminic receptors may produce further unwanted effects. Similarly, with the narcotic analgesics, interactions with a specific opioid receptor subtype (mu-receptor) probably produce the analgesia, but effects on other opioid receptors cause sedation, dysphoria, or hedonic effects which may lead to drug dependence. There is a clear need for drugs which act not only on specific receptor subtypes, but which also confine their effects to localized brain regions. Such drugs are gradually emerging and are mentioned where relevant.

This relative non-specificity of action of psychotropic drugs leads to difficulties of classification. For example, drugs usually classed as sedatives, hypnotics, or anxiolytics are here described in relation to their effects on arousal and sleep systems. Many of them, however, are also drugs of dependence, examples of which are discussed under reward and punishment systems. Similar difficulties occur with many of the other drug groups. In fact, the properties of psychotropic drugs overlap as much as the symptoms of psychiatric disease and for the same reasons.

Another recurring theme which emerges from consideration of the psychotropic drugs is that none of them are curative in any psychiatric disease. They may provide long-lasting symptomatic relief and allow time for natural remission to occur, but often only by introducing a further abnormality into an already disturbed system. A hypnotic may produce sleep in an insomniac, but the sleep is not normal sleep and may become yet more abnormal when the drug is stopped. An antidepressant may lighten mood in a depressive illness, but in some subjects it may precipitate mania. It is questionable whether further development of present-day psychotropic drugs will ever achieve cures in such conditions. In degenerative states, such as Alzheimer's dementia and perhaps chronic schizophrenia, present drugs cannot be expected to replace lost neurones. The new generation of psychotropic agents may perhaps include nerve growth factors or even neural implants which encourage the innate capacity of surviving neurones to grow, make new connections, and re-establish the integrity of functional systems of the brain. These possibilites are just appearing on the horizon.

Part I
Arousal and sleep

2
Arousal and sleep systems

All the general principles described in Chapter 1 apply to arousal and sleep systems. They interact with other functional systems and generate patterns of neural activity which may at times have an asymmetric hemispherical distribution. They utilize many transmitters and employ multiple redundant back-up systems. They are subject to malfunction, as manifested in anxiety neuroses and sleep disorders, and they are exquisitely sensitive to centrally-acting drugs. The neurological organization of these systems is described in this chapter; functional disorders and the effects of psychotropic drugs are discussed in Chapters 3 and 4.

Arousal systems

The ability to support consciousness is a fundamental attribute of the human brain. However, the degree of consciousness can vary from full alertness and vigilance, through a series of different levels and types of awareness, to deep sleep. These variable states of arousal, reactivity, or responsiveness, along with their somatic accompaniments, are largely controlled by the arousal systems of the brain.

There has been much discussion concerning the definition and measurement of arousal. Is it a behaviour or a psychological state? Can it be measured by its somatic accompaniments, such as motor activity or heart rate, or by its electrical correlates, such as the rate and degree of synchronization of electroencephalographic (EEG) activity? There are many instances in which these variables do not match (Vanderwolf and Robinson 1981). For example, high levels of presumed psychological arousal, induced by stimuli such as novel environments or central nervous stimulant drugs, are usually associated with the measurable behavioural effect of increased motility in laboratory animals such as rats, while low levels of arousal, occurring during sleep or after central nervous system depressant drugs, are associated with immobility. Yet sometimes in states of apparent extreme arousal provoked by a frightening stimuli, the behavioural response may be immobility (freezing behaviour). Similarly, low voltage fast activity on the EEG is usually associated with behavioural arousal, but such EEG activity can also occur during behavioural sleep, as in paradoxical sleep, after some drugs, and in human subjects in coma. Slow-wave EEG activity is usually correlated with low

11

levels of behavioural arousal, but may also occur during active behaviours such as lapping milk in cats, shivering in rats, and during concentration on mental tasks in humans. Such behavioural-EEG dissociations are discussed further below.

Even when behavioural and EEG arousal apparently match, the quality of arousal may vary widely: it may consist of generalized vigilance, concentrated selective attention, motor readiness or activity, and each of these conditions may be accompanied by variable emotional states. Arousal occurs during laughing, but also during crying, and in fear or anger. Arousal, though a convenient term, is clearly not a unitary phenomenon operating along a single dimension. It is a complex of different states of neural activity produced through a variety of combinations of several anatomical and functional subsystems, resulting in changeable patterns of brain and behavioural response to internal or external stimuli. Thus, it is not surprising that arousal cannot be measured in terms of any one variable, any more than 'emotionality' could be defined in terms of any one emotion. In referring to different states of arousal, it is necessary to specify which manifestations and which types of response are involved.

Arousal systems in the brain appear to include at least two closely integrated components (Routtenberg 1968): a general arousal sysem (Arousal System I), which exerts a tonic background control over central nervous system excitability, and a goal-directed or emotional arousal system (Arousal System II), which contributes phasic and affective components of arousal and is also concerned in selective attention. Both subsystems influence the somatic responses to external and internal stimuli. These systems allow for both very rapid (phasic) and for sustained (tonic) responses of the whole organism to the environment. The selection of the appropriate response to a stimulus is greatly influenced by activity in reward and punishment systems (Chapter 5), and by learning and memory (Chapter 8), but the state of readiness to respond, and the speed and degree of the response, is mainly determined by activity in arousal systems.

General arousal

The general arousal system is a non-specific system which exerts a tonic control on the degree of responsiveness of the cerebral cortex and many subcortical structures (Mountcastle 1974; Webster 1978; Brazier 1977; Stein 1982). A major neurological substrate is the brainstem reticular formation, a system of nerve cells and fibre tracts which links sensory information from the internal and external environment with the cortex and with effector-motor systems (Fig. 2.1) . The reticular formation receives an input, in afferent collaterals from the sensory pathways and via the spinothalamic tracts, from virtually all the sensory systems of the body. Its connections include fibres from pathways subserving pain, temperature, touch, pressure, from visceral

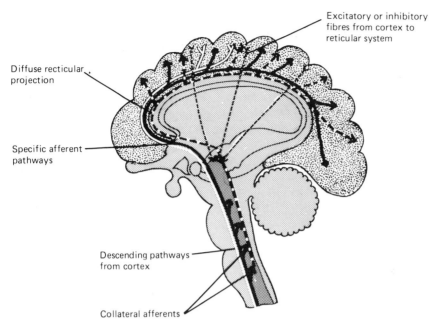

Excitatory or inhibitory fibres from cortex to reticular system

Diffuse recticular projection

Specific afferent pathways

Descending pathways from cortex

Collateral afferents

Fig. 2.1. Diagram of brainstem reticular formation and some connections involved in the general arousal system. Specific afferent pathways, ascending to localized cortical areas, also send inputs via afferent collaterals to the reticular formation. The output from the reticular formation is diffusely distributed to all cortical areas. Other outputs (not shown) are distributed to other parts of the brain and to the spinal cord. By this mechanism, a specific sensory stimulus not only excites a localized area of cortex but also, through the reticular formation, causes diffuse cortical excitation, allowing evaluation of the stimulus. Feedback systems, which may be either excitatory or inhibitory, also pass from cortex to reticular system. The appropriate behavioural response is then transmitted via descending pathways from the cortex.

sensory endings, from vestibular, auditory, olfactory and retinal pathways, and from brain areas concerned with thoughts and emotions. These connections are not specific for sensory modality since impulses from different sense organs impinge on the same reticular neurones. The output from the reticular formation is transmitted by long ascending fibres which are diffusely distributed to all cortical areas and also to other parts of the brain, and by descending motor fibres in the reticulospinal tracts.

The anterior part of the reticular formation, and also a central core of ascending fibres, carry mainly facilitatory influences to the cortex. This portion comprises the reticular activating system, which has long been thought to be of primary importance in maintaining consciousness. Electrical stimulation of this area in animals evokes immediate and marked cortical EEG activation, and will cause a sleeping animal to awake instantaneously

(Moruzzi and Magoun 1949). Furthermore, the neuronal activity provoked by reticular activating system stimulation is very widespread, including the whole cortex, thalamic nuclei, basal ganglia, hypothalamus, other portions of the brainstem, and the spinal cord. This diffuse activation continues for up to a minute after the initial stimulation.

The reticular activating system appears to provide a background level of stimulation which lowers the cortical threshold to excitation from other pathways, including the specific sensory tracts. Thus, for example, a visual stimulus excites not only the visual cortex through its specific afferent pathways, but also the whole cortex through non-specific pathways from the reticular activating system. The discrete, specific projections allow the cortex to discriminate the origin and type of stimulus, while the diffuse non-specific projections, along with intracortical connections, presumably allow other parts of the cortex to evaluate the significance of each specific sensory stimulus in relation to the present situation, memories of past events, associated sensory input, and other relevant factors. The effect of sensory information entering the cortex via the specific sensory pathways, and therefore the behavioural response to it, is in this way modulated by the non-specific input from the reticular activating system.

Normally, the activity of the reticular activating system is itself driven by sensory traffic in the afferent collaterals. However, the reticular activating system appears to possess an intrinsic tone, since in surgical preparations in which its afferent input is sectioned (encéphale isolé; Bremer 1935; (Fig.2.2) some cortical activity can still be maintained, as shown by the fact that such preparations show alternating patterns of sleep and wakefulness on the

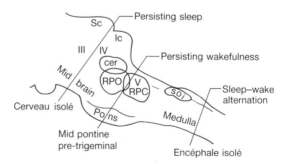

Fig. 2.2. Diagram of section through cat brain indicating location and effects of cerveau isolé, encéphale isolé, and midpontine pretrigeminal preparations. cer, Nucleus coeruleus; RPC, nucleus reticularis pontis caudalis; RPO, nucleus reticularis pontis oralis; sol, nucleus parasolitarius; Ic, inferior colliculus; Sc, Superior colliculus; III, oculomotor nucleus; IV, trochlear nucleus; V, trigeminal nucleus. (From Salamy 1976, by kind permission of John Wiley & Sons Inc., New York.)

electroencephalogram. On the other hand, if the brain is sectioned rostral to the reticular activating system (Bremer's cerveau isolé preparation) consciousness is lost and a state of perpetual sleep supervenes. Similar data is sometimes provided by disease. Thus, when the reticular activating system is damaged by haemorrhage, tumour, or infection, the patient loses consciousness even if the cortex is still intact.

Pharmacological evidence also attests to the importance of the reticular activating system in maintaining consciousness. Drugs which directly depress neuronal activity in the reticular activating system (low doses of barbiturates) decrease the level of consciousness, while drugs which directly stimulate activity at this site (amphetamines) have an alerting effect. However, drugs which depress activity in the afferent collaterals to the reticular activating system need not produce sleep or unconsciousness because they do not impair its intrinsic tone. Such an action appears to be exerted by low doses of the antipsychotic drug chlorpromazine which can have a calming effect with little depression in the level of consciousness. Some psychotomimetic drugs such as lysergic acid diethylamide (LSD), appear to facilitate transmission through the afferent collaterals, thus enhancing the effects of sensory stimulation and possibly accounting for some of the psychodelic effects. The differential sites of action of small doses of barbiturates, amphetamines, chlorpromazine, and LSD on the reticular activating system and its afferent collaterals were demonstrated by Bradley (1958) and Bradley and Key (1958; Fig. 2.3). The actions of these drugs are described in detail in Chapter 4 and 14.

The effect of reticular activating system activity on the cortex is modified by interacting feedback systems from cortex to reticular formation (Fig. 2.1). Descending cortico-reticular fibres may be either excitatory or inhibitory. Activity in excitatory pathways further stimulates the reticular activating system so that the arousing effect of the original stimulus is magnified. Conversely, when descending inhibitory pathways are activated, the effect of the original stimulus is damped down and limited. Thus, the brain exerts a selective control over its own sensory input so that the arousing effect of relevant stimuli is greater than that of irrelevant stimuli.

Vanderwolf and Robinson (1981) claim that neither the cortex nor the reticulocortical projections are essential for waking behaviour since alternating patterns of behavioural sleep and wakefulness continue in decorticated rats. Nevertheless, in the intact animal these connections are almost certainly involved in modulating arousal, and Sutherland et al. (1981) point out that decortication also removes the descending corticoreticular fibres and that control over behaviour is probably organized at each level in the nervous system, although the behavioural significance of the control processes may change from level to level. As pointed out in Chapter 8, associative learning can occur in a spinal preparation, but this does not imply that learning does not involve higher structures in intact animals.

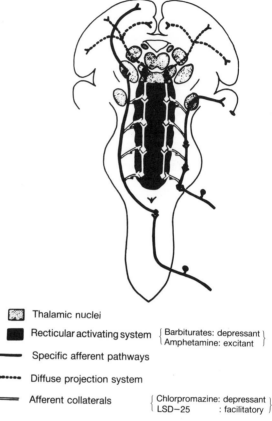

Thalamic nuclei

Recticular activating system { Barbiturates: depressant }
                             { Amphetamine: excitant }

Specific afferent pathways

Diffuse projection system

Afferent collaterals { Chlorpromazine: depressant }
                     { LSD–25   : facilitatory }

Fig. 2.3. Diagram showing sites of action of drugs affecting activity in the reticular activating system and its afferent collaterals. Drugs which directly affect activity in the reticular activating system (barbiturates, depressant; amphetamine, stimulant) alter the level of consciousness by effects on the diffuse cortical projection system. Drugs which depress activity in the afferent collaterals (chlorpromazine) do not impair consciousness because they do not affect the intrinsic tone of the reticular activating system. LSD-25 appears to facilitate transmission through the afferent collaterals, enhancing the diffuse cortical effects of sensory stimulation.
(From Bradley 1961, by kind permission of Oxford University Press.)

Goal-directed and emotional arousal

Closely connected with the general arousal system is a second arousal system which is more specific and goal-oriented. It appears to supply cortical responses with emotional 'colour' by imbuing them with such qualities as fear and anxiety, anger, pleasure, and aversion. To a large extent, this system determines the quality and strength of the response to any stimulus, and its activity adds a selective, goal-directed aspect to arousal behaviour (Routtenberg 1968).

The main anatomical basis for this aspect of arousal is the limbic system, a heterogeneous group of functionally-related structures surrounding the midbrain (Papez 1937; MacLean 1949, 1969; Isaacson 1974, 1982; Fig. 2.4). It includes tissues derived from the limbic lobe of the paleocortex (cingulate, parahippocampal, hippocampal and dentate gyri, induseum griseum, olfactory lobe and bulb), related subcortical nuclei (amygdaloid nucleus, anterior thalamic, septal and hippocampal nuclei), and fibre tracts (fornix, mammillothalamic tract, stria terminalis, and olfactory tract). The connections of the limbic system are complex and not fully delineated; recent findings have been reviewed by Iverson (1984). They include many interconnections between the different limbic structures and close connections to and from the thalamus, hypothalamus, and striatum. In addition, there are connections with the reticular activating system, and with the median forebrain bundle which links the brainstem, limbic system, and the entire neocortex.

Certain of the limbic nuclei appear to be directly involved in controlling emotional tone (Isaacson 1974, 1982). Electrical stimulation of some parts of the amygdala in many animal species produces rage, aggression, and attacking behaviour, while stimulation of other parts of the amygdala inhibits this behaviour (Siegel 1984; Koolhas 1984). Total bilateral destruction of the amygdala has a taming effect in rats and rhesus monkeys (Herbert 1984). There also seems to be a separation between fear and flight behaviour on the one hand and aggressive attacking behaviour on the other, depending upon which part of the amygdala is stimulated or sectioned. Stimulation of the septal region has a taming effect on various animals, including the possum and the monkey, and decreases most emotional responses, while destruction increases emotional and social responses. Interconnected with these limbic nuclei are nuclei in the lateral, ventromedial, and posterior hypothalamus, which appear to generate basic drives such as hunger, thirst, and sex.

All these nuclei also form part of the reward systems, described in Chapter 5. Electrical stimulation in many limbic areas appears to be highly rewarding in all animals species studied and it is thought that their activity contributes an element of incentive or motivation that leads to reward-seeking behaviour in arousal (Olds 1962; Stein and Wise 1969). Also of importance are 'punishment' areas where electrical stimulation is aversive. These appear to be involved in avoidance behaviour. At present, it is not possible to define exactly the neurophysiological substrates for separate emotions: presumably each emotion involves activation of a unique pattern of limbic and neocortical structures. The question is discussed further in relation to anxiety in Chapter 3 and to other emotions related to reward and punishment in Chapter 5. There is evidence of some right hemispherical specialization for the experience of emotions (Schwartz et al. 1975; Ross 1984; Geschwind 1983).

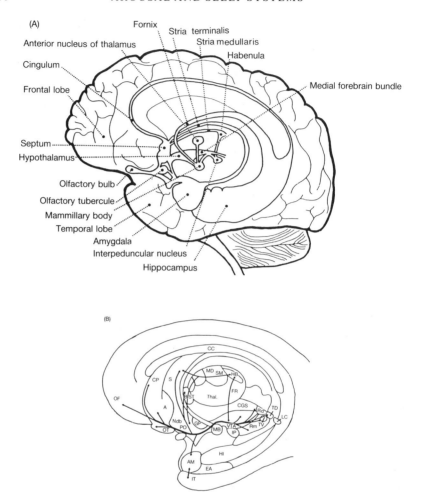

Fig. 2.4. Some structures and connections of the limbic system. (A) Schematic diagram of the classic limbic system proposed by Papez (1937) and MacLean (1949). (B) Diagram of limbic connections. VTA, ventral tegmental area; Rd, Rm, raphe nuclei; OF, orbital frontal cortex; CP, caudate-putamen; S, septum; OT, olfactory tubercle; A, nucleus accumbens CC, corpus callosum; Ndb, nucleus of the diagonal band; PO, preoptic area; FR, fasiculus retroflexus; SM, stria medullaris; HB, habenula; BST, bed nucleus ofstria terminalis; GP, globus pallidus; AM, amygdala; IT, inferotemporal cortex; HI, hippocampus; MB, mammillary body; IP, interpeduncular nucleus; MD, medio-dorsal nucleus of thalamus; Thal, thalamus; CGS, central grey substance; TV, ventral tegmental nucleus; TD, dorsal tegmental nucleus; LC, locus coeruleus; EA, entrorhinal area. The heavy line of fibre tracts passing from brainstem to forebrain is the medial forebrain bundle. (From Stinus et al. 1984.)

These emotional components of arousal contributed by the limbic system are integrated with the mechanisms for learning and memory, in which the hippocampus plays a vital role, as discussed in Chapter 8. Through learning and memory, the arousing effects of repeated stimuli can be either enhanced or extinguished.

The reticular and limbic arousal systems interact closely with each other. In many ways, they can be thought of as complementary, the general arousal system providing a tonic background of cortical responsiveness while the goal-directed system focusses attention onto factors relevant at the moment. However, Routtenberg (1968) proposes that in certain respects the systems are mutually inhibitory, activity in one tending to suppress activity in the other. He suggests that there is a dynamic equilibrium between the two systems, and it seems likely that maximally efficient behaviour under different circumstances requires a shifting optimal balance of activity between general and limbic arousal and their interactions with other cortical and subcortical systems.

Selective attention

As already mentioned, the brain exerts a selective control over its own sensory input. It is not a passive recipient of the multitude of environmental stimuli which impinge on it, but contains mechanisms which allow it to avoid distraction by irrelevant stimuli and to direct attention towards behaviourally relevant stimuli. Such selective attention is a complex process which includes several components such as vigilance, concentration, focussing, scanning, and exploration (Mesulam 1983). The process involves co-operative activity within the reticular and limbic arousal systems, and in connected cortical and subcortical sensory and motor structures.

Observations, reviewed by Mesulam (1983), on patients with the syndrome of unilateral neglect and related experiments with laboratory primates have shed some light on the brain structures involved in selective attention. The posterior parietal cortex appears to be of particular importance. Patients with lesions in this area tend to ignore sensory events occurring within the contralateral half of the sensory field. Effects are most pronounced if the damage is on the right side of the brain: such patients may neglect to dress the left side of the body, ignore objects on the left, and fail to read or write on the left half of a page. In the monkey, electrophysiological recordings have shown that individual neurones in the inferior parietal cortex increase their firing rate when the animal looks at or approaches motivationally relevant objects, such as food when the animal is hungry or water when it is thirsty. Detection of similar stimuli which have no motivational relevance does not increase the firing rate of the cells. It appears that these neurones are able to associate sensory information with internal drives and that increased firing in the neurones corresponds to a state of heightened selective attention. Most of these neurones are responsive to stimuli in the con-tralateral visual field; presumably damage to them accounts for the unilateral neglect observed clinically.

The connections of these posterior parietal neurones have been worked out in experiments on primates using horseradish peroxidase and are shown in Fig. 2.5a. They receive *sensory* information from higher order association cortex and from thalamic nuclei, *motor* information from the frontal eye fields, striatum and superior colliculus, *limbic* information from the cingulate and retrosplenial cortex and nucleus basalis, and *reticular* information from the locus coeruleus, brainstem raphe nuclei and intralaminar thalamus. They also send efferent connections to all these structures. Unilateral neglect has been shown to occur after lesions in several of these connections, including lesions in the thalamus and striatum in man, and in the hypothalamus and ascending monoaminergic pathways in animals.

Mesulam (1983) suggests that selective attention is regulated by this neural network which is proposed to contain three representations of the outside world (Fig. 2.5b): a sensory template, centred around the posterior parietal cortex; a motor map, centred around the frontal eye fields, which is used for scanning and exploration; and a motivational map, centred around the cingulate cortex, which focusses interest and expectancy. All these areas receive inputs from the reticular formation which regulate the level of acti-vation in the relevant region and supply the components of arousal and vigilance. Experimental evidence indicates that all these processes are rela-tively specialized in the right hemisphere. For example, right-sided lesions are more likely than left-sided lesions to lead to unilateral neglect; in 'split-brain' patients the right hemisphere is superior for vigilance tasks, and neuro-logically intact humans tend to pay slightly more attention to events on the left side of the body.

Somatic arousal

Both arousal systems give off efferent connections which activate body responses to arousal (Fig. 2.6). Descending fibres from the reticular for-mation in the reticulospinal tracts play a major role in regulating muscle tone and are also involved in posture and movement. Thus, part of the response to excitation of the general arousal system is increased muscle tone, increased reflexes, an alert posture and readiness for movement, while inhibition of this system produces muscular relaxation. Centres for autonomic control of cardiovascular, respiratory, and other responses are also situated in the reticular formation. The limbic system, through its hypothalamic connec-tions, is a major determinant of both autonomic and endocrine responses to arousal. Increased activity in the limbic arousal system results in increased sympathetic activity and increased output of anterior and posterior pituitary hormones, while decreased activity leads to a predominance of vegetative

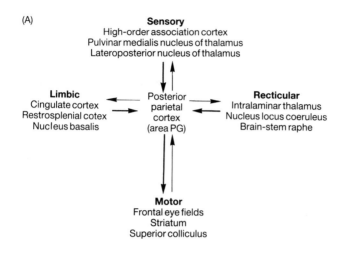

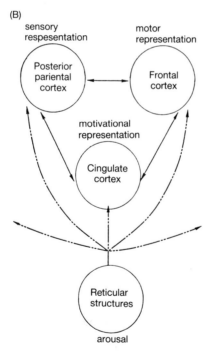

Fig. 2.5. Brain areas involved in selective attention. (A) Relevant connections of posterior parietal neurones. (B) Proposed representations of the outside world and their anatomical substrates (for explanation see text). (From Mesulam 1983.)

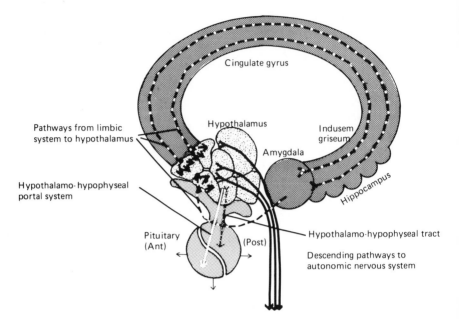

Fig. 2.6. Diagram of some central connections involved in peripheral arousal responses.

parasympathetic activity. There are also close interconnections between limbic and striatal structures (Mogenson *et al.* 1980; Mogenson 1984) and alterations in muscle tone normally accompany emotional responses. Different emotions may trigger different somatic responses: the pallor of fear, the purple of rage, the blush of shame (Lang *et al.* 1972). Different patterns of cardiovascular and electrodermal activity are evoked by rewarding as compared with frustrating conditions (Tranel 1983). However, reports from subjects with spinal cord injuries show that such peripheral responses are not essential for the subjective experience of emotion (Lang *et al.* 1972). Somatic changes occurring in states of arousal are described in Chapter 3.

Neurotransmitters and arousal

In view of the multiplicity of synaptic connections required for the integrated control of arousal, it is not surprising that several neurotransmitters are utilized. Cell bodies containing noradrenaline, dopamine, and serotonin are all present in the reticular formation, and cell groups containing cholinesterase, indicating cholinergic transmission, have also been demonstrated. Many of these neurones have overlapping projections to cortical and limbic areas, and it has therefore proved difficult to assign particular functions to individual cell groups (Webster 1978).

Cholinergic systems

The distribution of cholinergic pathways in the brain is still not fully delineated; recent findings are described by Cuello and Sofroniew (1984; Fig. 2.7). One pathway from the reticular activating system to the cortex appears to be cholinergic. Thus, stimulation of the reticular activating system produces both electroencephalographic and behavioural arousal, accompanied by increased release of acetylcholine from the cerebral cortex. The administration of cholinergic agents produces low voltage, fast activity in the EEG, characteristic of cortical activation, and abolishes slow wave activity characteristic of low arousal states. There is an increase in acetylcholine turnover in the cortex during arousal and a decrease in slow wave sleep.

An example of behavioural-EEG dissociation occurs with antimuscarinic drugs such as atropine. These drugs abolish the EEG effects of acetylcholine and produce slow wave activity, but with certain doses of atropine (5.0 mg/kg or more in rats) this 'low arousal' EEG activity occurs during behavioural wakefulness, especially when the animals are immobile though not asleep (Vanderwolf and Robinson 1981). Nevertheless, atropine-resistant fast EEG activity reappears during walking, changing posture, or struggling. This atropine-resistant fast activity may involve non-cholinergic reticulocortical pathways. Montplaisir (1975) concludes that 'tonic' EEG activation during arousal may be cholinergic at the cortical level even though other neurotransmitters may be involved. Mason and Fibiger (1979) demonstrated a functional interaction between cholinergic and noradrenergic systems in the

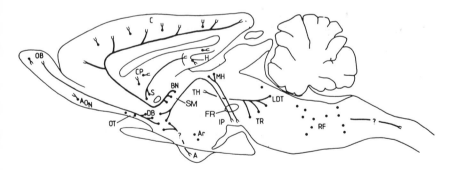

Fig. 2.7. Diagram of cholinergic cell groups and major cholinergic pathways in the rat brain. OB, olfactory bulb; AON, anterior olfactory nucleus; DB, nucleus of the diagonal band; S, septum; CP, caudate putamen; H, hippocampus; BN, nucleus basalis; A, amygdala; TH, thalamus; Ar, arcuate nucleus; TR, tegmental reticular system; LDT, lateral dorsal tegmental nucleus; RF, hindbrain reticular formation; C, cortex; IP, nucleus interpeduncularis; SM, stria medullaris; MH, medial habenula; OT, olfactory tubercle; FR, fasiculus retroflexus. Classical motor and autonomic preganglionic neurones are not represented. (From Cuello and Sofroniew 1984.)

brain, and suggest that cholinergic activity modulates activity in noradrenergic systems to influence the degree of behavioural arousal.

A system of cholinergic neurones with their cell bodies in various forebrain nuclei (nucleus of diagonal band, medial and lateral preoptic nuclei, nucleus basalis, and the extrapeduncular nucleus) project to all parts of the cerebral cortex. One of the functions of this system may be in learning and memory (Chapter 8). Cholinergic neurones in the periventricular system are involved in reward and punishment systems (Chapter 5). There are cholinergic pathways extending from neurones in the septum to the hippocampus and from the habenular nucleus to the interpeduncular nucleus (Iverson and Iverson 1981). High concentrations of acetylcholine are found in the interpeduncular nucleus, hippocampus, hypothalamus, basal ganglia, and cerebral cortex.

Both muscarinic and nicotinic cholinergic receptors are present in the nervous system, but the central functions of the two subtypes are obscure. Most central nervous system neurones exhibit an excitatory response to iontophoretically applied acetylcholine, but some are inhibited while others show excitation followed by depression.

Noradrenergic systems

Monoamine-containing cell groups in the reticular formation have been localized by histofluorescence techniques (Table 2.1) . Cell groups containing noradrenaline are designatad A_{1-7}. Groups A_{1-5} project to the spinal cord and hypothalamus, and may be involved in autonomic function. Groups $A_{6,7}$ constitute the locus coeruleus, a collection of only a few thousand

Table 2.1. Monoamine-containing cell groups in the reticular formation

Cell group	Transmitter	Nuclei	Projections
$A_{1,2}$	noradrenaline	various	spinal cord
$A_{3,4,5}$	noradrenaline	various	hypothalamus, preoptic area
$A_{6,7}$	noradrenaline	locus coeruleus and subcoeruleus	thalamus, neocortex, limbic system, cerebellum, spinal cord
$A_{8,9}$	dopamine	substantia nigra	corpus striatum
A_{10}	dopamine	ventral tegmentum	limbic system, frontal cortex
$A_{11,12,13}$	dopamine	various	hypothalamus, thalamus, median eminence
B_{1-9}	serotonin	raphe nuclei and several other nuclei	wide distribution in diencephalon and spinal cord

neurones with extremely diffuse projections to many areas including the cerebral cortex, limbic system and spinal cord (Fig. 2.8a). These cells have been much studied and are thought to be involved in general and limbic arousal (Jouvet 1972 1977; Webster 1978; Jacobs 1984), selective attention (Mason 1979; Clark *et al.* 1984), anxiety and fear reactions (Gray 1982; Chapter 3), affective and pain responses (Redmond 1982; Chapter 5), and cortical plasticity (Pettigrew 1978; Chapter 8). The extensive afferent and efferent connections of the locus coeruleus suggest that it may function (among other things) as an alarm relay system associated with attention, vigilance, and anticipation (Redmond 1982), and that it provides an important link between the general and limbic arousal systems.

Electrical stimulation of the locus coeruleus produces increased EEG arousal with behavioural signs of fear and anxiety, while bilateral destruction in animals produces loss of forebrain noradrenaline and continuous slow wave sleep. Direct recording from single noradrenergic neurones in the locus coeruleus in freely-moving cats, rats, and monkeys (Jacobs 1984) show that the firing of these cells is strongly state-dependent, the highest firing rates occurring during behavioural arousal and attention, and the lowest during sleep.

Adrenergic pathways in the median forebrain bundle are also involved in reward and reinforcement (Stein and Wise 1969; Stein 1968; Chapter 5) which contributes part of the goal-directed limbic arousal system. Noradrenergic pathways in general are thought to play a role in the mechanism of drive and aggression (Fuxe *et al.* 1970).

A role of catecholamines in arousal is further indicated by the observations that behavioural and EEG arousal is produced both in animals and humans by the injection of noradrenaline into the cerebral ventricles or directly into the substance of the brain and that L-dopa and sympathomimetic drugs produce increased arousal, while depletion of brain monoamines with reserpine causes EEG and behavioural de-arousal (Levitt and Lonowski 1975; Candy and Key 1977; Vanderwolf and Robinson 1981).

The effects of noradrenaline released by noradrenergic neurones in the reticular formation depend on the type of noradrenergic receptor activated. Adrenergic receptor subtypes are described in more detail in Chapter 11. They include post-synaptic $alpha_1$-receptors, which in general mediate excitatory effects, and post-synaptic beta-receptors, which generally mediate depressant effects in the central nervous system (Quarantotti *et al.* 1975; Bevan *et al.* 1977; Aghajanian and Rogawski 1983). Adrenergic $alpha_2$-autoreceptors exert an inhibitory modulatory control over noradrenaline release. The distribution of these receptors differs in different parts of the brain. The neocortex contains both $alpha_1$_ and beta-receptors, and may show either excitatory or depressant responses to noradrenaline. The locus coeruleus contains mainly $alpha_2$-receptors and the iontophoretic application of noradrenaline depresses the firing of neurones in this nucleus. The dorsal

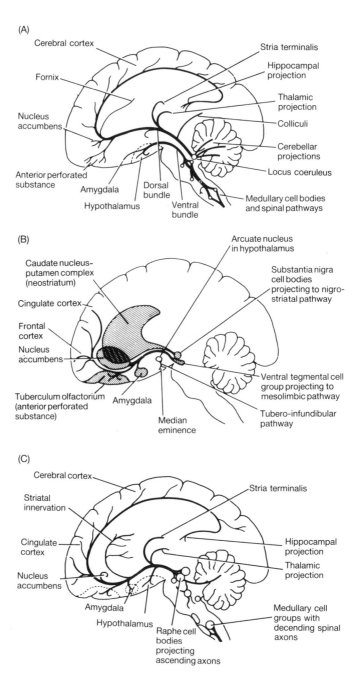

Fig. 2.8. Monoaminergic pathways in the brain. (A) Noradrenergic pathways. (B) Dopaminergic pathways. (C) Serotonergic pathways. Note wide distribution of noradrenergic and serotonergic pathways and more discrete dopaminergic projections. Diagrams are based on animal data. (From Kruk and Pycock 1979.)

raphe nuclei contain mainly alpha$_1$-receptors and are almost universally activated by the iontophoretic application of noradrenaline (Aghajanian and Rogawski 1983).

Aghajanian and Rogawski (1983) describe some unusual characteristics of alpha$_1$-mediated effects in the central nervous system. The post-synaptic neuronal response to noradrenaline exhibits a time course of at least 100 msec or possibly longer. This slow time course contrasts with conventionally described post-synaptic excitation, for example by acetylcholine, which lasts only tens of milliseconds. Furthermore, alpha$_1$-mediated adrenoceptor activation does not usually cause an action potential in the absence of a simultaneously applied excitatory drive. Instead, it enhances conventional excitatory synaptic activity, possibly by increasing general cellular excitability. Alpha$_1$-receptors thus seem to play a modulatory role in neural activity rather than participating in the rapid transmission of impulses. The role of monoamine systems in arousal may be related to this effect. Monoaminergic activity elicited by stimulation of the locus coeruleus appears to increase the signal-to-noise ratio in many brain areas and to form part of a generalized 'enabling' system (Karli 1984).

Dopaminergic systems

Cells of groups A$_{8-13}$ in the reticular formation contain dopamine (Table 2.1, Fig. 2.8b). Groups A$_{8,9}$ constitute the substantia nigra, project to the corpus striatum, and affect muscle tone. Group A$_{10}$, situated in the ventral tegmental area, consists of the cell bodies of the dopaminergic mesolimbic pathway. These cells project along the median forebrain bundle to limbic areas and to the frontal cortex. This pathway is involved in limbic-mediated arousal; its stimulation by application of dopamine to the nucleus accumbens produces intense arousal, hypervigilance, hyperactivity and exploratory behaviour in several animal species (Stevens 1979). Furthermore, the cell bodies of Group A$_{10}$ lie within the reward area found from self-stimulation experiments (Webster 1978; Chapter 5). Single unit recording of the activity of dopaminergic cells in the substantia nigra and ventral tegmental area (Jacobs 1984) show a stable rate of discharge with little variation between quiet waking and sleep. However, the discharge rate increases during movement and appears to be particularly related to purposive movements. Groups A$_{11-13}$ project to parts of the hypothalamus, thalamus, and median eminence; their functions are not clear, but they are involved in the release of hypothalamic and pituitary hormones. Dopaminergic systems involved in schizophrenia and in Parkinsonism, and dopamine receptor subtypes are described in Chapter 13.

Serotonergic systems

Cell groups B$_{1-9}$ in the reticular formation all contain serotonin (Table 2.1, Fig. 2.8b). Groups B$_{1-3}$ project to the spinal cord; the others have diffuse connections, passing along the median forebrain bundle, the whole cerebral cortex and also limbic and hypothalamic structures. The functions of these systems is largely unknown, but the upper and lower raphe nuclei which contain the cells of $B_{7,8}$ and B_{1-3} are involved in arousal and sleep in animals. Single unit recordings from the dorsal raphe nuclei in freely moving cats (Jacobs 1984) shows that the discharge rate of these serotonergic cells is closely related to the level of behavioural arousal: the highest rates of discharge occur during arousal, lower rates during slow wave sleep, and the cells become completely quiescent during paradoxical sleep. Their activity appears to be modulated, but not controlled, by noradrenergic activity. Serotonergic pathways in the median forebrain bundle may interact with noradrenergic and dopaminergic pathways in reward functions (Chapter 5), and other serotonergic pathways may be related to sensory perception and memory (Chapter 14). Jacobs (1984) suggests that the various monoaminergic systems subserve different but related functions in arousal: noradrenergic and serotonergic systems, with their widespread projections, may transmit information to the rest of the central nervous system concerning the animals' general behavioural state, while the more discretely projecting dopaminergic systems may be related to purposive movements and changes of muscle tone related to focussed attention. The cell bodies of noradrenergic, serotonergic, and dopaminergic neurones in the reticular formation all appear to be autoactive, showing regular spontaneous activity during quiet waking; this property may largely account for the intrinsic tone of the reticular activating system.

Present knowledge thus suggests that at least four transmitter systems, cholinergic, noradrenergic, dopaminergic, and serotonergic, are involved in various aspects of arousal. This list is unlikely to be exhaustive; for example, the dopaminergic pathway from the ventral tegmental area to the nucleus accumbens is subject to feed-back control in which the neurotransmitter is GABA (Stevens 1979), and there is growing evidence that various polypeptides are involved in arousal and sleep and that these may be co-secreted with monoamines (Johansson *et al.* 1981). Neurotransmitter systems involved in sleep are described later in this chapter. The locus coeruleus contains dopamine and opioids as well as noradrenaline and has receptors for GABA (Redmond 1982) and acetylcholine (Mason and Fibiger 1979). In addition, several amino acids (glutamic acid, glycine, taurine, aspartic acid) are released by the cortex following electrical stimulation of the midbrain reticular formation, and these may also modulate reticulo-cortical activation (Montplaisir 1975; Bandler 1984).

Performance and arousal

The relationship between the level of arousal and performance is complex. If, for example, performance is measured as reaction time and this is plotted

against an index of arousal such as subjective alertness, heart rate, or electrodermal activity, it is found that the speed of response becomes faster as
the subject becomes more alert, but at a certain point, when the subject
becomes over-aroused, the speed of response begins to decline. Such considerations led to the formation of the 'Yerkes-Dodson law' (Corcoran 1965),
which holds that the quality of performance is related in an inverted U-shaped
function to arousal level. Thus, performance is poor when subjects are
under-aroused, and also when they are over-aroused, with the optimal level
of arousal lying somewhere in the middle (Fig. 2.9). The situation is further
complicated by the fact that the particular level of arousal which is optimal
for performance depends on the nature of the task. In general, complex tasks,
especially those requiring fine motor co-ordination, are performed better at
relatively low levels of arousal, while less demanding tasks are performed
better at higher levels of arousal. Peak performance on a particular task
presumably reflects an optimal balance of activity between the general and
limbic arousal systems.

These relationships are important in determining the effects of drugs on
performance. Central nervous system stimulant drugs may improve performance in relatively under-aroused subjects. However, in moderately or

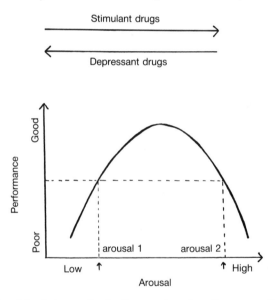

Fig. 2.9. Relationships between level of arousal and performance. Performance is
maximal when the level of arousal is optimal for a given task, but declines when the
level of arousal is below (arousal 1) or above (arousal 2) the optimal level. Central
stimulant drugs may improve performance in relatively under-aroused subjects, but
impair it in highly aroused subjects; central depressant drugs may have the opposite
effects. (From Ashton and Stepney 1982.)

highly aroused subjects, such drugs may impair performance by making them over-aroused. A similar dual effect on performance may occur with central nervous system depressants; the performance of highly aroused subjects may be enhanced when the arousal level is reduced, while that of relaxed subjects may be reduced in efficiency. Arousal levels of different subjects vary according to personality, circumstances and pathological states such as anxiety neuroses, and the effects of drugs on performance vary with individuals and cannot always be predicted. Such effects are of considerable importance insofar as they affect car driving, machine operating skills, and mental concentration at work. The relation of personality to activity in arousal and reward and punishment systems is discussed further in Chapters 3 and 5.

Electroencephalographic measures of arousal

Some aspects of arousal can be measured by behavioural testing, subjective report, and recording of peripheral autonomic activity (Chapter 3). However, the most direct and sensitive non-invasive method of measuring cortical activity is by mean of the electroencephalogram (EEG). Surface recorded brain potentials are thought to reflect local currents flowing in the dendrites of the superficial cortex and may be paced from the thalamus (Brazier 1977; Stein 1982). Characteristic patterns are generated in different states and both the amplitude and the frequency of surface waves are determined to a great extent by activity in the reticular activating system. Electroencephalography is of increasing importance in psychopathology and psychopharmacology, both for clinical assessment and for research. For this reason, a brief description is given here of encephalographic methods in current use.

EEG wave bands

EEG wave bands are conventionally divided into four frequency bands (Table 2.2).The division between bands is somewhat arbitrary and differs between different authors. Average values are: delta, 1–3 Hz; theta, 4–7 Hz; alpha, 8–13 Hz; beta, 14 to over 40 Hz. Although the exact designation of each frequency band is arbitrary, the different frequencies (although they may overlap) do not occur as a continuum from 1 to 40 Hz, but seem to reflect different types of brain activity (Fig. 2.10). Beta activity, which is characteristic of high arousal states (although it also occurs in paradoxical sleep and other states of low behavioural arousal), consists of low voltage relatively unsynchronized activity which may be superimposed upon or largely replace the more synchronized waves typical of lower arousal states. Alpha activity characterizes the relaxed state in awake subjects and consists of slower, higher voltage, more synchronized waves. It is prominent in normal subjects relaxing with eyes shut and may be replaced by faster activity by opening the eyes or by mental concentration (alpha-blocking). However, alpha activity can occur during mental concentration (Vanderwolf and

Table 2.2. Electroencephalographic wave bands

Wave band	Frequency (Hz)	Approximate amplitude (V)	Characteristic Associated activity*
delta	1–3	100	deep sleep central nervous depressant drugs
theta	4–7	100	some pathological states
alpha	8–13	50	awake relaxation
beta	14–40+	20	increased arousal,
beta$_1$	14–26		mental activity
beta$_2$	27–40		central nervous
beta$_3$	over 40		depressant drugs

* See text for fuller explanation.
References: Cooper *et al.* 1980, Stein (1982), Saletu (1980).

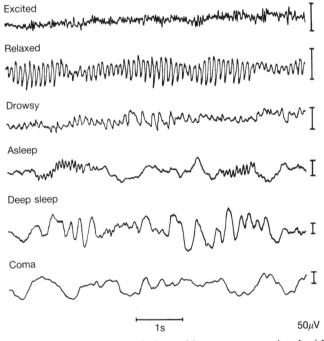

Excited

Relaxed

Drowsy

Asleep

Deep sleep

Coma

1s   50μV

Fig. 2.10. Characteristic electroencephalographic patterns associated with different states of arousal. Note that in certain circumstances, EEG and behavioural arousal may be dissociated (see text). (From Penfield and Jasper 1954, by kind permission of Little, Brown and Co.)

Robinson 1981). If the subject becomes drowsy even slower waves appear and in deep sleep high amplitude delta waves dominate the EEG. Different EEG patterns seen in different stages of sleep are described in the the next section. Theta activity in man occurs locally over cerebral lesions such as tumours or abcesses, but is not prominent in the normal EEG. However, increased theta activity is seen in certain pathological states such as schizophrenia, psychopathic personalities, hyperactive children, and children 'at risk' of schizophrenia (Chapter 13). In some animals (e.g. cats and rats), a pronounced theta rhythm related to the state of arousal is obtained from the hippocampus (Rawlins 1984; Vanderwolf and Robinson 1981), but this is much less marked in primates and humans.

Power-frequency spectrum

Recent technical advances have made it possible to analyse the power-frequency spectrum of the EEG. This technique gives a sensitive measure of shifts of frequency and/or amplitude in the EEG with changing conditions and over different electrode positions (Fink 1978). Generalized increased beta activity and a shift in the dominant alpha activity towards a higher frequency is associated with stress in normal subjects, and is also seen in anxiety neuroses (Chapter 3) and in patients with high neuroticism scores on the Eysenck Personality Questionnaire (Eysenck and Eysenck 1975). Increased frequency variability occurs in schizophrenia (Chapter 13). There are also hemispheric differences in frequency associated with different mental tasks in normal subjects: linguistic tasks tend to induce greater fast activity in the left hemisphere, while visuospatial tasks increase fast activity more in the right hemisphere. These hemispheric asymmetries may be shifted in schizophrenia.

EEG frequency is also extremely sensitive to the effects of centrally acting drugs. In general, hypnotics and sedatives tend to increase slow wave activity while central stimulants tend to increase fast wave activity. Anxiolytic drugs such as the benzodiazepines may increase both slow and fast wave activity; the increase in beta-activity is thought to be due to disinhibition. A wide range of psychotropic drugs give distinctive profiles on spectral analysis, and these have been of predictive value in developing new antidepressant and antipsychotic drugs (Chapters 12 and 14). Typical computer analysed EEG profiles of four classes of psychotropic drugs are shown in Fig. 2.11 (Itil and Soldatos 1980).

Cortical evoked potentials

Signal averaging techniques have made it possible to record cortical evoked responses to stimuli such as light (visual evoked potential), sound (auditory evoked potential), and somatic sensory stimuli (somatosensory evoked potential) (Fig. 2.12). The early, small amplitude, components of these potentials

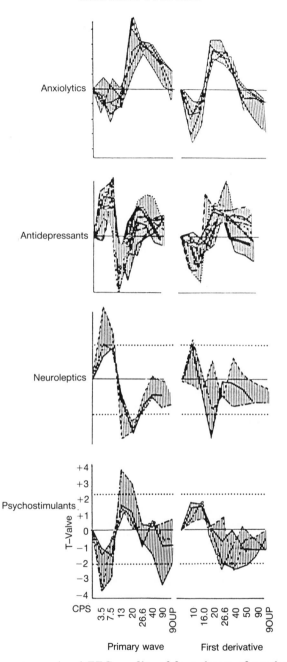

Fig. 2.11. Computer analysed EEG profiles of four classes of psychotropic drugs. Results of several studies using a variety of different drugs in each group. (From Itil and Soldatos 1980.)

(up to 10 ms after the stimulus) reflect the passage of impulses through the brainstem to the primary cortical sensory areas. The later components reflect more generalized cortical activation, and are thought to be associated with cortical cognitive and processing events. There are various conventions for measuring different peaks: a fairly robust measure is the amplitude of the N_1 and P_2 components, occurring in the region of 100 and 200 ms after the stimulus (Fig. 2.12). The amplitude of these peaks is, in general, increased and their latency shortened in states of increased attention and by central nervous system stimulant drugs, while drowsiness and central depressant drugs decrease their amplitude and increase their latency (Shagass and Straumenis 1978). Over a certain range, increased stimulus strength increases the amplitude of these components, but there are considerable individual differences in evoked potential response at high stimulus strengths (Buchsbaum 1976). Some components of evoked potentials also correlate with personality characteristics (Golding and Richards 1985; Ashton et al. 1985). A positive wave, occurring at about 300 ms post-stimulus (P300) appears to be associated with decision-making and stimulus/response uncertainty. For reviews of this fast developing field in relation to psychopathology, see Dongier et al. (1977) Shagass (1977), and Fenton (1984).

Event-Related slow cortical potentials

Various slow cortical potentials, occurring 500 ms or more post-stimulus, have been related to certain cognitive processes. The best known of these slow potentials is the contingent negative variation (CNV) (Walter et al. 1964), which consists of a slow negative potential developing in the period

Fig. 2.12. Cortical Evoked Potentials. (A) Auditory evoked potential (AER). (B) Visual evoked potential (VER). (C) Somatosensory evoked potential (SEP). Components such as N_1 and P_2, occurring approximately 100 ms and 200 ms post-stimulus, and later components, are thought to reflect cognitive processes (see text). The tracings represent the averaged response to 30 light flashes (A), 30 tones (B), 30 non-painful electrical stimuli to the skin over the median nerve at the wrist (C) in normal human subjects. (D) Contingent negative variation (CNV). Average of 10 responses to a warning stimulus, S_1 (light flash) and an imperative stimulus, S_2 (brief tone) requiring a motor response. CNV is calculated as the area xyz in which B is drawn through the prestimulus baseline and P is a perpendicular to the baseline at a point immediately after S_2. CNV magnitude is expressed in μVs. VER and AER: visual and auditory evoked responses to S_1 and S_2. The CNV is thought to reflect certain cognitive processes including expectancy and its magnitude is related to the level of arousal (see text).

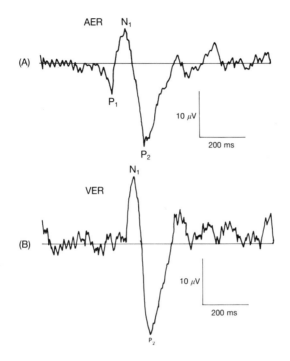

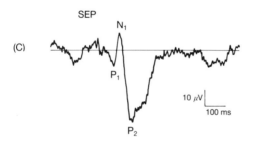

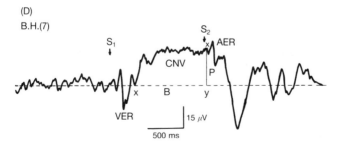

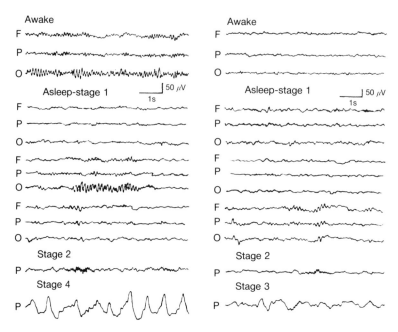

Fig. 2.13. EEG characteristics of orthodox sleep stages in two subjects. Locations of leads: F, frontal; P, parietal; 0, occipital. (From Dement and Kleitman 1957.)

between a warning stimulus and a subsequent imperative stimulus, usually requiring a motor response such as pressing a button (Fig. 2.12). The CNV includes an early component consisting of an orienting response, and a later motor-readiness component, immediately preceding the motor response. Possibly other components concerned with cognitive processes such as expectancy sustain the negativity in the intermediate period. The genesis of the CNV is not fully understood, but it may be initiated by activity in the reticular and limbic arousal systems (Rebert 1973) and appears to involve both cholinergic and catecholaminergic systems (Thompson *et al.* 1978). The magnitude of the CNV is thought to be related linearly to attention and non-monotonically (inverted U) to arousal (Tecce *et al.* 1978). CNV magnitude is in general increased by central stimulant drugs and decreased by central depressant drugs, but many centrally active drugs have dose-related biphasic effects (Ashton *et al.* 1974, 1976, 1980, 1981). CNV magnitude is altered in various psychopathological states including anxiety, depression and schizophrenia (Dongier *et al.* 1977; Shagass 1977). Other slow potentials, including the post-imperative negative variation (Timsit-Berthier 1981) also appear to have psychopathological correlates.

Sleep systems

Towards the lower extreme of the arousal spectrum lies the phenomenon of sleep, itself an expression of two distinct levels of arousal. The two types of sleep, orthodox and paradoxical, are conventionally described in terms of their EEG accompaniments (Oswald 1980; Hartmann 1976; Salamy 1976; Koella 1981a,b).

Orthodox sleep

Orthodox sleep is somewhat arbitrarily divided into four stages which merge into one another, and represent a continuum of decreasing cortical and behavioural arousal (Fig. 2.14). Stage 1 is a transient phase, occurring at the onset of sleep, in which the EEG shows a tendency towards synchronization, predominant alpha activity (8–13 Hz) and a general flattening of the trace. Stage 2 consists of low amplitude waves, punctuated by sleep spindles which are bursts of synchronized electrical activity at 12–15 Hz. Stages 3 and 4 are associated with increasing amounts of high voltage synchronized delta waves at 1–3 Hz. These latter stages represent the deepest level of sleep and are also termed slow wave sleep (SWS).

Somatic accompaniments of orthodox sleep include decreased peripheral sympathetic activity, as evidenced by a slow and regular heart rate, low and steady blood pressure, slow respiration, and reduction of body temperature. Blood flow to the brain is reduced and its distribution is altered: in the waking state the rate of flow is high in anterior parts of the hemispheres and lower in the occipital, parietal, and temporal regions; in SWS blood flow to the anterior parts decreases and a rise occurs in the temporal regions (Ingvar 1979). The eyes show slow rolling movements and the pupils are constricted. Some degree of tone is preserved in the skeletal muscles and the tendon reflexes are usually present although they may be depressed in Stage 4. However, co-ordinated movements such as turning over in bed, occur in

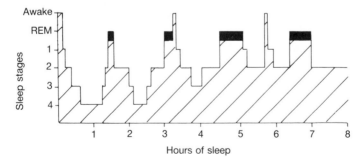

Fig. 2.14. Distribution of sleep stages during a night in normal young adults. (From Horne, 1976.)

Stage 2. Considerable endocrine activity occurs during SWS and there is a large output of growth hormone (Adam and Oswald 1977). Prolactin, and in early puberty luteinizing hormone and testosterone also show sleep dependent secretion (Oswald 1976).

Paradoxical sleep

Paradoxical sleep or rapid eye movement sleep (REMS) has quite different characteristics. The EEG shows low voltage, unsynchronized fast activity similar to that found in the alert conscious state. The eyes show rapid jerky movements which can be recorded on the electro-oculogram. The jaw muscles relax at the onset of REMS and the tone of the skeletal muscles is completely lost, with absence of tendon reflexes. However, this state is periodically interrupted by spasmodic jerky movements of the limbs with hypertonus and momentarily increased tendon reflexes. These limb movements are like the rapid eye movements and quite unlike the more co-ordinated movements seen in orthodox sleep or in the waking state. Peripheral autonomic activity is increased: the heart rate becomes irregular with bursts of tachycardia, the blood pressure fluctuates, respiration becomes irregular, sweating and penile erection occurs, and there is an increased output of adrenaline and free fatty acids. There is an increase in blood flow to the brain which may reach levels above those of wakefulness (Oswald 1976); maximal rates of flow occur in the frontal and parietal regions (Ingvar 1979).

It has been claimed that dreaming is closely associated with REMS. Aserinsky and Kleitman (1953) woke subjects after REMS and orthodox sleep periods and found that reports of dreaming occurred in 74 per cent of wakenings from REMS and in only 17 per cent wakenings from orthodox sleep. However, subsequent research has shown that if subjects are asked simply to recount mental experiences during sleep there is an almost equally high rate of recall from orthodox sleep as from REMS (Freeman 1972). The mental experiences during REMS are often more vivid and perceptual, involving a sense of active participation, while those during orthodox sleep tend to be conceptual, mundane, and inactive (Salamy 1976). Nevertheless, dramatic and often frightening dreams are not uncommon at the onset of orthodox sleep and Vogel (1975, 1978) states that dreaming indistinguishable from REMS dreams can occur in all sleep stages. It seems clear that some form of mentation and therefore cortical activity occurs at all stages of sleep.

The distribution of orthodox and REMS during a night's sleep in normal young adult subjects is shown in Fig. 2.13. Orthodox sleep makes up about 75 per cent of total sleeping time. Early in the night there is a predominance of SWS (Stages 3 and 4) while Stage 2 sleep predominates later. The first REM episode occurs about 90 min after the onset of sleep, lasting only a few minutes. REM episodes recur approximately every 90 min and last longer as the night progresses. There are normally between four–six episodes of REMS per night. One or two brief awakenings also commonly occur during the night. The sleep pattern is influenced by age, the amount and proportion of both SWS and REMS being greater in infants and smaller in the aged. Changes in sleep patterns produced by disease and drugs are mentioned in later sections.

Neural mechanisms of sleep

It is now generally accepted that both types of sleep are largely the result of active processes promoted and maintained by neural mechanisms in the lower brainstem, basal forebrain, pons, and vestibular nuclei and parts of the limbic system. Electrical stimulation of the lower brainstem and areas in the basal forebrain produces EEG synchronization and behavioural sleep in intact animals, and records from single neurones in these areas show that they begin to discharge 1–2 min before the onset of natural sleep (Block and Bonvallet 1960; Bremer 1970). Conversely, complete transection of the brainstem rostral to the bulbar portion, isolating the brain from the lower portion of the reticular formation, causes marked insomnia in cats with desynchronization of the EEG and ocular signs of increased wakefulness (Batini *et al.* 1959; Fig. 2.2). Thus, the lower portion of the reticular formation contains mechanisms for activating orthodox sleep by means of inhibitory fibres to the reticular activing system and, probably via relays in the thalamic nuclei, to the cortex.

The neural mechanisms for REMS appear to originate in the pons, brainstem, and vestibular nuclei. Stimulation and section experiments have demonstrated separate centres in these areas which control EEG desynchronization and flaccid paralysis on the one hand and the superimposed phasic events of clonic limb and eye movements on the other (Jouvet 1967, 1973; Pompeiano 1967; Chase and Morales 1984). REMS appears to be a subcortical phenomenon since it can occur after decortication; SWS on the other hand depends on the integrity of the cortex (Jouvet 1973).

The mechanisms which promote both orthodox and REMS are thought also to have reciprocal inhibitory connections with the active waking system, so that activation of the sleep mechanism at the same time inhibits awakening, and vice versa. Thus, both awakening and sleep result from the combination of active waking or sleeping mechanisms and passive de-waking or de-sleeping mechanisms (Koella 1974, 1981a,b).

Neurotransmitters and sleep

Several neurotransmitters, neuromodulators, and hormones appear to interact in a highly complex manner in the sleep-wakefulness cycle. These include serotonin (and possibly melatonin), noradrenaline, dopamine, acetylcholine, GABA, and probably various polypeptides and hormones. The role of these substances in sleep has been reviewed by Gaillard (1983), Koella (1981a,b), and Monnier and Gaillard (1981).

Serotonergic systems

There is considerable evidence that serotonergic mechanisms are of prime importance in sleep in animals. These are mediated by ascending fibres from the anterior raphe nuclei which terminate throughout wide regions of the telencephalon and diencephalon, and have connections with the limbic system and frontal lobe (Kostowski 1975) and by descending fibres from cell groups B_7 and B_9 which project to the cervical spinal cord (Bowker 1984). Depletion of brain serotonin by *para*-chloro-phenylalanine (*p*-CPA), which inhibits serotonin synthesis, is followed in cats by marked insomnia, the degree of which is proportional to the decrease in cerebral serotonin. This insomnia is reversed by small doses of the serotonin precursor 5-hydroxytryptophan. Similarly, surgical destruction of the mesencephalic and pontine raphe system produces severe insomnia proportional to the decrease in serotonin in the nerve terminals. In intact animals, parenteral injection of 5-hydroxy-tryptophan or the injection of small doses of serotonin into the carotid artery or fourth ventricle induce behavioural sleep with EEG synchronization, while the administration of serotonin receptor blockers decreases sleep. Electrical stimulation of serotonergic nerves in the solitary tract nucleus produces EEG synchronization, and hippocampal and midbrain levels of serotonin and its metabolite 5-hydroxyindoleacetic acid (5HIAA) have been shown to increase during sleep (Koella 1974, 1981a,b; Jouvet and Pujol 1974; King 1974).

There is general agreement that serotonergic mechanisms promote SWS in animals; Koella (1974, 1981a,b) views serotonin as a transmitter both for active 'pro-sleep' and as an 'anti-waking' agent, by inhibition of arousal systems. The role of indole amines in REMS is more controversial. Henrikson *et al.* (1974) and Koella (1974) suggest that serotonin actively inhibits REMS and also prevents the obtrusion of REMS phenomena into waking activity. Recordings from single neurones in the raphe dorsalis of the cat show that they have maximal rates of firing during wakefulness, lower rates during SWS, and are silent during REMS episodes (McGinty and Harper 1976; Jacobs 1984). It is possible that some raphe cells may be involved in initiating REMS even if they are quiescent once it occurs, and Monnier and Gaillard (1980) point out that the results of lesioning experiments suggest that there is some specialisation in the raphe system, the anterior part being concerned with SWS and the posterior part possibly with the priming of REMS. Furthermore, other neurones in the raphe nuclei contain acetylcholine and several polypeptides, and it seems likely that these may also be involved in modulation of ascending and descending influences during the sleep-waking cycle (Bowker 1984).

In man, the role of serotonin in sleep is even less clear. L-tryptophan has been found to increase slow wave sleep in several studies reviewed by Hart-mann (1979), although the effects on REMS are variable. Conflicting results are mentioned by Oswald *et al.* (1982) and Spinweber *et al.* (1983). 5-hydroxy-tryptophan and *p* -CPA affect mainly REMS (Wyatt and Gillin 1976). In a small study over nine nights, of four patients with dementia, Wyatt *et al.* (1974) showed that cerebral ventricular fluid concentrations of 5HIAA were highest during slow wave sleep, lower during waking, and lowest during REMS. The levels of 5HIAA were thought to reflect corresponding activity of central serotonergic neurones, and suggested that, in man as in animals, serotonin is involved in waking, slow wave sleep, and REMS.

Melatonin is synthesized from serotonin in the pineal gland but may also occur in other parts of the brain, notably the hypothalamus (Koslow 1974). Pineal melatonin concentration is well known to be responsive to environ-mental light and darkness, and a role for melatonin in sleep is suggested by observations that it induces sleep in chicks, cats, and rats (Holmes and Sugden 1982). Melatonin also seems to be a potent sleep-inducer in man, intravenous doses of 50 mg producing sleep with normal patterns of orthodox and REMS (Cramer *et al.* 1974). However, its physiological role in sleep is not known.

Noradrenergic and dopaminergic systems

It seems likely that the serotonin-containing cells of the raphe nuclei are connected anatomically with the noradrenaline-containing cells of the locus coeruleus and with dopamine-containing cells in the ventral tegmental area, and that the functional relationship between these systems is important in the sleep-waking cycle (Koslowski 1975; Stevens 1979). While serotonergic activity, as described above, appears to promote slow wave sleep and possibly prevents REMS and waking, the catecholamine system tends to act in reverse to promote waking and to inhibit SWS and allow REMS (Wyatt and Gillin 1976; Key and Krzywoskinski 1977; Koella 1981a,b). These effects are due to mutually inhibitory feedback loops whereby the raphe nuclei inhibit the catechol amine systems and these reciprocally inhibit the raphe nuclei (Kos-lowski 1975).

Enhancement of central catecholamine activity produces behavioural and EEG arousal and inhibits sleep. This effect can be produced by drugs such as amphetamine, L-dopa, cocaine (Herning *et al.* 1985), or, in animals, electrical stimulation of the locus coeruleus (which results in increased release of nor-adrenaline). Conversely, reduction of central catecholamine activity (with 6-hydroxydopamine, tryosine hydroxylase inhibitors, methyldopa, reserpine and alpha$_2$ stimulants) induces a state of behavioural and/or EEG sedation (Koella 1981a,b).

While it is clear that catecholamines promote waking and inhibit SWS, their role in REMS is not known (Gaillard 1983; Monti 1983; Koella

1981a,b). Lesioning, electrophysiological, and pharmacological investigations have given conflicting and often apparently incompatible results. For example, Chu and Bloom (1973) reported that the firing rates of adrenergic neurones in the locus coeruleus of cats were high during wakefulness and REMS but low during drowsiness and SWS, while McGinty *et al.* (1974) and Jacobs (1984) found that the firing rates of both noradrenaline and serotonin-containing cells decreased or even ceased during REMS. Nevertheless, catecholaminergic activity does seem to be related in some way to REMS and Koella (1981a,b) suggests that some optimal level of activity is required. In support of this, REMS is decreased in cats and rats by the alpha$_2$-receptor stimulant clonidine (which decreases noradrenaline release), the alpha$_1$-receptor antagonist phenoxybenzamine, the beta-receptor antagonist propranolol, and selective beta$_1$-antagonists (Leppavuori and Putkonen 1980; Gaillard 1983; Monti 1983; Lanfumey *et al.* 1985). Alpha$_1$-, alpha$_2$-, and beta-adrenoceptors, as well as serotonin and dopamine receptors may all be involved in the generation of REMS, and Gaillard (1983) emphasizes the importance of collateral inhibition in cell populations and of changes in receptor sensitivity in sleep/waking cycles.

In man, REMS is also decreased by clonidine and increased by the alpha$_2$ antagonist yohimbine (Kanno and Clarenbach 1985). On the other hand, chronic administration of drugs which deplete central monoamine systems or block adrenergic receptors (reserpine, methyldopa) increase REMS, while drugs which increase central monoamine activity (L-dopa, amphetamine, monoamine reuptake blockers, monoamine oxidase inhibitors) decrease REMS (Hartmann 1976; Kay *et al.* 1976; Wyatt and Gillin 1976). These apparent divergences between animal and human studies may be due to differences in drug dosage or duration. In addition, in manic-depressive and schizophrenic psychoses there are profound abnormalities in REMS which may be related to abnormal central monoamine function, (Schultz *et al.* 1978) (Chapters 11 and 13).

Cholinergic systems

Present evidence suggests that cholinergic mechanisms, as well as producing arousal, induce or facilitate paradoxical sleep. The rate of liberation of acetylcholine from the cerebral cortex (Jasper and Tessier 1971) and corpus striatum (Gadea-Ciria *et al.* 1973) of the cat is increased during REMS compared with slow wave sleep. Injection of acetylcholine or carbachol in the region of the locus coeruleus induces REMS in animals (George *et al.* 1964), and atropine (Jouvet 1969) and the intraventricular administration of hemicholinium-3 (Hazra 1970) reduce REMS in cats. In man, anticholinergic drugs such as atropine and scopolamine suppress REMS, while anticholinesterases appear to increase REMS. Thus, nightmares and excessive dreaming are common symptoms of anticholinesterase poisoning and industrial workers exposed to organophosphates have been found to have longer REM periods than normal or reduced latency of REMS (Wyatt and Gillin 1976).

Although cholinergic activity is evidently important in paradoxical sleep, the extent to which it contributes to the various components is not clear. While it may account for the tonic components, such as EEG desynchronization, it is likely that an interaction with other systems is involved in the phasic components, such as the rapid fluctuations in muscle tone and autonomic activity. Probably muscarinic receptors are involved in REMS; stimulation of nicotine receptors leads to arousal (Monnier and Gaillard 1981).

GABA-ergic systems

The general inhibitory actions of GABA are likely to be involved in sleep. Jasper *et al.* (1965) showed that the release of GABA from the cat's cerebral cortex is increased during EEG synchrony; infusion of GABA induces cortical synchronization and behavioural sleep (Godschalk *et al.* 1977); and increasing brain levels of GABA in rats by aminooxyacetic acid decreases behavioural arousal (Benton and Rick 1976). In man, benzodiazepines, which enhance GABA activity in the central nervous system (Guidotti *et al.* 1978), promote Stage 2 orthodox sleep and inhibit REMS and slow wave sleep (Kay *et al.* 1976). In addition, GABA-ergic systems in several parts of the brain exert an inhibitory control over the release of neurotransmitters associated with arousal, including noradrenaline, dopamine and acetylcholine (Benton and Rick 1976).

Polypeptides

The possibility that various polypeptides are somehow involved in sleep has been investigated for many years. These studies are reviewed by Drucker-Colin (1981), Inque *et al.* (1982), and Koella (1983). For example, Kornmuller *et al.* (1961) showed in cross-circulation experiments in dogs that a blood-borne substance from a sleeping donor induced EEG synchrony in the recipient. Monnier and Hosli (1965) obtained a dialysate from the venous blood draining the brain in sleeping rabbits which would induce SWS in recipient rabbits. The sleep-inducing agent was subsequently isolated and identified as a polypeptide containing eleven amino acids, with a molecular weight of approximately 800; it was named delta sleep inducing peptide (DSIP). This substance was later found also to increase REMS in cats (Inque *et al.* 1982) and to be present in the human brain (Schoenenberger and Schneider-Helmert 1983). Pappenheimer and his colleagues (1967) collected the cerebrospinal fluid of sleep-deprived goats and isolated a tetrapeptide (molecular weight approximately 500) that induced SWS on intraventricular injection in several animal species. A similar tetrapeptide was isolated in Japan from the brainstem of sleep-deprived rats (Nagasaki *et al.* 1974; 1976). Difficulties in the interpretation of such studies were discussed by Drucker-Colin (1981) who concluded that the existence of a specific sleep-inducing peptide in animals was not yet proved conclusively.

In man, circulating polypeptides do not appear to be critical for sleep induction since conjoined twins with shared circulations have independent cycles of sleep, waking, REMS and orthodox sleep (Lenard and Schulte 1972). However, peptide sleep-promoting factors produced in the brain may be part of a multitude of hypnogenic or de-awaking substances signalling sleepiness in states of sleep deprivation (Koella 1983), and they may also be involved in the circadian rhythmicity so characteristic of sleep (Inque *et al.* 1982). It is possible that they have a therapeutic potential for insomnia and anxiety (Schneider-Helmert *et al.* 1981). Schoenenberger and Schneider-Helmert (1983) report some preliminary clinical studies with DSIP. Injections of this substance induced sleep in normal subjects and restored normal sleep in insomniac patients as well as in one patient with a central nervous depressant withdrawal syndrome.

Certain polypeptide hormones may also play a part in the modulation of sleep. For example, it has been suggested that the release of growth hormone during SWS early in the night triggers the subsequent appearance of REMS (Stern and Morgane 1977). Growth hormone induces a dose-dependent increase of REMS in cats, rats, and humans (Drucker-Colin 1981). It is possible that this effect is an indirect result of increased protein synthesis induced by the hormone, and studies showing that protein synthesis inhibitors such as chloramphenicol decrease REMS rebound following REMS deprivation or amphetamine withdrawal would tend to support this idea. Drucker-Colin (1981) studied the effects of specific antibodies against proteins obtained from the cat's midbrain reticular formation during REMS and found that such antibodies had similar effects to protein synthesis inhibitors: like chloramphenicol, they blocked the phasic aspects of REMS. The importance of protein synthesis and of anabolic hormones in regulating or inducing sleep has yet to be assessed; Jouvet (1977) pointed out that total hypophysectomy does not seriously alter the sleep-waking cycle. However pituitary hormones and brain polypeptides including substance P, cholecystokinin, somatostatin, neurotensin, endogenous opioids, arginine vasopressin, vasoactive intestinal polypeptide, hypothalamic releasing factors as well as steroid hormones including oestrogens have all been implicated as possible neuromodulators of sleep processes (Cooper *et al.* 1978; Thomson and Oswald 1977; Byck 1976; Drucker-Colin 1981; Koella 1983; Bowker 1984).

Sleep deprivation

Insomnia is a common complaint, but major deleterious effects of sleep deprivation have been difficult to demonstrate experimentally. Total sleep deprivation leads to impairment of performance in tasks requiring vigilance, since there is an increasing tendency for subjects to snatch 'microsleeps'. In continuous prolonged tasks, a marked deterioration in performance begins after about 18 h (Mullaney *et al.* 1983). However, performance in short tasks remains remarkably normal. After 60 h total sleep deprivation, performance in games of darts and table tennis remained at 97 per cent and 100 per cent of pre-deprivation values in one study reported by Wilkinson (1965). Neurological and psychological changes occur including visual disturbances, tremor, slowness of speech, nystagmus, misperceptions, visual hallucinations, and depersonalization, increased suggestibility, subjective lassitude, anxiety, and decreased pain tolerance (Horne 1976a; Oswald 1980; Wilkinson 1965; Mullaney *et al.* 1983). Total sleep deprivation combined with isolation has been used in 'brain washing' techniques.

Recovery from total sleep deprivation is charcteristized by a rebound of SWS and later of REMS, usually at the expense of Stages 1 and 2 sleep which appear to be more 'expendable'. Kales *et al.* (1970), in a study of 205 h of total sleep deprivation, found that in the first three recovery nights SWS increased 350, 250, and 200 per cent, respectively, from pre-deprivation levels. REMS showed a smaller and delayed rebound, increasing 30, 60, and 20 per cent over the same nights. Total sleeping time was increased during recovery nights, with an increase is 50 per cent on the first night, smaller increases on succeeding nights, and a return to normal on the fourth night.

Healthy young adults appear to adjust remarkably well to moderate total sleep limitation (e.g., from 8 to 6 h for 6 weeks). A greater percentage of time is devoted to SWS, at the expense of Stages 1 and 2 and REMS, and few adverse effects have been demonstrated (Horne 1976b; Horne and Wilkinson 1985). Naturally occurring short sleepers have comparatively large amounts of SWS and small amounts of Stages 1 and 2 and REMS (Jones and Oswald 1968).

Early reports of severe psychological effects after selective deprivation of REMS (Dement 1960) have not been supported by later work and numerous studies have reported only mild disturbances after REMS deprivation for up to 14 consecutive nights. These include irritability, anxiety, increased appetite, difficulty in concentration, possibly some disturbance of memory function, but normally little impairment in psychometric tests (Vogel 1975; Horne 1976b; Agnew *et al.* 1967; Faber and Havrdova 1981; Fowler *et al.* 1973). On recovery nights, there is a rebound with an increase in REMS time, increased vividness of dreams and sometimes nightmares (Oswald 1980). More marked and longer-lasting changes occur after drugs which reduce both REMS and SWS (Oswald 1980; Chapter 4).

Selective deprivation of SWS has been less studied. However, Agnew *et al.* (1967) reported that deprived subjects became depressed and lethargic, physically inactive and less responsive to the environment. Johnson *et al.* (1974) found impairment in vigilance tasks similar to that after total sleep deprivation. Rebound in SWS occurs on recovery nights. Comparisons of selective sleep state deprivation in animals and man suggest that REMS deprivation leads to increased cortical excitability while SWS deprivation leads to decreased cortical excitability (Vogel 1975).

Function of sleep

Despite growing information on the mechanisms which generate and regulate sleep, its function remains enigmatic. The overwhelming desire to sleep when deprived, and the rapid restoration of SWS and REMS after deprivation suggest that both types of sleep are necessary in man. Since orthodox and paradoxical sleep are so different physiologically, it is assumed that their functions also differ.

Orthodox Sleep

It is generally accepted that sleep is necessary for growth in the young and that it performs restorative functions in the adult, although the precise nature of these functions is only beginning to become clear. Much evidence (quoted by Adam *et al.* 1977; Adam and Oswald 1977; Oswald 1976) now supports the idea that SWS is connected with anabolic activity throughout the body. Anabolic hormones, including growth hormone, prolactin, luteinizing hormone, and testosterone are released during SWS. Growing animals and humans sleep more than adults, and sleep deprivation in the young stunts growth. SWS and growth hormone secretion appear to increase in adults after physical exercise and other factors which increase cerebral metabolic rate, including body heating and sustained, demanding attention (Horne 1983). SWS is correlated with changes in body weight: acute starvation and hyperthyroidism, in which there is increased protein catabolism during the day, are associated with increased SWS and growth hormone output during the night, while in hypothyroidism SWS is decreased. In addition, a wide range of body tissues in animals and man show increased rates of protein synthesis or mitoses during sleep. Adam *et al.* (1977) propose that SWS favours energy-yielding (ATP-producing) compared with energy-using (ATP-depleting) processes throughout the body, and such alteration in metabolic state is believed to favour protein synthesis for growth and repair.

SWS, in which the majority of cortical neurones have reduced firing rates and cortical responsiveness is at its lowest, may be of particular importance for anabolic processes in the brain. Increased concentrations of ATP and RNA and increased rates of protein synthesis have been found in the brains of rats, cats, and golden hamsters during sleep, and lower concentrations during sleep deprivation. Other workers have related SWS to memory consolidation (Fowler *et al.* 1973; Broughton and Gestaut 1973; Stern and Morgane 1977; Ekstrand *et al.* 1977) and to cognitive processes related to daytime visual load (Horne 1976a,b), both of which may require protein synthesis in the brain. However, none of these results can yet be regarded as conclusive and it is still not clear in man exactly what sleep achieves that cannot be achieved by relaxed wakefulness (Horne 1979).

Paradoxical sleep

The function of REMS is even less clear than that of SWS; nor is it known whether the separate tonic and phases of REMS subserve different functions. In evolution, REMS seems to have appeared before SWS, and it is thought to be a more 'primitive' form of subcortical sleep. It seems possible that one of the functions of REMS in some mammals is to conserve heat and energy (Horne 1977). During REMS, peripheral vasoconstriction occurs in the heat-dissipating vascular organs of rabbits, cats, and other mammals, suggesting a thermoregulatory function. Furthermore, the amount of REMS is greater in small mammals, who can conserve relatively more energy during sleep, than in larger mammals, and is more abundant in rodents that hibernate than in non-hibernating rodents of similar size. Sleep in general, including hibernation, appears to have originated as an adaptive process in response to environmental factors such as difficulty in finding food and low temperatures. It may also serve to protect some animals from predators.

However, these considerations do not appear to apply to primates, and it is quite possible that REMS, like other subcortical processes, has further evolved to perform different or more complex functions. Among apes, the amount of REMS is no longer negatively correlated with size, but is more abundant in larger species; man has more REMS than the chimpanzee and chimpanzees have more REMS than the rhesus monkey. On another evolutionary path, some dolphins (Dall's porpoise) appear never to sleep at all, while the bottle-nosed dolphin and the pilot whale sleep with one hemisphere at a time, possibly alternating sleep stages between hemispheres and experiencing SWS in one hemisphere and REMS simultaneously in the other (Durie 1981).

It has been suggested that REMS may in some way be necessary for normal psychological functioning in man. Although, as mentioned above, REMS deprivation in general leads to only mild psychological changes, there may be some important, if subtle, effects. Irritability is common after REMS deprivation and Shaw *et al.* (1982) report that normal emotional responses to horrifying films become blunted in deprived subjects. In schizophrenia and depression, on the other hand, REMS time may be increased and REMS deprivation may be beneficial. There are close anatomical and functional interactions between brain structures promoting REMS and limbic structures subserving emotional and motivational functions. In rats, REMS deprivation lowers the threshold for and increases the response rate of (rewarding) intracranial self-stimulation and increases sexual behaviour (Vogel 1975). Such links may well persist in man and may be evidenced in the highly emotional content of some REMS dreams. What function, if any, such links perform for mental health in man remains obscure.

Many investigations have sought to establish a link between REMS and memory. Sleep in general seems to improve memory and learning in animals and man, while sleep deprivation, especially REMS deprivation, impairs these processes. Thus, it has been suggested that sleep, especially REMS, is necessary for some memory processes. In particular, the connection between REMS and motivational systems would tend to strengthen memory consolidation. However, interpretation of the many conflicting results is difficult and, in a critical review Vogel (1975) concludes that an effect of REMS deprivation on learning and memory is not established. Horne (1979) suggested that although REMS may facilitate certain types of memory in animals and man, it is the integrity of the total orthodox-paradoxical sleep cycle which is most important for learning and memory in general.

Circumstantial evidence often adduced in support of a connection between REMS and memory includes the observations that learning and memory defects in old age, Korsakoff's and Alzheimer's dementias, other brainstem lesions, and mental retardation are associated with decreased amounts of REMS while infants and children have increased amounts of REMS. These observations would support equally the work suggesting that REMS, as well as SWS, is concerned with growth and protein synthesis in the brain (Oswald 1976; Adam et al. 1977; Drucker-Colin 1981). Possibly brain protein synthesis and consolidation of memory are associated, in so far as learning requires alterations in or strengthening of synaptic connections throughout the brain. Adam et al. (1977) point out that REMS periods are too short in most animal species to provide for major protein synthesis. However, oscillations in the rate of protein synthesis in the brain may underlie orthodox sleep and REMS cycles, and explain why both sleep stages seem to be involved in memory.

REMS has also been closely connected with dreaming, although it now appears that dreams can occur in both sleep stages. The observations of increased cerebral blood flow and a rapid rate of firing of most cerebral neurones during REMS give evidence of a particularly high level of brain activity. Current thinking suggests that dreams may be a by-product of this activity, which is related as much to forgetting as to remembering. Thus, Moiseeva (1979) suggested that during REMS the brain is 'editing' information received during the day and maintaining or establishing some synaptic connections by rehearsal while inhibiting others. Crick and Mitchison (1983) made the similar suggestion that 'unlearning' occurs during REMS, in which unwanted memory traces are removed and strong ones reinforced. Dreams presumably appear as fragments of these processes which happen to reach consciousness.

Further investigations of the tantalising connections between REMS, dreaming, memory, and temporal lobe epilepsy are discussed in Chapter 9. Alterations of sleep in psychotic states are described in Chapters 11 and 13, and drug effects on SWS and REMS are mentioned in Chapters 4, 12, and 14.

3
Disorders of arousal and sleep systems

Since the organization of sleep and wakefulness is highly elaborate and their function much influenced by external events, it is not surprising that disorders of these systems are common. As discussed in Chapter 2, sleeping and waking mechanisms operate together as a homogeneous functional unit, the final output of which determines the level of arousal. Thus, disorders of one mechanism inevitably tend to affect others: anxiety is accompanied by insomnia; poor night-time sleep is associated with daytime sleepiness. However, for convenience the disorders are divided here into those which are mainly manifested in the waking state (e.g., anxiety syndromes) and those whose main characteristic is sleep disturbance (e.g., insomnia and hypersomnia). Sleep disturbances in chronic pain syndromes, depression, and schizophrenia are discussed in later chapters.

Anxiety states

Anxiety is a normal adaptive response to certain types of stress; it increases 'drive' (Shaw *et al.* 1982; Chapter 5) and, at optimal levels, improves behavioural efficiency (Chapter 2). The manifestations of clinically described anxiety states are similar to those experienced by normal subjects exposed to anxiety-provoking situations and any psychophysiological differences appear to be quantitative rather than qualitative (Lader 1978, 1980). Thus clinical anxiety has been defined as 'anxiety which is more severe, more persistent or more pervasive than the individual is accustomed to or can bear' (Lader 1980, p. 226). It occurs when the degree of stress to which an individual is exposed overcomes his ability to adapt to it efficiently (Gelder *et al.* 1983). Vulnerability to stress appears to be linked to certain genetic factors such as trait anxiety (Eysenck 1957; Roth 1984) and to environmental influences. Difficulties in the current classification of clinical anxiety states are discussed by Tyrer (1985). In normal subjects anxiety symptoms may be induced by severe stress; certain drugs (including caffeine, amphetamine, psychotomimetics, lactate, or adrenaline infusions); withdrawal from central nervous system depressant drugs (narcotics, hypnotics, anxiolytics); and by hypoglycaemia, hypercarbia, starvation, or prolonged sleep loss. Anxiety may accompany hormone-secreting tumours such as phaeochromocytoma or carcinoid, and psychiatric disorders such as schizophrenia and depression.

Clinical manifestations

Symptoms

Both psychological and somatic symptoms occur in anxiety states (Gelder *et al.* 1983). A major psychological symptom is a pervading sense of apprehension and fear, usually without apparent or sufficient cause. Other psychological symptoms include restlessness, difficulty in concentration, and specific phobias. Somatic symptoms may be related to almost any body system: cardiovascular (palpitations, chest pain); respiratory (tightness in the chest, dyspnoea, overbreathing); gastrointestinal (dry mouth, poor appetite, dysphagia, epigastric discomfort, gaseous distension, diarrhoea, or urgency); urogenital (frequency and urgency of micturition, menstrual disorders, impotence, loss of libido); central and autonomic (insomnia, nightmares, tinnitus, blurred vision, dizziness, faintness, paraesthesiae, sweating); and neuromuscular (tremor, weakness, increased muscle tension with stiffness and pain, headaches).

Somatic changes

The symptoms of anxiety are accompanied by somatic alterations. Since the pioneering work of Cannon (1936) and Selye (1956) on the profound neuroendocrine changes induced by stress, much research has been devoted to identifying and quantitating somatic variables in anxiety. The results of many such studies have been reviewed by Lader (1978, 1980), Mason (1972), Lang *et al.* (1972), and the several anatomical linkages in the brain by which neural and presumably psychological stimuli can influence many autonomic and endocrine systems have been outlined by Mason (1972). In general, the somatic changes associated with anxiety are similar in normal subjects and anxious patients. Patients with anxiety syndromes are characterized not so much by abnormal resting levels of neuroendocrine activity, as by enhanced responsiveness to stressful stimuli and slower than normal rates of habituation to repeated stimuli.

Cardiovascular changes Tachycardia and an increase in blood pressure occurs in normal subjects exposed to stress (Taggart *et al.* 1973; Taylor and Meeran 1973). In anxious patients, resting heart rate and blood pressure may be normal or raised but both tend to be more variable and to show greater than normal increases in response to stressful procedures. Furthermore, stress-induced tachycardia or hypertension are maintained for longer in patients with anxiety syndromes than in normal subjects (Lader 1980).

Sweat gland activity A number of studies have compared sweat gland activity in normal subjects and patients with a variety of anxiety disorders (Lader and Wing 1964, 1966; Lader 1967; Bond *et al.* 1974; Horvath and Meares

1979; Ohman *et al*. 1974). In general, anxious patients show a greater number of spontaneous fluctuations in skin conductance, and a slower rate of habituation in the skin conductance response to auditory and other stimuli than normal subjects. Frequency of spontaneous fluctuations has been found to correlate positively and rate of habituation negatively with psychiatric ratings of anxiety.

Respiration Respiratory rate normally increases during stress and is often raised in anxious patients (Lader 1980); panic attacks are commonly accompanied by hyperventilation, which may induce respiratory alkalosis, carpopedal spasm and many symptoms including dizziness, tinnitus, headache, and paraesthesiae. Blood gas analysis may show alterations in acute cases but may be normal in chronic cases (Lum 1981; Bonn *et al*.1984; Hibbert 1984).

Muscle activity Muscle tension, particularly in the neck and jaws, is increased by anxiety. Electromyographic studies have shown greater than normal activity in the masseter, forearm, frontalis, and neck muscles in anxious patients, and a greater response to stimuli such as white noise (Lader 1980; Goldstein 1972). Prolonged muscle tension may give rise to occipital or frontal headache, backache, and tooth or jaw ache, symptoms seen commonly in anxiety neurosis. Finger, hand, and jaw tremor are common in anxiety states and presumably result from sympathetic hyperactivity since they respond to beta-adrenergic antagonists. James *et al*. (1977) reported that oxprenolol improved performance under stress in stringed instrument players, while propranolol is used in anxiety states associated with tremor and other somatic complaints (Tyrer and Lader 1974).

Catecholamines Numerous studies in animals (reviewed by Anisman *et al*. 1981) have shown that stress increases the synthesis and utilization of catecholamines and serotonin. In normal human subjects exposed to a variety of stressful situations, the urinary excretion of adrenaline and noradrenaline increases (Mason 1972; Lader 1980; Bloom *et al*. 1963). Plasma catecholamine concentrations may also be raised in stressful situations, and in anger and after laughing (Lader, 1980). Taggart *et al*. (1973) found raised plasma concentrations of noradrenaline, but not adrenaline, in normal subjects stressed by public speaking. Intravenous infusion of a mixture of noradrenaline and adrenaline (0.28 mg of each over 36–41 minutes) produced palpitations, tremor, restlessness, apprehensiveness, tension, and dyspnoea in six of eleven normal subjects studied by Frankenhaeuser and Jarpe (1962). Normal subjects receiving catecholamine infusions tend to report feeling 'as if ' they were anxious, while in subjects with anxiety neurosis such infusions reproduce their morbid anxiety-syndrome (Lader 1980).

There have been relatively few studies of catecholamines in patients with anxiety states. In 11 anxious patients, urinary adrenaline excretion increased following a psychiatric interview (Elmadjian et al. 1957), and there was a positive correlation between plasma catecholamine concentrations and anxiety ratings in a group of 13 patients with anxiety/depression (Wyatt et al. 1971b). Several other studies (reviewed by Mason 1972) have shown increased urinary catecholamine secretion in psychiatric patients especially during periods of stress. Significant correlations have been reported between anxiety and adrenaline excretion, while aggressiveness appears to be associated more with noradrenaline excretion (Cohen et al. 1961).

Sodium lactate infusion Intravenous infusion of sodium lactate may induce feelings of anxiety in some subjects. The mechanism for this reaction is not clear, although some authors have suggested that it might be due to catecholamine release (Lader 1978). Shader et al. (1982) review studies showing that some anxious patients, but not normal subjects, developed panic reactions when infused with sodium lactate (0.5M, 10 mg/kg body weight for up to 20 min). Anxious patients did not develop a similar reaction when infused with a glucose solution or normal saline. The panic reaction was diminished or abolished by adding calcium to the lactate solution or by pretreatment with imipramine or monoamine-oxidase inhibitors; pretreatment with propranolol had no effect on the subjective symptoms, and the alpha$_2$-agonist clonidine diminished the effect only temporarily. No differences were found between normal and anxious patients in plasma calcium ion concentration, but plasma noradrenaline concentrations, heart rate, and diastolic pressure were higher in patients who panicked. After symptomatic recovery from their anxiety states and withdrawal from treatment, patients were able to tolerate sodium lactate infusion without developing panic reactions.

Some clinicians, particularly in the United States, distinguish between generalized anxiety disorders, which respond to benzodiazepines, and panic disorders (including agoraphobia), which respond to antidepressant drugs. Patients with the latter type of syndrome are particularly prone to develop panic reactions on sodium lactate infusion. This technique may therefore be of importance in deciding on treatment, and also provides an opportunity to study a psychopathological syndrome under laboratory conditions (Rifkin and Siris 1984).

Corticosteroids In normal subjects, acute or chronic stress increases the urinary output of 17-hydroxycorticosteroids (Lader 1980; Mason 1972; Tecce et al. 1965). In psychoneurotic patients, greater than normal increases in 17-hydroxycorticosteroid excretion and in plasma 17-hydroxycorticosteroid concentration, and raised plasma concentrations of cortisol and ACTH have been observed, especially during emotional crises and panic episodes (Mason 1972; Lader 1980). However, Shader *et al.* (1982) reported that there was no further increase in plasma cortisol concentration in anxious patients during panic attacks induced by sodium lactate infusion.

It is clear that the pituitary-adrenalcortical and sympathetic nervous systems respond sensitively to psychological influences and to stress. Anticipation, novelty, uncertainty, and unpredictability seem to be particularly potent stimulating factors for both catecholamine and corticosteroid secretion (Mason 1972). There does not appear to be a clear differention for particular emotional states; Mason (1972) suggests that adrenal cortical hormone output may be stimulated in anticipation of activity or coping and that there may be some dissociation between the proportions of noradrenaline and adrenaline secreted during fear and anger. Marked difference between individuals have been noted in both corticosteroid and catecholamine responses to stress. The output of other steroid hormones and of polypeptides including oxytocin and endogenous opioids is also increased by stress (Mason 1972; Anisman *et al.* 1981; Hughes 1983), but these have been less systematically studied in relation to anxiety states.

Electroencephalographic changes The characteristic general hyperactivity, insomnia, and heightened somatic reactivity of anxiety all suggest increased cortical arousal, and objective confirmation has been found in many electroencephalographic studies. Anxious patients tend to have less alpha activity than normal subjects, a significantly faster alpha frequency, and even faster beta activity (13–35 Hz). Cortical evoked potentials in anxiety are reviewed by Shagass *et al.* (1978). The magnitude of the slow cortical potential, the contingent negative variation, is decreased in anxious patients compared with control subjects, especially in anxiety-provoking situations and distraction, and is slower to habituate (McCallum and Walter 1968; Walter 1964; Klorman and Ryan 1980). Negativity following the contingent negative variation is prolonged in neurotics compared to control subjects (Dongier 1973; Timsit-Berthier 1973). Visual and auditory evoked potentials tend to show greater than normal amplitude, shorter latency and slower recovery in anxious patients (Bond *et al.* 1974; Tyrer and Lader 1976; Shagass *et al.* 1978). There is some evidence that cortical activation during stress is normally lateralized to the right hemisphere, and that high levels of anxiety may affect hemisphere processing and interhemispheric functioning (Tucker *et al.* 1977, 1978).

Mechanisms of anxiety
The clinical syndromes of anxiety have been widely regarded as states of over-arousal, and indeed the symptoms and signs are compatible with increased activity in all arousal systems (Chapter 2). While the subjective

emotion of anxiety is relatively specific in that it is readily distinguishable from other emotions, most of the somatic changes also occur in other states of increased arousal, both pleasant and unpleasant. Thus, while there is little doubt that anxiety states are attended by enhanced levels of arousal, hyperarousal by itself is too broad a concept to encapsulate anxiety. Accordingly, attempts have been made to define particular neurological systems in which hyperactivity or dysfunction is specific to anxiety.

In general terms, a number of brain structures are likely to be interdependently involved in anxiety: these include cortical areas, which recognize and evaluate anxiety-provoking stimuli, and limbic areas which generate affective components and, along with the reticular formation and hypothalamic nuclei, activate the autonomic and endocrine concomitants of stress and arousal. Within the limbic system there is evidence that parts of the amygdaloid nucleus are particularly concerned with anxiety, since stimulation of some parts of this nucleus evokes fear responses in many animal species and severe anxiety in humans, while lesions of the amygdala in animals (rats and Rhesus monkeys) have a taming effect with increased placidity (Shaw *et al.* 1982; Herbert 1984; Isaacson 1974, 1982). Kapp and Gallagher (1981) suggest that the amygdala is specifically involved in fear reactions to the threat of painful stimuli (Chapter 8). Redmond (1982) suggests that both normal anxiety and anxiety states may result from increased noradrenergic activity in the locus coeruleus. Gray (1981a, 1982), as discussed below, places particular emphasis on the septo-hippocampal system, and its afferent connections from the locus coeruleus and raphe nuclei. Thalamic and hypothalamic regions appear to be involved in flight mechanisms in animals (Malmo 1972; Shaw *et al* 1982). Biochemical mechanisms involved in anxiety appear to include at least noradrenaline and serotonin (Gray 1981, 1982) and endogenous opioids (Kapp and Gallagher 1979) and probably many others.

Various hypothetical models suggesting ways in which these various systems function together to produce anxiety have been proposed. Lader (1978, 1980) suggests a general model of anxiety, outlined in Fig. 3.1. In this model, external and internal stimuli impinge upon the brain at various conscious and unconscious levels, where they are evaluated for possible threats to the individual. If a potential threat is detected, activity in certain parts of the brain, including the limbic system and the dorsal adrenergic bundle, is increased, producing further cortical and somatic arousal and an affect which is appropriate to the stimulus (fear and anxiety). The widespread physiological effects of the arousal are relayed back to the brain, constituting a positive feedback loop.

On this model, pathological trait anxiety is regarded as an extreme deviation at the upper end of the continuum of personality anxiety. Genetic factors and experience which affect the internal 'drives' may interact to render some

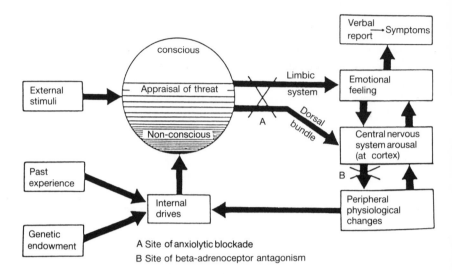

Fig. 3.1. General model of anxiety. External and internal stimuli impinging on the brain are evaluated for potential threat. If threat is detected, increased activity in limbic structures and dorsal bundle causes heightened emotional, cortical and somatic arousal. Sites of action of anxiolytic drugs (Chapter 4) are also indicated. (From Lader 1978, by kind permission of Raven Press, New York.)

individuals more susceptible than others to anxiety under minimal stress. Cognitive factors may also be important: if the anxiety-provoking stimuli are not consciously perceived, then the emotional reaction may seem excessive or inappropriate, and itself engender further anxiety. This scheme draws together several other theories of anxiety and some clinical observations but makes no attempt to specify in neurophysiological terms how threats to the individual are assessed or how such threats engender anxiety instead of other emotions such as depression and hostility.

Koella (1981a), in a study of EEG correlates of anxiety, also implicates the reticular activating system and dorsal adrenergic bundle and suggests from indirect evidence that in anxious individuals there is an excess of activity in general arousal systems (ascending reticular arousal system) and local goal-directed arousal systems (presumably limbic system) and an imbalance of activity between the two systems. Claridge (1967) had earlier proposed such a dissociation between a postulated tonic arousal system controlling general arousal and an arousal modulating system which suppressed or facilitated the arousing effects of incoming information.

Gray (1981a, 1982, 1985) has proposed a more detailed psychophysiological model of anxiety, which is defined as a 'central state elicited by threats of punishment, frustration or failure, and by novelty or uncertainty' (Gray

1981a, p. 194). These stimuli activate a postulated behavioural inhibition system (BIS) (Fig. 3.2) which in turn produces behavioural inhibition, an increment in arousal, and increased attention. On this hypothesis, 'activity in the BIS constitutes anxiety' (Gray 1981a, p.194).

The evidence for Gray's hypothesis rests largely on observations of the effects of anxiolytic drugs on animal behaviour (Gray 1977). In general, drugs which have anxiolytic effects in man counteract specifically the behavioural effects in animals of the classes of stimuli on the left of Fig. 3.2: stimuli associated with punishment or with the omission of expected reward, and novel stimuli. Moreoever, they produce similar effects in all animal species studied, from goldfish to chimpanzees. Hence, Gray concluded that anxiety and its neural basis are phylogenetically ancient and that the animal studies may therefore be applicable to men.

One example of the animal tests employed to assess anxiolytic drugs is the immediate punishment test (Geller–Seifter procedure) a type of conflict test (Iverson 1980). If rats are trained to press a lever for food reward, and then given an electric shock to the feet every time they respond and obtain the reward, their lever-pressing behaviour becomes severely depressed. Drugs which have anxiolytic effects in man reverse this behavioural inhibition; the rats start responding again despite receiving the 'punishment' of electric shocks. This release of punishment behaviour appears to be specifically related to anxiolytic actions since it is exerted by benzodiazepines, barbiturates, meprobamate, and alcohol, but not by major tranquillizers such as chlorpromazine with prominent central nervous system depressant effects, analgesics such as morphine, or stimulants such as amphetamine.

The effects of anxiolytic drugs on animal behaviour in these and a variety of other tests led Gray (1981a, 1982) to conclude that the drugs acted to reduce

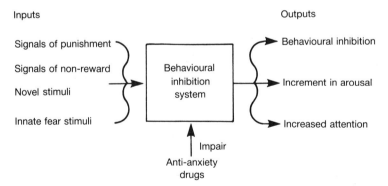

Fig. 3.2. Behavioural inhibition system. The system responds to any of its adequate inputs with all of its outputs. On this model, activity in the behavioural inhibiton system constitutes anxiety and anxiolytic drugs act by depressing such activity. (From Gray 1982, by kind permission of Oxford University Press.)

activity at a common site, the proposed behavioural inhibition system. Both an anatomical and a biochemical basis for this system is proposed. The anatomical location is suggested to be in the limbic system and to involve the septo-hippocampal system or its connections. Two pathways appear to be important: the noradrenergic afferents from the locus coeruleus to the septo-hippocampal system and the serotonergic afferents from the raphe nuclei.

Destruction of noradrenergic neurones in the pathway from the locus coeruleus via the dorsal ascending noradrenergic bundle to the septo-hippocampal system by locally injected 6-hydroxydopamine releases punishment behaviour in rats and produces electrophysiological changes in the septo-hippocampal system that are characteristic of anxiolytic drugs. Similarly in primates, surgical lesions or pharmacological suppression of locus coeruleus activity produces relaxation, while electrical stimulation or pharmacological activation of noradrenergic activity at this site produces physiological and behavioural signs of stress (Redmond 1982). Stress increases the firing rate of locus coeruleus neurones and noradrenergic activity in the dorsal bundle, while all anxiolytic drugs including barbiturates, meprobamate, ethanol, and benzodiazepines impair impulse conduction and noradrenergic activity in this pathway, especially under stress.

Depletion of brain serotonin by parachloraphenylalanine in rats also releases punished behaviour, which can then be reinstated by raising brain serotonin concentration with 5-hydroxytryptophan. Depletion of brain serotonin with the neurotoxin 5,7-dihydroxytryptamine administered into the ascending serotonergic pathways at the level of the median forebrain bundle produces similar effects. Serotonergic antagonists such as methysergide and cinanserin also increase punished responding in cats and pigeons (Iverson 1980; Sepinwall and Cook 1980). The pathways involved may be the serotonergic systems from the dorsal raphe nuclei to the amygdala and hippocampus (Iverson 1980).

From this evidence, Gray (1981a) proposes that a critical action of antianxiety agents is to depress noradrenergic and serotonergic impulses to the septo-hippocampal system under conditions of stress: it is this action that is responsible for the anti-anxiety, as distinct from the sedative, anticonvulsant or other effects of these drugs. The effects may be indirect, mediated through a primary action at the GABA receptor complex (Quintero et al. 1985; Chapter 4), and there is evidence for GABA-ergic terminals both in the locus coeruleus and in the raphe nuclei (Gray 1982).

This hypothesis of the mode of action of anxiolytic drugs forms the basis of a more general theory of anxiety in which the septo-hippocampal behavioural inhibition system is envisaged to interact with several interconnected limbic structures, including other areas of the hippocampus, mammillary bodies, anterior thalamus, and cingulate, temporal and prefrontal cortex. The system is envisaged to act as a match/mismatch comparator whose general function is to compare actual with expected stimuli. Gray (1981a, 1982) proposes that the system functions in two modes. If actual stimuli match expected stimuli, a 'checking' mode is operated and behaviour, controlled by other brain systems, is not affected. If, however, a mismatch occurs between predicted and actual stimuli, or if predicted stimuli are aversive, a 'control' mode comes into operation, in which the system takes over direct control of behaviour. Operation of the 'control' mode in turn activates the three outputs of the behavioural inhibition system shown on the right of Fig. 3.2. Ongoing motor behaviour is immediately inhibited; general arousal is enhanced, and increased attention is devoted to checking the environment. These effects are probably mediated, not at the point of motor output, but at high-level brain systems involved in the planning and overall execution of motor functions. The behavioural inhibition system is envisaged to be continuously active, but its greatest activity occurs in the event of a mismatch or threat, which is also the time that anxiety is greatest.

This theory can accommodate many observations in relation to human anxiety. For example, obsessive/compulsive neurosis can be interpreted as an excessive checking of potential environmental hazards, while phobic symptoms can be attributed to inhibition of motor programmes. Anxiolytic agents would decrease activity in the system, especially in 'control' mode when it is most active, while the success of behavioural therapy could result from maximizing the rate of habituation in the hippocampus. The prefrontal and cingulate areas of the neocortex appear to play a particularly important role in human anxiety. These neocortical areas not only supply information to the septo-hippocampal system about motor programmes, but also provide a connection between cortical language systems and the limbic system. Thus, in humans the 'control' mode of the behavioural inhibition system can be activated, and anxiety triggered, by purely semantic stimuli. Some psycho-surgical treatments for severe anxiety have been directed towards interrupting the connections between the prefrontal cortex and the limbic system (Beaumont 1983). Finally, the theory can be extended to cover trait anxiety by proposing that the greater the innate reactivity of the behavioural inhibition system, the more susceptible is the individual to anxiety.

The postulated comparator function of the septo-hippocampal system, which is supported by other authors (O'Keefe and Nadel 1978; Norton 1981; Rawlings 1984) is also related to learning and memory (Chapter 8) and to reward seeking and punishment avoidance behaviour (Chapter 5). In relation to anxiety, the details of Gray's theory have been questioned (Wilbur and Kulik 1981), but the hypothesis remains the most coherent and specific yet proposed.

At the cellular level, Kandel (1983), and Kandel and Schwartz (1982) suggest that anxiety may be a learned response involving changes in the strength of certain synaptic connections, with enhanced (excitatory) neurotransmitter release: a process akin to the sensitization demonstrated in aplysia on repeated noxious stimulation (Chapter 8). The implications of this suggestion for human anxiety is discussed by Roth (1984). It has also been suggested that anxiety states in man may represent a malfunction of central GABA-ergic systems (Leonard 1985; Chapter 4).

Sleep disorders

Sleep disorders are reviewed by Hartmann (1980), Parkes (1977, 1981) and Scott (1981). Some appear to result from over-activity in arousal systems, others may represent specific disturbances of REM or orthodox sleep mechanisms, while many are mixed. A concise neurophysiological classifiction is difficult, and here they are discussed under the clinical categories of insomnia, hypersomnia, and episodic sleep disturbances.

Insomnia

Individuals show great variability in their sleep requirements. Although most people allowed to sleep *ad libitum* do so for 7–8 h a day, some normal subjects require less than 3 h, and others over 12 h (Parkes 1981). Hartmann (1980) estimates that up to 30 per cent of the population at some time complain of difficulty in sleeping. Insomnia can be caused by any factor which increases the activity of the general or limbic arousal system or which decreases the activity of the brainstem and forebrain sleep systems (Chapter 2); many causes act on both systems. An attempt to relate some of the causes of insomnia to these systems is shown in Fig. 3.3.

Increased sensory stimulation of any kind tends to activate reticular arousal systems, resulting in difficulty in falling asleep. Common causes include pain or discomfort and external stimuli such as noises, bright lights, or extremes of temperature. Anxiety from any cause may also delay sleep onset. Here, the arousal presumably results from increased activity in limbic arousal systems. Conditions associated with generalized hyperactivity such as manic states and hyperthyroidism may also hinder the onset of sleep. Hyperkinetic children appear to need relatively little sleep.

Drugs are an important cause of insomnia. Difficulty in falling asleep may result directly from the action of central nervous system stimulants such as tea, coffee, sympathomimetic amines and some antidepressants, especially monoamine oxidase inhibitors. Drug withdrawal after chronic use of hypnotics, tranquillizers, narcotics, and alcohol commonly causes a rebound syndrome with hyperexcitability, anxiety, and insomnia (Chapter 6). Rapidly metabolized central depressants such as alcohol, short-acting benzodiazepines, and barbiturates after enzyme induction has occurred (Chapter 4) may, on the other hand, cause early waking.

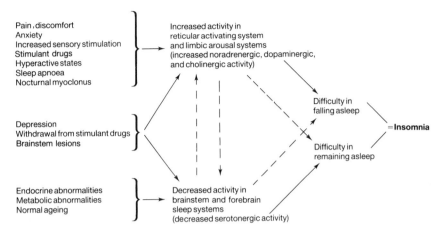

Fig. 3.3. Some causes of insomnia: relation to arousal and sleep systems. (Adapted from Hartmann 1982, by kind permission of Macmillan Ltd.)

Difficulty in staying asleep is characteristic of certain types of depression. Patients typically complain of early waking but sleep records show many awakenings during the night, reduced Stage 4 sleep, increased time spent in REMS, and an abnormal distribution of sleep stages (Schultz *et al.* 1978). Such changes have been ascribed in some cases to alterations of cortisol secretion, or to more general abnormalities in circadian rhythmn. Some depressed patients, in contrast, have hypersomnia. Alteration of sleep stages, increased dreaming, and nightmares may also occur in schizophrenia. Interference with circadian rhythms in normal subjects may cause difficulty in falling asleep or early waking.

Frequent arousals from sleep are associated with nocturnal myoclonus, 'restless legs syndrome', muscle cramps, bruxism, and head-banging. The aetiology of these conditions is in most cases unknown. The EEG often shows a normal sleep pattern and the repetitive movements usually occur during orthodox sleep (Hartmann 1980). However, myoclonus resulting from cortical or diencephalic lesions may arise in any sleep stage while myoclonus due to spinal lesions is usually more apparent in orthodox than REMS (Parkes 1981). Nocturnal myoclonus is common in patients with sleep apnoea, narcolepsy, and chronic renal failure and it may also occur in patients taking L-dopa or clomipramine (Parkes 1981).

Other conditions associated with insomnia but also giving rise to daytime sleepiness are described in the next section. There remains a group of 'poor sleepers' who seek medical help and whose complaints of poor sleep are supported by polygraphic studies (*British Medical Journal* 1984), but in whom usually no particular cause is found.

Hypersomnia

The term hypersomnia is usually taken to include not only excessive total sleep, but also attacks of unwanted sleep and excessive daytime sleepiness. The latter symptom may occur in any type of insomnia.

Narcoleptic syndrome

The narcoleptic syndrome is the commonest cause of excessive daytime sleep, with an incidence of perhaps 20,000 in the United Kingdom (Parkes 1977). The mean age of onset is 24 years, and the frequency and symptoms tend to increase with age. Both sexes are equally affected and there is a positive family history in 46 per cent of cases (Parkes 1977, 1981); a genetic basis for the disease has been confirmed by Langdon *et al.* (1984).

The most prominent complaint is of *sleep attacks* (narcolepsy): periods of sudden, irresistible sleep which may occur at any time and are sometimes emotionally triggered. The attacks occur several times a day and usually last for some minutes, but may continue for hours or even days (Parkes 1977). *Cataplexy* (attacks of muscle weakness during which the patient may fall, although he feels fully conscious) may occur in combination with sleep attacks or independently. It is often precipitated by emotions such as anger or laughter. Attacks of *sleep paralysis* may occur with or without narcolepsy and cataplexy. These are associated with the onset or end of sleep and consist of complete inability to perform voluntary movements despite full consciousness. Characteristically, they include loss of the sense of passage of time and can be very frightening. *Hypnagogic hallucinations*, auditory or visual, which are sometimes experienced by normal subjects on falling asleep, may be particularly frequent and vivid in the narcoleptic syndrome. *Daytime dreams* often occur during narcoleptic attacks. Over 90 per cent of narcoleptics have disordered night sleep with extreme restlessness and many awakenings; a few patients have frequent nightmares. About 25 per cent of narcoleptics display *automatic behaviour* during waking hours. During these episodes, which can occur several times daily and last for minutes to hours, the subject appears drowsy or only half-awake and displays inappropriate, repetitive, or nonsensical behaviour. Loss of the sense of the passage of time is again typical and there is a subsequent complete or partial amnesia covering the period of the episode. The automatic behaviour seen in the narcoleptic syndrome is similar to that which occurs in transient amnesic attacks which may be associated with epilepsy, migraine, and psychogenic states (Chapter 9). In narcoleptic subjects there is also evidence of a central disturbance in autonomic control (Levander and Sachs 1985).

Polygraphic recordings in show abnormalities in the timing of REMS (Hartmann 1980). During cataplexy there is an immediate or almost immediate onset of REMS; in sleep attacks a REMS period starts within a few minutes, and night-time sleep in most narcoleptics is characterized by unusually short

REMS latency. The narcoleptic syndrome appears to be the only known condition in which REMS occurs immediately or within minutes from sleep onset, the usual latency of REMS in normal subjects being about 90 min (Hartmann 1980). Thus narcolepsy appears to be a disorder of REMS and it has been suggested that it results from an inability to inhibit REMS, or that it is akin to epilepsy, so that the symptoms are essentially fits of REMS. Some narcoleptics have attacks which are similar to those of temporal lobe epilepsy. In addition, narcoleptic subjects appear to have lower than normal levels of both tonic and phasic arousal (Levander and Sachs 1985).

Narcolepsy is sometimes precipitated by high carbohydrate foods, an observation which suggests an inborn error of carbohydrate metabolism, possibly a deficiency of cerebral glucose-6-phosphate (Parkes 1977). Abnormalities of central monoamine (especially noradrenergic) activity have also been suggested although no specific abnormality has been found (Hartmann 1980; *Lancet* 1975; Scott 1981). However, narcolepsy partially responds to treatment with sympathomimetic amines (amphetamine, methyl phenydate) and monoamine reuptake blockers (clomipramine, imipramine). Benzodiazepines and gamma hydroxybutyrate are also sometimes effective (Scott 1981). The possibility that narcolepsy is an immune related disease is discussed by Parkes et al. (1986).

Idiopathic hypersomnolence

Narcolepsy may merge with the condition of idiopathic hypersomnolence and the two syndromes may co-exist. Idiopathic hypersomnolence is less common, with a prevalence of about 4000 patients in the United Kingdom (Parkes 1981). It has a similar age of onset, sex distribution, and familial incidence to the narcoleptic syndrome and may be lifelong and disabling. However, there are differences in many respects. In idiopathic hypersomnolence the onset of daytime sleep tends to be gradual rather than sudden and can be resisted. Sleep does not occur suddenly in unusual circumstances although it may be precipitated by travelling, monotonous circumstances, comfort, and food. The somnolence differs from normal drowsiness only in its frequency and persistence. Patients with idiopathic hypersomnolence complain of recurrent daytime sleepiness and regularly take lengthy naps. Automatic behaviour is even more frequent (45 per cent) than in the narcoleptic syndrome and, like all the symptoms, tends to be worst in the morning. It may persist for 30–120 min after waking (sleep drunkenness) and is associated with a high incidence of traffic, household, and occupational accidents.

Night time sleep in idiopathic hypersomnolence is characterized by rapid sleep onset (1–3 min), a normal sleep pattern, a low incidence of reported dreams, few awakenings, and prolonged orthodox sleep. Total sleep time is usually 8–12 h and morning arousal is excessively difficult, the patients sleeping through alarms loud enough to wake their neighbours (Parkes 1981). This sleep pattern contrasts with the poor nights, frequent interruptions, and early waking of narcoleptics.

Idiopathic hypersomnolence appears to result from the excessive occurrence of orthodox sleep and may be due to increased activity or decreased inhibition of orthodox sleep-promoting structures in the brain. The fact that narcolepsy and idiopathic hypersomnolence are sometimes seen in the same patient suggests that the two disorders may have a similar pathology. Serotonergic mechanisms may possibly be involved in idiopathic hypersomnolence since it sometimes responds strikingly to the serotonergic receptor blocker methysergide, which is of no value in narcolepsy. Other drugs acting on serotonergic mechanisms including pizotifen, cyproheptadine, and mianserin are sometimes helpful. Clonazepam at night is occasionally effective in both idiopathic hypersomnolence and cataplexy, perhaps because of its anticonvulsant effect. Stimulants such as dextroamphetamine and other sympathomimetic drugs, even in high dosage, produce little improvement in idiopathic hypersomnolence although they are useful in the narcoleptic syndrome.

Kleine–Levin syndrome

In this rare syndrome, periods of hypersomnolence appear at intervals of days or weeks and last for a similar time. It occurs chiefly in adolescent males and tends to resolve in a decade or two. Attacks consist of cycles of hyperphagia with irritability, hallucinations, headaches, and signs of autonomic and sexual hyperactivity, followed by hypersomnia lasting several days with irritability on awakening. The aetiology is unknown, but in view of the disturbance of sleep, sexual behaviour, and appetite, a hypothalamic disturbance seems likely (Scott 1981). There is no established treatment, but lithium salts may prevent attacks in some patients (Hartmann 1980).

Sleep apnoea syndromes

These syndromes, defined by Guilleminault *et al.* (1973) and Guilleminault and Tilkian (1976), consist of frequent and prolonged apnoeic periods during nocturnal sleep. Apnoea lasting up to 10 s occurs normally during REMS, but in sleep apnoea airflow through the oropharynx ceases for 20–120 s, 30 to several hundred times a night (Hartmann 1980). Waking usually terminates each period of apnoea, with the result that sleep is seriously disturbed and the most prominent symptom is usually of excessive daytime sleepiness. Most patients are chronically tired and have frequent short sleep episodes during the day, sometimes resembling narcolepsy (which may co-exist); others have prolonged daytime sleep periods, and some have difficulty in morning arousal with episodes of automatic behaviour, similar to idiopathic hypersomnolence (Parkes 1981).

Sleep apnoea occurs predominantly in subjects over 40 (though it can occur in children and infants) and is much more common in men than women (Parkes 1981). Two types have been described: central and obstructive sleep apnoea, although some patients have both types. In *central sleep apnoea* the respiratory movements of the diaphragm cease during the apnoeic periods. This type probably results from damage to brainstem centres or other neurological structures controlling respiration and is seen in bulbar poliomyelitis, bilateral cordotomy, Ondine's curse, Shy–Drager syndrome, musclar dystrophy and several other disorders (*Lancet* 1979a). In *obstructive sleep apnoea* inspiratory movements continue during the apnoeic periods, which are caused by occlusion of the upper airway. The causes include acromegaly, Down's syndrome, enlarged tonsils adenoids, and obesity, and snoring itself which is inordinately loud in this condition. The syndrome of obesity with obstructive sleep apnoea and excessive daytime sleepiness has been termed the Pickwickian Syndrome.

Sleep apnoea usually though not exclusively occurs in REMS. In normal REMS, the automatic control of breathing is depressed and the respiratory response to increasing hydrogen ion and CO_2 concentration is decreased. This lack of respiratory response may be exaggerated in sleep apnoea. Cessation of breathing without reawakening can occasionally result in coma and death. Substantial falls of arterial oxygen saturation can occur during each apnoeic episode, and such recurrent periods of hypoxaemia may cause chronic progressive illness with intellectual deterioration, polycythaemia, and respiratory and cardiovascular failure (Parkes 1981; Guilleminault *et al.* 1984).

Treatment of obstructive sleep apnoea involves removal of the obstruction where possible (*Lancet* 1979a,b; Hartmann 1980; Parkes 1977; Sullivan *et al.* 1981). There is no specific treatment for central apnoea but stimulant drugs are sometimes of value. Hypnotic drugs are contra-indicated in both types of sleep apnoea, because of the respiratory depression they produce.

Other organic sleep disorders

A number of organic lesions, often involving the reticular formation or posterior and lateral hypothalamus, can give rise to a variety of sleep disorders.

Encephalitis lethargica and other forms of encephalitis may cause narcolepsy, sleep reversal with profound drowsiness or sleep by day and alertness at night, or prolonged sleep or stupor lasting several weeks. The sites involved appear to be the midbrain tegmentum or posterior hypothalmus (Scott 1981). Hypersomnolence is a feature of fever due to bacterial infections. Some bacteria, including the pneumococcus, contain muramyl peptides. These have been shown to act as sleep-promoting agents, possibly by interfering with serotonergic systems since they bind to serotonin receptors. It has been suggested that this mechanism could explain the sleepiness that accompanies pneumococcal and related infections (Root-Bernstein and Westall 1983;

Masek and Kadlec 1983). Trypanosomiasis can in its later stages cause sleep reversal and hypersomnolence. This presumably results from involvement of brain tissue by nests of parasites colonising the choroid plexus (Parkes 1977). Severe head injury, brain tumours, uraemia, hepatic encephalopathy, anorexia nervosa, chronic alcoholism, other drugs, cerebrovascular disease, and dementia can all cause sleep disorders including insomnia, sleep reversal, prolonged sleep stupor, or coma.

Sleep reversal is particularly common in the elderly in whom it may be associated with cerebrovascular disease or Alzheimer-type dementia. However elderly subjects tend to require less sleep at night but take daytime naps: these normal changes may lead to complaints of insomnia. A special problem in the elderly is iatrogenic insomnia, often resulting from overprescription of hypnotic drugs, especially benzodiazepines, which may cause or aggravate nocturnal confusion and disorientation, and automatic behaviour during the day.

Episodic sleep disturbances

Some sleep disturbances reviewed by Hartmann (1980) and Scott (1981) are characterized by sudden episodes during the night. They may all occur occasionally in normal subjects, but may constitute a clinical problem if they appear in exaggerated forms.

Occasional sleepwalking occurs in 15 per cent of children and 1–6 per cent of adults, and is associated with stage 4 orthodox sleep. There is usually complete amnesia for the event. Rarely somnambulists walk considerable distances and can injure themselves, e.g. by falling out of windows. In most cases sleepwalking occurs in isolated episodes and no particular treatment is required. Sleep talking can occur at any stage of sleep but is most frequent during Stage 2.

Secondary nocturnal enuresis after a period of controlled micturition occurs in 2.6 per cent of girls and 3.6 per cent of boys, and may occasionally persist to adulthood (Scott 1981). In a few cases an abnormality of the urinary tract, epilepsy, diabetes, or a large fluid intake may account for the symptom, but usually no organic cause can be found. The enuretic episode typically occurs about 1–3 h after the onset of sleep during stage 3 or 4 orthodox sleep, often before the first episode of REMS; it can occur during REMS (*British Medical Journal* 1968). Enuresis may occur during a brief arousal from sleep but usually there is complete amnesia for the event on awakening. Drug treatment is not usually required although imipramine is useful in some cases.

Night terrors occur mainly in children and are common during the early school years. The child suddenly sits up in bed, screams and appears terrified but usually there is no detailed associated dream. Sympathetic activity is increased as evidenced by tachycardia and increased respiratory rate. Sometimes the child stares wildly and appears to be hallucinating; usually he is inaccessible and difficult to wake. There is total amnesia for the event next day. Night terrors are usually said to occur during Stage 3 or 4 sleep (Hartmann 1980; *British Medical Journal* 1971), but Scott (1981) states that the EEG shows a marked REMS pattern during such episodes. Night terrors usually resolve spontaneously after a time and no specific treatment is required.

In contrast with night terrors, nightmares are vivid, unpleasant dreams, associated with strong emotions of fear, with evidence of increased sympathetic activity. Not uncommonly, a sense of muscle paralysis or suffocation is present. They usually occur towards the end of a long period of REMS (Hartmann 1980), frequently cause awakening, and are remembered. Increased frequency of nightmares occurs in narcolepsy and in psychiatric states including anxiety syndromes, depression, and schizophrenia. Hartmann (1980) reports that a group of adults complaining of frequent nightmares had personality profiles suggestive of schizoid personality traits, and some had a history of schizophrenic episodes. Several groups of drugs cause nightmares including cholinomimetic drugs, psychotomimetic drugs, and propranolol (*Drug Newsletter* 1986). Nightmares are common during the withdrawal syndrome from central nervous system depressant drugs and after general anaesthetics. They may also occur in starvation, fevers, or after prolonged sleep loss. In short, any factor leading to increased REMS may cause nightmares, which appear to consist of particularly intense periods of REMS with increased limbic (emotional) and autonomic activity.

However, Vogel (1975, 1978) and Stein (1982) point out that frightening dreams can occur in orthodox sleep. Stein claims that 'in fact, the terrifying experience of the worst nightmares—being crushed, burnt, suffocated or pushed over the edge of a precipice—probably occur in ..... SWS and not REMS' (Stein 1982, p. 305).

4
Drugs acting on arousal
and sleep systems

Nearly all psychotropic drugs act at some point on arousal and sleep systems in the brain. Central nervous system stimulants and depressants are classified according to whether they increase or decrease cortical arousal; anxiolytics and tranquillizers are designated by their effects on emotional arousal; antipsychotic drugs and antidepressants have specialized effects on arousal and sleep systems, and these systems are also affected by a wide range of other drugs from antihistamines to antihypertensive agents. This section considers some drugs used therapeutically for their effects on arousal: central nervous system depressants, classed as hypnotics, sedatives, and anxiolytics; and certain stimulants, the sympathomimetic amines and xanthines. The effects of other psychotropic drugs on arousal and sleep are discussed in later chapters: narcotic analgesics, alcohol, and cocaine (Chapter 7), drugs affecting memory (Chapter 10), antidepressants (Chapter 12), antipsychotic and psychotomimetic drugs (Chapter 14).

Hypnotics, sedatives, anxiolytics

Benzodiazepines

The drug explosion in the 1950s, which gave rise to antidepressants and antipsychotic drugs, also produced minor tranquillizers, now chiefly represented by the benzodiazepines. These became by the 1970s the most commonly prescribed of all drugs in the western world. Lader and Petursson (1981) estimated that one in ten of all men and one in five of all women in the United Kingdom were taking tranquillizers or hypnotics for some time each year, usually for several weeks, and many patients had taken them for years. Levels of prescribing have been discussed by Trethowan (1975), Marks (1978, 1983), and Skegg *et al.* (1979). Recently, there has been some decline in benzodiazepine prescriptions in the United Kingdom and the number of benzodiazepines available on the National Health Service has been limited (DHSS Publication 1985).

When they first appeared, the benzodiazepines, more than most new drugs, appeared to be 'Wonder Drugs' . They calmed the mind, relaxed the muscles, controlled insomnia, helped people to tolerate life-stresses, and were also useful anticonvulsants. At the same time they were extremely safe and it seemed that their dependence-producing potential was much lower than that of the barbiturates. However, it is now clear that these drugs are not without adverse effects, especially with chronic use. On the other hand, investigation of their mode of action is beginning to lead to a further understanding of GABA receptors in the brain and of the neurological mechanisms underlying anxiety.

Pharmacokinetics

The pharmacokinetics of the benzodiazepines are reviewed by several authors (Greenblatt *et al.* 1981, 1983; Breimer and Jochemsen 1981; Fawcett and Kravitz 1982; Jack 1981). All benzodiazepines have similar actions, and pharmacokinetic rather than pharmacodynamic factors account for most of the clinically important differences between the individual drugs.

Benzodiazepines are generally well absorbed when given by mouth although at variable rates. The rate of absorption determines the speed of onset of pharmacological effects after a single dose and is of clinical importance. Rapid absorption is clearly desirable when the drugs are used as hypnotics, but less so when they are used in multiple dosage as anxiolytics.

Plasma concentrations of benzodiazepines initially decline rapidly after a single dose because of tissue redistribution (alpha half-life). There is a fast uptake into the grey matter of the brain followed by a slower phase of redistribution into the white matter and adipose tissue. The rate of redistribution is variable and depends on the lipid solubility of the different drugs. This phase is followed by a more gradual decline in plasma concentration due to the beta phase of drug elimination (beta half-life, elimination half-life). This phase shows an even greater variability between different benzodiazepines, ranging between about 2 h for triazolam to up to 200 h for the pharmacologically active metabolite desmethyldiazepam (Table 4.1). Benzodiazepines with long elimination half-lives accumulate in the body if taken chronically.

Virtually all the benzodiazepines undergo hepatic metabolism in the body via oxidation or conjugation and some form pharmacologically active intermediary metabolites. Oxidation of benzodiazepines is decreased in the elderly, in patients with cirrhosis of the liver, and in the presence of enzyme-inhibiting drugs. The elimination half-lives and residual effects of benzodiazepines which are oxidized are prolonged in elderly patients (Cook 1979; Murphy *et al.* 1982). Benzodiazepines which are conjugated include oxazepam, lorazepam, and temazepam. Conjugation is less influenced by age and disease than oxidation, and it has been suggested that these benzodiazepines might be more suitable for elderly or compromised patients (Greenblatt *et al.* 1983).

Table 4.1. Pharmacokinetic properties of some benzodiazepines

Drug	Clinically important metabolites	Beta half-life in fit young subjects (h)
Chlordiazepoxide		5–30
	desmethylchordiazepam demoxepam	36–200
Clobazam		12–60
	desmethylclobazam	36–200
Diazepam		20–100
	desmethyldiazepam	36–200
Alprazolam		6–20
Flunitrazepam		25–30
Lorazepam		10–20
Nitrazepam		15–38
Oxazepam		4–15
Temazepam		8–22
Midazolam		2–8
Triazolam		2–5

Actions

The actions of all the benzodiazepines are broadly similar and are mainly on the central nervous system. They exert four major therapeutic effects: sedative/hypnotic, anxiolytic, muscular relaxant, and anticonvulsant. As hypnotics, and particularly as anxiolytics, they have largely replaced other agents because they are more effective, much safer in overdose, less likely to interact with other drugs, and until recently have been thought to be less likely to induce dependence (Petursson and Lader 1981b). Benzodiazepines are also used as preoperative medication in which their hypnotic, anxiolytic and muscle relaxing effects have a combined therapeutic value, as well as an amnesic effect which probably results from the hypnotic action (Chapter 8).

Sedative/hypnotic effects The benzodiazepines are effective hypnotics. A major site of this action is probably the brainstem reticular formation which is of central importance in wakefulness and sleep (Chapter 2). The reticular formation is very sensitive to depression by benzodiazepines; small doses decrease both spontaneous activity and responses to afferent stimuli and block cortical EEG arousal evoked by stimulation of the reticular formation (Harvey 1980; Baldessarini 1980; Haefely *et al.* 1981). In man, small doses of benzodiazepines also reduce the amplitude and prolong the latency of cortical evoked potentials, which are thought to be modulated by the midbrain reticular formation (Saletu *et al.* 1972; Ashton *et al.* 1974, 1976, 1978). However, because of their interaction with the major central inhibitory transmitter GABA, discussed below, the benzodiazepines also cause widespread central nervous system depression. Probably through an interaction with GABA, the benzodiazepines decrease the turnover of acetylcholine, noradrenaline, dopamine, and serotonin in many regions of the brain (Harvey 1980; Haefely *et al.* 1981).

It is still not clear whether the sedative/hypnotic effects are separate from the other actions. In small doses, the benzodiazepines produce mainly anxiolytic effects but increasing dosage leads to sedation and, as dosage is increased, to hypnosis and stupor (Harvey 1980). The changes in the waking EEG are similar to those produced by other sedative/hypnotic drugs: there is a decrease and slowing of alpha activity and an increase in low voltage fast activity especially in the beta range (Fig. 2.9). The changes mainly affect frontal and rolandic areas (Fink 1969; Pfeiffer *et al.* 1964).

(i) Effects on sleep. The effects on sleep are reviewed by Hartmann (1976), Kay *et al.* (1976), Baldessarini (1980), Harvey (1980), and Wheatley (1981). In general, benzodiazepines hasten sleep onset, decrease nocturnal awakenings, increase total sleeping time, and often impart a sense of deep or refreshing sleep. However, the sleep induced by benzodiazepines differs from normal sleep in the duration of the various sleep stages (Fig. 4.1). Stage 2 sleep is prolonged and mainly accounts for the increased sleeping time. By contrast, the duration of slow wave sleep (Stages 3 and 4) is usually decreased although the normal nocturnal peaks in plasma concentrations of growth hormone, prolactin, and luteinizing hormone, are little affected. REMS is altered in several ways: latency to the first REM episode is increased; total REMS time is reduced; eye movements during REM sleep are decreased; nightmares and bursts of tachycardia during REM episodes are also reduced, but there may be an increase in the number of REM episodes, especially late in the night.

These changes may occur with most benzodiazepines in normal subjects but there are considerable variations in response, depending on dosage, duration of treatment, individual benzodiazepines, and clinical state. The increase in total sleeping time is greater in patients with insomnia than in normal subjects and greatest in patients with the shortest baseline sleep. In neurotic patients, Stage 3 sleep may be prolonged although Stage 4 is reduced. Small doses of benzodiazepines may produce less marked alterations in sleep stage proportions; for example, several benzodiazepines in low dosage did not alter REMS in some studies (Kay *et al.* 1976) although shortening SWS and prolonging Stage 2 sleep. REM latency may be decreased rather than increased in some insomniac neurotics. Some benzodiazepines, notably nitrazepam, have been reported to increase the amount of REMS in schizophrenia with depression, endogenous depression, neuroses, and in normal subjects working alternating shifts. With triazalam, possibly because of its short half-life, REMS is diminished early in the night but increased later.

(ii) Tolerance. The general mechanisms and types of drug tolerance are described in Chapter 6, to which the reader is referred for a full discussion.

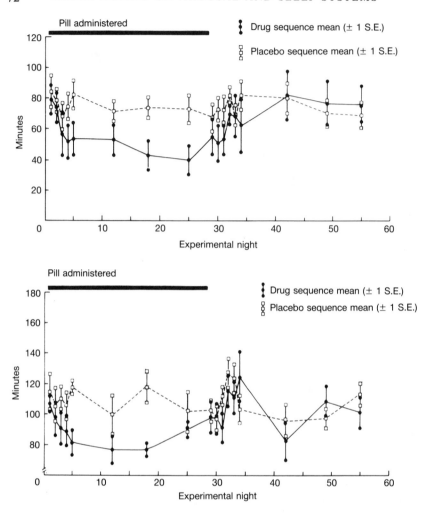

Fig. 4.1. Effect of chlordiazepoxide on slow wave sleep (SWS) and rapid eye movement sleep (REMS). Open symbols and dotted lines, placebo; filled symbols and solid line, chlordiazepoxide. Upper trace, effects on total SWS (N = 9) Lower trace, effects on total REM time (N = 9). (From Hartmann 1976, by kind permission of John Wiley & Sons Inc., New York.)

Tolerance to the hypnotic effects of benzodiazepines develops with chronic use (Petursson and Lader 1984) and may lead to escalation of dosage. Sleep latency, Stage 2 sleep, SWS, REMS, and intrasleep awakenings all tend to return towards pretreatment levels after some weeks (Adam *et al.* 1976a,b; Kay *et al.* 1976; Hartmann 1976a,b; Harvey 1980; Kales *et al.* 1978). However, Oswald *et al.* (1982) found that self-ratings of sleep quality and delay quality and delay to sleep onset remained stable in 97 poor sleepers taking nightly doses of lormetazepam (2 mg) or nitrazepam (5 mg) for 24 weeks. The number of self-reported dreams may increase on continued use but the dreams are less bizarre than before medication. In rats tolerance develops both to the hypnotic effects of benzodiazepines (Sepinwall and Cook 1979) and to the effects on brain noradrenaline (but not serotonin) turnover, suggesting that at least part of the hypnotic effects are mediated by inhibition of noradrenergic systems (Harvey 1980; Iverson 1980).

(iii) Rebound insomnia. Rebound insomnia commonly occurs on withdrawal of benzodiazepines. This is seen most dramatically when the drugs have been taken in high doses or for long periods (Adam *et al.* 1976a,b) but can probably occur after only a week of low dose administration (Kales *et al.* 1978; Nicholson 1980a,b). There is often a marked rebound in sleep latency, which becomes longer than the premedication level, and in intrasleep awakenings, which become more frequent than before medication. There may also be an increase in slow wave sleep. REM sleep also shows a rebound pattern with decrease in REM latency, increase in total REM time, eye movements, and intensity of dreaming. Nightmares may occur and add to the frequent awakenings. These symptoms, which occur both in normal subjects and in patients with insomnia, are most marked on cessation of benzodiazepines with short or moderately short half-lives (e.g., triazolam, nitrazepam, lorazepam) and may last for many weeks. With triazolam, which has the shortest duration of action, some rebound effects may occur during the latter part of the night, even on continued administration. Kales *et al.* (1978) note that rebound insomnia can occur even after low doses of flunitrazepam which are ineffective for either inducing or maintaining sleep. With long acting benzodiazepines (e.g. flurazepam) slow wave sleep and REM sleep may remain depressed for several weeks and then slowly return to baseline, sometimes without a rebound. These rebound effects are probably a reflection of pharmacodynamic tolerance (Chapter 6). They lead to continuation of usage and contribute to the development of dependence.

(iv) 'Hangover' effects. The hypnotic efficacy and residual effects of benzodiazepines are reviewed by Bond and Lader (1981), Nicholson (1980a), Roth *et al.* (1980), Johnson and Chernick (1982) and Dordain *et al.* (1980). The short-acting benzodiazepines temazepam (10–20 mg) and triazolam (0.125–0.25 mg) appear in some studies to be effective hypnotics free from residual sequelae. However Bond and Lader (1981) considered that 0.5 mg was the minimum effective hypnotic dose of triazolam, and at this dose performance was impaired at 16 h after administration. Oxazepam exerts few residual effects but its efficacy is doubtful, while lorazepam (2–5 mg) impairs performance in some tests after 12 h. Diazepam (5 and 10 mg) produces few residual effects when used occasionally, but chronic use leads to accumulation and performance was impaired in anxious patients taking 25 mg daily. Nitrazepam (5–10 mg), has prolonged residual effects and produces subjective 'hangover' after single doses but these became less marked after several days treatment. Bond and Lader (1981), and Johnson and Chernik (1982) comment on the large individual variations in response to different benzodiazepines and on the fact that the results of single dose studies in normal subjects cannot necessarily be extrapolated to multiple dosing in anxious insomniacs. It is still not known whether hypnotic treatment in insomniacs improves or worsens their performance the next day.

Anxiolytic effects The benzodiazepines are potent anxiolytic agents. In contrast to barbiturates, anxiolytic effects are exerted at low doses which produce minimal sedation. Of the many clinical trials demonstrating their efficacy and safety, one of the most recent is that by Cohn (1981) who noted the superiority of diazepam and alprazolam over placebo in a multicentre trial of 976 outpatients with moderate to severe anxiety symptoms of at least 1 month's duration. However, in minor affective disorders presenting to general practitioners, benzodiazepines appear to be no more effective that brief counselling (Catalan and Gath 1985). Anxiolytic effects have been reported in normal subjects with high trait-anxiety, but in those with low trait-anxiety personalities, benzodiazepines may produce paradoxical increases in anxiety feelings (Parrott and Kentridge 1982). Similarly, benzodiazepines may improve the performance of normal subjects subjected to experimental stress, but worsen it in low stress conditions (Parrott and Davies 1983). In preoperative dental patients, O'Boyle *et al.* (1986) found that temazepam relieved anxiety in patients with high anticipatory state anxiety but not in those with low state anxiety

Benzodiazepines also alleviate experimentally induced anxiety behaviour in animals. The major site of this action is believed to be the limbic system. Benzodiazepines suppress electrical activity in the septal region, amygdala, hippocampus, and hypothalamus (Tsuchiya and Kitagawa 1976; Robinson and Wang 1979) and decrease the turnover of acetylcholine, noradrenaline, serotonin, and dopamine in these areas (Iverson 1980; Harvey 1980; Baldassarini 1980; Agarwal *et al.* 1977; Haefely *et al.* 1981; Dannenberg and Weber 1983). The anti-anxiety effects may be mediated by suppression of serotonin or noradrenaline output, or both, in certain limbic pathways as discussed in Chapter 3.

The effects of benzodiazepines on monoaminergic systems are probably mediated through a primary action at GABA receptors which results in the enhancement of the actions of GABA, as discussed below. There is evidence for GABA-ergic terminals both in the locus coeruleus and in the raphe nuclei (Gray 1982); the involvement of these structures in anxiety is discussed in Chapter 3. Haefely *et al.* (1981) point out that the effect of benzodiazepines in reducing noradrenergic activity at the locus coeruleus and dopaminergic activity in the mesolimbic pathway is most marked under conditions of high activity induced by stress. Both GABA receptors and benzodiazepine receptors, however, are widely distributed throughout the brain and it is still not clear why benzodiazepines should have relatively selective anxiolytic actions at low dosage. An interaction with endogenous opioids may also be involved in their anxiolytic actions of (Millan and Duka 1981; Cooper 1983).

Tolerance to the anxiolytic effects seems to develop less readily than to the hypnotic effects (Petursson and Lader 1981b). In clinical use, most patients reporting initial drowsiness find that it wears off in a few days, while the anxiolytic effect remains, for weeks or months. However, it has been claimed that benzodiazepines are no longer effective in the treatment of anxiety after 1-4 months of continuous treatment (Drug and Therapeutics Bulletin 1980; Burrows and Davies 1984). Some patients appear to become tolerant to the anxiolytic effects and steadily increase their dosage even when stresses contributing to anxiety are relieved.

Muscular relaxant effects Benzodiazepines induce skeletal muscle relaxation in doses which do not affect locomotion. They are useful for relieving spasticity due to upper motorneurone lesions, degenerative neurological disease, muscle pain and spasm, tetanus, and some neuromuscular disorders (Speth *et al.* 1980). The musclar relaxation adds to the therapeutic effects when benzodiazepines are used as hypnotics, anxiolytics, and for preoperative medication. The main site of this action is probably supraspinal, by enhancement of GABA activity in the reticular formation. The effect of electrical stimulation of the medullary reticular formation on spinal neurones is suppressed by small doses and the tonic facilitatory influence of the reticular formation on spinal gamma neurones is attenuated (Harvey 1980). It is possible that polysynaptic inhibition in the spinal cord is also enhanced. Some degree of tolerance develops to the muscular relaxant effect.

Anticonvulsant effects Benzodiazepines exhibit anticonvulsant activity in man and animals. In animals they inhibit seizures induced by pentylenetetrazol or picrotoxin, but seizures induced by strychnine or electroshock are suppressed only in maximal doses which impair locomotor activity. They prevent seizures elicited by repeated electrical stimulation of the amygdala, and prevent photic seizures in baboons. The action appears to be due to suppression of the spread of electrical activity rather than to a local effect on the site of epileptic discharge, and is probably a result of enhancement of the inhibitory actions of GABA. In both animals and man, tolerance to the anticonvulsant effect develops quickly. Nevertheless, benzodiazepines are the treatment of choice in status epilepticus, in fits induced by a variety of drugs and poisons associated with withdrawal of alcohol and other depressants, and in pre-eclampsia. They are sometimes of value in psychomotor and myoclonic epilepsy. Probably most benzodiazepines have anticonvulsant activity, but diazepam, clonazepam, lorazepam, and nitrazepam are said to be more selective in this respect (Harvey 1980; Rall and Schleifer 1980; Speth *et al.* 1980; Rogers *et al.* 1981).

Mechanisms of action

Benzodiazepine and GABA receptors The anxiolytic effects of the benzodiazepines were at first attributed to a relatively selective depressant effect on the limbic system (Dannenberg and Weber 1983). Their mechanism of action became clearer with the discovery of specific benzodiazepine binding sites in the rat brain (Mohler and Okada 1977; Squires and Braestrup 1977). These sites have a high stereospecific and selective affinity for benzodiazepines, and are unevenly distributed, being most concentrated in the cortex, limbic system and cerebellum. They have since been found in the brain of many vertebrate species including fish (Nielsen *et al.* 1978) and man (Mohler and Okada 1978). Their characteristics are reviewed by Speth *et al.* (1980). Other benzodiazepine binding sites, including lower affinity binding sites in rat brain membranes and peripheral binding sites, have also been demonstrated (File and Pellow 1983; Pellow and File 1984) but their pharmacological importance is unknown.

Sepinwall and Cook (1979) discussed the evidence suggesting that there was a relation between brain high affinity benzodiazepine binding sites and anxiety. The binding affinity of different benzodiazepines shows a significant positive correlation with the potency of their antianxiety effects in several animal tests. Different strains of rats and mice with high and low emotionality show differences in density of specific brain benzodiazepine binding sites, fewer binding sites being present in more emotional animals. Some non-benzodiazepine compounds which bind to the benzodiazepine sites also attenuate anxiety. Stressful manipulations of animals which lead to anxiety decreases the number of specific binding sites.

Growing evidence reviewed by Speth *et al.* (1980) also links central benzodiazepine binding sites with GABA. The distribution of GABA receptors is similar to that of benzodiazepine binding sites. Occupation of these sites by benzodiazepines enhances the actions of GABA, and the actions of the benzodiazepines require the presence of GABA. However, the benzodiazepines do not affect GABA synthesis, release, or uptake.

The benzodiazepine binding site reflects not only the site where the drugs are bound but is also the site where they produce their effects; it is therefore a benzodiazepine receptor (Speth *et al.* 1980). Braestrup and Nielsen (1980) suggested that the benzodiazepine receptor is a membrane protein which makes up part of the complex of the post-synaptic GABA receptor (Fig. 4.2). This receptor is a multimolecular unit; it includes a number of functionally related macromolecules forming a cluster defined as the GABA supra-

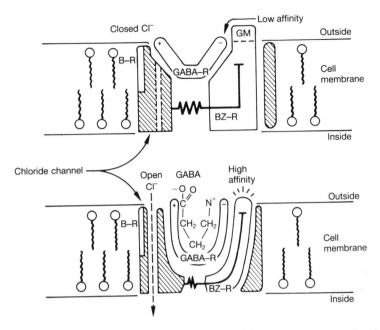

Fig. 4.2. Diagram of the postulated post-synaptic GABA A receptor complex. BZ-R, benzodiazepine receptor; B-R, barbiturate receptor; GABA-R, GABA recognition site; GM, GABA modulin. Occupation of the GABA recognition site by GABA leads to configurational changes causing opening of chloride channels in the neuronal membrane, with consequent hyperpolarisation. The affinity of this site is proposed to be controlled by GABA modulin. Occupation of the benzodiazepine receptor site by benzodiazepines may cause phosphorylation of GABA modulin, favouring the high affinity state of the GABA receptor and enhancing the inhibitory actions of GABA. Occupation of the barbiturate receptor sites by barbiturates causes prolonged opening of the chloride channel. (For fuller explanation, see text). (Modified from Braestrup and Nielsen 1980.)

molecular receptor assembly, or GABA receptor unit (Toffano *et al.* 1980). Its constituents include: (1) a GABA recognition site, (2) a chloride channel, (3) a benzodiazepine binding site, (4) a binding site for barbiturates and some convulsants, (5) one or more enzymes, and (6) a protein that modulates affinity for GABA. This unit, the GABA A receptor, is different from some other GABA receptors. The GABA B receptor, for example does not control a chloride channel (Harrison and Simmonds 1983).

As illustrated in Fig. 4.2, occupation of the GABA recognition site by GABA causes configurational changes in the GABA-receptor which lead to opening of the chloride channels in the neuronal membrane. Chloride ions enter the cell, hyperpolarizing it and making it resistant to excitation. This is the mechanism of GABA-mediated post-synaptic inhibition. [Pre-synaptic GABA receptors probably cause inhibition by depolarization (Enna 1981)].

The post-synaptic GABA receptor is assumed to exist in two states: a high affinity state which favours reaction with GABA, and a low-affinity state which discourages GABA occupation. It is proposed that the affinity for GABA is controlled by a protein on the membrane surface which has been termed GABA-modulin (Toffano et al. 1980; Guidotti et al. 1983). This protein has been isolated and characterised. It exists in two molecular forms, one of MW 15 000 and one of MW 400-800. It is a protein kinase Type II inhibitor, loosely embedded in the lipid membrane, and appears to mask the high affinity binding of GABA by limiting the extent of phosphorylation at the recognition site (Toffano et al. 1980). The benzodiazepine receptor site is closely linked to GABA-modulin and occupation of the benzodiazepine receptor by benzodiazepines may cause phosphorylation of GABA-modulin (Costa 1981; Guidotti et al. 1983). This favours the high affinity state of the GABA receptor, allows more molecules of GABA to react with it, and thus enhances the normal inhibitory actions of GABA.

The receptor site for barbiturates and for some convulsants is directly linked to the chloride channel and does not immediately involve the GABA-recognition apparatus. Occupation of this site by barbiturates prolongs the opening of the chloride channel, causing a long-lasting neuronal inhibition. This prolonged effect may partially explain why respiratory depression and narcosis are much more profound with barbiturates than with benzodiazepines. Some convulsants (e.g. picrotoxin) also interact at this site, but keep the chloride channel closed, favouring excitation.

The evidence so far discussed leads to the conclusion that benzodiazepines enhance the action of GABA by favouring the high-affinity state of the GABA receptor and suggests that the effects of benzodiazepines might be explicable in terms of GABA-enhancement in various systems of the brain. Since GABA is a universal inhibitory transmitter, present in the 30-50 per cent of brain synapses, which directly inhibits neurones and also inhibits activity in certain cholinergic, noradrenergic, dopaminergic, and serotonergic pathways (Haefely et al. 1981), this hypothesis apears at first sight attractive. Thus, GABA enhancement in the hippocampus and cortex might to lead to anticonvulsant effects; in the reticular formation and cerebellum, to muscular relaxation; in arousal systems to sedative/hypnotic effects, and in the limbic system to anxiolytic effects.

However, such an interpretation is undoubtedly over-simplified. There is reason to believe that the effects of benzodiazepines are not all mediated in the same way. For example, in both animals and man tolerance develops to the sedative and anticonvulsant effects, but much less to the antianxiety effects (Sepinwall and Cook 1979), and tolerance appears to develop at different rates for difference psychomotor functions affected by benzodiazepines (Aranko *et al.* 1983). Some GABA antagonists, such as muscimol, are not anxiolytic, although they are anticonvulsant and cause muscular relaxation. There is also evidence that some of the muscular relaxant effects of the benzodiazepines may be exerted through an interaction with presynaptic GABA receptors in the spinal cord (Iverson 1978a,b). Some non-benzodiazepines which bind to benzodiazepine receptors, such as zopiclone, are anxiolytic but devoid of other actions (Sepinwall and Cook 1979). Thus, it appears that there may be several types of benzodiazepine receptors mediating separate actions, and there are undoubtedly several types of GABA receptors. Evidence relating to benzodiazepine receptor subtypes is at present sparse and has been discussed by Gray (1982), Gee and Yamamura (1982), File and Pellow (1983) and Pellow and File (1984). GABA receptor subtypes are discussed by Costa (1981), Enna (1981), Enna and Andree (1982), Johnstone and Willow (1982), Iverson (1978), Harrison and Simmonds (1983). It is possible that the multiple types of GABA - benzodiazepine receptors are conformational variants of the same amino acid sequence and that different conformations subserve different physiological functions (Squires 1983).

Benzodiazepine receptor ligands The existence of benzodiazepine receptors in the body implies that there is a natural substance (or substances) with which they normally interact. Hence, there has been a search for endogenous benzodiazepine receptor ligands. Mohler (1981) and Speth *et al.* (1980) considered several substances including inosine, hypoxanthine, nicotinamide, thromboxane A_2, ethyl-beta-carboline-3-carboxylate, and GABA modulin, but none were considered to fulfil this role. Costa *et al.* (1983) isolated a polypeptide from rat brain which displaces benzodiazepines from their high affinity binding sites. This substance may be a precursor of an octadecaneuropeptide (ODN) with anxiogenic activity proposed as an endogenous benzodiazepine receptor ligand (Ferrero *et al.* 1984). Sandler (1982) isolated from human urine a beta-carboline (tribulin) which apeared to be related to stress. He suggested that this might be an endogenous ligand since other beta-carbolines which are potent benzodiazepine receptor ligands induce anxiety in human volunteers (Braestrup *et al.* 1980). If either ODN or tribulin are physiologically active benzodiazepine receptor ligands, the natural mechanism for regulating anxiety would appear to be not by means of an anxiolytic agent like the benzodiazepines but via an anxiogenic agent. It is possible that there are two sets of endogenous ligands, one mimicking the anxiolytic properties of benzodiazepines and the other mimicking the anxiogenic properties of beta-carbolines (Costa *et al.* 1983) and that some anxiety states are characterized by dysfunction of these GABA-regulating systems.

The recent development of a series of synthetic compounds which bind selectively to central high affinity benzodiazepine receptors may lead to further information on this question. These substances are reviewed by Hunkeler *et al.* 1981; Skolnick *et al.* 1982; Braestrup *et al.* 1983; Gallagher and Tallman 1983; Pellow and File 1984; Martin 1984, and some are shown in Table 4.2.

Some of these compounds are agonists: non-benzodiazepines such as zopiclone and some triazopyridazines produce classical benzodiazepine-like effects. Others including imidazodiazepines, pyrazaloquinolines, and beta-carbolines comprise a spectrum of partial agonists and competitive antagonists. They have some benzodiazepine-like actions but not others, antagonize one or more benzodiazepine effects, or combine agonist and antagonist properties. Yet others are termed 'inverse agonists' (Braestrup *et al.* 1983); they bind to benzodiazepine receptors, but produce opposite, anxiogenic, stimulant, and convulsant effects. The spectrum of activity exerted by this series of benzodiazepine receptor ligands suggests that the various actions of benzodiazepines may be separable and that it may be possible to develop compounds with specific anxiolytic, anticonvulsant, sedative or muscular relaxant properties.

Of the benzodiazepine agonist/antagonists, the most studied is RO 15-1788, an imidazodiazepine with little agonist activity (Hunkeler *et al.*

Table 4.2. Some benzodiazepine receptor ligands

Receptor activity	Ligands	Effects
Agonists	benzodiazepines zopiclone triazopyridazines	anxiolytic; anticonvulsant; hypnotic; muscle relaxant
Partial agonists/ competitive antagonists	imidazodiazepines pyrazoloquinolines some beta-carbolines	some benzodiazepine actions, but not others; antagonize one or more benzodiazepine effects; combine agonist and antagonist properties
Antagonists	RO 15–1788 (imidazodiazepine)	reverse benzodiazepine effects; almost no intrinsic effects
Inverse agonists[1]	some beta-carbolines[2] some polypeptides[3]	anxiogenic convulsant stimulant

[1] Braestrup *et al.*(1983).
[2] E.g., tribulin (Sandler, 1982).
[3] E.g. octadecaneuropeptide (Ferrero *et al.* 1984.)

1981). In animals it reverses the behavioural, biochemical, and electrophysiological effects of benzodiazepines and precipitates withdrawal signs in benzodiazepine-dependent animals (Cummin *et al.* 1982). In man, oral RO 15-1788 antagonizes diazepam effects on psychomotor performance without decreasing bioavailability and reverses benzodiazepine effects on REMS (Darragh *et al.* 1982 1983; Gaillard and Blois 1983). Given intravenously, it reverses sedation and impaired psychomotor performance induced by intravenous doses of benzodiazepines (Ziegler and Schalch 1982). It is almost devoid of intrinsic effects in man in oral doses up to 600 mg (Darragh *et al.* 1983); mild stimulant effects have been reported after intravenous (Schopf *et al.* 1984) and oral (Higgitt *et al.* 1986) use, suggesting slight inverse agonist activity. File and Pellow (1986) reviewed the effects of RO 15-1788 in animals and man and concluded that it does have some intrinsic activity and can produce both agonist and inverse agonist actions at central benzodiazepine receptors. Possible clinical applications of this compound are reviewed by Ashton (1985b).

At present two beta-carbolines have been identified with the properties of inverse agonists. Possible mechanisms of their interaction with GABA receptors are discussed by Braestrup *et al.* (1983) and Gallagher and Tallman (1983). It will be interesting to see if inverse agonists are found for other receptor sites such as those for endogenous opioids, since in many axons GABA coexists with polypeptides such as enkephalin, with which it may be co-released (Guidotti *et al.* 1983).

Adverse effects

The acute toxicity of the benzodiazepines is low but when used chronically they can exert a wide range of undesirable effects (Ashton 1986).

Oversedation When given as day time treatment, drowsiness, fatigue, and psychomotor impairment may occur as dose-related extensions of the pharmacological activity of the drugs. However, tolerance develops to these effects in a few days at therapeutic dosage. With increased doses, ataxia, dysarthria, motor inco-ordination, diplopia, muscle weakness, vertigo, mystagmus, and mental confusion or apathy develop. When used as hypnotics, these effects may not be noticed, but many benzodiazepines give rise to a subjective 'hangover' , and after most of them, even those with short elimination half-lives, psychomotor performance may be impaired the next day. Their possible contribution to traffic accidents is discussed by Skegg *et al.* (1979), Betts and Birtle (1982), and Ashton (1983a), although in anxious patients benzodiazepines may actually improve psychomotor performance (Oblowitz and Robins 1983). Oversedation from benzodiazepines is most marked in the elderly. Drowsiness, incoordination and ataxia leading to falls, poor memory and acute confusional states may result even from small doses (Baldessarini 1980). Some patients chronically treated with benzodiazepines have been noted to have abnormal CAT scans with a higher ventricle/brain area than controls (Lader *et al.* 1984). The clinical significance of these findings is not clear, but the possibility has been raised that the cognitive impairment caused by chronic benzodiazepine usage is related to structural brain damage.

Disinhibition: paradoxical effects Occasionally, benzodiazepines produce apparently stimulant effects. Clonazepam, given as an anticonvulsant, can sometimes produce aggressive and hyperactive behaviour and seizures may be exacerbated (Rall and Schleifer 1980). Some anxious patients report an increase in anxiety, insomnia, hypnogogic hallucinations on induction of sleep, nightmares, and irritability (Baldessarini 1980; Rogers *et al.* 1981). Patients on low doses of benzodiazepines may sometimes commit uncharacteristic antisocial acts such as shoplifting and sexual offences, while higher doses may produce outbursts of rage and violent behaviour, usually in anxious patients (Lader and Petursson 1981). Benzodiazepine usage has been suggested as a contributory cause of baby-battering. Triazolam in high doses (0.5 and 1 mg) has produced a syndrome consisting of severe anxiety, paranoia, hyperacusis, altered smell and taste, and paraesthesiae, (*Drug and Therapeutics Bulletin* 1979). As mentioned above, benzodiazepines cause increased EEG beta activity. suggesting excitatory effects in some pathways. These paradoxical effects of benzodiazepines have been attributed to disinhibition of behaviour previously suppressed by social restraints, fear or other anxiogenic stimuli (Speth *et al.* 1980).

Affective reactions Benzodiazepines can aggravate depression and provoke suicidal tendencies in depressed patients (Baldessarini 1980), and chronic benzodiazepine use can cause depression or 'emotional anaesthesia' in patients with no previous history of depressive disorder. On the other hand some patients experience euphoria, at least initially, and it is of interest that benzodiazepines have been found to have reinforcing properties in animals (Yanagita 1981; Pilotto *et al.* 1984; Chapter 5) and have abuse liability when used intravenously and orally in man (Strang 1984; Griffiths *et al.* 1984; Bergman and Griffiths 1986). In the presence of organic brain disease, benzodiazepines can cause tremulousness, crying, impaired concentration, nocturnal confusion, and agitation (*Drug Newsletter* 1983; Rogers *et al.* 1981; Lader and Petursson 1981).

Adverse effects in pregnancy The adverse effects on the foetus and neonate of benzodiazepines administered to the mother during pregnancy have been reviewed by Ashton (1985b). Their teratogenic potential in humans appears to be extremely low, if present at all (Schardein 1976; Beeley 1978). However, there is a theoretical risk of 'behavioural teratogenesis' due to faulty development of transmitter systems in the brain (Lewis 1978). Benzodiazepines readily traverse the placenta, are concentrated in foetal tissues since metabolism by the foetal liver is minimal, and can cause neonatal depression if given in late pregancy (Stirrat and Beard 1973; Singh and Mirkin 1973). Infants exposed *in utero*, may develop benzodiazepine withdrawal symptoms appearing 2–3 weeks after birth. The drugs are also present in the mother's milk for some days after administration.

Metabolic, endocrine, and autonomic effects. Benzodiazepines may affect the central control of endocrine function. Grandison (1983) reported that benzodiazepines altered the secretion of anterior pituitary hormones in rats, possibly due to an action on the central nervous regulation of pituitary function. Peripheral benzodiazepine receptors in the anterior pituitary can modulate prolactin secretion. Beary *et al.* (1983) found that the administration of temazepam (20 mg) as a single oral dose to normal women caused a significant decrease in plasma cortisol concentration and a rise in plasma prolactin concentration. These changes were ascribed to an action on pituitary or hypothalamic GABA receptors. Similar effects were found in males after oral administration of oxazepam. Petursson and Lader (1984) reported a significant increase in growth hormone secretion following diazepam administration to normal subjects. Endocrine and autonomic symptoms reported during benzodiazepine administration include menstrual irregularities, breast engorgement, galactorrhoea, hypotension, constipation, diarrhoea, incontinence, and impotence.

Overdose and drug interactions Taken alone, benzodiazepines rarely produce serious acute effects and patients have recovered spontaneously without permanent sequelæ after taking doses of several grams (Mathew and Lawson 1979). In patients with obstuctive pulmonary disease, however, benzodiazepines in moderate doses can increase alveolar ventilation and cause carbon dioxide narcosis (Harvey 1980). Although depression of consciousness occurs after overdose, consciousness returns while blood concentrations are still very high, presumably because of the rapid development of tolerance, as in the case of alcohol (Chapter 6). Rebound insomnia and other benzodiazepine withdrawal effects occur during recovery from acute benzodiazepine overdose (Haider and Oswald 1970).

Benzodiazepines potentiate the depressant effects of other central nervous system depressants. The effects are mainly additive at the sites of action although some authors suggest that synergistic effects may also occur especially with alcohol which probably also acts on GABA receptors (Ticku 1983; Speth *et al.* 1980; Paul and Whitehouse 1977; Hockings and Ballinger 1983). The potentiation of other central nervous system depressants can aggravate or precipitate respiritory failure especially in the elderly or those with pulmonary disease; they may also add to hypotension and occasionally cause fatal hypothermia in myxoedema (Proudfoot 1982; Rogers *et al.* 1981). Benzodiazepines are involved in about 40 per cent of self-poisonings in the United Kingdom usually in combination with other drugs (Proudfoot 1982). Under these circumstances their additive effects may be clinically important (Ashton 1985b).

Benzodiazepine dependence Drug dependence in general is discussed in Chapter 6, and dependence on narcotic analgesics, alcohol, nicotine, and cocaine are described in Chapter 7. Benzodiazepine dependence is described here since it is closely related to the anxiolytic and hypnotic actions of the drugs.

Early experience with benzodiazepines suggested that drug dependence was rare (Marks 1978, 1983). It has since become clear, however, that dependence on benzodiazepines occurs readily and quickly in some patients and is not uncommon. Such patients develop a reliance on the drug to maintain psychological comfort and suffer withdrawal symptoms if the drug is stopped or dosage reduced. Owen and Tyrer (1983) estimate that about one-third of patients taking benzodiazepines for six months become dependent, and some do so after only a few weeks of treatment (Murphy *et al.* 1984), while Kales *et al.* (1978) showed that withdrawal symptoms in the form of rebound insomnia can occur after administration of triazolam as a hypnotic for only 1 week. Some patients gradually escalate their dosage over time, but others become dependent while maintaining their original therapeutic dosage (Owen and Tyrer 1983). Very few patients compulsively seek large doses of benzodiazepines in order to obtain euphoric effects. Present estimates suggest that perhaps half a million people in this country are now dependent on benzodiazepines, and two or three million in the world (Salkind 1982; Owen and Tyrer 1983). Nearly 70 per cent of these are women. However, some studies suggest that perhaps 50 per cent of patients experience no withdrawal reactions despite regular treatment for years (Owen and Tyrer 1983; Tyrer and Owen 1983; Tyrer *et al.* 1982, Tyrer 1983). At present it is not possible to predict which patients are likely to become dependent, apart from those with a history of dependence on other drugs (Marks 1978). Tyrer and Owen (1983) suggest that patients with a 'passive-dependent' personality type are vulnerable, and Ashton (1984) noted high scores for neuroticism in patients dependent on benzodiazepines. Previous psychiatric history is not necessarily related to the development of dependence.

(i) Benzodiazepine withdrawal syndrome. Drug withdrawal, or reduction in dosage, in patients who have become dependent on benzodiazepines gives rise to a definite abstinence syndrome, which can be of considerable severity and has similarities to the withdrawal reactions of other central nervous system depressant drugs which cause dependence (Chapter 6). The syndrome has been described by Petursson and Lader (1981a,b, 1984), Lader and Petursson (1981), Salkind (1982), Tyrer and Owen (1983), Owen and Tyrer (1983), and Ashton (1984). Some of the common symptoms are shown in Table 4.3; most dependent patients undergoing withdrawal experience many or most of these symptoms, numerous though they are.

Table 4.3. Symptoms associated with benzodiazepine withdrawal

Psychological	Gastrointestinal
Drowsiness, fatigue	Nausea, vomiting
Excitability	Abdominal pain
Unreality, depersonalisation	Diarrhoea or constipation
Poor memory, concentration	Appetite, weight change
Perceptual distortions	Dry mouth
Hallucinations	Metallic taste
Obssessions	Dysphagia
Agoraphobia, phobias	Cardiovascular and respiratory
Panic attacks	Flushing, sweating
Depression	Palpitations
Paranoid thoughts	Hyperventilation
Rage, aggression	Urogenital and endocrine
Craving	Thirst
Acute psychotic episodes	Frequency, polyuria
Central nervous system	Incontinence
Headache	Menorrhagia
Pain (limbs, back, neck)	Mammary pain or swelling
Pain (jaw, teeth)	Loss of libido, impotence
Paraesthesiae (limbs, face)	Miscellaneous
Stiffness (limbs, back, jaw)	Skin rash/itching
Formication	Stuffy nose, sinusitis
Weakness	influenza-like symptoms
Tremor	
Muscle twitches, fasiculation	
Ataxia	
Dizziness, lightheadedness	
Blurred or double vision	
Tinnitus	
Speech difficulty	
Hypersensitivity (light, sound, taste, smell)	
Insomnia, nightmares	
Convulsions, temporal lobe fits	

References: Ashton (1984); Petursson and Lader (1981a, b); Hallstrom and Lader (1981); Owen and Tyrer (1983); Tyrer and Owen (1983).

The onset of the syndrome is related to the pharmacokinetic properties of the particular benzodiazepine involved. Withdrawal symptoms appear sooner on withdrawal from benzodiazepines with short elimination half-lives and are delayed after withdrawal from those with long half-lives. The time course of the withdrawal syndrome is often characterized by the early appearance of acute anxiety and psychotic symptoms (1–2 weeks after withdrawal) (Murphy *et al.* 1984) followed by a prolonged period of gradually diminishing mixed psychological and somatic symptoms (Ashton 1984).

The exact mechanism of the benzodiazepine withdrawal syndrome is not clear, but it seems likely that many of the symptoms result from underactivity of GABA-ergic systems in the brain. As discussed on in Chapter 6, it is known that chronic exposure of receptors to raised concentrations of their agonists can give rise to compensatory decreases in receptor sensitivity. Since benzodiazepines cause enhancement of GABA activity, a degree of sub-sensitivity to GABA would be expected to develop on chronic exposure to benzodiazepines. Tolerance to many of the effects of benzodiazepine occurs in man and animals, and there is some evidence in animals for a decrease in GABA-receptor density, diminished response to GABA agonists, and decreased density of benzodiazepine binding sites after chronic benzo-diazepine treatment (Cowen and Nutt 1982; Crawley et al. 1982). Decreased benzodiazepine receptor binding has been observed in rats after chronic administration of clonazepam (Crawley et al. 1982) and barbiturates (Ho 1980) and slight reductions in benzodiazepine receptor density have been observed after high doses of lorazepam (60 mg/kg) (Braestrup et al. 1979) and flurazepam (150 mg/kg) (Chiu and Rosenberg 1978). Diazepam given chronically in high or low doses (3–90 mg/kg orally) did not appear to alter specific binding in the rat brain although it did dramatically reduce striatal GABA receptor binding (Braestrup et al. 1979; Mohler et al. 1978). With-drawal of benzodiazepines after such changes have occurred would lead to a marked decrease in GABA activity, both because of GABA subsensitivity and because GABA activity would no longer be enhanced (Snyder 1981a). Consequently, a decrease in the direct inhibitory effects of GABA and a surge in output of other neurotransmitters in some areas of the brain (nor-adrenaline, serotonin, dopamine, acetyl choline, substance P, and opioid pep-tides) normally inhibited by GABA would be expected.

The role of these neurotransmitters in arousal and sleep systems, and in anxiety have already been discussed (Chapter 3). The same transmitters are also involved in reward and punishment systems (Chapter 5), and their activity is altered in affective disorders (Chapter 12), and psychotic states (Chapter 13). It seems likely that disturbances in neurotransmitter activity could contribute to the benzodiazepine withdrawal syndrome, although at present these can be envisaged only in the most general way. Noradrenaline and serotonin activity may be critical in the pathways from the locus coeru-leus and raphe nuclei to parts of the limbic system which appear from animal work to be involved in anxiogenesis (Chapter 3). Increased dopaminergic and serotonergic activity may be involved in the psychotic reactions which are similar to those seen in schizophrenia and produced by some psycho-tomimetic drugs such as LSD (Chapter 14). However, none of these pos-tulated central transmitter changes have been fully investigated in patients undergoing benzodiazepine withdrawal. Some of the metabolic and endo-crine effects may be due to changes in pituitary benzodiazepine receptors (Beary et al. 1983).

In many patients regularly taking benzodiazepines, symptoms of withdrawal occur while they are still taking the drugs without reduction in dosage (Ashton 1984). Thus, some patients complain simultaneously both of adverse effects attributable to benzodiazepine use and of benzodiazepine withdrawal phenomena. Possibly, such a merging of the symptomatology reflects uneven development of tolerance to the various actions of benzodiazepines, with some types of benzodiazepine or GABA receptors undergoing adaptive changes more quickly than others.

Since dependence takes time to develop, it is best prevented by limiting the duration of benzodiazepine use. Severe withdrawal effects are uncommon if the drugs have been used for less than 2 weeks (Owen and Tyrer 1983), and it would seem advisable to restrict regular benzodiazepine administration to periods of 7–14 days. The optimal method of withdrawing benzodiazepines in patients who have become dependent has not yet been determined; probably different regimes suit different patients and the management needs to be individually tailored. Various methods of slow dosage reduction combined with symptomatic treatment are described by Salkind (1982), Smith and Wesson (1983), Ashton (1984), and in *Drugs Newsletter* (1983, 1985).

Barbiturates

The barbiturates are used as anaesthetic agents (short acting barbiturates), anticonvulsants (phenobarbitone and its derivatives), and rarely as hepatic enzyme inducers. They have a long history as sedative/hypnotics, but such a use is no longer recommended because of serious disadvantages including low therapeutic index, frequency of death from overdose, rapid development of tolerance with loss of effectiveness, high incidence of drug dependence, and frequency of drug interactions. Nevertheless, a large poplulation of patients, perhaps over half a million in the United Kingdom (Rogers *et al.* 1981), most of them elderly, still regularly take barbiturates as hypnotics.

Pharmacokinetics

The pharmacokinetics and actions of barbiturates are described by Harvey (1980) and by Rogers *et al.* (1981). The sodium salts are well absorbed from the gut and can be given intravenously. Barbiturates are widely distributed in the body but the rate of distribution depends on their lipid solubility. Highly lipid soluble thiobarbiturates given intravenously produce peak central nervous system depressant effects within 30 s, when they reach maximal concentrations in the most vascular areas of the brain (grey matter). Their action is terminated within 30 m by redistribution to other tissues, the rate of uptake by different tissues being determined by blood flow. They become concentrated in the relatively poorly perfused fatty tissues over an hour after administration. Elimination from this site is relatively slow, with the result that anaesthesia is followed by residual central nervous system depression.

When less lipid soluble barbiturates such as phenobarbitone are given intravenously, the peak depressant effect is delayed for about 15 m, probably because of slow penetration of the blood-brain barrier. The duration of action of these barbiturates is determined by the rate of metabolism and excretion rather than by redistribution. Elimination half lives of some barbiturates are shown in Table 4.4.

Metabolism of barbiturates is mainly by hepatic microsomal enzymes and consists largely of oxidation reactions which produce pharmacologically inactive hydroxides and aldehydes. The rate of metabolism varies between individuals and is influenced by genetic factors. Repeated administration of barbiturates rapidly causes hepatic enzyme induction which leads to pharmacokinetic tolerance (Chapter 6) and may also give rise to drug interactions. Renal excretion of unchanged barbiturate is only significant for phenobarbitone (30 per cent) and barbitone (65-90 per cent), which have low lipid solubility and are relatively highly ionized. The other barbiturates are excreted as metabolites.

Table 4.4.   Some barbiturates and non-barbiturate hypnotics

Drug	Elimination half-life (H)	Hepatic enzyme induction
Barbiturate hypnotics		
Hexobarbitone	3–7	++
Heptabarbitone	6–11	++
Amylobarbitone	17–34	++
Quinalbarbitone	19–35	++
Pentobarbitone	21–46	++
Butobarbitone	34–42	++
Phenobarbitone	48–144	++
Barbiturate intravenous anaesthetics		
Sodium thiopentone	6	
Methohexitone	70–125 min	
Non-barbiturate hypnotics		
Chloral derivatives	8*	+*
Chlormethiazole	1–4	○
Glutethimide	5–20	++

* Trichlorethanol: common metabolite of chloral derivatives.

Actions

Sedative/hypnotic effects Barbiturates are potentially depressants of all excitable tissues. However, the central nervous system is the most sensitive to this effect and the drugs can therefore produce central nervous system depression in doses which have little peripheral effect. Depending on dosage, any degree of central depression can be produced, from mild sedation to general anaesthesia, coma, and death. Within the central nervous system, the reticular formation appears to be most sensitive to barbiturates and small doses, which hardly affect transmission in primary sensory pathways, depress reticular formation responses to sensory stimuli and raise its threshold to direct electrical stimulation (Bradley and Key 1958; Sharpless 1970). Barbiturates also inhibit some reticulo-limbic pathways (Tsuchiya and Kitagawa 1976). These actions reduce activity in both general and limbic arousal systems. The barbiturates appear to produce anxiolytic effects in animals (Gray 1981, 1982; Iverson 1980), but their effects on anxiety in man are inseparable from their sedative actions and they are inferior to benzodiazepines as anxiolytic agents. In spite of the exquisite sensitivity of the reticular formation, barbiturate effects on the brain are fairly unselective and only slightly larger doses also depress medullary vital centres. For this reason, the barbiturates have a low therapeutic index. Pain sensation, however, is relatively spared until the moment of unconsciousness, and in small doses barbiturates are hyperalgesic; hence they are not reliable hypnotics in the presence of pain. In some circumstances low doses can induce paradoxical excitment, probably due to suppression of inhibitory pathways.

(i) Effects on the EEG. The effects of barbiturates on the EEG are reviewed by Brazier (1977) and Harvey (1980). In small doses, barbiturates decrease low frequency EEG activity and increase fast activity (beta activity, 13–35 Hz). Fast activity starts in the frontal cortex and spreads to the parietal and occipital cortex. During this phase, the threshold for electrical arousal from the reticular formation may be transiently lowered. Clouding of consciousness and sometimes euphoria accompany the phase of fast activity, but pain responses are retained. As dosage is increased and consciousness is lost, high amplitude slow waves (5–15 Hz) appear on the EEG. Further dose increase produces delta activity (1–3 Hz) and this stage is accompanied by a loss of pain response suitable for surgical procedures. As the level of anaesthesia deepens, the slow EEG waves decrease in amplitude and occasional periods of electrical silence appear. Cortical evoked responses and event related slow potentials of the brain are in general reduced by barbiturates in a dose-related manner (Shagass and Straumenis 1978).

(ii) Effects on sleep. Hypnotic doses of barbiturates invariably produce dose-dependent alterations in sleep stages (Harvey 1980; Kay et al. 1976; Evans et al. 1968; Oswald 1980). The changes are similar to those produced by benzodiazepines and consist of a decrease in sleep latency, decrease in number of awakenings, and prolonged sleeping time (unless the duration of action of the drug has been reduced by enzyme induction). The duration of Stages 3 and 4 (SWS) is usually reduced, REMS latency prolonged, and total

REMS activity decreased. In some anxious patients and normal subjects SWS may, however, be prolonged. Plasma growth hormone concentrations are not altered during barbiturate administration, but plasma corticosteroid concentrations during sleep are reduced; there is a rebound increase in plasma levels of these hormones on drug withdrawal (Ogunremi *et al.* 1973). Tolerance to the hypnotic effects of barbiturates develops rapidly and in the study by Evans *et al.* (1968) REMS returned to baseline values after 5 nights in two normal subjects given 200 mg of sodium amylobarbitone *nocte*. Barbiturates used in anaesthesia can cause similar alterations in sleep stages.

(iii) Rebound insomnia. Rebound insomnia, which may last for several weeks, occurs on discontinuation of barbiturates after regular use. The symptoms are similar to those described for benzodiazepines and include a decrease in total sleep time, increased number of wakenings, and nightmares or vivid dreams associated with increased REMS activity. As with benzodiazepines, these rebound effects lead to continuation of use and form part of the withdrawal syndrome in barbiturate-dependent subjects. With short acting barbiturates, a compensatory rebound occurs in the latter part of each night while the drug is still being taken.

(iv) Hangover effects. Since most of the barbiturates have long elimination half lives, hangover effects and residual psychomotor impairment are common. Impairment of skills relating to aircraft flying and motor car driving have been shown to persist for 19-22 h in normal subjects given usual hypnotic doses of various barbiturates (Borland and Nicholson 1975; Clarke and Nicholson 1978). More subtle psychomotor changes, impairment of judgement, and irritability may also persist into the following day. Residual effects are most marked in the elderly who may develop depression, confusion and ataxia; chronic barbiturate usage is associated with falls and femoral fractures in the elderly (Macdonald and Macdonald, (1977).

Anaesthetic effects The anaesthetic effects of barbiturates are an extension of the sedative/hypnotic effects. Barbiturates depress respiration in a dose-related manner: at hypnotic concentrations, respiration is depressed but probably little more than during normal sleep (Harvey 1980); at anaesthetic concentrations, the respiratory response to both carbon dioxide and to hypoxia are reduced (Marshall and Wollman 1980). Barbiturates also depress cardiovascular centres in the medulla and have ganglion blocking effects. In sufficient concentration, they depress myocardial tissue. Anaesthetic doses of thiopentone in normal subjects cause a transient fall in blood pressure and a decrease in cardiac output. However, in hypovolaemic states such doses of thiopental may result in hypotension, circulatory collapse, and cardiac arrest. There is a reduction of sympathetic activity and cerebral blood flow and metabolic rate are reduced.

Anticonvulsant effects Most barbiturates have anticonvulsant properties but phenobarbitone and its congener primidone exert maximal anticonvulsant effects in subhypnotic doses and are therefore suitable for the treatment of epilepsy. They are effective in general tonic, clonic, and cortical focal seizures. Barbiturates limit the spread of seizure activity in the brain and also elevate seizure threshold. It is not clear whether the mechanism of the anticonvulsant effects (Rall and Schleifer 1980) is different from the mechanism of the hypnotic effects, which are discussed below.

Mechanisms of action

It now appears likely that many of the effects of barbiturates are explained by their interaction with specific binding sites on the GABA A post-synaptic receptor complex (Fig. 4.2; Braestrup and Nielson 1980; Toffano *et al.* 1980; Barker and Mathers 1981). The barbiturate binding site is directly linked to the chloride channel; occupation by barbiturates prolongs the opening of this channel, causing a long-lasting post-synaptic neuronal hyper-polarization. This mechanism might explain the observation that barbiturates are particularly effective against repetitive activity in a number of central nervous system pathways, having little effect on the initial impulse in a train but greatly depressing the response to subsequent impulses (Harvey 1980). Competition between barbiturates and GABA-antagonist convulsants (e.g. picrotoxin) at this site suggest that at least part of the anticonvulsant action of barbiturates is exerted here (Bowery 1976; Harrison and Simmonds 1983). Barbiturates also appear to inhibit the actions of some excitatory transmitters such as glutamate (Richards and Smaje 1976), acetylcholine, noradrenaline, and serotonin (Martin 1982).

Since barbiturates and benzodiazepines interact at closely associated sites on GABA receptors, it is to be expected that they have many similarities. Both enhance GABA activity in the brain and decrease the turnover of central noradrenaline, dopamine, serotonin and acetyl choline (Harvey 1980; Tsuchiya and Kitagawa 1976). However, while benzodiazepines appear to favour repetitive occupation of post-synaptic GABA receptors by GABA, barbiturates tend to prolong the inhibitory post-synaptic hyperpolarization produced by activation of these receptors. It may be for this reason that barbiturates are less selective than benzodiazepines in their depressant effects, showing no differentiation between anxiolytic and sedative effects, and depressing respiration in doses only slightly above hypnotic doses. Bar-biturates, like benzodiazepines, may also have presynaptic actions by mech-anisms which are at present not clear (Nicoll 1975, 1978; Richards 1972); they inhibit the release of noradrenaline and glutamate from rat synap-tosomes (Martin 1982). At high concentrations they also interfere with cal-cium uptake by nerve cell membranes (Blaustein and Ector 1975), but the relevance of this effect to depressant actions is not known.

Adverse effects

Oversedation Hypnotic doses of barbiturates commonly produce hangover effects with psychomotor impairment especially in the elderly, as mentioned above. Excessive dosage results in ataxia, slurred speech, nystagmus and impaired intellectual function.

Paradoxical effects, affective reactions Paradoxical excitment occurs in some patients, both young and elderly or debilitated, and in patients with pain. Euphoria or irritability sometimes accompany this disinhibitory effect, but depression may follow chronic barbiturate ingestion. The chronic use of barbiturates is sometimes associated with musculoskeletal pain, particularly in the neck, shoulder girdle, and upper limbs.

Hypersensitivity, idiosyncracy Allergic reactions of various types may occur, especially in atopic individuals. Crises may be precipitated in patients with porphyria since barbiturates enhance porphyrin synthesis.

Adverse effects in pregnancy Barbiturates freely cross the placenta and are rapidly distributed in the foetus where they are concentrated in the midbrain (British Medical Journal 1972). When given in late pregnancy, these drugs can depress vital functions and also cause withdrawal symptoms in the neonate (Ashton 1985a). These factors can be important in epileptic mothers taking barbiturates and in barbiturate addicts, and should be considered when barbiturates are maternally administered for the purpose of foetal enzyme induction.

Drug interactions Drug interactions with barbiturates are common, largely because of hepatic enzyme induction. The activity of drugs metabolized by these enzymes is reduced (e.g., other barbiturates, coumarins, phenytoin, chlorpromazine, cortisol, testosterone, vitamin D_3, tricyclic antidepressants, and oral contraceptive agents). Conversely, the metabolism of barbiturates may be slowed by enzyme inhibition with monoamine oxidase inhibitors. Barbiturates also have additive effects with other central nervous system depressants. Further drug interactions are mentioned by Rogers *et al.* (1981).

Overdose Despite a decrease in the number of prescriptions over the past 10–15 years (Johns 1977), barbiturate overdose still accounts for about 10 000 hospital admissions and 1500–2000 deaths each year in the United Kingdom. These fatalities represent about 50 per cent of the total deaths due to self-poisoning (Rogers *et al.* 1981). Barbiturates have a low therapeutic index and the hypnotic dose is only about a tenth of that required to produce fatal respiratory depression. Furthermore, tolerance to the respiratory depressant effects develops to a lesser degree than to the sedative/hypnotic effects, so that as tolerance increases, the therapeutic index becomes even lower. Death usually occurs from respiratory failure, often with associated cardiovascular collapse and renal failure. The ingestion of additional central nervous system depressants, especially alcohol, adds to the likelihood of a fatal outcome.

Tolerance, dependence, abuse Pharmacokinetic tolerance to barbiturates, due to hepatic enzyme induction, has already been mentioned. Pharmacodynamic tolerance (Chapter 6) also occurs and is probably more important in relation to drug dependence. Acute pharmacodynamic tolerance develops extremely rapidly, even after a single dose, and with chronic dosing tolerance continues to develop for some weeks or months. In contrast, enzyme induction reaches its peak over a period of days (Harvey 1980). Tolerance to the sedative/hypnotic effects develops to a greater extent than to anticonvulsant and lethal effects. At maximum tolerance the clinically effective dose may be increased about six times; the lethal dose, much less. Cross-tolerance to other depressant drugs including meprobamate, glutethimide, methaqualone, general anaesthetics, opiates, phencyclidine, and benzodiazepines has been shown to occur (Harvey 1980).

The development of tolerance leads to a tendency to escalate barbiturate dosage and to abstinence symptoms on drug withdrawal. In these circumstances barbiturate dependence rapidly develops. It has been estimated that the equivalent of 400 mg of quinalbarbitone used regularly for 2 months produces marked dependence. This is probably a conservative estimate and it is likely that at least a sixth of the 600 000 regular consumers of prescribed barbiturates in the United Kingdom are to some degree dependent (Rogers *et al.* 1981).

In addition, barbiturates are frequently abused, although the incidence of this practice is hard to estimate. The number involved probably considerably exceeds that of opiate abusers. Barbiturate abuse often coexists with abuse of opiates, other sedatives, benzodiazepines and amphetamines and cocaine. Like other drugs of abuse (Chapter 6), barbiturates have reinforcing properties in animals and can produce euphoria in man, especially when injected intravenously. Patterns of abuse are described by Jaffe (1980); they range from irregular short sprees of gross intoxication to the prolonged compulsive daily use of large doses. Chronic intoxication resembles alcohol intoxication, with general sluggishness, ataxia, dysarthria, irritability, and aggressiveness.

Withdrawal of barbiturates from dependent individuals produces an abstinence syndrome, the severity of which depends on previous dosage and degree of tolerance. Rebound insomnia, and psychological symptoms, such as anxiety and difficulty in concentration, are common and have been reported in many studies after only about 5 weeks of therapeutic doses (Oswald 1980; Evans *et al.* 1968; Ogunremi *et al.* 1973). These symptoms may persist for some weeks. More severe withdrawal symptoms include anxiety, restlessness, hallucinations, weakness, hypotension, gastrointestinal symptoms, delirium, and cardiovascular collapse or status epilepticus which may be fatal. The syndrome is similar to the alcohol withdrawal syndrome (Chapter 7) and is described more fully by Jaffe (1980).

Other drugs used in insomnia and anxiety

Hypnotics and sedatives

The pharmacological properties of a number of other commonly used sedative/hypnotics differ little from those of barbiturates and benzodiazepines. They are all general central nervous system depressants with similar hypnotic effects, including alterations in sleep stages, and may all produce dependence with an abstinence syndrome on withdrawal. Many of them have long elimination half lives, induce hepatic enzymes and give rise to drug interactions (Table 4.4). They all have additive effects with other central nervous system depressants. Some have anticonvulsant activity. Their mechanisms of action have not been studied in detail, but it is likely that many of them, like benzodiazepines and barbiturates, enhance GABA activity in the brain (Cowen and Nutt 1982).

In contrast, L-tryptophan and gamma-hydroxybutyrate are naturally occurring substances which are being explored as 'physiological hypnotics' that appear to produce normal sleep patterns without rebound efects or drug dependence. These drugs, although theoretically promising, have not been submitted to large scale controlled trials.

Chloral derivatives (chloral hydrate, triclofos, dichloralphenazone) In therapeutic doses, these are effective hypnotics, but cause respiratory and cardiovascular depression in overdose.

Chlormethiazole Chlormethiazole has hypnotic and anticonvulsant properties. Because of its short half-life, it is relatively free of hangover effects and has been recommended for use in the elderly. It has also been used in the management of alcohol and narcotic withdrawal, but there appears to be a considerable danger of dependence, especially when large doses are used (Exton-Smith and McLean 1979; Wheatley 1981). An action on the GABA A receptor site, similar to that of barbiturates, has been demonstrated (Harrison and Simmonds 1983).

Piperidinediones (glutethimide, methylprylone) These are effective sedative/hypnotics, but cardiovascular and respiratory depression occurs more readily than with the barbiturates.

Promethazine Promethazine is a phenothiazine derivative which is a histamine (H_1) receptor blocker and has antipruritic, anticholinergic, and sedative effects. It sometimes causes excitement rather than sedation. Some phenothiazines with antipsychotic actions also have hypnotic effects (e.g. chlorpromazine); these drugs do not alter normal sleep stages and do not appear to cause rebound on withdrawal, but their general use as hypnotics is limited by adverse effects.

L-*tryptophan* Unlike other hypnotics, L-tryptophan is not a general central nervous system depressant. However, it has been shown in several small studies to have hypnotic effects in man without disruption of sleep stages or rebound insomnia (Schneider-Helmert and Spinweber 1986). Oral doses of 5–15 g have been reported to reduce sleep latency, prolong SWS and to produce either no change or an increase in REMS in normal subjects and insomniacs (Wyatt *et al.* 1970; Wyatt and Gillin 1976; Hartmann 1971, 1979; Wheatley 1981). L-tryptophan is a precursor of serotonin, but the mechanism of its hypnotic action is not known. The role of serotonin in sleep is discussed in Chapter 2 and alterations in plasma tryptophan concentration during normal sleep have been studied by Chen *et al.* (1974). The use of L-tryptophan in depression is discussed in Chapters 11 and 12. L-tryptophan has a bitter taste and has caused nausea and vomiting in short term studies; its long-term effects are not known.

Gammahydroxybutyrate Gammahydroxybutyrate is found in maximum concentrations in the midbrain and hippocampus. It has been investigated as a hypnotic in a few small studies and in oral dosage of 1–3 g it appears to increase SWS and REMS in insomniac subjects without toxic effects or rebound in withdrawal (Mamelak *et al.* 1973). When injected intravenously, gammahydroxybutyrate has anaesthetic properties but may produce abnormal muscle movements, nausea and vomiting, bradycardia, and respiratory depression (Martindale 1982).

Other drugs used in anxiety

Beta-adrenoceptor antagonists Many of the somatic manifestations of anxiety, such as palpitations and tremor, are due to increased sympathetic activity with excessive activation of peripheral beta-adrenoceptors. These symptoms can be reduced by beta-adrenoceptor antagonists in normal subjects under stress (James *et al.* 1977; Taggart *et al.* 1973; Taylor and Meeran 1973; *Lancet* 1985) and in patients with anxiety syndromes (Tyrer and Lader 1974; Turner 1976). In low to moderate doses, beta-blockers appear to reduce somatic symptoms without much effect on psychic anxiety (Tyrer and Lader 1974). Furthermore, beta-blockers such as practolol, which do not enter the central nervous system in appreciable quantities, are as effective as propranolol and oxprenolol (Bonn *et al.* 1972). Thus it seems likely that the effect is peripheral.

However, high doses of some beta-blockers (e.g. 480 mg oxprenolol) may have additional central effects (Farhoumand *et al.* 1979). Beta-blockers have been used in many types of anxiety, including that due to withdrawal of other drugs such as benzodiazepines and alcohol (Bonn *et al.* 1972; Ashton 1984; Lancet 1973). By controlling peripheral sympathetic overactivity, they can sometimes interupt the vicious circle by which somatic symptoms reinforce psychic symptoms, but they have little effect on the subjective emotion of anxiety and should be reserved for patients with predominantly somatic complaints (Tyrer and Lader 1974). On the other hand, many patients with anxiety complain of both central and peripheral symptoms and combinations of beta-blockers with benzodiazepines are sometimes used (Turner 1976).

Clonidine Redmond (1982) suggested that pathological anxiety can result from functional overactivity of the locus coeruleus. Clonidine, which decreases the firing rate and release of noradrenaline from locus coeruleus neurones by stimulation of alpha$_2$-noradrenergic receptors, has been used with some success in treating anxiety associated with opiate, alcohol, and benzodiazepine withdrawal (Lal and Fielding 1983; *Lancet* 1980; Ashton 1984; Keshavan and Crammer 1985). Preliminary studies, reviewed by Redmond (1982) suggest that clonidine may also reduce clinical anxiety associated with depression, generalized anxiety disorders, and phobic-panic anxiety, although further trials are required to establish optimal dosage and indications. Clonidine does not affect anxiety ratings in normal non-anxious subjects.

Antidepressants A number of antidepressant drugs have additional sedative or anxiolytic effects. These are sometimes used in anxiety syndromes and are also of value in depressive states associated with anxiety. Tricyclic antidepressants with sedative effects include imipramine, amitriptyline, and butriptyline. Antidepressants claimed to have additional anxiolytic effects include dothiepin, doxepin, dibenzepin, and iprindole (Rogers *et al.* 1981). Monoamine oxidase inhibitors are sometimes used in phobic and panic disorders (Shader *et al.* 1982; Rifkin and Siris 1984). However, the rate of relapse in phobic disorders treated with antipressants is high (Gelder *et al.* 1983). In terms of Gray's (1981, 1982) theory of anxiety discussed in Chapter 3, it is difficult to understand how antidepressants which are not sedative can be effective in anxiety. Since they increase adrenergic and serotonergic activity at central synapses, they might be expected to aggravate anxiety (Wilbur and Kulik 1981). On theoretical grounds, it is also arguable whether antidepressants and benzodiazepines should be used together, but in psychiatric practice such a combination is not infrequent. Antidepressants are discussed further in Chapter 12.

Antipsychotic drugs Some of the antipsychotic drugs, such as chlorpromazine and haloperidol, have sedative, anticholinergic, and anxiolytic effects and may on occasion be of use in severe anxiety disorders associated with panic, anxiety provoked by psychotomimetic agents, and autonomic and anxiety symptoms associated with the abstinence syndromes of central nervous system depressants. These drugs are discussed in Chapter 14. GABA agonists are at present under investigation for chronic anxiety but their place is not established (Hoehn-Saric 1983). Buspirone, a drug with dopamine receptor agonist/antagonist activity also appears to have anxiolytic effects (Rubenstein and Norman 1984).

Drug treatment in insomnia and anxiety

As discussed in Chapter 3, insomnia has many causes, and hypnotic drugs are not always, perhaps rarely, indicated (Hartmann 1980). Marks and Nicholson (1984) reported the results of a conference on drugs and insomnia held at the National Institutes of Health, Bethesda. It was suggested that for purposes of practical management insomnia can be considered as transient, short-term, or chronic. Transient insomnia is due to an alteration in sleep conditions. Only occasionally is a hypnotic required; a rapidly eliminated preparation, used on a couple of occasions only, is recommended. Short-term insomnia may be due to emotional or physical stress. A hypnotic may be given for preferably not more than a week or two and ideally taken intermittently rather than regularly. A rapidly eliminated drug is usually appropriate, although a longer acting drug such as diazepam may be better if there is marked daytime stress. Chronic insomnia is usually secondary to other conditions, but in selected cases with no apparent cause the use of a hypnotic may be considered, in combination with general measures for improving sleep hygeine. Longer-acting benzodiazepines are thought to be most useful, but dosage should be intermittent (one night in three) and temporary (not more than a month).

The same principles apply to the drug treatment of anxiety. Anxiety coexisting with schizophrenia and depression is probably better treated with antipsychotics or antidepressants, although many psychiatrists add benzodiazepines. However, long-term treatment with anxiolytic drugs is 'inappropriate and positively harmful in chronic anxiety' (Rogers *et al.* 1981; p. 213). Benzodiazepines tend to lose their anxiolytic effects after long periods of chronic use and they may even aggravate or induce anxiety symptoms while also producing dependence (Ashton 1984). Initially, they have undoubted anxiolytic actions, and short, intermittent courses, in combination with other supportive measures, may be helpful during acute phases or temporary exacerbations of anxiety. Diazepam is suitable for intermittent use, but should not be given regularly for more than 2 weeks. Nevertheless,

the problem is difficult and the treatment of anxiety states remains unsatisfactory (Rogers *et al.* 1981).

Central nervous system stimulants

It may be significant that, compared with depressants, central nervous system
stimulants are little used clinically. Yet stimulants in the form of tea, coffee,
and caffeinated drinks are taken regularly by almost the whole population
from childhood onwards. Chronic use of some central nervous system stimulants can lead to drug dependence. This may occur with amphetamine and to
some extent with caffeine. Cocaine and nicotine are described in Chapter 7.

Directly acting sympathomimetic amines
Directly acting sympathomimetic amines act as central nervous system stimulants by activating receptors in the widely distributed noradrenergic pathways
concerned in arousal (Chapter 2). *Adrenaline, noradrenaline, and isoprenaline*
do not readily enter the brain when administered systemically in therapeutic
doses, but may nevertheless produce restlessness and apprehension. Large
amounts of noradrenaline are secreted in phaeochromocytoma and patients
with this tumour may complain of attacks of acute anxiety. The potent
peripheral cardiovascular and metabolic effects of these drugs may contribute
to their subjective effects.

Indirectly acting sympathomimetic amines
These drugs act largely by releasing endogenous catecholamines; their actions
are similar to directly acting agents but they penetrate the brain more readily.

Amphetamine
Amphetamine is a powerful central nervous system stimulant; the *d*–isomer
(*dextamphetamine*) is more potent in this respect than the *l*-isomer.
Methamphetamine and *methyl phenidate* are structurally related to amphetamine and are pharmacologically similar.

Pharmacokinetics
Amphetamine is well absorbed from the gastrointestinal tract and is partly
excreted unchanged in the urine, the rate of excretion being faster under acid
conditions. At a urinary pH of 5, the elimination half-life is 5 h. The apparent
volume of distribution is greater in addicts, who may develop an increased
tissue affinity for the drug. Some of the metabolites of amphetamine are
pharmacologically active and may possibly add to the psychotic symptoms
which occur in chronic users (Rogers *et al.* 1981).

Actions on the central nervous system The psychological actions of amphetamine in man depend greatly on dosage, individual personality chacteristics, and the prevailing mood and expectations at the time of administration. Typically, a single oral dose of 10–30 mg produces a feeling of increased alertness with heightened self-confidence, and increased motor and speech activity. There is often an elevation of mood which may proceed to elation and euphoria (high doses and especially intravenous administration produces a 'high' which may encourage drug abuse; Chapter 7). However, some subjects experience confusion, anxiety, dysphoria, or even transient drowsiness (Tecce and Cole 1974). Feelings of fatigue are postponed and the desire for sleep reduced.

Effects on performance are variable. In mental or psychomotor tasks, responses may be more rapid, concentration improved and errors reduced; sometimes, however, errors are increased in spite of more rapid performance; memory may be improved or impaired. Physical activity in sport may be improved and fatigue postponed. The enhancing effects on performance are more marked in the presence of fatigue or sleep deprivation. Large doses or chronic usage may reverse all these effects and be followed by mental depression and prolonged fatigue.

The effects of amphetamine on the waking EEG consist of desynchronisation and a shift towards faster frequencies. The effects on sleep consist of a considerable reduction in REMS, a reduction in SWS, and a decrease in total sleep time. On discontinuation, there is a marked rebound, especially in REMS, which may last for many weeks (Oswald 1980).

Amphetamine has a potent analeptic effect and will reverse the effects of central nervous system depressants. It also stimulates the medullary respiratory centre. It depresses appetite and has been used as an anorectic in the treatment of obesity. However, tolerance occurs rapidly and the effect in short-lived.

Sites and mechanisms of action Amphetamine has stimulant effects throughout the nervous system. It facilitates monosynaptic and polysynaptic transmission in the spinal cord and stimulates the medullary respiratory centre and lateral hypothalamic areas concerned with the control of feeding behaviour. It also stimulates the reticular activating system, where it lowers the threshold for arousal by electrical stimulation and reverses the depressant effects of barbiturates (Bradley and Key 1958; Fig. 2.3). In addition, it produces cortical desynchronization when injected into the reticular formation (Candy and Key 1977).

These effects are thought to be largely due to release of catecholamines from nerve terminals since they can be attenuated by depletion of monoamine stores with reserpine or 6-hydroxydopamine and by drugs which prevent catecholamine synthesis (Candy and Key 1977). Amphetamine may also have some direct stimulant action on noradrenergic receptors and some reuptake-blocking effect. In addition to releasing noradrenaline, amphetamine releases dopamine from dopaminergic nerve terminals. Some of its effects, for example increased locomotor activity, stereotyped behaviour in animals, and some psychotic symptoms in man, including aggravation of schizophrenic symptoms (Chapter 14), may be due to increased dopaminergic activity. There is evidence in animals that the rewarding effects are mediated in the nucleus accumbens (Carr and White 1986). In high doses, serotonin is also released and this may account for perceptual disturbances and add to psychotic symptoms.

Adverse effects Acute overdose with amphetamine produces a toxic psychosis with extreme restlessness, tremor, insomnia, panic, confusion, irritability, and delerium. Psychotic features such as paranoia, hallucinations, and aggressiveness with suicidal or homicidal tendencies may be prominent. Cardiovascular effects include headache, pallor or flushing, palpitations, cardiac arrhythmias, anginal pain, and hyper- or hypotension with cardiovascular collapse. Gastrointestinal symptoms include dry mouth, nausea, vomiting, diarrhoea, and abdominal cramps. Death may occur from coma, convulsions, or cerebral haemorrhage. Chronic intoxication may produce a schizophreniform psychosis similar to that produced by cocaine (Chapter 7).

Tolerance develops to the anorexic and euphoric effects of amphetamines and may lead to increasing dosage. Chronic abusers develop tolerence to the lethal effects and daily dosage of 1700 mg has been reported (Weiner 1980*a,b*). Nevertheless, tolerance to the psychic effects is much less and a toxic psychosis often appears after weeks or months of continued use. Chronic use of high doses of amphetamine may produce microvascular damage, chromatolysis of adrenergic neurones in the brain, and long-lasting or irreversible depletion of dopamine in the caudate nucleus. The latter change is associated with the development of exaggerated startle reactions, dyskinaesias, and postural abnormalities, possibly resulting from secondary supersensitivity of dopamine receptors in the caudate nucleus (Jaffe 1980). Cessation of amphetamine use produces a withdrawal syndrome characterized by depression, hypersomnia with increased REMS, hyperphagia, and debility. Amphetamine dependence is similar to cocaine dependence and is discussed further in Chapter 7.

Clinical use.   The main use of amphetamines is for narcolepsy, in which they prevent narcoleptic attacks and often improve cataplexy. Tolerance does not seem to occur when dextroamphetamine is used for this purpose in doses of 5–60 mg daily. Hyperkinetic children, apparently paradoxically, may become calmer when given amphetamines. The drugs are occasionally useful for combating excessive sedation induced by barbiturates in epileptics. Methylphenidate and methamphetamine have similar uses.

Anorectic agents A number of congeners of amphetamine have anorectic effects and have been used in the management of obesity. These include *diethyl-propion, phentermine, fenfluramine, and mazindol*. The actions of these drugs are similar to those of amphetamine and the anorectic effect is due to an action on hypothalmic centres where these drugs cause release of monoamines and also have a reuptake blocking effect. Fenfluramine mainly releases serotonin and on chronic use can cause central serotonin depletion. Mazindol appears to release mainly dopamine. The drugs also have general stimulant effects on the brain and cardiovascular system, although less than amphetamines. They all, to a greater or lesser extent, affect sleep and mood, and can give rise to tolerance, dependence, and a withdrawal syndrome although this is much less likely than with amphetamine. Fenfluramine has been shown to reduce REMS and SWS, increase intrasleep restlessness and to cause rebound effects on sleep and depression of mood on withdrawal (Lewis *et al.* 1971; Oswald *et al.* 1971). Nightmares appear with increasing dosage (Mullen and Wilson 1974).

Pemoline is a structurally unrelated drug which has a central stimulant action; it has been used for reversing the effects of central nervous system depressants, for minimal brain dysfunction in children, and for improving alertness in senile dementia.

Xanthines

Theophylline, caffeine. Theophylline and caffeine are chemically related plant alkaloids which are well absorbed from the gut and metabolized by the liver. They are potent central nervous system stimulants and have in addition many peripheral actions. Caffeine has virtually no theraputic uses, although it is widely taken in coffee and coca cola, and is incorporated into several 'over the counter' preparations. Theophyline preparations are mainly used in medicine for their effects on the respiratory system and effects on the nervous system are usually unwanted.

The central actions of caffeine include an increased feeling of alertness (Bruce *et al.* 1986), increased capacity for sustained intellectual performance, decreased reaction time, and increased magnitude of cortical event related potentials (Ashton *et al.* 1974). Typists are said to work faster with fewer errors, but some tasks requiring fine psychomotor skills may be adversely affected by doses equivalent to one to three cups of coffee or 85–250 mg caffeine (Rall 1980). With increasing doses and in sensitive subjects xanthines cause more pronounced central nervous stimulation with anxiety, restlessness, insomnia, tremor, and hyperaesthesia. Stimulant effects on the heart, decreased peripheral vascular resistance, diuresis, and relaxation of bronchial smooth muscle are among the peripheral actions, especially of theophylline.

Sites and mechanisms of action Sites of action in the brain include the reticular formation, in which increases in neuronal firing rates have been noted after administration of caffeine in rats, and the medullary respiratory centres, in which sensitivity to the stimulant efects of carbon dioxide is enhanced and the respiratory depressant effects of barbiturates and opioids reversed. The xanthines also produce emesis by a central effect. These stimulant effects may result from an increased turnover of monoamines in the brain (Rall 1980). The cellular basis of this action is controversial. It used to be thought that the xanthines inhibit the enzyme nucleotide phosphodiesterase, thus decreasing the breakdown of cyclic AMP and enhancing the central and peripheral actions of this nucleotide. However, although this effect is undoubtedly produced by high concentrations of xanthines, its importance at therapeutic dosage is doubtful and it now seems likely that the clinical effects are mainly mediated by block of receptors for adenosine (Rall 1980; Snyder 1981a,b). Williams (1984) suggests that adenosine, a nucleoside with hypnogenic actions, may be a physiological modulator of central arousal systems. Effects on the translocation of intracellular calcium are also produced but only by high concentrations, above the therapeutic range.

Adverse effects Acute toxic effects include signs of intense central nervous system stimulation with excitement, delirium, sensory disturbances, and focal and general convulsions which may be refractory to anticonvulsant agents. Vomiting is prominent and cardiovascular effects, including cardiac arrhythmias may occur. Such toxicity is rare with caffeine but less so with theophylline. The chronic ingestion of moderate to large amounts of coffee may occasionally give rise to headaches and somatic and psychological reactions similar to anxiety neurosis (Greden 1974). Heavy caffeine consumers (over about 4 g caffeine daily) were found by Gilliland and Andress (1981) to have higher ratings of anxiety and depression, and a poorer academic performance than abstainers, but a causal relationship was not established. Some tolerance occurs and a mild withdrawal syndrome with headache, lethargy, nervousness and lack of concentration has been reported (Rogers *et al.* 1981).

Part II
Reward and punishment

5

Reward and punishment systems

The idea of a goal-directed arousal system in the brain (Chapter 2) implies the existence of some mechanism for selecting appropriate goals, for initiating the behaviours required to achieve them, and for signalling when they have been attained. If a goal proves favourable for survival in the prevailing circumstances, it is advantageous to reinforce behaviour leading to it; if the goal proves to be unfavourable, behaviour leading to it must be suppressed and avoidance action taken in future. Such a signalling system may be provided by certain 'reward' and 'punishment' pathways in the brain discovered by Olds and Milner (1954). These are closely integrated with arousal systems and with learning and memory, and appear to be fundamental for motivation, and for goal-seeking and avoidance behaviour. They are thought to form the basis for instinctive drives such as hunger, thirst, and sex, and are probably the substrate of more complex emotional/cognitive states such as hope and disappointment.

Reward systems

Intracranial self-stimulation

Olds and Milner (1954), and Olds (1956, 1977) reported a series of experiments showing that rats will work to obtain electrical stimulation at specific sites in the brain. Rats which had been stimulated through intracranial electrodes implanted at some locations were observed to return repeatedly to that part of the cage where they had received the stimulation. When allowed to stimulate themselves by pressing a lever, they would sometimes do so at the rate of over 100 times a minute for hours on end. The animals appeared to like the stimulation and it seemed that activity in certain parts of the brain generated a pleasurable or rewarding sensation. Furthermore, motivation for self-stimulation was so strong that the rats would learn to perform various tasks such as traversing complex mazes in order to obtain it. This behaviour was similar to learning for food reward. When food reward and the opportunity for intracranial self-stimulation were both restricted, animals preferred the stimulation, even at the cost of starvation (Routtenberg 1978). Such findings suggested that the effects of intracranial self-stimulation and food reward were similar and that rewarding stimulation sites were located in neural pathways subserving reinforcement of goal-directed behaviour in the natural state (Redgrave and Dean 1981).

The above type of self-stimulation behaviour was elicited most strikingly when the electrodes were implanted in the lateral hypothalamus, an area known to be related to feeding mechanisms. However, self-stimulation appears to be a variable phenomenon and stimulation at other sites may induce different behaviours. At some locations animals may stimulate themselves by pressing a lever but will not learn to traverse a maze to obtain the stimulation. Some areas elicit relatively weak responses, the animals sustaining self-stimulation for only short periods, or preferring food to self-stimulation when sufficiently hungry. With some electrode placements, responses are only obtained if the rats are motivated by sexual arousal rather than by hunger. If multiple sites for stimulation are provided, there is a tendency to alternate the self-stimulation from electrode to electrode and preferred sites may change depending on whether the animals are hungry or thirsty (Olds 1977; Redgrave and Dean 1981; Routtenberg 1978).

Sites which support intracranial self-stimulation have been found in all vertebrate species studied, including man, and patients describe different sensations according to electrode locations (Heath 1964; Levitt and Lonowski 1975; Redgrave and Dean 1981). These results suggest that there may be a complex of rewarding pathways in the brain subserving different types of reinforcement behaviour.

Anatomical sites

Anatomical locations from which various types of self-stimulation behaviour can be obtained have been mapped in many investigations reviewed by Redgrave and Dean (1981) and Routtenberg (1978). Table 5.1 shows many of the large number of sites which have been implicated; Fig. 5.1A shows the diverse locations of some of them.

It is clear that self-stimulation sites are distributed widely in the brain, from the frontal lobes to the medulla, and that they include areas of very different function, from sensory processing (olfactory bulb and nucleus of the tractus solitarius) to motor activity (cerebellum and motor nucleus of the trigeminal nerve). Self-stimulation is also supported from sites in the fibre tracts connecting many of these areas, notably the median forebrain bundle. This runs in the lateral hypothalamus and carries ascending projections from the brainstem nuclei, including the locus coeruleus and raphe nuclei, to the diencephalon and telencephalon, as well as descending projections from the median forebrain. Routtenberg and Santos-Anderson (1977) stress the importance of fibre systems from the frontal lobe. They cite experiments by Rolls and Cooper (1973, 1974) showing that prefrontal cortex neurones in rats are activated during self-stimulation at many sites but not by stimulation in neutral areas, and that local anaesthetization of certain areas of prefrontal

Table 5.1. Some sites which support intracranial self-stimulation in various animal species

Brain area	Sites which support self-stimulation	
Forebrain	frontal cortex olfactory nucleus; nucleus accumbens; septal area; amygdaloid nucleus; hypothalamus	entorhinal cortex caudate nucleus; entopeduncular nucleus; hippocampus; ventral and medial thalamus; median forebrain bundle; dorsal noradrenergic bundle
Midbrain and brainstem	ventral tegmental area; raphe nuclei; superior cerebellar peduncle; mesencephalic nucleus of trigeminal nerve	substantia nigra; nucleus coeruleus; periaqueductal grey matter
Cerebellum	deep cerebellar nuclei	other cerebellar areas
Medulla	motor nucleus of trigeminal nerve; nucleus of tractus solitarius	

cortex decreases the rate of self-stimulation from other sites and raises the electrical threshold required to produce self-stimulation. Routtenberg and Santos-Cooper (1977) suggest that the prefrontal cortex may be vital to the intracranial self-stimulation system and point out that it is the origin of fibre tracts which run through many self-stimulation loci throughout the neuraxis and that these pathways intermingle with the median forebrain bundle at the level of the hypothalamus. At least five well established areas for self-stimulation lie in the path of the frontal cortex descending fibre system (Fig. 5.1A).

Most, if not all, of the sites which support self-stimulation have anatomical connections with limbic structures, where the emotional, autonomic, and motor responses appropriate to reward may be generated. Many of these same pathways are also involved in arousal and in learning and memory systems. The discovery of brain rewarding areas seems to hold the key for understanding the normal processes of motivation, reinforcement, and learning. Nevertheless, Routtenberg and Santos-Anderson (1977) point out that intracranial self-stimulation itself remains an enigma: the anatomical circuitry of no single site has yet been worked out, let alone the integration between sites, and it may be premature to speculate too far on the properties common to all sites (Redgrave and Dean 1981).

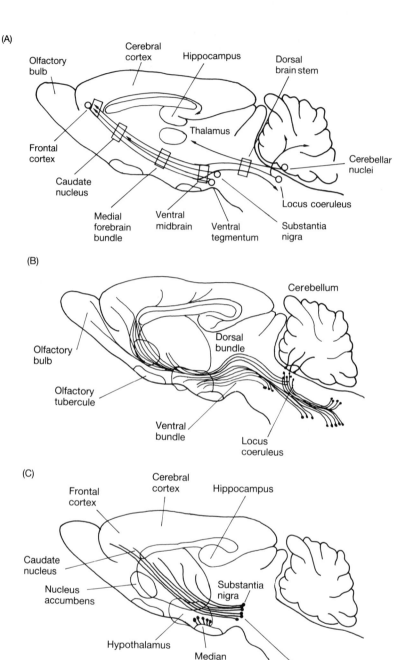

Fig. 5.1. (A) Pathways of reward in the rat brain. Circles: location of cell bodies; rectangles: regions where reliable self-stimulation is obtained. (B) Noradrenergic systems in reward pathways. (C) Dopaminergic systems in reward pathways. (From Routtenberg 1978, by kind permission of W. H. Freeman and Company.)

Neurotransmitters

Noradrenaline

There is strong experimental evidence for the involvement of catecholamines in brain stimulation reward. At first it seemed likely that noradrenaline was the most important of the catecholamine neurotransmitters. Sites which elicit self-stimulation coincide with histological maps of noradrenergic nerve distribution (Stein *et al.* 1977; Stein 1978). In particular, a dorsal noradrenergic pathway originates in the locus coeruleus (A_6 noradrenaline cell group) and innervates the neocortex, cerebellum, hippocampus, and thalamus. A ventral pathway originates from noradrenaline containing cells in the medulla and pons (cell groups A_1, A_2, A_5, A_6 and A_7) and innervates the hypothalamus and ventral parts of the limbic system (Fig. 5.1B). A periventricular pathway originates from various noradrenergic cell bodies and innervates the median regions of the thalamus and hypothalamus. All these pathways, and the locus coeruleus itself, support self-stimulation, although the role of the central pathway has been disputed (Stein *et al.* 1977; Routtenberg 1978). Electrical stimulation of rewarding areas in the median forebrain bundle results in an increased liberation of noradrenaline and its metabolites from the lateral hypothalamus, while stimulation of neutral areas does not (Stein and Wise 1969).

Pharmacological evidence also suggests a role for nordrenaline. Drugs which release catecholamines (amphetamine, nicotine) enhance self-stimulation behaviour and lower the threshold for self-stimulation. Many of these drugs are self-administered by animals and taken compulsively by man (Chapter 6). Drugs which deplete stores, block receptors, or inhibit the synthesis of catecholamines (reserpine, chlorpromazine, alpha-methyl-paratyrosine) supress self-stimulation. Selective block of noradrenaline synthesis by inhibition of dopamine-beta-hydroxylase, abolishes self-stimulation, while local instillation of noradrenaline restores this behaviour (Stein 1978; Stein *et al.* 1977). It also appears that self-stimulation is mediated by alpha- rather than beta-adrenergic receptors since intraventricular injections of the alpha-blocker phentolamine (50 μg) decreases the rate of self-stimulation in rats while injections of the beta-blocker propranolol (50 μg) does not (Stein *et al.* 1977).

Some of the conclusions concerning the role of noradrenaline in self-stimulation have been questioned. For example, Routtenberg (1978) and Routtenberg and Santos-Anderson (1977) showed that complete destruction of the locus coeruleus had little effect on the rate of self-stimulation from an electrode in the dorsal brainstem in rats. At present the status of noradrenaline is uncertain: it seems to play a part in self-stimulation reward but it does not appear to be the only transmitter involved. Furthermore, as discussed in Chapter 3, high levels of noradrenergic activity are aversive and are probably involved in the generation of anxiety. In line with this view is the observation that small doses of central nervous system stimulants, such as amphetamine, are hedonic, but dysphoria and acute psychotic reactions occur with higher doses.

Dopamine

Although there are many self-stimulation sites in the brain which are not near a dopaminergic system (Wise 1980), it seems likely that dopamine is a transmitter in some reward pathways. There are dopaminergic fibres in the median forebrain bundle. These include the nigrostriatal pathway from substantia nigra to caudate nucleus and the mesolimbic pathway from the ventral tegmental area to the nucleus accumbens, olfactory tubercle, septal area, and frontal cortex (Redgrave and Dean 1981; Fig. 5.1C). Neuronal mapping and stimulation studies of ventral tegmental and substantia nigra areas seem to indicate that self-stimulation is uniquely associated with dopamine containing cells (Wise 1980). However, Arbuthnott (1980) points out that some non-dopaminergic cells have a similar distribution and other work suggests that the conduction velocities of axons which support self-stimulation in the median forebrain bundle are too high to be the fine non-myelinated fibres of dopaminergic systems (Redgrave and Dean 1981). Destruction of dopaminergic neurones with 6-hydroxydopamine gives conflicting results: some studies have shown a severe reduction in self-stimulation behaviour after this procedure but others have shown only temporary effects, depending in the sites of stimulation.

Pharmacological evidence supports the involvement of dopamine in reward systems (Wise 1980; Stein 1978; Routtenberg 1978; Redgrave and Dean 1981). Drugs which inhibit dopamine synthesis or block dopamine receptors disrupt intracranial self-stimulation from a number of sites, even at the locus coeruleus, a predominantly noradrenergic structure. When dopamine blockade is limited to one hemisphere, self-stimulation responses are suppressed for that hemisphere but not for the other. Dopamine blockade also raises the electrical threshold for self-stimulation in a dose-dependent manner. Conversely, drugs which release dopamine (amphetamine) or stimulate dopamine receptors (apomorphine) sometimes increase rates of self-stimulation. Furthermore, in rats with indwelling intravenous catheters, apomorphine is avidly self-administered even after catecholamine depletion, and apomorphine self-administration is blocked by the dopamine receptor antagonist pimozide. Wise (1980) concludes that dopamine receptor activation can itself be rewarding.

Royall and Klemm (1981) observed that small intraperitoneal doses of apomorphine and haloperidol (which did not affect general performance) respectively increased or decreased the rewarding effects of saccharine in rats and suggested a dopaminergic role in the perceived hedonic quality of natural reinforcers. At present it is generally accepted that dopamine plays some, probably important, role in brain reward pathways.

Endogenous opioids

Both noradrenaline and dopamine have general effects in heightening arousal and increasing goal-seeking behaviour. However, reward can also be identified with reduction of arousal when the goal is achieved and satisfaction results. Stein (1978) suggests that the latter aspect of reward may be mediated by enkephalin or a related opioid peptide. In line with this suggestion is the observation that pharmacological agents which are apparently rewarding include not only stimulants such as amphetamine and cocaine, which release catecholamines, but also depressants such as morphine and opiate narcotics, which are now generally agreed to act on endogenous opioid receptors (Hughes *et al.* 1975; Chapter 7).

In many brain areas the distribution of cell bodies containing endogenous opioids and of opioid binding sites overlaps very closely with that of catecholamine-containing cell areas, and rewarding sites (including the amygdala, locus coeruleus, pontine central grey, zona compacta of the substantia nigra, bed nucleus of the stria terminalis, and nucleus accumbens) contain beta-endorphin and other polypeptides as well as catecholamines (Elde *et al.* 1976; German and Bowden 1974). Thus, it seems likely that stimulation of the same rewarding areas releases both classes of neurotransmitters or modulators, and that both play an essential part in reward mechanisms. Stein (1978) reports experiments in which rats were found to work for injections of various opiates and opioids, including morphine and enkephalin, directly into the cerebral ventricles. The response was blocked by the specific opioid antagonist naloxone and also by noradrenaline depletion. Cooper (1984) notes that rats will also work to self-inject morphine specifically into the ventral tegmental area, and that this behaviour can be blocked by haloperidol, a dopamine receptor antagonist, or by 6-hydroxydopamine lesions of ascending dopaminergic pathways. Opiate-based reinforcement may therefore operate through catecholaminergic links.

It seems reasonable to conclude that reward processes are regulated by the joint actions of dopamine, noradrenaline, and endogenous opioids, and Stein (1978) suggests that a normal action of endogenous opioids is to bring successful reward-seeking behaviour to a satisfying termination. A particular role for endogenous opioids in mediating social reward has been postulated by Panksepp (1981) and is discussed in Chapter 11.

Integration of transmitter systems

The evidence discussed above suggests that the normal operation of reward systems involves a number of neurotransmitters. Stein (1978), following the analysis of Olds (1975), suggests that rewards act in several ways to influence behaviour: to motivate, to steer, and eventually to terminate the rewarded response. He further suggests that motivation, which mobilizes approach responses in the animal and increases the general readiness to act, is largely mediated by dopaminergic neurones. There is evidence that dopamine is normally involved in food and water rewards in animals and several workers have suggested that it is particularly concerned with motivational and incentive aspects of reward response (Wise 1980; Crow 1972; Herberg *et al.* 1976). Noradrenergic pathways may, at least in part, mediate steering of behaviour (i.e., selecting among a choice of possible behaviours), which depends on reinforcement of certain responses by past memories. Although noradrenaline does not seem to be essential for memory (Chapter 8), it may favour consolidation of experiences which are accompanied by emotional arousal and catecholamine release. Such a learning function would be important in guiding behaviour towards responses that had previously been found to be rewarding and in steering it away from responses remembered to be aversive. Oomura and Auo (1984) reached somewhat similar conclusions from experiments in macaque monkeys in which behaviour related to food reward was correlated with the activity of single cells in the orbitofrontal cortex after the local electrophoretic application of catecholamine agonists and antagonists. It appeared that dopaminergic pathways were involved in the motor processes of obtaining the reward while noradrenergic pathways were activated in anticipation (memory) of reward. Finally, attained rewards terminate reward-seeking behaviour by gratification and this function may be subserved in part by an opioid peptide, such as enkephalin. A hypothetical synthesis of the function of the three neurotransmitters/modulators that, from intracranial self-stimulation experiments, appear to be involved in reward systems is shown in Table 5.2. It appears that electrical stimulation falsely activates the systems in place of natural rewards.

In the present state of knowledge, it is difficult to explain exactly how the results with intracranial stimulation fit into this scheme, or indeed to relate the results of pharmacological manipulation in general with those of intracranial self-stimulation. For example, why should drugs, which are apparently themselves rewarding and which increase noradrenergic, dopaminergic, or enkephalinergic activity in the brain, increase intracranial self-stimulation behaviour? It might be expected that such drugs, by biochemically stimulating reward systems, would decrease the need or desire for additional electrical stimulation. Yet the drugs appear to make electrical stimulation even more rewarding: they increase the rate of self-stimulation and lower the electrical threshold required to induce the behaviour (Chapter 6). Both drug and intracranial self-stimulation experiments suggest that the behaviours hypothetically mediated by dopaminergic and adrenergic systems (pursuit behaviour and selected responses leading to gratification) are themselves rewarding. Possibly expectation of reward generates pleasurable emotions discussed

Table 5.2. Different roles of reward

Role	Behavioural effect	Putative neurotransmitter
Incentive (motivation, drive)	Initiate and facilitate pursuit behaviour	dopamine
Reinforcement (learning)	Guide response selection via knowledge of response consequences	noradrenaline
Gratification (drive-reduction)	Bring behavioural episode to satisfying termination	enkephalin

From Stein 1978 (by kind permission of Raven Press, New York.)

below. In addition, activity in reward systems is influenced by that in reciprocally connected punishment systems.

Punishment systems

Anatomical pathways

Activity at certain sites in the brain appears to generate sensations that are strongly aversive; animals will work as avidly to avoid stimulation at these sites as they will to obtain stimulation at rewarding points (Olds and Olds 1963; Delgado *et al.* 1954). A major anatomical pathway subserving aversive effects appears to be the periventricular system, a group of fibres running between the midbrain and thalamus with extensions into the hypothalamus, basal ganglia, limbic system, and cerebral cortex (Stein 1968; Fig. 5.2A). The median forebrain bundle and periventricular system probably interact, since they distribute fibres to various common sites along their paths (Levitt and Lonowski 1975; Criswell and Levitt 1975). A further pathway subserving aversion may originate in the dorsal raphe nuclei and distribute to periventricular regions of the brain, but some fibres run in the median forebrain bundle and terminate in various parts of the limbic system (Stein and Wise 1974; Fig. 5.2B). Destruction of either of these pathways results in a generalized defect in passive avoidance so that an animal will no longer suppress behaviour that precipitates an aversive stimulus such as an electric shock to the feet.

It has been suggested that these pathways act as a 'punishment' system favouring avoidance behaviour and also selecting the appropriate reward behaviour that will terminate a particular aversive state, for example, feeding in hunger, drinking in thirst, etc. (Stein 1971, 1982). The interaction between reward and punishment systems allows for many dimensions of reward and

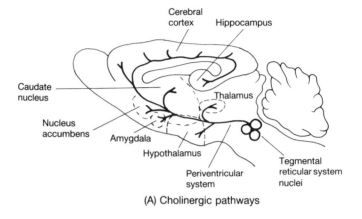

(A) Cholinergic pathways

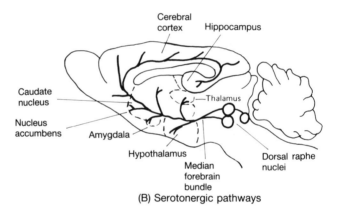

(B) Serotonergic pathways

Fig. 5.2. Punishment pathways in the rat brain. (A) Cholinergic pathways. (B) Serotonergic pathways

punishment. Activity in reward systems not only engenders active reward, but also inhibits activity in punishment systems. Conversely, activity in punishment pathways is positively aversive and also inhibits activity in reward pathways. Presumably, there can be innumerable degrees of partial inhibition or excitation in the different pathways, resulting in finely graded shades of reward/punishment activity. The arrangement appears to be similar to that described for the reciprocally connected arousal and sleep mechanisms in the brain (Chapter 2) which include active waking and sleeping mechanisms, and passive de-waking and de-sleeping mechanisms. Reward and punishment systems are also closely integrated with learning and memory systems (Chapter 8). Thus, lack of expected reward, as well as active punishment, is unpleasant; similarly, lack of expected punishment, as well as active pleasure, is rewarding. The hippocampal comparator system described in relation to anxiety neurosis (Chapter 3) is thought to be involved in forming the expectation of reward or punishment as a result of learning.

Neurotransmitters

Acetylcholine

The periventricular system appears to be at least partly cholinergic (Stein 1968; Fig. 5.2A). The deficit of passive avoidance resulting from destruction of this system can be reversed by local instillation of cholinergic drugs such as carbachol or acetylcholine, while the local application of anticholinergic drugs such as atropine produces similar effects to surgical destruction.

Cholinergic systems are also closely involved in learning and memory (Chapter 8), and it is likely that certain aspects of these functions which require suppression of behaviour (such as suppression of incorrect response during learning, extinction of learned responses when they become inappropriate, and habituation to environments which have become familiar) are mediated through the periventricular system (Criswell and Levitt 1975). As already mentioned, the periventricular system communicates with the limbic circuit, and many limbic structures receive innervation from both the periventricular system and the median forebrain bundle. Thus together the two systems can be envisaged to promote the seeking of reward and the suppression of punished behaviour.

Other neurotransmitters may also mediate aversive effects in periventricular structures. From experiments involving the local injection of various agonists and antagonists into the central grey and medial hypothalamus, Schmitt *et al.* (1984) conclude that GABA, excitatory amino acids, and opioids may all interact to modulate aversive reactions (flight behaviour) in the rat.

Serotonin

The fibres from the raphe nuclei which run in the median forebrain bundle are serotonergic (Fig. 5.2B). Stein and Wise (1974) suggest that this system acts antagonistically to the median forebrain bundle reward system and that goal-directed behaviour is reciprocally regulated through noradrenergic and serotonergic pathways here. Thus, rewarding intracranial self-stimulation in the lateral hypothalamus is facilitated by the intraventricular injection of noradrenaline, but suppressed by serotonin. Self-stimulation is also facilitated by inhibition of serotonin synthesis (by *para*-chloro-phenylalanine) and suppressed when brain concentrations of serotonin are increased (by treatment with 5-hydroxytryptophan and a monoamine oxidase inhibitor). Likewise, passive avoidance behaviour is antagonized by noradrenaline, by blockade of serotonin synthesis, and by the serotonin-receptor blocker methysergide, and facilitated by alpha-adrenergic blockade, by serotonin agonists (such as alpha-methyltryptamine), and by some doses of serotonin. Ogren (1981) describes further evidence that serotonin is involved in avoidance learning. These results were obtained in various animal species including rats and pigeons, but Stein (1971) cites some evidence that similar systems may operate in man.

The effects of drugs which alter brain concentrations of noradrenaline and serotonin on the performance of animals in the Geller–Seifter test, a conflict test which involves both punishment and reward, have been discussed in Chapters 3 and 4. It is thought that the anxiolytic effects of benzodiazepines and other anxiolytic drugs are exerted at least partly by decreasing activity in serotonergic punishment pathways, and that activity in these pathways is increased in anxiety.

Emotional components of reward and punishment

Reward and punishment systems are thought to be involved not only with certain types of behaviour, but also with their subjective accompaniments or mood. Thus, rewarding events may presumably elicit a range of pleasurable feelings (joy, contentment, hope, repletion), and aversive events a range of unpleasant feelings (pain, fear, disgust, guilt, depression). Omission of expected rewards or punishments may result in other emotions (disappointment, relief). Some emotions that may be elicited by the presentation or omission of a reward or punishment following an operant behaviour such as pressing a lever have been suggested by Stein *et al.* (1977) and a modification of these ideas is shown in Table 5.3. This table is not intended to be comprehensive. The various neurotransmitters presumably interact in complex ways and through different pathways to involve particular emotions after naturally occurring rewarding or punishing events, such as food or pain. The limbic pathways involved have not yet been fully worked out, but it is noteworthy that a similar array of neurotransmitters (catecholamines, serotonin, GABA, and opioid polypeptides) are involved in the nervous central of appetite (Morley and Levine 1983) and of pain (Terenius 1981).

Personality and reward/punishment and arousal systems

Innate, genetically determined, individual structural and functional characteristics of arousal and of reward and punishment systems probably account to a large extent for the major dimensions of personality: extraversion/ introversion, neuroticism/stability, and psychoticism (Eysenck and Eysenck 1963, 1975). Present understanding of this question is considered by Eysenck (1981). A considerable body of physiological, behavioural, pathological, and pharmacological evidence supports Eysenck's (1957, 1967) hypothesis that introverts are characterized by a greater intrinsic activity in arousal systems

Table 5.3. Effects of presenting or withholding a rewarding or punishing event as a consequence of an operant behaviour

	Reward	Lack of reward
Transmitters	catecholamines, opioids	serotonin, acetylcholine
Emotion		
anticipation of event	'hope'	'hope'
occurrence of event	'joy', 'contentment'	'disappointment'
Operant behaviour	facilitated	suppressed
	Punishment	Lack of punishment
Transmitters	serotonin, acetylcholine	catecholamines, ?opioids
Emotion		
anticipation of event	'fear', 'anxiety',	'fear', 'anxiety',
occurrence of event	'pain', discomfort', 'panic'	'relief'
Operant behaviour	suppressed	facilitated

Reference: Stein *et al.* (1977).

than extraverts. Gray (1981b), in a critique of Eysenck's hypothesis, marshals equally strong evidence for a biological explanation of several dimensions of personality in terms of individual differences in susceptibility to reward and punishment (Fig. 5.3).

These theories of individual personality differences have major implications for variations in response to psychotropic drugs and for vulnerability to dysfunction of arousal and reward/punishment systems, such as occur in anxiety syndromes, depressive states, schizophrenia, chronic pain syndromes, drug dependence and other types of compulsive behavior. Anxiety syndromes and anxiolytic/sedative drugs have been described in Chapters 3 and 4; disorders of reward and punishment systems and psychotropic drugs with major actions on these systems are discussed in Chapters 6 and 7.

Pain systems

A large component of the punishment mechanisms must be provided by the systems responsible for signalling pain and nociception. These are reviewed by Bowsher (1978a), Zimmerman (1981), Yaksh and Hammond (1982), Jessell (1982), and outlined by Shaw *et al.* (1982) and Stein (1982).

Pain sensation

Pain is a complex experience resulting from variable interactions between physical, emotional, and rational components (Melzack 1973). The physical

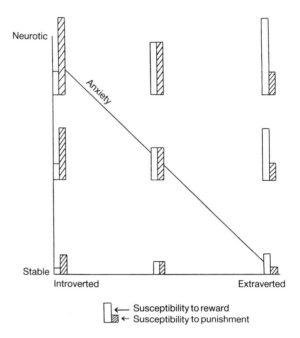

Fig. 5.3. Hypothetical relationships between personality dimensions and susceptibility to reward and punishment. On this model, extraverts are more susceptible to reward than to punishment, while the converse holds for introverts. Anxiety is characterized by increasing degrees of susceptibility to punishment (see also Chapter 3). (From Gray 1970.)

component (sensory-discriminative) is supplied by the nociceptive system described below; the emotional component (motivational-affective) involves the limbic system, including the punishment pathways; the rational component (cognitive-evaluative) is derived from the cerebral cortex. Excitatory and inhibitory feedback systems link all components.

Two types of physical pain sensation are recognized: (a) *first pain* is sharp or pricking, rapid in onset and brief in duration, well localized, and can only be elicited from the skin, and (b) *second pain* is burning in character, delayed in onset (up to 1 s after the stimulus) but prolonged, poorly localized, and may be elicited from both skin and deep structures. The reflex response to first pain is a phasic withdrawal reaction, whilst that to second pain is a slowly developing tonic muscular contraction (guarding or rigidity). First pain is responsible for withdrawal reflexes and protects the body from injury; second pain probably only occurs in the presence of tissue damage and may serve to splint or rest the affected part. It is interesting that potent analgesic drugs such as morphine have little effect on first pain in subanaesthetic doses.

In clinical and experimental settings, it is important to distinguish between *pain threshold* and *pain tolerance* . The intensity of a stimulus required to be perceived as painful (threshold) is variable, but the intensity of a painful stimulus that a subject will tolerate is even more variable and depends on personality and on social, educational, cultural, and environmental factors. Analgesic drugs and procedures have differing effects on pain tolerance and pain threshold. A further important clinical distinction is that between *acute pain* and *chronic pain* (Chapter 6).

Neuroanatomy of nociceptive pathways

The basic anatomical organization of pain pathways is shown dia-grammatically in Fig. 5.4.

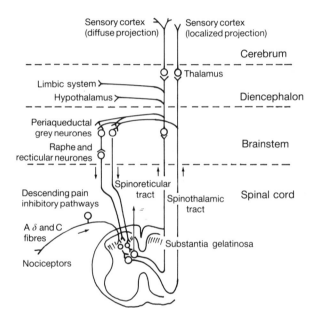

Fig. 5.4. Diagram of the organisation of pain pathways. For explanation see text. (References: Thompson 1984a,b; Zimmerman 1981.)

Nociceptors

Peripheral nociceptors are situated at the terminals of afferent neurones whose cell bodies lie in the dorsal root ganglia. These nociceptors are of two types: (a) high threshold mechanoreceptors connected to myelinated A delta axons which are relatively large diameter (1–5 μm) and fast-conducting (5–10 m/s), and (b) polymodal nociceptors, consisting of the bare terminals of C fibres which are unmyelinated, small diameter (0.5–2 μm) and slow conducting

(0.5–2m/s; Swett and Bourassa, 1981). These different nociceptors largely underlie the two types of cutaneous pain (first and second pain), but the central connections are also important in determining the responses to stimulation (Bowsher 1978a).

Substantia gelatinosa

The central axons of these sensory neurones enter the dorsal horns of the spinal cord where they give off branches which run up and down the cord for one or two segments. Many collaterals penetrate the substantia gelatinosa and terminate there on Golgi Type II cells. These cells also receive connections from adjacent spinal regions and from descending pathways from the brain. The interneurones of the substantia gelatinosa are probably important sites for the gating mechanism of pain described below.

Spinothalamic tract

The axons of the substantia gelatinosa interneurones terminate in the chief nucleus of the dorsal horn and synapse with the second order afferent neurones. These cross to the opposite side of the spinal cord and ascend in the lateral spinothalamic tract. In the brainstem, the spinothalamic tracts from each side merge and pass through the brainstem as the spinal lemniscus before terminating in the ventral posterior nucleus of the thalamus. From here, third order sensory axons pass to discrete localized projections on the sensory cerebral cortex. This system apears to be primarily responsible for well localized, sharp first pain.

Spinoreticular pathways

In addition to the specific sensory pathways of the spinothalamic tract, impulses in nociceptive fibres are projected centrally through diffuse connections. Small spinal nerve root fibres connect, partly directly and partly through interneurones in the substantia gelatinosa, with cells in the dorsal horn of the spinal cord. These give rise to spinoreticular axons which ascend in crossed and uncrossed multisynaptic pathways, making numerous connections with the medullary reticular formation, to the intralaminar thalamic nuclei, the hypothalamus, and limbic areas. From the thalamus, diffuse, non-specific projections pass to widespread areas of the cortex of both hemispheres, probably mediating the poorly localized second pain. The intralaminar thalamic nuclei also give off more localized projections to the corpus striatum, which may be concerned with the reflex motor responses to painful stimuli. The hypothalamic projections connect with autonomic centres which supply the autonomic concomitants of pain, while the limbic connections are probably responsible for the emotional components. These spinoreticular pathways, with connections to reticular formation, limbic system and cortex, are also closely concerned in the arousal systems of the body (Chapter 2).

Descending inhibitory pathways

Inhibitory pathways descend from the periventricular and periaqueductal grey matter, and from the nucleus raphe magnus, the giant cell nucleus and other structures in the reticular formation, to the spinal cord. In the dorsal horn, these axons terminate on the endings of the first sensory neurones or on the connected interneurones in the substantia gelatinosa. These descending inhibitory pathways contribute to the spinal pain gate mechanisms.

Spinal gate-control mechanisms in pain regulation

The original gate-control theory of Melzack and Wall (1965) has been modified in the light of later experimental findings (Wall 1978). However, the basic concept that, due to local inhibitory control mechanisms, not all nociceptive impulses which reach the spinal cord are transmitted to the brain, remains unchallenged. It appears that the propagation of nociceptive impulses can be inhibited at spinal cord level by at least three systems, all of which probably interact with short interneurones in the substantia gelatinosa (Fig. 5.5)

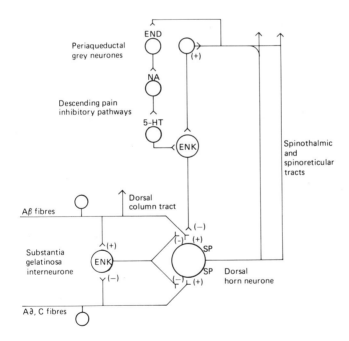

Fig. 5.5. Gate-control mechanisms in pain regulation. SP, substance P; ENK, enke-phalin; END, endorphin; NA, noradrenaline; 5-HT, serotonin. For explanation see text. (Reference: Thompson 1984a.)

Inhibition by afferent stimulation The responses of dorsal horn neurones to peripheral nociceptive stimuli can be inhibited by simultaneous stimulation of large A fibre afferents (for example, A beta-fibres from low threshold mechanoreceptors). One mechanism for this inhibition is activation by the large A fibres of short substantia gelatinosa interneurones, which then presynaptically inhibit the dorsal horn spinothalamic cells. Such inhibition can be obtained not only from A beta-fibres but also from A delta-fibres which contain nociceptor afferents. The effect of the presynaptic inhibition is to block the onward transmission of spinothalamic impulses resulting from nociceptor stimulation of dorsal horn cells, particularly those from small C fibre primary afferents. The degree to which potentially painful stimuli are propagated to higher centres thus depends on the relative proportions of small and large fibre activity. Stimulation of A fibres is thought to be an important mechanism of the analgesic action of transcutaneous electrical nerve stimulation, acupuncture, massage, and other counter-irritation procedures. As discussed below, substance P may be the excitatory transmitter from C fibre afferents to dorsal horn cells, and enkephalin may be the inhibitory transmitter liberated by the short interneurones in this system. There are in addition other mechanisms, including post-synaptic inhibition, for gating of pain by afferent stimuli, and for the excitatory and inhibitory effects of different spinal cord neurones (Stein 1982; Wall 1978).

Inhibition from periaqueductal grey and medullary raphe nuclei Firing of dorsal horn cells in response to noxious stimuli can also be inhibited, and profound analgesia produced, by electrical stimulation of the periaqueductal grey matter in the brainstem or of the raphe nuclei in the medulla, to which it projects. Such stimulation decreases the slope of the curve relating stimulus intensity to response rate of the neurone and can be regarded as a gain control of the spinal system for the transmission of pain information (Zimmerman 1981) (Fig. 5.6). It is achieved by descending impulses from the medullary region impinging on dorsal horn cells or interneurones through pathways which are probably serotonergic but may involve an enkephalinergic link (Bowsher 1978a).

Inhibition from lateral reticular formation A further descending inhibitory system appears to originate from structures in the lateral reticular formation. Electrical stimulation of this area also produces deep analgesia and decreases the firing rate of dorsal horn cells in response to noxious stimuli. The characteristic effect on the relation between stimulus intensity and neuronal response rate is to raise the threshold of response and to produce a parallel displacement of the curve to the right (Zimmerman 1981) (Fig. 5.6). This system is believed to be separate from the periaqueductal grey system and to

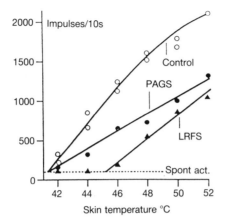

Fig. 5.6. Effects of descending pain inhibitory pathways on response of dorsal horn cells. PAGS, periaqueductal grey stimulation; LRFS, lateral reticular formation stimulation; number of action potentials elicited by heat stimulation (ordinate) plotted against temperature of heat stimulus (abcissa) in an anaesthetized cat. PAGS decreases the slope of the curve while LRFS raises the threshold of response and produces a parallel displacement of the curve to the right. For fuller explanation see text. (From Zimmerman 1981, by kind permission of Sandoz Ltd., Basle.)

involve a catecholamine neurotransmitter, probably noradrenaline (Wilson and Yaksh 1980).

These pain gate control systems in the spinal cord provide another example of the way in which the nervous system controls its own sensory input, as discussed in relation to arousal (Chapter 2). In fact, the system is undoubtedly closely related to arousal systems, and pain sensation and responses are largely modulated by the degree and type of activity in arousal systems. For example, potentially painful stimuli may pass unnoticed during the excitement of sporting activities or may be greatly aggravated by fear of its consequences or by depression. Numerous other examples are given by Melzack (1973) and by Beecher (1959). Learning and memory are equally closely involved in pain, and fear of a previously experienced pain can generate similar responses to those evoked by the pain itself. Thus, limbic and cortical gate control mechanisms can add to those operating at spinal cord level.

Pain neurotransmitters and neuromodulators

Chemical mediators at sensory nerve endings

Nociceptors are stimulated by strong mechanical and thermal stimuli and are also sensitive to a number of chemical agents. Certain types of clinical pain, notably that of inflammation, probably derive from chemical activation of nociceptors. Endogenous algesic agents include serotonin, histamine, kallikrein, bradykinin, adenophosphates, pepsin, trypsin, potassium, and hydrochloric acid. Some of these are released after tissue injury. In addition, prostaglandins potentiate the effects of the other algesic agents. These substances are also present in the central nervous system where they may act as transmitters or modulators, but their central functions are not understood. Chemical mediators of pain at sensory nerve endings are reviewed by Bond (1979), Zimmermann (1981), and Terenius (1981).

Substance P

Substance P is a undecapeptide which acts both as a neurotransmitter and a neuromodulator in various body systems (Henry 1980; Otsuka and Konishi 1983; Oehme and Krivoy 1983). Its major role in pain appears to be as an excitatory neurotransmitter at primary nociceptive nerve endings in the dorsal horn of the spinal cord. Substance P is present in small peripheral nerve fibres, their dorsal root ganglion cells, and in synaptic vesicles at their terminals in the substantia gelatinosa. It is released in a calcium-dependent manner in response to stimulation of nociceptive neurones but not after stimulation of large diameter afferents alone. When iontophoretically applied to the spinal cord or trigeminal nucleus caudalis, it excites only those neurones which respond to noxious stimuli. Intrathecal injection of substance P produces hyperalgesia, while depletion of spinal cord substance P (with capsaicin) or the application of substance P antagonists produces analgesia. Substance P may produce slow excitatory postsynaptic potentials in dorsal horn neurones (Otsuka and Konishi 1983) lasting over 30 s, much longer than the transitory action potentials produced by excitatory neurotransmitters such as glutamate. Although substance P is 200 times more potent than glutamate as a stimulant at some synapses, it is possible that it acts as a modulator of neuronal excitability rather than as a neurotransmitter. It may be co-released from primary afferent nerve terminals with some other, as yet unidentified, fast-acting transmitter. At present glutamate and ATP appear to be possible candidates for this role.

In certain circumstances, substance P can produce analgesia; Oehme and Krivoy (1983) reported that low doses inhibit and high doses facilitate synaptic transmission. Analgesia may be due to an induced release of opioid peptides while hyperalgesia is likely to be due to direct stimulant effects on nociceptive pathways.

Under physiological conditions, the release of substance P may be controlled, at least partly, by the presynaptic actions of short interneurones containing the endogenous opioid pentapeptide enkephalin (Fig. 5.7). The distribution of enkephalin in the spinal cord and brain is similar to that of substance P, and enkephalinergic interneurones project presynaptically onto the terminals of substance P-containing primary afferent fibres. Release of

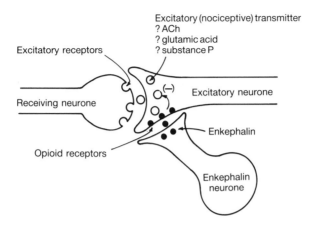

Fig. 5.7. Presynaptic inhibition by short enkephalinergic neurones. Stimulation of opioid receptors by enkephalin inhibits release of excitatory transmitters such as substance P. Opioid receptors may also be stimulated by narcotic analgesics such as morphine (Chapter 7).

enkephalin from the interneurones is believed to reduce the release of substance P, possibly by hyperpolarizing the presynaptic terminals and reducing the calcium flux across the synaptic membrane (North and Williams 1983). However, Duggan (1983) suggests that the inhibitory effects of enkephalin on dorsal horn neurones may be exerted through a post-synaptic action. Whether pre- or post-synaptic, the interaction between substant P-containing and enkephalinergic neurones is probably one of the mechanisms for the gate control of pain in the spinal cord.

However, both peptides also act at other sites and are present in various locations in the brain, and their actions are not confined to nociceptive systems. One other action of substance P which may have a general connection with its nociceptive role is that it appears to play a part in the general adaptation to prolonged stress. The administration of substance P to rats can normalize the disturbances in sleep, learning, blood pressure, and heart rate that result from the stress of immobilization, noise, or electric footshocks applied for 3–5 weeks (Oehme and Krivoy 1983).

The release of substance P is also antagonized by morphine in a concentration-dependent, stereospecific, naloxone-reversible manner. This antagonism occurs only at the sites of termination of nociceptive primary afferent fibres and not at other sites rich in substance P (such as the substantia nigra). Part of the analgesic effect of morphine and other opioid agents is thought to result from this action, in which the drugs combine with pre-synaptic enkephalin receptors and mimic the actions of the enkephalinergic interneurones. Actions on opioid receptors in the limbic system at the same time modulate the emotional responses to pain. The actions of the these drugs are described in Chapter 7 and endogenous opioid systems are discussed further below.

In addition to substance P, other non-opioid polypeptides, including somatostatin, neurotensin, angiotensin II, and cholecystokinin, may be involved in pain modulation in the spinal cord and brain (Sweet 1980; Luttinger *et al.* 1983).

Monoamines

The supraspinal descending inhibitory systems which modulate nociceptive transmission in the spinal cord appear to be mediated by monoamine neurotransmitters. The analgesia produced by electrical stimulation of the periaqueductal grey and the medullary raphe nuclei is accompanied by release of serotonin in the spinal cord (Wilson and Yaksh 1980). This analgesia is blocked by decreasing serotonin synthesis with *para*-chloro-phenylalanine (Zimmerman 1981). Application of serotonin to the spinal cord in rats produces an analgesia which is blocked by serotonin antagonists (methysergide, cyproheptadine) and enhanced by agents which increase synaptic concentrations of serotonin (monoamine oxidase inhibitors and serotonin reuptake blockers, such as clomipramine).

A serotonergic link in the analgesia produced by opiates is suggested by the observation that the intrathecal administration of methysergide blocks the analgesic effect of morphine injected into the periaqueductal grey. Bowsher (1978a) suggests that enkephalinergic neurones in the periaqueductal grey excite cells in the nearby dorsal raphe nucleus whose serotonergic axons stimulate further serotonin-containing neurones in the nucleus raphe magnus in the lower brainstem. The axons of these cells descend to the substantia gelatinosa in the spinal cord where they may activate inhibitory enkephalinergic interneurones (Fig. 5.5). The analgesia produced by periaqueductal stimulation is naloxone-reversible; tolerance and cross-tolerance to morphine develop after repeated stimulation (Lewis and Liebeskind 1983). Beta-endorphin may also contribute to this pain suppression system (Bolles and Fanselow 1982). Similar opioid and serotonergic pathways have been implicated in the anaesthesia produced by acupuncture (Han and Terenius 1982). It is possible that dopamine is also involved, since the analgesia produced by stimulation of the periaqueductal grey is potentiated by agents which increase concentrations of dopamine (Sweet 1980) and blocked by dopamine antagonists (Lewis and Liebeskind 1983).

Electrical stimulation of the lateral reticular formation, on the other hand, produces an analgesic effect which appears to be mediated by noradrenaline. This analgesia is accompanied by release of noradrenaline in the spinal cord and is not affected by manipulation of serotonin concentrations (Zimmerman 1981). Direct application of noradrenaline and alpha-adrenergic stimulants to the spinal cord produces analgesia which is not affected by opioid or serotonin antagonists. Noradrenaline also appears to be involved in the analgesia produced by opiates (Yaksh 1982) and acupuncture (Han and Terenius 1982). Histamine and acetylcholine may also mediate some pain suppression pathways (Lewis and Liebeskind 1983; MacLennnan *et al.* 1983).

The involvement of noradrenaline and serotonin as neurotransmitters in pain-suppressive systems, and at the same time in systems which promote anxiety (Chapter 3) seems at first sight paradoxical. However, it should be noted that the anatomical pathways diverge and also that the level of monoaminergic activity may be critical. At high levels of stimulation, as in threatening conditions, pain suppression along with anxiety, leading to escape behaviour, may be adaptive (see Chapter 6). Pain suppression is only one of a number of general bodily responses to stress. For example, activity in noradrenergic pain-suppressive pathways in linked with cardiovascular responses (Duggan 1982). The noradrenergic system appears to be tonically active while the serotonergic and opioid-mediated pain-suppressive systems may be mobilized only at certain levels of activity.

Amino acid neurotransmitters

Several amino acid transmitters have putative roles in nociception. The possibility that glutamate may be an excitatory transmitter for primary nociceptive afferents has already been mentioned. GABA may have both peripheral and central effects in pain transmission. Desarmenien *et al.* (1984) demonstrated the existence of two types of GABA receptor (GABA A and GABA B) on the membranes of A delta and C dorsal root ganglion neurones, respectively. Activation of GABA A receptors depolarized the nociceptive neurones, while activation of GABA B receptors shortened the calcium component of action potentials. GABA-containing neurones are also widely distributed in the brain, and evidence that it may be involved in central antinociceptive systems is reviewed by de Feudis (1982). Increases in cerebral GABA concentrations in animals enhance the analgesic actions of opiates, and GABA-agonists, GABA-transaminase inhibitors and GABA-uptake inhibitors produce analgesia. This analgesia is not reversed by naloxone and must therefore be induced by a different mechanism from that produced by opiates. GABA applied to the nucleus raphe magnus also produces analgesia which is not reversed by naloxone, and Lovick and Wolstencroft (1983) suggest that it is involved in stimulation-produced analgesia. Glycine, which, like GABA, inhibits the firing of dorsal horn cells (Wilson and Yaksh 1980), beta-alanine, and taurine (de Feudis 1982) may also play a role in analgesia.

Endogenous opioid polypeptide systems

Until recently, understanding of the physiological role of endogenous opioid peptides has been confused by the discovery of multiple opioids and opioid receptors in the body. The picture is now becoming clearer and a brief outline is given here of the present state of knowledge of these peptides in relation to pain.

Endogenous opioids are reviewed in the *British Medical Bulletin* (1983), and much of the information is encapsulated briefly by Thompson (1984). The term opioid refers to directly acting compounds whose actions are specifically antagonized by naloxone; effects that are not antagonised by naloxone are by definition not mediated by opioid receptors. *Opiates* are products derived from opium and the the term is generally applied to morphine derivatives. *Narcotic analgesics* (Chapter 7) are agents which act on opioid receptors to produce naloxone-reversible analgesia (Hughes and Kosterlitz 1983).

Endogenous opioids Of the endogenous opioid polypeptides, three classes appear to be of major physiological importance: *enkephalins* derived from the precursor pro-enkephalin A; *dynorphins* derived from pro-enkephalin B; and *endorphins*, derived from pro-opiomelanocortin (Hughes 1983; Table 5.4). These opioids are closely related structurally but differ in the length of their peptide chains. They function as short-acting neurotransmitters (shorter-length peptides) or long-acting neuronal or hormonal modulators (longer-length peptides) at their respective opioid receptors. Many of them interact with more than one receptor, probably because of their structural flexibility which allows them to take up different conformations (Terenius 1980). There are several other endogenous opioids, including peptide E, alpha- and beta-neoendorphins, and others, whose function is less clearly understood.

Opioid receptors There appear to be at least three distinct opioid receptor subtypes, although these may be interconvertible. Like alpha- and beta-adrenoreceptors, these have different pharmacological profiles, different tissue distributions, different binding properties, and probably mediate different though overlapping actions (Table 5.4). *Mu-receptors* are the main sites of action of the narcotic analgesics. The enkephalins and beta-endorphin also act as agonists, but are not specific for mu-receptors. Naloxone and nalorphine are antagonists. Mu-receptors are almost certainly involved in analgesia but their role in other peptidergic functions is not clear. *Delta-receptors* are activated by enkephalins, which have a greater affinity for them than for mu-receptors, and by beta-endorphin which has equal agonist activity at mu- and delta-receptors. Naloxone has less antagonist activity at delta than at mu-receptors. These receptors are also involved in antinociception and probably in limbic functions. It is possible that mu- and delta-receptors represent high and low affinity states of a unitary receptor (Atweh and Kuhar 1983). *Kappa-receptors* respond to dynorphin and also to the synthetic analgesics ketazocine, pentazocine and buprenophine. Naloxone has some antagonist

Table 5.4. Endogenous opioids and receptors

(a) Endogenous opioids

	Enkephalins	Dynorphins	Endorphins
Precursor Peptides	pro-enkephalin A (met) enkephalin (5) (leu) enkephalin (5) peptide E (25)	pro-enkephalin B dynorphin (17) beta-neoendorphin (9) dynorphin (1–8) dynorphin (1–9)	pro-opiomelanocortin beta-endorphin (31)
Function at receptors			
long-acting at mu	?peptide E	?dynorphin	beta-endorphin
long-acting at delta	?	?beta-neoendorphin	beta-endorphin
long-acting at kappa	?	dynorphin beta-neoendorphin	—
short-acting at mu	(met) enkephalin	—	—
short-acting at delta	(leu) enkephalin	—	—
short-acting at kappa	—	dynorphin 1–8 or 1–9	—

(b) Opioid receptors

	mu	delta	kappa	?sigma
Agonists	narcotic analgesics	enkephalin	nalorphine	N-alkylnormetazocine (SKF 10047)
	enkephalins beta-endorphin	beta-endorphin	dynorphin ketazocine pentazocine buprenorphine	cyclazocine phencyclidine
Antagonist	naloxone nalorphine	naloxone (less than at mu receptors)	naloxone (less than at mu receptors)	naloxone (less than at mu receptors)
Some biological responses (?)	analgesia euphoria respiratory depression cough supression endocrine effects	analgesia motor functions euphoria endocrine effects	analgesia sedation miosis	dysphoria- hallucinations respiratory and motor stimulation

References: Hughes and Kosterlitz (1983); Morley (1983); Atweh and Kuhar (1983); Jaffe and Martin (1980).

activity. These receptors appear to be involved in certain types of pain in animals. It has been suggested that mu-, delta- and kappa-receptors are interchangeable forms of a single opioid receptor complex (Barnard and Demoliou-Mason 1983). *Sigma-receptors* were originally categorized by *in vivo* pharmacological studies, but they have not been demonstrated by binding studies. Agonists for these receptors include N-alkylnormetazocine (SKF 10047), cyclazocine and possibly phencyclidine (Simon 1981; see Chapter 7).

It has been suggested that activation of these receptors accounts for the hallucinogenic properties of these drugs. However, sigma receptors may not be true opioid recptors (Paterson *et al.* 1983). *Eta-receptors* have also been described, but their significance is not known.

Like other receptors, the opioid receptors consist of a recognition site, to which drugs bind, and a translating mechanism which ultimately produces the biological response. The response is generally one of cellular inhibition which is achieved by membrane hyperpolarization due to opening of potassium channels, and by depression of transmitter release (Wouters and Van den Bercken 1980; Henderson 1983; North and Williams 1983). The endogenous opioid system as a whole appears to operate in the body as a widespread and complex inhibitory signalling mechanism in which selectivity is achieved by particular combinations of opioid peptides and receptors (Thompson 1984a,b).

Distribution and function The distribution of opioid peptides and receptors in the nervous system is described by Cuella (1983), Atweh and Kuhar (1983), and Khachaturian *et al.* (1985) and summarized in Table 5.5. The distribution of the peptides differs somewhat from that of the receptors, and the distribution of each different opioid peptide is distinct. Within the central nervous system, opioid peptides and their associated receptors are found most often in association with sensory, limbic and neuroendocrine systems. Enkephalinergic systems consist mainly of short neurones diffusely distributed; dynorphin systems have longer neurones, also widespread; endorphins are largely found in endocrine cells, but some neurones project as far down as the spinal cord. Enkephalins are co-stored with catecholamines in chromaffin tissue, while dynorphins are co-stored with vasopressin and endorphins are co-synthesized with corticotrophin in the hypothalamus and pituitary.

(i) Nociceptive systems. Opioid receptors and peptides are closely associated with systems subserving pain sensation at several levels and are probably of physiological importance in pain modulation. Their interaction with substance P and with monoaminergic antinociceptive systems has already been mentioned, and is further reviewed by Gebhart (1982). Enkephalins appear to control the responses of dorsal horn neurones; they may also modulate pain at higher sites in the central nervous system, but they are rapidly destroyed *in vivo* by enkephalinases and their physiological analgesic effects are short-lived. Beta-endorphin is less rapidly degraded in the body and has more enduring analgesic effects. Injection of beta-endorphin into the cerebrospinal fluid produces a long-lasting analgesia (Oyama *et al.* 1980, 1982); stimulation of periaqueductal grey also produces prolonged analgesia and is accompanied by the release of beta-endorphin as well as enkephalins. The analgesia following electroacupuncture and transcutaneous electrical stimulation may outlast the period of stimulation by several hours; this

Table 5.5.   Distribution of opioid peptides and receptors

Distribution of opioid peptides (areas of highest concentration)

Methionine enkephalin	corpus striatum, caudate putamen, globus pallidus
	limbic system: olfactory bulb, tubercle, septum,
	  nucleus accumbens, hippocampus
	hypothalamus
	medulla, pons, spinal cord: periaqueductal grey,
	  substantia gelatinosa.

Beta-endorphin	hypothalamus, pituitary
Dynorphin	hypothalamus

Distribution of opioid receptors

Location	Effect mediated

Spinal cord: dorsal horn, lamina I and II
Trigeminal nerve? substantia gelatinosa
Periaqueductal grey, medial and
  intralaminar thalamic nuclei,
  ?striatum
	Analgesia
	  spinal (body)
	  trigeminal (face)
	  supraspinal

Nuclei of tractus solitarius,
  commisuralis, ambiguxus,
  locus coeruleus, parabrachial,
  area postrema, superior colliculus,
  pretectal.
	Autonomic reflexes
	  cough suppression, orthostatic
	  hypotension, inhibition of gastric
	  secretion, respiratory depression,
	  nausea and vomiting, meiosis

Posterior pituitary, hypothalamus,
  accessory optic system, ?amygdala
	Endocrine effects
	  inhibition of vasopressin secretion,
	  hormonal effects

Amygdala, nucleus stria terminalis,
  hippocampus, cortex, medial thalamic
  nuclei, nucleus accumbens,
  ?basal ganglia
	Behavioural and mood effects

Striatum	Motor rigidity

References: Cuello 1983; Atweh and Kuhar 1983.

long-term effect is thought to be due to the release of beta-endorphin (Clement-Jones and Besser 1983). The role of dynorphin in pain modulation is still not clear.

While enkephalinergic systems in the spinal cord and elsewhere may be tonically active in pain modulation, the beta-endorphin system and further enkephalinergic activity appear to be triggered into action by noxious stimuli and other stresses. Thus, naloxone does not usually cause hyperalgesia unless the subject already has pain or has been subjected to prolonged pain (Buchsbaum *et al.* 1983). A variety of stresses appear to induce the release of endogenous opioids. These include electric footshock, which produces a six-fold increase in circulating concentrations of beta-endorphin in rats (Bowsher 1978a), pregnancy (Sicuteri 1981), various types of severe pain (Sicuteri 1981), depressive disorders (Terenius 1982; Almay *et al.* 1980), and endotoxic, haemorrhagic, and spinal shock (Holaday and Faden 1982). In these conditions beta-endorphin may be co-released with ACTH, and enkephalins with adrenaline from the adrenal medulla and noradrenaline from peripheral nerves (Hughes 1983), as part of the general reaction to stress. Endorphins may also be involved in placebo analgesia (Fields and Levine 1984). The responsivity of an individual's endogenous opioid systems may affect his vulnerability or sensitivity to pain and stress.

(ii) Limbic system. Very high concentrations of opioid receptors are found in the amygdala and in the corpus striatum, especially the globus pallidus. Delta-receptors are located on presynaptic dopaminergic terminals in the corpus striatum and their action is to inhibit dopamine release. Mu-receptors are found in the same areas, but are not associated with dopaminergic terminals. Opioid receptors and peptides are also present in the hippocampus and cortex although in relatively low concentrations. In the cortex they tend to be distributed in polysensory association areas rather than in primary sensory cortex.

The opioid systems in limbic areas may play a role in mood and behaviour (Koob and Bloom 1983). Opioid receptors are found in rewarding areas, such as the ventral tegmental area, amygdala, and locus coeruleus (where opioids are co-secreted with monoamines), and opioid agonists such as morphine, are potent reinforcers in animals and support intracranial self-stimulation. The role of opioids in reward systems has been discussed above; their possible role in affective disorders is considered in Chapter 11. Limbic opioid systems are probably also involved in modulating the emotional components of pain, especially during arousal and stress, and they may also be involved in memory (Chapter 8). Thus, they appear to be intimately concerned in 'the whole pleasure-pain modality' (Bolles and Fanselow 1982, p. 26). Their presence in cortical association areas suggests that they subserve an integrative role on sensory and behavioural function, rather than a direct influence on sensory transmission (Atweh and Kuhar 1983).

(iii) Endocrine and autonomic areas. Endogenous opioids also have important modulating actions in the endocrine system, especially on posterior pituitary and hypothalamic functions, and associated autonomic functions. These actions are closely integrated with pain modulation and limbic activity, especially under stress, and may be involved in the endocrine abnormalities found in depression (Chapter 11).

It is clear that, like other complex functional systems, the nociceptive system utilizes a multitude of chemical mediators which together modulate nociceptive information at all levels from peripheral nociceptor to cerebral cortex to produce the final resultant sensation of pain. The interactions of this apparent plethora of transmitters and modulators seem particularly intricate. However, of all the sensations pain is perhaps the one most immediately important for survival and is of fundamental importance in arousal, reward and punishment, and learning and memory. It is possible that several overlapping back-up systems have developed during the course of evolution (Sweet 1980).

Of particular interest is the existence of multiple neurochemically and anatomically discrete pain suppressive systems. It appears that the physiological trigger for some of these systems is stress and that they represent an adaptation to certain emergency conditions in which pain suppression rather than feeling favours optimal coping behaviour. The particular pain suppression system activated appears to depend on the type of stress. Thus, in rats prolonged intermittent electrical footshock causes an opioid-mediated analgesia which is naloxone reversible, and manifests tolerance and cross-tolerance with morphine, while continuous footshock of the same intensity produces analgesia which is not affected by opioid or monoamine agonists or antagonists, but which is blocked by the centrally acting anticholinergic agent methylscopolamine, and attenuated by monoamine depletion and the antihistamine diphenhydramine (Lewis and Liebeskind 1983).

Despite the elaborate organization of pain suppression systems, malfunction appears to occur in some chronic pain syndromes described in Chapter 6 and pain perception is altered in a number of psychiatric conditions, such as depression, anxiety, and schizophrenia.

6

Disorders of reward and punishment systems

Reward and punishment systems, described in Chapter 5, clearly serve adaptive functions in promoting behaviours which increase the chances of survival and preventing behaviours that lead in the opposite direction. In certain conditions, however, activity in these systems appears to be maladaptive, and these can be regarded as disorders of reward and punishment systems. Drug dependence and disorders of pain sensation are considered here in this category. Depressive syndromes, in which reward and punishment systems are also centrally involved, are discussed in Chapter 11.

Drug abuse and dependence

Reinforcing properties of drugs

Present evidence suggests that the biological basis for drug abuse lies in the reward systems of the brain. The same drugs which are abused by man have been shown to act as reinforcers in animals: animals will learn to self-inject or inhale these drugs or to administer them by intragastric tube and will work either to continue self-administration or to avoid the administration of antagonists. A large number of drugs have been found by many authors (reviewed by Woods 1978) to have positive reinforcing properties in several animal species (Table 6.1). These include central nervous system stimulants, opiates, alcohol, hypnotics, benzodiazepines (Yanagita 1981), gaseous anaesthetics, organic solvents, nicotine (Deneau and Inoki 1967; Spealman and Golderg 1982), and cannabis (delta 9-tetrahydrocannabinol) (Kaymakcalan 1972). Negative reinforcement, the active avoidance of drug injection, occurs with the opiate antagonists naloxone and nalorphine in opiate-dependent monkeys.

Deneau et al., (1969) observed that animals' patterns of drug-taking are often similar to those of human drug-takers. For example, ethanol-reinforced responding in monkeys, like that of human alcoholics, often takes the form of episodes of severe intoxication followed by abstinence-induced withdrawal states. Under certain conditions (including the use of large intravenous doses, schedules of continuous reinforcement, and continuous drug access) corresponding patterns are found betweeen drug-reinforced responding in animals and human drug abuse (Woods 1978; Griffiths et al. 1983; Villarreal and Salazar 1981).

Table 6.1. Some drugs which act as reinforcers* in animals

Drug	Route	Species
Amphetamines	IV	monkey, rat, baboon, others
Cocaine	IV, IM	monkey, rat, baboon, others
Procaine	IV, IM	monkey, rat, baboon, others
Pipadrol	IV	monkey
Methyl phenidate	IV	monkey
Phemetrazine	IV	monkey, baboon
Apomorphine	IV	rat
Diethylpropion	IV	baboon
Clotermine	IV	baboon
Chlorphentermine	IV	baboon
Codeine	IV	monkey
Methadone	IV	monkey
Morphine	IV, IM	monkey
Pentazocine	IV	monkey
Propiram	IV	monkey
Propoxyphene	IV	monkey
Phencyclidine	IV, inhalation	monkey
Barbiturates	IV, inhalation	monkey
Either	inhalation	monkey
Chloroform	inhalation	monkey
Lacquer, thinners	inhalation	monkey
Nitrous oxide/oxygen	inhalation	monkey
Nicotine	inhalation, IV	rat, monkey, ape, dog
Alcohol	inhalation, IV	rat, monkey, ape, dog
Marihuana	inhalation	rat, monkey
Benzodiazepines	IV, intragastric	monkey

* Animals will voluntarily self-administer these drugs after suitable priming, depending on dose, schedule, route of administration, and species.

Woods (1978) noted that drug-seeking and drug-taking are, like intra-cranial self-stimulation, examples of operant behaviour, maintained and influenced by the learned consequence of the behaviour and the current environmental conditions, in the same way as other reinforcement behaviours. It seems likely that all such behaviours are centrally mediated by the same neural pathways. In view of the compulsive nature of intracranial self-stimulation behaviour, it is not surprising to find it linked with the self-administration of drugs. Numerous observations show that drugs which are reinforcing can also enhance the rate of self-stimulation via electrodes implanted in reward pathways. Enhanced self-stimulation behaviour, usually after an initial period of depression, has been shown after the administration of suitable doses of morphine, heroin, barbiturates, benzodiazepines, amphetamine, nicotine, and other drugs in the rat (Bush et al. 1976; Lorens 1976; Olds and Travis 1960; Larson and Silvette 1975; Stein, 1978; Haefely, 1978). Drugs which do not affect, or which reduce self-stimulation, such as naloxone and chlorpromazine, have consistently been found not to be reinforcing in self-injection experiments. The precise localization of the intra-cranial electrodes appears to be important for drug effects on self-stimulation, suggesting that drugs act at very specific loci in the brain (Nelson *et al.* 1981).

Drugs which enhance self-stimulation behaviour also lower the stimulus intensity at which electrical stimulation becomes rewarding. Kornetsky *et al.* (1979) found a close relationship between the abuse potential of a series of drugs in humans and their ability to lower the threshold for rewarding brain stimulation in rats (Chapter 7, Table 7.2). At the same time there was an increased threshold (decreased sensitivity) to stimulation of a punishment area in the reticular formation. Recordings of EEG activity were also made and it was found that the administration of morphine in rats caused EEG activation in the reward pathway located in the median forebrain bundle-lateral hypothalamic area, and simultaneously EEG synchronization (deacti-vation) in a punishment area in the reticular formation. Similar findings have been reported in humans. For example Heath (1972) studied EEG activity during cannabis smoking in a patient with implanted intracranial electrodes and reported bursts of activity from limbic areas (septum, temporal cortex and hippocampus) which coincided with 'rushes' of euphoria and died down as the 'rushes' subsided.

Animal studies are in general validated in human work, and Jasinski *et al.* (1984) describe methods to assess abuse liability of drugs in drug abusers by quantitating their hedonic effects ('liking scores') and withdrawal symptoms. Their results support the hypothesis that the prime attribute of drugs liable to abuse is the ability to activate brain reward systems and/or to depress punishment systems. The exact mechanisms are not clear, but it is noteworthy that all reinforcing drugs can influence one or more of the putative trans-mitters involved (dopamine, noradrenaline, enkephalins or endorphins, acetyl-choline, serotonin, Chapter 5) or act upon the corresponding receptors. All drugs of abuse can produce hedonic effects; indeed drug dependence can be viewed as an 'addiction to pleasure' (Bejerot 1980). In addition, such drugs relieve the hypophoria (poverty of affective reactions, poor self-image, feelings of not being liked by others) characteristic of drug abusers (Martin *et al.* 1978). At the same time, they reduce other needs by acting, for instance, as analgesics, anorexiants, or sexual depressants; this action may be of importance in certain types of drug-taking sociopaths who may have ex-aggerated needs such as to avoid pain, for sex or for food (Martin *et al.* 1978).

The total phenomenon of drug dependence in man is no doubt complex and a host of other factors discussed further below—pharmacological, con-stitutional, environmental, and social—all make variable contributions to the final goal-directed, drug-seeking behaviour (see *Theories of Drug Abuse* 1980, for a review). In its broadest sense, dependence or addiction has been defined as 'an emotional fixation... acquired through learning, which intermittently or continually expresses itself in a purposeful, stereotyped behaviour with the character and force of a natural drive, aiming at a specific pleasure or the avoidance of a specific discomfort' (Bejerot 1980, p. 254). This definition includes non-drug-orientated behaviours, such as compulsive sexual behaviour, gambling, overeating (Jonas and Gold 1986), excessive indulgence in athletic pursuits, and many others which may all depend upon activity in brain reward systems. Of the pharmacological factors, the development of drug tolerance and of drug withdrawal effects require special mention.

Drug tolerance

The responsiveness to a given blood or tissue concentration of a centrally acting drug (natural tolerance) varies widely between individuals and depends on many factors including personality, environment, state at the time of administration, and expectations (Schachter 1971; Eysenck 1967; Ashton *et al.* 1981). Drug tolerance in an individual is a state of diminished responsiveness of the body to a previously administered drug, so that a larger dose is required to elicit an effect of similar magnitude or duration. Tolerance develops to many drugs and, although it occurs with most drugs of abuse, it is not in itself a sufficient condition for drug dependence. For example, many people become tolerant to alcohol without apparently coming to crave its regular use (Madden 1979); with nicotine the range of tolerated dosage is smaller although the dependence-producing potential is probably much greater (Russell 1978).

The degree of tolerance developed to a drug is not uniform throughout body systems. With the narcotics a high degree of tolerance develops to the respiratory depressant and analgesic effects, yet much of the hedonic effects appear to remain (Herz *et al.* 1980b). With barbiturates, tolerance to the respiratory depressant effects is less marked than that to the sedative effects and with benzodiazepines, tolerance develops more rapidly to the sedative than to the anxiolytic effects. For nicotine, parts of the brain appear to retain their sensitivity in chronic smokers and very small doses can still cause changes in cortical evoked potentials (Ashton *et al.* 1980), although the nausea and vomiting of the neophyte smoker no longer occurs. With some drugs, tolerance to some effects can occur at the same time as sensitization to other effects. This heterogeneity is perhaps not surprising in view of the multiple mechanisms involved in tolerance and the fact that several operate simultaneously in various parts of the body.

Pharmacokinetic tolerance

The development of drug tolerance probably reflects a continuum of body adaptations from first exposure to long continued use, and involves pharmacokinetic and pharmacodynamic factors. Pharmacokinetic tolerance is usually the result of an increase in the rate of metabolism due to induction of hepatic drug metabolizing enzymes by the drug. It occurs most strikingly with barbiturates and some other hypnotics but is also seen with nicotine and with other drugs which are not abused (Smith and Rawlins 1973, Table 6.2). This type of tolerance develops over a period of several days and then reaches plateau. On cessation of the drug, enzyme activity declines over a period of 6–8 weeks. Enzyme induction has little effect on the peak intensity of drug action, but decreases the duration of action. There is not usually more than a three-fold decrease in sensitivity (Jaffe 1980) and pharmacokinetic tolerance is of lesser importance in the development of drug dependence than pharmacodynamic tolerance.

Table 6.2.   Some enzyme-inducing substances

Barbiturates	DDT
Glutethimide	gamma-benzene hexachloride (Lindane)
Meprobamate	Phenothiazines
Phenylbutazone	Aldrin, Dieldrin, Endrin
Phenytoin	Phenazone
Ethanol	Griseofulvin
Cigarette smoking	Rifampicin

Reference: Rogers *et al.* 1981.

Pharmacodynamic tolerance

Pharmacodynamic tolerance appears to result from a variety of tissue adaptations which decrease the response to a given concentration of a drug at its site of action. *Acute tolerance* can develop very rapidly: it can be demonstrated within minutes of a single administration of alcohol in the drug-naïve animal or non-alcoholic human (Cicero 1978). In man and animals the sedative/hypnotic effects of alcohol, barbiturates, and benzodiazepines are greater, at the same blood concentrations, immediately after drug administration when the blood concentration is rising than during recovery when the blood (and tissue) concentration is falling (Cicero 1978; Iverson and Iverson 1981). Acute tolerance tends to disappear within days if the drug is not repeated (Iverson and Iverson 1981; Triggle 1981). The mechanisms involved are not clear. With some drugs, acute tolerance may be due to tachyphylaxis, caused by persistent occupation of receptors (nicotine) or by depletion of readily available transmitter stores (indirectly acting sympathomimetic amines; Bowman *et al.* 1968). However, it is possible that acute tolerance can also result from changes in receptor affinity for a drug, since receptor molecules may undergo conformational changes which allow alteration between active and inactive states (Triggle 1981).

Chronic tolerance occurs when drug administration is continued over a period of time. It has long been known that chronic exposure to central nervous system depressants results in a compensatory increase in the activity of excitatory systems which to some extent balances the depressant effects of the drug. Conversely, with central nervous system stimulants, a compensatory increase in inhibitory activity occurs. Within limits, these changes allow the animal to adapt to the continued presence of a drug in its body and to function relatively normally. These homeostatic changes may result from alterations in the output or turnover of excitatory or inhibitory neurotransmitters or neuromodulators, and/or to changes in the sensitivity and density of receptors. Such changes tend to occur over a time-course of the order of weeks rather than hours or days; they may last for months or even years after the cessation of some drugs such as alcohol (Cicero 1978).

Littleton (1983), in discussing alcohol, distinguishes two degrees of central nervous system tolerance (Fig. 6.1). In *decremental tolerance*, adjustment is made so that increasing doses of alcohol have less depressing effect on brain function than in the non-tolerant state, but function is normal in the absence of alcohol. This adaptation would be appropriate when an organism is intermittently subjected to a range of drug concentrations, as in alcoholic binges. In *oppositional tolerance*, the response of the brain to a given concentration of alcohol is also decreased, but its activity in the absence of alcohol is increased. This type of tolerance would be adaptive for an organism exposed

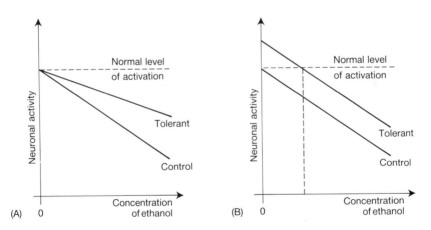

Fig. 6.1. Model of decremental and oppositional tolerance to alcohol in the central nervous system. (A) Decremental tolerance: increasing doses of ethanol exert a lesser depression of neuronal activity in tolerant subjects, but activity in the absence of ethanol is normal. (B) Oppositional tolerance: neuronal activity is less depressed by ethanol in tolerant subjects, but activity in the absence of alcohol is increased above normal levels. (From Littleton 1983.)

to a constant concentration of alcohol, but would give rise to abstinence symptoms if the drug was withdrawn.

Receptor modulation

Much recent work has shown that tissue receptors for neurotransmitters and neuromodulators exhibit plasticity: they are dynamic structures capable of making adaptive changes depending on the supply of agonist or antagonist (Fig. 6.2). For example, decreasing the supply of an agonist at a synapse (either by cutting the presynaptic nerve or blocking the receptor with an antagonist) results after a time in an increase in receptor sensitivity, the so-called denervation supersensitivity. Conversely, a chronic increase in

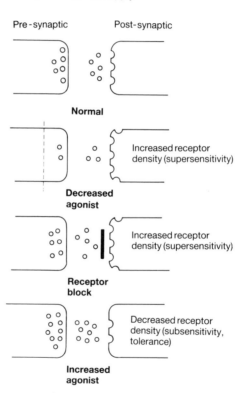

Fig. 6.2. Adaptive changes in receptor density in response to chronic exposure to receptor agonists and antagonists. Chronic decrease in concentration of agonist at a synapse, or blockade of receptors, may result in increased receptor density and supersensitivity; chronic increase in agonist concentration may lead to decreased receptor density and subsensitivity.

exposure to agonist results in a compensatory decrease of receptor sensitivity. Thus receptors are capable of tuning their receptivity up or down to compensate for changes in agonist supply. The result of such changes is a return towards normal function, or tolerance to the new conditions.

One mechanism by which receptor sensitivity can be altered is by changes in receptor density, as indicated in Fig. 6.2. Other mechanisms involve changes in receptor affinity or in the cascade of biochemical events within the cell initiated by the formation of the drug/receptor complex. Recent work on the modulation of receptor sensitivity has been described by Sulser (1981), Berridge (1981), Triggle (1981), Perkins (1982), Johnstone and Willow (1982a,b), Costa (1981), Creese and Snyder (1980), Barnes 1981, and Hoffman and Lefkowitz (1980).

Since many drugs act as agonists or antagonists at receptor sites, it is not surprising that alterations of receptor sensitivity have been found to occur after chronic drug administration. A major effect appears to be on receptor density, and changes in the number of receptors have been demonstrated by a variety of methods (binding studies combined with electrophysiological and behavioural methods) following chronic dosing with many classes of drugs. These changes affect not only post-synaptic receptors, which mediate the effects of neurotransmitters, but also pre-synaptic receptors, which modulate neurotransmitter release (Langer 1977). Thus, noradrenaline and some antidepressant drugs, cause decreases in density (down-regulation) of pre- and post-synaptic adrenergic receptors (Sulser 1981; Langer and Dubocovich 1977; Creese and Sibley 1981; Svensson 1980). Isoprenaline and some doses of amphetamine cause down-regulation of post-synaptic beta-receptors (Creese and Sibley 1981; Perkins 1982). In some systems the receptors appear to be actually lost from the membranes, perhaps by internalisation (Hoffman and Lefkowitz 1980). Conversely, increases in density of adrenergic receptors occur with beta receptor antagonists (Perkins 1982) and reserpine (Creese and Sibley 1981), while increased density of pre- and post-synaptic dopamine receptors develops during chronic treatment with dopamine receptor antagonists including many antipsychotic drugs (Creese and Snyder 1980). The effects and clinical significance of receptor modulation resulting from antidepressant and antipsychotic drugs is discussed in Chapters 12 and 14, but it is clear that the phenomenon is not confined to dependence-producing drugs.

Information on receptor changes induced by addictive drugs is at present relatively sparse. Decreases in GABA receptor density have been shown in some studies after chronic administration of benzodiazepines, barbiturates and alcohol (Cowen and Nutt 1982; Braestrup et al. 1982; Mohler et al. 1978). Decreased binding at benzodiazepine and barbiturate sites on the GABA receptor has also been shown after chronic dosing with these drugs (Crawley et al. 1982; Ho 1980) in some but not all studies. With amphetamine, certain doses appear to cause down-regulation of beta-adrenoceptors, but cocaine appears to lead to an increase in beta-receptor binding (Creese and Sibley 1981). In the case of opiates, the evidence at present suggests that these drugs do not cause changes in affinity or sensitivity in opiate receptors (Herz *et al.* 1980b), but Creese and Sibley (1981) suggested that this question should be reinvestigated in the light of the discovery of multiple types of opiate receptors. In addition, receptor modulation in response to drugs appears to be regionally distributed, being apparent in some parts of the brain but not in others.

The action of central nervous system stimulants and depressants on their target receptors also affects the release and turnover of other neuro-transmitters; this effect may indirectly cause changes in density in the receptors of such transmitters. Thus, beta-adrenoceptor supersensitivity has been demonstrated after chronic administration of alcohol and opiates; increased density of muscarinic cholinergic receptors occurs after alcohol and barbiturates, and alcohol also appears to lead to down regulation of dopamine receptors (Creese and Sibley 1981). In general, it would appear that the response of the brain to central nervous system depressants is down regulation of receptors for inhibitory neurotransmitters and up-regulation of those for excitatory transmitters, while the response to stimulants is the opposite. However, the responses may be limited to certain sites and to certain types of receptors.

Transmitter release

The control of transmitter release is highly complex. One complication is introduced by the multiplicity of pre-synaptic receptors. For example, Langer (1977) has described the many different receptor types that can be found at noradrenergic synapses in the peripheral nervous system and most of these have also been identified in the central nervous system. As shown in Fig. 11.4, not only are there pre-synaptic alpha$_2$- and beta-adrenoreceptors but also receptors for prostaglandins, enkephalin, dopamine, acetylcholine, adenosine and angiotensin, all of which modulate noradrenaline release. In addition, there are multiple post-synaptic receptors which modulate the effects of released noradrenaline; and other transmitters, for example dopamine, can stimulate post-synaptic alpha- and beta-adrenoceptors. A similar multiplicity of pre- and post-synaptic receptors exists at serotonergic, dopaminergic, and other synapses, and many neurones release more than one neurotransmitter or modulator.

Because of this elaborate and dynamic arrangement, it is almost impossible for a chronically administered drug to exert actions limited to one neuro-transmitter system or to one function of a system. A drug which acts on the nervous system, whether or not it induces changes in receptor sensitivity, is likely to affect transmitter release—which is in turn often linked by feed-back mechanisms to transmitter synthesis and turnover. Thus barbiturates, opiates, benzodiazepines, and alcohol have been shown to affect the release and/or turnover of acetylcholine, noradrenaline, dopamine, serotonin, and GABA (Okamoto 1978). Prolonged dosage with opiates decreases the synthesis and release of some endogenous opioids (Herz *et al.* 1980a; Herz 1981; Ho *et al.* 1980). Similar multiple changes in the release and turnover of neurotransmitters and modulators have been shown after long-term treatment with numerous other drugs. Such effects are by no means confined to drugs with dependence-producing potential and they may help to explain the rebound withdrawal effects which occur with many types of drugs.

Cross-tolerance

The development of tolerance to one drug may confer a degree of tolerance to other drugs to which an animal has not been exposed. Such cross-tolerance can result from pharmacokinetic or pharmacodynamic factors. Administration of an enzyme inducer will speed the metabolism of other drugs degraded from the same pathways. This type of *pharmacokinetic cross-tolerance* can give rise to drug interactions. Barbiturates, for example, increase the rate of metabolism of several other drugs including warfarin and phenytoin, and also of other barbiturates.

Pharmacodynamic cross-tolerance occurs between drugs which act similarly at the same receptor sites. Thus, tolerance to one barbiturate or benzodiazepine is associated with tolerance to all other barbiturates or benzodiazepines; tolerance to amphetamine confers tolerance to the effects of other sympathomimetic amines and to the anorectic effect of cocaine in animals (Jaffe 1980). Similar cross-tolerance occurs between opiates and opioids which act as agonists on the same opiate receptors. Sensitivity to antagonists acting on these receptors is however, greatly increased (Way and Glasgow 1978).

Secondly, cross-tolerance occurs between drugs which induce the same homeostatic body reactions. Alcoholics, for example, exhibit tolerance to many other central nervous system depressants including general anaesthetics, other sedative/hypnotics, and to some actions of tetrahydrocannabinol. Individuals tolerant to barbiturates are also tolerant to other depressant drugs including meprobamate, glutethimide, methaqualone, general anaesthetics, and the hypnotic (but not the musclar relaxant) effects of benzodiazepines. There is also some degree of cross-tolerance between opioids and phencyclidine.

Hoffman and Lefkowitz (1980) describe a form of heterologous desensitization or tolerance occurring in cells which have receptor sites for more than one neurotransmitter/modulator. For example, a cell which responds to catecholamines through a beta-adrenoceptor mechanism and to prostaglandins through a separate prostaglandin receptor might after exposure to catecholamines become less responsive both to these and to prostaglandins. This type of desensitization has been demonstrated in many cell types.

Reverse tolerance

Reverse tolerance, the development of increased sensitivity to the effects of a previously administered drug, has been reported in some cases. A course of a neuroleptic drug sometimes leads to increased susceptibility to extra-pyramidal effects during a second course (Sovner and diMascio 1978) and some dopamine receptor agonists (amphetamine, cocaine, bromocriptine) may increase the sensitivity to subsequent challenge with directly or indirectly acting dopamine receptor agonists (Post 1978). These effects may be due to differential actions of the drugs on pre- and post-synaptic dopamine receptors.

Behavioural tolerance

Present evidence of synaptic changes resulting from chronic drug admin-istration, as outlined above, does not appear to account for all the observed phenomena of tolerance, particularly for drugs of dependence. For example, rats learn to overcome the ataxic effects of alcohol if they receive the drug before performing tasks in which the absence of ataxia is rewarded or its presence punished, while rats given equal or greater doses of alcohol after the task, or who are not exposed to the task, do not overcome the ataxia to the same extent, although they become equally tolerant to other alcohol effects (Cicero 1978; Jaffe 1980). Similarly, tolerance to amphetamine anor-exia is contingent, occuring only if the drug is given before and not after food (Carlton and Wolgin 1971). The concept of behavioural tolerance (critically reviewed by Demellweek and Goudie 1983) suggests that an important com-ponent of drug tolerance is through adaptations of behavioural responses through learning and memory processes, including operant and classical conditioning (Siegel 1975, 1983; Bierness and Vogel-Sprott 1984; Chapter 8). No particular neurochemical mechanisms are assumed, but presumably they are the same as those which underlie learning and memory (Chapter 8). Thus, drugs may produce adaptative changes not only at their primary sites of action, but also in the pathways subserving the particular behaviours which they influence. However, the nature of these latter changes has yet to be demonstrated. It is possible that some cases of reverse tolerance (such as that observed with cannabis) is due to learning of a drug's rewarding effects, so that, after previous exposure, a smaller dose will trigger these effects in the manner of a conditional response.

Dosage escalation

The development of tolerance may lead to escalation of dosage in an attempt to obtain the original drug effect in the face of the counteracting body defences. Thus, narcotic addicts may exceed a dose that would produce fatal respiratory depression in a naive subject, and alcoholics may retain their composure at blood alcohol concentrations that would fell a teetotaller. However, there appears to be a maximal limit to tolerance (Cicero 1978) and this varies considerably between different classes of drugs. Petursson *et al.* (1981) point out that tolerance does not necessarily lead to escalation of dosage of benzodiazepines, and gross escalation of nicotine dosage does not occur with smokers (Ashton and Stepney 1982). Whether or not dosage has increased, cessation of drug use in subjects who have become tolerant generally leads to withdrawal effects.

Withdrawal effects: abstinence syndrome
Relation to tolerance

When compensatory pharmacodynamic changes have taken place in the body in response to the presence of a drug, its sudden withdrawal can give rise to a number of adverse effects. These appear to represent an overswing or rebound of activity in the systems affected by the drug and are largely the opposites of the original drug effects. In general, the abstinence syndrome of central nervous system depressant drugs is characterized by agitation and hyperexcitability, while that of a stimulant drug is characterized by fatigue, inertia, and general depression. Withdrawal effects occur not only with drugs which are abused, but also with other drugs which induce adaptive changes in the body. Thus, withdrawal of long-term neuroleptics is sometimes followed by exacerbation of tardive dyskinaesia, thought to be due to hypersensitivity of post-synaptic dopamine receptors in the corpus striatum (Chapter 14). Other examples are discussed by Grahame-Smith (1985). Withdrawal symptoms occurring on sudden cessation of chronically administered drugs are, in general, related to the development of tolerance and seem to be explicable in terms of the pharmacodynamic mechanisms described above. The distribution, duration, and severity of the symptoms depend on the particular body systems which have undergone adaptive modulations and the degree of adaptive changes induced. Withdrawal effects are reversed by an apppropriate dose of the drug which restores the *status quo*.

Clinical manifestations
The most dramatic abstinence syndromes occur on withdrawal, after tolerance has developed, of drugs which have potent reinforcing or rewarding effects. These drugs when used chronically cause widespread, though uneven, adaptive changes affecting the entire neuraxis and withdrawal effects can be demonstrated throughout the autonomic and central nervous system. The particular features of individual drug withdrawal syndromes are described in the sections on each drug.

A prominent withdrawal symptom from both depressants and stimulants which exert hedonic effects is a marked craving for the drug. This craving appears to be directly related to the degree to which the drug activates reward systems in the brain, and (in animals) supports self-administration and lowers the threshold for intracranial self-stimulation. Craving is a marked feature of opiate and alcohol withdrawal, but it occurs to a lesser extent during withdrawal from drugs which have weaker intrinsic hedonic effects. Thus, it is not severe during withdrawal from benzodiazepines in spite of the presence of other widespread withdrawal symptoms (Ashton 1984) and is absent on withdrawal from drugs such as chlorpromazine which do not support self-stimulation in animals. Craving is usually drug-specific. However, if the drug is not available, withdrawal symptoms of some drugs may be partially alleviated by other drugs with similar actions (see cross-dependence, below). Substitution of other, more readily available, drugs for the original drug of dependence by addicts may lead to multiple drug abuse.

Craving is possibly the result of down-regulation of receptors in reward systems in the brain. It may lead to compulsive drug use and escalation of dosage as tolerance develops in these systems. On drug cessation, aversive symptoms may result from relative overactivity of punishment systems, leading to goal-directed, drug-seeking behaviour. In drug abusers, the initial motivation for reward may become gradually displaced to varying degrees by motivation to avoid the punishment of withdrawal. Such a shift has been described in the development of alcoholism (Royal College of Psychiatrists 1979) and in cigarette smoking (Ashton 1983a,b; Ashton and Stepney 1982; Fig. 6.3).

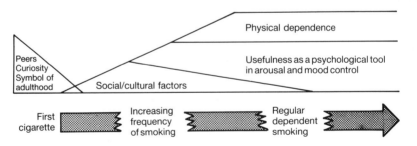

Fig. 6.3. Changes over time in importance of factors motivating cigarette smoking behaviour. (Adapted from Ashton and Stepney 1982.)

Physical and psychological dependence

A distinction is often made between physical and psychological dependence. Physical dependence is said to have occurred when withdrawal of the drug produces physical effects. Such dependence can be so severe that sudden drug withdrawal is lethal, as with barbiturates and alcohol, but it can exist to a variable extent and can occur, as already mentioned, with drugs such as chlorpromazine which are not usually addictive. Psychological dependence is said to occur when withdrawal symptoms are mainly limited to psychological effects such as anxiety or craving without life-threatening physical symptoms, and the term is often aplied to amphetamine or cocaine dependence. However, there can be no true distinction between physical and pscyhological dependence since psychological symptoms clearly result from physicochemical events in the brain.

Cross-dependence

Withdrawal effects caused by abstinence from one drug may often be partially alleviated by other drugs, a phenomenon known as cross-dependence. Thus, the manifestations of withdrawal from heroin can be partially suppressed by other opioids such as methadone, and one barbiturate can substitute for another in reversing the barbiturate withdrawal syndrome. Partial cross-dependence also occurs between drug groups, and is seen between alcohol and barbiturates, and between sedative/hypnotics and anxiolytics. This phenomenon is probably similar to pharmacodynamic cross-tolerance described above. It has important clinical implications and forms the basis of substitution treatment of physical dependence.

Time relationships

The time it takes for dependence to develop varies with drugs, dosage, and dosage schedule and also with the criteria used for defining dependence. However, the process is initiated by the first dose and can develop very rapidly. Mild withdrawal effects in the form of REMS rebound can occur within a week after short-acting hypnotics given in therapeutic doses once nightly (Kales *et al.* 1978) and the opiate antagonist naloxone can precipitate withdrawal effects in subjects given therapeutic doses of morphine, heroin or methadone 8-hourly for 2 or 3 days. The degree of dependence increases over time with continued drug use and it is usually estimated that marked dependence to most central nervous system depressants has developed within 2–4 months at therapeutic doses.

The time of appearance, severity, and duration of the withdrawal syndrome is influenced by pharmacokinetic factors. With rapidly eliminated drugs, withdrawal symptoms appear earlier and are more intense than with more slowly eliminated drugs. Abrupt displacement of opiates from their receptors by naloxone precipitates almost immediate symptoms, while discontinuation of long-acting opiates such as methadone produces withdrawal symptoms that are delayed, gradual in onset, and generally less severe. With rapidly eliminated drugs, withdrawal effects may develop between doses, increasing the motivation for continued drug use. The relief by the drug of the withdrawal effects acts as a further reinforcer of drug-using behaviour. This cycle of events is seen with short-acting benzodiazepines, especially the widely used lorazepam, and with amphetamines and nicotine. Many drug withdrawal regimes are based on the substitution of a long-acting preparation, for which there is cross-dependence.

The duration of withdrawal syndromes has probably been generally under-estimated. Acute, severe physical symptoms do not usually last for more than a matter of weeks, but physical and psychological symptoms including sleep disorders, muscle pains, and anxiety can certainly continue for many months after benzodiazepine withdrawal (Ashton 1984) and craving can continue for a similar time after stopping cigarette smoking (Ashton and Stepney 1982). Prolonged withdrawal symptoms are also described for cocaine (Chapter 7). Prolonged withdrawal effects after other drugs would probably be found if they were specially investigated.

Interacting factors

The relationships between the reinforcing properties of drugs, tolerance, dependence, and compulsive drug use are complex. Patients receiving nar-cotics for pain relief, although developing tolerance, do not usually have problems in withdrawing these drugs when they no longer have pain and they rarely become compulsive drug users or exhibit compulsive drug-seeking behaviour. The majority of people who drink alcohol regularly have become tolerant and may experience some withdrawal symptoms if deprived, yet do not become compulsive drinkers. Another often quoted example is that of American soldiers in Vietnam, many of whom became heroin dependent, but were able subsequently to stop drug-taking without serious difficulty or medi-cal help (Alexander and Hadaway 1982). It appears that many non-pharmacological factors including sociological and constitutional variables are important in drug abuse.

Sociological influences on drug-taking are discussed by Jaffe (1980) and Levison (1981) and the importance of learning and conditioning in narcotic dependence is discussed by Siegel (1978) and Lal et al. (1976). Of the con-stitutional factors, twin and family studies have suggested a genetic element in some forms of drug abuse (Eysenck and Eaves 1980; Goodwin et al. 1978). Personality variables have also been investigated in relation to several drugs. Compulsive drug users tend to exhibit personality characteristics largely encompassed within the dimension of psychoticism (Eysenck and Eysenck 1975; Martin et al. 1978). These characteristics include risk-taking, impul-sivity, sensation or stimulus-seeking, rebelliousness, aggressiveness, and intolerance of frustration. Some drug abusers also have high scores for neuroticism and extraversion (Eysenck and Eysenck 1963) and these factors are predictive for cigarette smoking (Cherry and Kiernan 1976), while tran-quilliser users may be high in neuroticism, but low in extraversion (Ashton 1984; Golding et al. 1983). Compulsive users of drugs with reinforcing properties may have brain systems which are particularly susceptible to reward and punishment. This possibility has been discussed in relation to anxiety by Gray (1970, 1977, 1981b) and in relation to smoking by Ashton and Stepney (1982). Thus, there may be individuals who are particularly vulnerable to compulsive drug use and to relapse after withdrawal. However, there does not appear to be a clearly defined trait or constellation of traits that describes all varieties of compulsive drug users or predicts their liability to relapse (Jaffe 1980; Levison 1981).

The basic pharmacological characteristics of drugs which are compulsively used appear to include: (1) an action on brain reward and punishment systems which either produces a pleasurable effect or allays discomfort, (2) the development of pharmacodynamic tolerance, and (3) the appearance of psychologically uncomfortable withdrawal effects on abstinence. These pharmacological factors, no combination of which is necessarily sufficient to produce drug dependence, interact with constitutional and environmental factors, influencing behaviour. With some drugs, the pharmacological influences may be extremely strong. For example, Villarreal and Salazar (1981) observe that all animals in experimental groups from seven different species will spontaneously self-administer amphetamine-like drugs when put in conditions in which they can, at first accidentally, operate a device that injects the drug. Allowed unlimited access to such drugs, monkeys will spontaneously continue self-administration to the point of death. With other drugs, such as cannabis and LSD, and possibly opiate narcotics (Alexander and Hadaway 1982), environmental factors may be more important, at least in humans; while with alcohol genetic influences may play a major part. Whatever the precipitating or aggravating factors, compulsive drug use is clearly a reward-seeking behaviour, mediated by reward and punishment systems in the brain, and directed towards obtaining repeated administrations of the drug.

Disorders of pain sensation

Acute pain clearly subserves a useful function in protecting the body from injury, both by evoking an immediate withdrawal reaction and by providing an aversive stimulus which (via learning and memory) promotes future avoidance behaviour to noxious stimuli. The somatic reaction to acute pain is one of generalized arousal, with cortical, autonomic, motor, and endocrine activation. This response is well adapted to fight or flight behaviour. If circumstances require sustained physical activity, it may also be adaptive to inhibit pain sensation and, as discussed in Chapter 5, powerful pain suppressive systems are temporarily activated by stress. More persistent pain, resulting from tissue injury, excites the further response of skeletal muscle spasm or rigidity around the site of injury which may help to rest and protect the affected tissue and so hasten recovery. Some forms of chronic pain, however, do not appear to be adaptive, while diminished sensitivity to pain exposes the body to damage. These conditions constitute disorders of pain sensation.

Decreased pain sensitivity

Insensitivity to pain may result from lesions in pain pathways at any site from the peripheral nerves to the brain (Bowsher 1978b). It also occurs rarely as a congenital condition which may sometimes be associated with overactivity of opioid systems (Dehen *et al.* 1977; Yanagita 1978). States of lowered arousal due to drugs or disease, and some psychiatric abnormalities such as hysteria or schizophrenia may produce indifference to pain, and reactivity to noxious stimulation is reduced in profound mental deficiency (IQ less than 20) (Bond 1979).

Chronic pain syndromes

Chronic pain can arise from structural or functional disease of most organs of the body and may be of varying duration. However, there are some heterogeneous disorders which have come to be grouped as chronic pain syndromes, partly because they are difficult to diagnose and treat and hence become longstanding, and partly because, whatever the underlying cause, they present a similar pattern of behaviour.

The physiological accompaniments of chronic pain are quite different from those of acute pain (Table 6.3). In place of acute sympathetic responses, so-called vegetative signs emerge including sleep disturbances, irritability, and lowered pain tolerance (Sternbach 1981). Deprivation of SWS and REMS may add to the symptoms produced by continuous pain and Moldofsky (1982) suggests that both rheumatic pain and migraine may be provoked or aggravated by sleep disturbance. The psychological features of acute pain, which resemble anxiety, tend to be replaced in chronic pain by

Table 6.3. Some somatic and psychological features of clinical pain

Acute pain	Chronic pain
tachycardia	sleep disturbance
increased cardiac output	irritability; aggression
increased blood pressure	appetite disturbance
pupillary dilation	constipation
palmar sweating	psychomotor retardation
hyperventilation	lowered pain tolerance
hypermotility	social withdrawal
escape behaviour	abnormal illness behaviour
anxiety state	(masked) depression

Reference: Sternbach 1981.

signs characteristic of depression. Conversely, many of the somatic symptoms of chronic pain also occur in depression, and there is a considerable overlap between the two conditions.

There are various classifications of chronic pain syndromes, of which one based on that of de Felice and Sunshine (1981), which does not claim to be exhaustive, is shown in Table 6.4. The causes are diverse, and include pain resulting from organic causes and pain in which no organic cause can be found. Many of cases are intermediate in that an organic cause may be present but does not appear to be sufficient to account for the degree of pain complained of. Perhaps 50 per cent of patients have no adequate physical basis for pain, while many patients with apparently adequate lesions do not complain of pain (Sternbach 1981). Hence it can be a difficult clinical problem to decide how much of a patient's pain is physical and how much is psychogenic in origin. Whatever the background, however, chronic pain can lead to a characteristic behaviour pattern in which the pain becomes the dominant feature of the patient's existence, vegetative symptoms are present, the patient becomes socially withdrawn and assumes the role of an invalid, and depression develops, either in the form of depressed mood or masked as somatic symptoms (Sternbach 1981). Nevertheless, not all patients with the conditions listed in Table 6.4 develop the chronic pain syndrome.

Table 6.4. Some disorders which may be associated with chronic pain syndromes

---

Concealed organic causes
  carcinomatosis, invasion/compression syndromes due to cancer
Neurological disorders
  nerve entrapment syndromes
  reflex sympathetic dystrophies (causalgia)
  myofascial syndromes
  phantom limb pain
  neuralgias (trigeminal, glossopharyhgeal, post-herpetic)
  spinal arachnoiditis or cord damage
  thalamic pain
  headaches (various)
Psychiatric disorders
  depression, hysteria, compensation neurosis
Unknown aetiology
  idiopathic chronic pain

Reference: deFelice and Sunshine 1981.

Neurological disorders

Neurological disorders producing pain are reviewed by Bowsher (1978b), Bond (1979), and Lance and McLeod (1981).

Peripheral nerve lesions Various lesions of peripheral nerves can produce neuropathic pain which is burning, shooting, or indescribably unpleasant. In all cases the pain probably results largely from interference with gate-control mechanisms due to damage to low-threshold mechanoreceptor fibres. If impulses from these large fibres do not reach the spinal cord, they cannot activate inhibitory interneurones which would normally suppress the input from small fibres; hence pain sensation is enhanced. In addition to interference with gate-control, pain may result from altered neurophysiological properties of damaged peripheral nerves which may generate spontaneous impulses and show unusual sensitivity to mechanical disturbance (Lance and McLeod 1981). Furthermore, the activity of pain suppressive systems in the brain, including affective components, may be altered in states of persistent pain.

(i) Causalgia. Partial damage to peripheral nerve trunks may give rise to causalgia, a particularly intense, but diffuse burning pain, accompanied by altered autonomic activity in the affected part. Raised emotional tension aggravates the pain and this may be through abnormal activity in higher autonomic centres which are also linked with emotional responses (Bond 1979).

(ii) Phantom limb pain. Amputation or deafferentation of a limb (or other parts of the body) is regularly associated with persistence of the body image or phantom of the affected part. The phantom may be painful or painless and tends to shrink and eventually to disappear over time. Phantom limb pain occurs in about 30 per cent of patients after amputation and persists in 5-10 per cent (*British Medical Journal* 1975). The pain may be aggravated or triggered by stimulation of neighbouring parts of the body, by visceral activity such as micturition, or by emotional arousal. The pain may be perceived in definite parts of the phantom, which may seem to move or feel as if it is fixed in an uncomfortable position or as if it is distorted.

Several mechanisms probably contribute to phantom limb pain. Loss of gate-control, as in other peripheral nerve lesions, probably results from the deafferentation and may be combined with decreased activity in supraspinal pain suppression systems. Howe (1983) suggests that reafferentation of deafferented small fibre dorsal horn neurones by low-threshold primary afferents from adjacent or distant dermatomes may be an important mechanism, at least in brachial plexus avulsion. Phantom limb pain is more likely to occur if the limb was painful before amputation and its incidence may be related to certain personality characteristics discussed later (Bond 1979).

Dorsal root lesions Irreversible damage to the cell bodies of large afferent fibres in the dorsal root or trigeminal ganglia may occur as a result of herpes zoster and give rise to post-herpetic neuralgia. Stimulation of small fibres gives rise to intense, burning pain similar to causalgia, presumably because of loss of gate-control mechanisms as in peripheral nerve lesions (Bowsher 1978b). There may be an associated depression, as with other types of chronic pain. Damage to dorsal roots can be caused by compression in disease of the vertebral column and occurs in some neuropathies such as tabes dorsalis in which it may account for the typical 'lightning' pains.

Spinal cord and brainstem lesions Lesions involving the spinothalamic tracts, for example in multiple sclerosis, may initiate burning pain on the opposite side of the body below the lesion. Anaesthesia dolorosa after posterior inferior cerebellar artery thrombosis is probably due to interference with the descending inhibitory reticulospinal system. Trigeminal and glossopharyngeal neuralgia resemble 'lightning pains' : the pain is repetetive, fleeting, severe, and occurs in paroxysms. These neuralgias have been ascribed to epileptiform discharges of the cranial nerve nuclei (Bowsher 1978b) or to demyelinization of the sensory neurones or mechanical irritation at the sensory root entry zone by tortuous cerebral arteries (*Lancet* 1984b). They may be triggered by afferent stimuli from peripheral areas supplied by the same nerve, for instance by speaking, chewing or swallowing. Some cases respond to anticonvulsant drugs such as carbamazepine, phenytoin, and clonazepam, and to surgical destruction of the nerve roots (Hayward 1977). Similar symptoms occur in idiopathic trigeminal neuralgia, the pathology of which remains obscure, and may temporarily follow structural damage to cranial nerve nuclei in multiple sclerosis.

Lesions in the thalamus and cerebral cortex
Damage to the ventroposterior thalamic nuclei, usually as a result of a cerebrovascular accident, may produce the thalamic syndrome, in which partial sensory loss and hemiparesis is combined with a burning pain and autonomic changes similar to causalgia. The pain is continually present but aggravated by slight stimuli to the painful areas. The pain may be due to irritation of thalamic and autonomic pain pathways, loss of gating mechanisms at thalamic level, or both (Bowsher 1978b). Rarely, the sensory cortex may be the origin of pain which may accompany focal epileptic attacks arising in this area (Lance and McLeod 1981).

Migraine and other headaches The typical features of migraine are well known (Hayward 1977). The attack may be preceded by an aura (often visual) and, the ensuing headache is often unilateral, throbbing in quality, and accompanied by nausea, vomiting, photophobia, hyperaesthesia, irritability, and autonomic disturbances. Many clinical variants of greater or lesser severity are seen. One of the most severe is migrainous neuralgia, or cluster headaches, in which the pain is throbbing and exceptionally intense but not accompanied by gastrointestinal symptoms. At the other extreme, migrainous headaches merge into tension headaches associated with anxiety, headaches associated with depression, and generalized psychogenic pain in other parts of the body—panalgesia (Sicuteri 1981). In certain individuals, headaches form part of the chronic pain syndrome.

A vascular aetiology for migraine is suggested by the fact that constriction and dilatation of certain blood vessels accompany different phases of the attack. The aura is associated with intracranial vasoconstriction, as shown by angiographic and isotopic blood flow studies (Rogers *et al.* 1981), and is presumably due to cerebral ischaemia, but the initial stimulus to vasoconstriction is unknown. During the attack, dilatation of the superficial temporal artery may be observed, and the headache is usually ascribed to dilatation of the external carotid artery and other extracerebral vessels. Both the vasodilatation and the headache may respond to the vasocontrictor drug ergotamine. However, vasodilatation by itself does not produce headache in normal subjects, although headache can be induced by agents which also stimulate peripheral nociceptors (e.g., histamine, bradykinin, prostaglandins). The release of these agents has not been consistently shown to be increased in migraine, although an initial increase in the concentration of circulating serotonin followed by a sharp drop as the headache develops has been reported (Hayward 1977). Many of the peripheral manifestations of the attack appear to be mediated by serotonin, and the serotonin receptor blocking drug methysergide is sometimes effective as a prophylactic agent. Ergotamine also has serotonin blocking effects.

However, although serotonin stimulates nociceptors peripherally, it has antinociceptive effects centrally since, as already noted, it is a major transmitter in descending pain-suppressive pathways. Sicuteri (1981) argued that migraine and related syndromes may represent functional disorders of pain suppressive systems. He suggested that decreased activity in descending inhibitory serotonergic pathways results from a primary deficiency of interacting endogenous opioid mechanisms in the brain and spinal cord (Chapter 5). He pointed to the clinical similarities between migraine and the narcotic abstinence syndrome, in which nausea, vomiting, irritability, and hyperaesthesia are also prominent, and presented a model of migraine as a 'quasi-abstinence syndrome' (Sicuteri 1981, p. 123). In support of this hypothesis, concentrations of endogenous opioids in the cerebrospinal fluid have been shown to be abnormally low in migraine and cluster headaches and in the narcotic abstinence syndrome (Chapter 7). There is also indirect evidence that central serotonergic activity in some areas may be decreased during migraine attacks, since cerebrospinal fluid concentrations of the precursor tryptophan rise, suggesting decreased serotonin turnover. The mechanism proposed for the precipitation of migraine and other headaches is that repeated stress in individuals with fragile pain-suppressor systems leads to exhaustion of these systems.

This provocative hypothesis for the aetiology of migrainous headaches remains to be substantiated. It does not attempt to explain the migrainous aura or the localization of the pain. It is discussed further below in relation to general mechanisms of chronic pain syndromes. However, the theory carries implications for the treatment of migraine with drugs (other than opiates) which potentiate central serotonergic activity such as lisuride, pizotifen, and cinnarizine (Sicuteri 1981). Pearce (1984a; 1985) also argued in favour of a primary neural cause for migraine, which then causes a secondary disorder of the microcirculation, and Geaney *et al.* (1984) reported that patients with migraine, like those with depression (Chapter 11) appear to have a defect in serotonin uptake systems in platelets and possibly in the brain. Other causes of headache are reviewed by Hayward (1977).

Psychogenic factors

Certain personality characteristics (reviewed by Bond 1979; 1980) are associated with increased susceptibility to pain. At the same time, personality variables affect the behavioural response to pain. These factors can lead to a variety of interactions between patients with pain and their families, friends and medical attendants. A number of 'pain games' can be played, with the patient using his pain to assume the role of home tyrant, pain professional, analgesic drug addict, or confounder of medical knowledge (Bond 1980). Personality traits and pain may also merge with mental illness, and pain may be a prominent feature in several mental disorders, especially anxiety neurosis and depression (Bond 1979; Sternbach 1981).

Psychological and psychiatric states can add to the experience of pain resulting from organic disease and also produce psychogenically determined pain, so that most clinical pain syndromes are an inextricable mixture of psychological and somatic components. In terms of conscious experience, there is probably no difference between organic and pscyhogenic pain, although each may perpetuate and enhance the other. In clinical situations, the affective components of pain are usually paramount; intellect plays a far less important role than emotion in the experience of pain (Bond 1979). This is in marked contrast to experimentally-induced pain, in which cognitive strategies rather than personality variables determine pain tolerance (Lukin and Ray 1982).

Anxiety Individuals prone to anxiety under stress have increased sensitivity to pain and complain of greater severity of pain when ill than more stable individuals. The dimension of neuroticism interacts with extraversion/ introversion. In general, pain threshold is lower in introverts, but extroverts complain more of pain although they have a higher pain threshold. Studies in patients with cancer pain and during childbirth show that patients most likely to complain of pain are those who score highly on both neuroticism and extraversion. Gray (1981a,b) has suggested that vulnerability to punishment is greater in neurotic than in more stable individuals, due to increased activity in septo-hippocampal punishment pathways (Chapter 3). However, anxiety is more common in acute than in chronic pain and relief of pain is accompanied by a fall in neuroticism scores, suggesting that anxiety can be both the result and the cause of pain experience (Bond 1980).

In anxiety neurosis (Chapter 3), pain is a common complaint. Pains are often musclar and electrophysiological studies reveal increased muscle tension which may be the cause of the pain. In some patients, exquisitely tender nodules (possibly localized areas of muscle spasm) act as trigger spots for inducing widespread pain.

Hysteria Hysterical personality traits are associated with exaggeration of symptoms, poor tolerance of pain, and demanding and manipulative behaviour. Such behaviour may be seen in some patients with chronic pain (of organic or psychogenic origin) who appear to use their pain to dominate or tyrannize their families. In hysterical neurosis, pain may be regarded as a conversion symptom, a mental defence mechanism of dissociation which prevents distressing emotions reaching consciousness (Bond 1979). The disability may produce secondary gains such as increased attention, liberation from responsibility, or financial gain. The characteristic feature of patients with hysterical pain is the discrepancy between the apparent severity of the pain and the degree of concern displayed.

Hypochondria Patients with hypochondriacal or obsessional personality traits commonly complain of pain. Such patients may become preoccupied with pain and fear of disease and demand constant explanation and reassurance.

Schizophrenia In some schizophrenic patients, pain is a prominent symptom: such pain is usually ill-defined and may be described in bizarre terms (Bond 1979). Other schizophrenic patients appear to be abnormally insensitive or tolerant to pain. They may maintain apparently uncomfortable positions for long periods of time and fail to react normally to painful external stimuli. Shallowness of affect is characteristic of schizophrenia and it seems likely that altered pain responses are at least partly due to disturbances in the limbic control of affective components of pain. There may also be alterations of endogenous opioid systems in schizophrenia, as well as cognitive disturbance and dissociation of cortical and autonomic arousal responses (Chapter 13).

Depression Of all psychological states, depression is most closely linked to chronic pain. Pain accentuates depression of mood in individuals with depressive personality traits, and in turn such individuals experience more pain than those who are less prone to depression (Bond 1979). Significant depression (as assessed by psychiatric and psychological tests) occurs in a high proportion of chronic pain patients Tyrer *et al.* (1986), while over half of patients hospitalized for depression complain of pain as a major symptom (Sternach 1981). Thus, it appears that chronic pain can cause depression and that depression can cause the psychological experience of pain. The two conditions can become linked in a self-perpetuating circuit.

Chronic pain can occur in both neurotic and endogenous depression. Von Knorring *et al.* (1983), in a series of 161 depressed patients, found that pain was commoner in neurotic reactive depression than in other diagnostic subgroups, and that it was more frequent in females than males. Patients complaining of pain had significantly more muscle tension, autonomic disturbances, and hostile feelings than those without pain, and there was no relationship between pain and feelings of sadness or signs of inhibition/retardation.

In patients with pain secondary to depression and in those with depression secondary to pain, there is a tendency towards somatization, so that depression is masked and the major symptoms are physical (Sternbach 1981). It has been suggested that such masked depression serves as a coping mechanism whereby attention is deflected from intolerable mental suffering to less intolerable physical suffering (Bond 1979). De Benedittis and De Gonda (1985) found that patients with psychogenic pain tended to show greater right hemisphere EEG activation than those with somatogenic pain, and that psychogenic pain occurred more frequently on the left side of the body. These findings are interesting since emotional functions appear to involve predominantly the right hemisphere (Chapter 8) and there is some evidence of right hemisphere dysfunction in depression (Wexler, 1980; Chapter 11). The site of pain in depressive disorders varies but lumbar and abdominal pain, headache and facial pain are all common.

Depressive facial pains Two types of chronic psychogenic facial pain appear to be particularly associated with masked depression (Hayward 1977; Bond 1979; Feinmann *et al.* 1984). In facial arthromyalgia (Costen's syndrome, temporomandibular joint dysfunction syndrome), the pain is localized to the region of the temporomandibular joint and its musculature. It is described as a dull ache, often with acute severe exacerbations. In atypical facial pain, the pain is felt deep in the soft tissues or bone and varies from a dull ache to severe throbbing. It may be localized to the teeth or involve the gums and tongue. There may be associated hypersensitivity of the teeth, oral dysaesthesia, and disturbance of taste. Both these syndromes are seen most commonly by dentists and they may be attributed to dental abnormalities such as malocclusion; however they are not improved by occlusal adjustment. A depressive aetiology is suggested by the observation that they often respond to long-term treatment with tricyclic antidepressant drugs. However, the study by Feinmann *et al.* (1984), pain relief with dothiepin appeared to be independent of antidepressant effect. Only 35 per cent of 93 patients with facial pain were considered to have a depressive neurosis. Psychiatric symptoms when present disappeared in both placebo and dothiepin groups when pain subsided, and did not recur with the recurrence of pain when treatment was stopped.

Idiopathic chronic pain

There remains a residue, which may amount to a significant proportion of patients, who have no detectable organic lesion, no discernible increase in nociceptive input, and no known psychiatric disorder (de Felice and Sunshine 1981). The pain may take a variety of forms; one such obscure pain is proctalgia fugax, a paroxysmal pain felt deeply within the anal canal (Lance and McLeod 1981), but any part of the body may be affected. Such patients show the characteristic behaviour pattern of chronic pain syndromes and adopt a life-style centring on the pain. They are usually singularly unresponsive to medical or surgical treatment, but may occasionally benefit from psychotherapy, hypnosis, acupuncture or transcutaneous electrical stimulation.

Mechanisms of chronic pain syndromes

While most types of pain due to organic disease can be reasonably well explained in terms of increased nociceptive stimulation or disruption of gate control systems, it is more difficult to pinpoint the mechanisms which lead to psychogenic pain and which produce the mixture of symptoms seen in chronic pain syndromes.

The close relationship between chronic pain and (possibly masked) depression has led to the suggestion that the underlying basis for both conditions may be similar. Several observations indicate that a linking factor may be activity in certain central serotonergic systems. Thus, brain concentrations of serotonin are decreased in some types of depression (Asberg *et al.* 1976) (Chapter 11) and depletion of brain serotonin in certain brain areas is associated with increased pain sensitivity and spontaneous pain (Moldofsky 1982; Johansson and von Knorring 1979). Conversely, increased brain serotonin activity is accompanied by decreased pain reactivity in animals (Moldofsky 1982), and treatment with antidepressants which increase central serotonergic activity can relieve both chronic pain and depression in man. It is possible that these drugs have analgesic actions which are independent of their antidepressant effects (Steinbach 1981; Feinmann *et al.* 1984), and tricyclic antidepressants have been shown to potentiate the analgesic effects of morphine (Biegon and Samuel 1980).

Sternbach (1981) has suggested that the chronic pain syndrome results from depletion of brain serotonin, especially in the dorsal raphe nuclei, leading to decreased activity in the serotonergic descending pain suppression systems. Central serotonergic under-activity is postulated also to cause sleep disturbance and depression. Possibly, the depletion is a consequence of prolonged over-activity resulting from the initial pain or stress. Another theoretical possiblity is that prolonged serotonergic activity might lead, not to serotonin depletion, but to tolerance to serotonergic effects in the body. At present there is no direct support for this attractive and simple hypothesis, despite undeniable evidence relating serotonin both to pain and to depression. However, the anatomical and physiological link between pain in depression and depression in chronic pain is likely to be found in limbic punishment systems, in which serotonergic mechanisms interact with a number of other transmitter systems.

More complex biochemical interactions are likely to be involved since serotonergic antinociceptive pathways are probably linked to opioid systems, as discussed in Chapter 5. There is strong evidence that serotonergic pain suppression systems are activated by opiates and endogenous opioids (Yaksh and Rudy 1978). For example, the analgesia produced by electrical stimulation of the periaqueductal grey, which is accompanied by release of serotonin in the spinal cord (Wilson and Yaksh 1980), is reversible by naloxone (Lewis and Liebeskind 1983) as well as by serotonin depletion or antagonism. Similar analgesia produced by injection of morphine or beta-endorphin into the periaqueductal grey is blocked by serotonin antagonists (Yaksh 1982) as well as by naloxone. Opiates and endogenous opioids may also exert a more direct analgesic action by inhibition of nociceptive neurones in the brain and spinal cord (Yaksh and Rudy 1978), and by inhibition of limbic pathways concerned with the affective components of pain (Henderson 1983). Morphine has been shown to decrease the responses to nociceptive stimuli of individual neurones in the thalamic nuclei in the cat (Nakahama et al. 1981). Endogenous opioids such as beta endorphin are powerful analgesics and probably exert their actions through both direct and serotonergic mechanisms (Chapter 7). These and other observations have led to the suggestion that a primary causative factor in chronic pain syndromes might be an abnormally low concentration or activity of endogenous opioids, particularly of beta-endorphin.

An interesting feature of the analgesia produced by electrical stimulation of the periaqueductal grey is that, although profound, it is short-lived. With repeated stimulation, tolerance to the analgesic effect occurs, and cross-tolerance to the analgesic action of morphine also develops (Lewis and Liebeskind 1983). Similar naloxone reversible analgesia can be induced by intermittent electrical fotshocks in rats; this too shows tolerance and cross-tolerance with morphine (Lewis and Liebeskind 1983). Thus, it seems possible that chronic pain syndromes may result from the development of tolerance to endogenous opioid analgesics.

In this context, attempts have been made to ascertain whether concentrations of endogenous opioids are abnormal in chronic pain syndromes, and whether they are altered by measures which affect the pain. The answers to these questions are by no means clear-cut for many reasons. There have been major technological difficulties in identifying separate endogenous opioids; several endogenous opioids may be affected differentially in chronic pain; changes in opioid concentrations in blood or even cerebrospinal fluid may not reflect changes in activity in critical brain or spinal cord sites; and chronic pain syndromes are aetiologically heterogeneous.

Clement-Jones et al. (1979), using a specific radioimmunoassay technique, found no significant difference in lumbar cerebrospinal fluid concentrations of beta-endorphin and methionine enkephalin between a group of 10 patients with recurrent pain from diverse organic causes and six pain-free control subjects. However, beta-endorphin concentrations were much more variable in the patients with pain, and the mean concentration was higher. Low frequency electroacupuncture alleviated the pain in the 10 patients, and this was associated in all cases with a rise in beta-endorphin concentrations, but no change in methionine enkephalin. In ventricular cerebrospinal fluid, Akil et al. (1978a,b) found reduced or undetectable concentrations of both beta-endorphin and metenkephalin in similar patients with recurrent pain.

Terenius (1982) and Almay et al. (1980) measured endorphin-like activity ('Fraction I') in chronic pain syndromes. Fraction I contains unidentified polypeptides which bind to opioid receptors but are distinct from both beta-endorphin and enkephalins. The concentration of these peptides in the cerebrospinal fluid was decreased, compared with normals, in patients with organically caused chronic pain (mainly due to neurological disease) but increased in patients with depression and psychogenic chronic pain. The patients with organic pain also had very low concentrations of substance P and of the serotonin metabolite 5-hydroxy-indoleacetic acid, in the cerebrospinal fluid, suggesting low activity in nociceptive and pain modulatory pathways generally. Low frequency electroacupuncture was found to relieve pain and to increase Fraction I concentrations in these patients. The relatively high concentration of endorphin-like activity in the depressed patients with pain was in line with other observations showing increased Fraction I concentrations in manic-depressive patients (von Knorring et al. 1978), although a subgroup of depressed patients with low cerebrospinal fluid concentrations of 5-hydroxy-indoleacetic acid may also have low concentrations of Fraction I polypeptides (Almay et al. 1980).

In patients with migraine, Sicuteri (1981) found extremely low or undetectable concentrations of morphine-like factors (mainly represented by methionine enkephalin) in the cerebrospinal fluid during migrainous attacks, but normal concentrations during headache-free periods. In patients with cluster headaches, morphine-like immunoreactivity in cerebrospinal fluid was undetectably low both during headaches and in headache-free periods. It was suggested that migraine and cluster headaches are due to deficiency or increased inactivation of endogenous opioids. The apparent opioid deficiency possibly leads to under-activity of serotonergic pain-suppressor systems since plasma and platelet serotonin concentrations were also found to be lowered during migraine atacks, while plasma and cerebrospinal fluid concentrations of tryptophan (the precursor of serotonin) were increased. Sicuteri (1981) draws attention to some similarities between the migrainous state as well as other chronic pain syndromes (panalgesia) and the opioid withdrawal syndrome (Chapter 7). In both conditions there appears to be a deficiency of endogenous opioids and a hypersensitivity to serotonin and catecholamines.

The results of these and many other investigations indicate that (as with most clinical syndromes) it is unlikely that a single abnormality will be found to account for the manifestations of chronic pain syndromes. These can occur in the presence of low, normal, or high cerebrospinal fluid concentrations of various endogenous opioids and are sometimes but not always associated with low serotonergic activity. The role of other neurotransmitters or modulators of pain, such as acetylcholine (MacLennon et al. 1983), neurotensin (Luttinger et al. 1983), dopamine and noradrenaline (Sicuteri 1981), have yet to be explored. The greatest stimulus to the pain suppressive systems is stress (Chapter 5), which may be involved both as a cause and a result of chronic pain syndromes, but whether prolonged stress can produce exhaustion of, or tolerance to, intrinsic pain modulation systems has not yet been ascertained. The picture of the chronic pain sufferer as an individual who has depleted or developed tolerance to his own opioid system, and hence manifests the reward-seeking behaviour of the deprived narcotic addict, is nevertheless an intrigueing one.

From the practical point of view, it has become clear that conventional analgesic drugs do not represent the only pharmacological means for treating pain. A number of psychotropic drugs (reviewed by Bond 1979) may, in some circumstances, have analgesic actions or add to the effects of analgesics, usually because of their actions on affective pain components. These include neuroleptics, antidepressants, and occasionally benzodiazepines, which are discussed in other chapters. The ability of placebos to attenuate pain has been known for some time; more recently it has appeared that some of their effects may involve endogenous opioid systems (Butler et al. 1983; Clement-Jones and Besser 1983). Non-drug procedures such as acupuncture, transcutaneous nerve stimulation, and possibly hypnosis may also activate endogenous pain suppressive systems (Clement-Jones and Besser 1983). Of various surgical procedures (Bond 1979; Miles 1977), electrical stimulation of the periventricular and periaqueductal grey is of particular theoretical interest in view of the part these areas probably play in physiological pain modulation (Lewis and Liebeskind 1983). Practical aspects of chronic pain management are reviewed by Twycross and Lack (1983).

7

Drugs acting on reward and punishment systems

The drugs described in this section exert major actions on reward and punishment systems (Chapter 5) and are all drugs of dependence (Chapter 6). Some have potent effects on pain systems and are of therapeutic importance (narcotic analgesics), but all are also used as recreational agents because of their rewarding properties. Other drugs which induce dependence, but are used therapeutically for their actions on arousal systems (central nervous systems depressants and stimulants) are described in Chapter 4. Antidepressant drugs and drugs which induce depression also affect reward and punishment systems, and these are discussed in Chapter 12. Psychotomimetic drugs are described in Chapter 14.

Narcotic analgesics, opiates, opioids

Narcotic analgesics, opiates, and opioids all act on endogenous opioid receptors (Chapter 5). The terminology relating to these drugs has been clarified by Hughes and Kosterlitz (1983). Narcotic analgesics are agents which act on opioid receptors to produce naloxone-reversible analgesia; opiates are drugs derived from opium; the term opioid describes any compound whose direct actions are specifically antagonized by naloxone.

Morphine
Morphine is the main active ingredient of opium and remains the standard agent against which other agents are measured. Other opioid agonists (Table 7.1) have generally similar actions.

Pharmacokinetics
Morphine is well absorbed from peripheral sites and can be given by subcutaneous, intramuscular, intravenous, and epidural injection. Absorption after oral administration is irregular and extensive first-pass hepatic metabolism occurs so that a higher dosage is required to obtain an equivalent effect by this route. Peak analgesic effects occur approximately 1 h after intramuscular injection and 2 h after ingestion, and last 3–4 h or longer, depending on dose and route of administration. The free base is rapidly distributed and concentrated in peripheral body tissues, but compared to

Table 7.1. Some opioid agonists, agonist/antagonists, and antagonists

Drugs	Oral potency* ratio	Duration of analgesic effect (h)	Main site of opioid receptor interaction
Opioid agnoists			
morphine	1	4	mu
codeine	1/6	4	mu
dihydrocodeine	1/3	4	mu
dextropropoxyphene	1/6–1/9	10	
pethidine	1/8	2	mu
heroin	1.5	3–4	mu
dextromoramide	2	2	mu
methadone	3–4	8	mu
levorphanol	5	6	mu
Mixed agonist/antagonists			
nalorphine	2/3	1–4	mu, kappa, sigma
pentazocine	1/18	3	mu, kappa, sigma
buprenorphine	25[1]	8	mu
Antagonist		Antagonistic effect	
naloxone	–	1–4	mu (delta, kappa, sigma)

* Oral potency ratio = oral dose of morphine/oral dose required for equivalent analgesic effect.
[1] Sublingual buprenorphine.
References: Rogers *et al.* 1981; Jaffe and Martin 1980; Houde 1979; Twycross and Lack 1983.

other opium alkaloids (codeine, heroin) morphine crosses the blood/brain barrier rather slowly and reaches the brain in relatively small quantities, despite its potent central effects. Detoxification of morphine is by hepatic metabolism and the metabolites are mainly excreted in the urine. The elimination half-life is 18–60 h. Some enzyme induction occurs with chronic morphine administration, but tolerance is mainly due to pharmacodynamic factors.

Actions

Central nervous system The main actions of morphine on the central nervous system are *analgesia*, *drowsiness*, *mood changes*, and *mental clouding*. Morphine is a powerful analgesic, affecting both the sensory and affective components of pain. Pain sensation is selectively depressed in doses which leave other sensations unaltered. Continuous dull pain and visceral pain are relieved at lower doses than sharp intermittent or cutaneous pain. Many patients report that pain is still present, but is less distressing after morphine.

Experimental pain is less affected; morphine may produce little change in pain threshold although there is usually an increase in pain tolerance.

Morphine can exert potent analgesic effects with little effect on the level of consciousness or motor reflex activity, but as the dose is increased subjects become drowsy, experience a feeling of pleasant indifference and warmth, and may sleep. The effect on the EEG is a shift towards low frequency, high voltage activity. Chronic dosing reduces REMS and SWS and increases Stage 2 sleep.

Some patients experience a euphoria after morphine, and this is pronounced in morphine-dependent subjects. Rapid intravenous injection in addicts produces an intense 'thrill' lasting about 45 s, accompanied by warmth and flushing of the skin. This is followed by a period of sustained euphoria or 'high'. However, dysphoria may occur, especially in normal subjects, who may complain of inability to concentrate, difficulty in mentation, and general lethargy.

Other central nervous system effects include nausea and vomiting, depression of cough reflexes, respiration and cardiovascular reflexes, and pupillary constriction. Tolerance develops to these effects, and also to the analgesic and euphoric actions. High doses of morphine can cause muscle rigidity, convulsions, and death from respiratory depression. Neuroendocrine effects include increased output of ACTH, prolactin, and growth hormone, and decreased output of thyrotropin and luteinizing hormone. Depression of luteinizing hormone leads to a decreased plasma concentration of testosterone and testicular atrophy in men, and amenorrhoea in women may occur after prolonged opiate use.

Peripheral effects Morphine produces generalized arteriolar and venous dilatation with marked vasodilatation in the skin. The lowered peripheral resistance may lead to postural hypotension. The effect on blood vessel tone is partly due to peripheral histamine release and partly due to central suppression of adrenergic tone. The vasodilator and sedating effects are utilized in the treatment of acute left ventricular failure. There is a reduction in gastric, biliary, and pancreatic secretions, in gastric and intestinal motility, and a generalized increase in smooth muscle tone. Spasm of the biliary and pancreatic tracts, and of the anal sphincter may occur; the tone of the ileocaecal valve is increased. Propulsive peristalsic waves throughout the small and large intestines are decreased, and water absorption from the intestinal contents is increased. These factors combine to produce marked constipation. Similar changes are seen in the smooth muscle of the urinary tract. The effects are partly due to direct actions on peripheral opioid receptors, but there may also be central effects since the injection of minute amounts of morphine into the cerebral ventricles causes a naloxone-reversible inhibition of gastrointestinal propulsive activity (Jaffe and Martin 1980).

Mechanisms of action

Morphine is a selective agonist of opioid mu-receptors, having only slight activity at delta- and kappa-receptors (Chapter 6). It has a certain structural similarity to endogenous opioids and receptor selectivity is probably due to the rigidity of the morphine molecule (Terenius 1980). Most of its effects result from interactions with endogenous opioid systems. It mimics many of the actions of enkephalins and beta-endorphin, but is not so rapidly destroyed and so has a more prolonged effect.

The analgesic action results from stimulation of opioid receptors at several levels in the central nervous system. In the spinal cord morphine has a direct depressant effect on cells in the substantia gelatinosa which respond to noxious peripheral stimuli (Duggan *et al.* 1977a,b). It also inhibits the release of substance P and other excitatory nociceptive neurotransmitters (Chapter 5). Administration of morphine and other opiates into the lumbar sub-arachnoid space of rats produces a stereospecific, dose-dependent, naloxone-reversible analgesia, with no motor impairment and no sensory alteration to non-noxious stimuli (Wilson and Yaksh 1980). In man, cervical and lumbar intrathecal single doses of morphine (0.5-1 mg) can produce pain relief lasting for 12-24 h. Similar effects are produced by epidurally administered morphine and pethidine (Behar *et al.* 1979; Cousins *et al.* 1979).

In the brain, electrical stimulation or microinjection of morphine, enke-phalins or beta-endorphin into certain areas, including the periaqueductal grey matter, dorsal raphe nuclei, periventricular grey matter and some thal-amic and medullary loci, produces behavioural analgesia in rats and primates (Yaksh and Wilson 1980; Jaffe and Martin 1980). The analgesia may endure for hours and is largely reversible by naloxone. Cross-tolerance between elec-trical stimulation and opiate or opioid injection may develop. This analgesia appears to be partly mediated by descending serotonergic and/or nor-adrenergic pain-suppressive pathways (Chapter 5). The apparent activation of these descending fibres by morphine may be due to disinhibition, since the action of opioid peptides and morphine on nerve cells is mainly depressant (Henderson 1983). Morphine and endogenous opioids depress the release of several neurotransmitters at several sites in the brain. Release of acetylcholine, noradrenaline and substance P is decreased, and there are alterations in release of dopamine and GABA (Jaffe and Martin 1980; Wood and Stotland 1980; Gold *et al.* 1979a; Jhamandas and Sutak 1976).

A further locus of the analgesic action of morphine in the brain is in the limbic system. It is probably by an action here that it obtunds the affective components of pain. As already noted, the limbic system is richly endowed with mu as well as other opioid receptors, particularly in the amygdala and many other areas including the locus coeruleus. Opioids and opiates depress the firing rate of locus coeruleus cells in a sterospecific, naloxone-reversible manner, probably by a direct action on the neurones (Gold *et al.* 1979a;

Henderson 1983). Release of noradrenaline from the widespread projections of the locus coeruleus is blocked and this effect may underlie the reduction of anxiety and the feeling of pleasant indifference evoked by morphine. Opiate actions on thalamic nuclei decrease the cortical release of acetylcholine (Jhamandas and Sutak 1976; Wood and Stotland 1980); this may diminish the arousing effects of painful stimuli and lead to drowsiness.

The hedonic effects of morphine presumably also result from actions on opioid receptors at limbic sites. Morphine is directly rewarding to animals who will work to receive injections of the drug into the cerebral ventricles or ventral tegmental area; it also enhances intracranial self-stimulation at several brain sites. These actions are reversed by naloxone, and sometimes by dopamine receptor antagonists, suggesting an opioid-dopamine link (Cooper 1984). However, destruction of mesolimbic dopamine neurones in the nucleus accumbens does not attenuate heroin self-administration in rats (Pettit et al. 1984). Marczynski and Hackett (1976), and Marczynski and Burns (1976) have also shown that morphine enhances, in a dose-dependent, naloxone-reversible manner, certain electrocortical responses (post-reinforcement EEG synchronization and the reward-contingent positive variation) associated with reward in the cat. Dysphoric effects may possibly result from actions at other receptors.

At a cellular level, the mode of action of morphine and other opioid receptor agonists is still not clear. Direct depressant effects may be due to hyperpolarization associated with opening of potassium channels (Henderson 1983). Pre-synaptic inhibition (Fig. 5.7), decreasing the release of other neurotransmitters, may also explain some actions. For example, release of hypothalamic and pituitary hormones from dopaminergic inhibitory control may account for some of the neuroendocrine effects. Complex interactions with dopaminergic and GABAergic mechanims may be involved in some effects such as the muscle rigidity in man and catalepsy, circling, and stereotyped behaviour in animals observed after high doses. High doses may block the release of GABA, resulting in the convulsant effects (Breuker et al. 1976). The emetic effect of morphine is not naloxone-reversible and therefore presumably not mediated by opioid receptors; it is thought to be due to stimulation of the dopaminergic medullary chemoreceptor trigger zone and is blocked by dopamine receptor antagonists such as chlorpromazine.

Adverse effects

Gastrointestinal effects Nausea and vomiting are relatively uncommon in recumbent patients but nausea occurs in 40 per cent and vomiting in 15 per cent of ambulant patients. In clinical use, these can largely be prevented by the use of dopamine receptor antagonists. Addicts develop a high degree of tolerance to the emetic effects.

Constipation is common in patients taking morphine therapeutically but may usually be controlled by the use of purgatives. Little tolerance develops to this effect and morphine addicts are usually constipated. Biliary and ureteric spasm may be partially alleviated by anticholinergic drugs such as atropine. Acute retention of urine due to spasm of the bladder sphincter may occur in patients with prostatic enlargement.

Respiratory depression Morphine has a direct depressant effect on brainstem respiratory centres, discernible at doses which do not alter consciousness. The sensitivity of the respiratory centre to increases in carbon dioxide tension is decreased and the centres regulating respiratory rhythm are depressed, resulting in irregular or periodic breathing. Death from morphine overdose is nearly always due to respiratory arrest. Patients with reduced respiratory reserve are particularly vulnerable to these effects.

Effects in pregnancy Morphine crosses the placenta and is taken up by the foetus which is more sensitive than the adult to its depressant effects. Maternally administered morphine in late pregnancy and labour may depress respiration in the neonate. In addition, morphine dependence can develop *in utero* and a withdrawal syndrome develop after birth (Ashton 1985).

Drug interactions Phenothiazines, monoamine oxidase inhibitors, and tricyclic antidepressants may all exaggerate and prolong the central nervous system depressant effects of morphine. Some phenothiazines appear to enhance the analgesic effects of morphine; such a combination is sometimes valuable in the management of severe chronic pain (Thompson 1984a,b).

Hypersensitivity, idiosyncracy Allergic reactions occur occasionally in the form of skin rashes, probably related to histamine release. Anaphylaxis has been reported rarely following intravenous injections and it is possible that it occasionally accounts for sudden death in addicts. Asthma can be precipitated by opiates in anaesthetized patients. Patients with hepatic disease are vulnerable to drug accumulation and relative overdose.

Abuse, dependence, tolerance Many of the opiates, particularly heroin, have a high dependence-producing potential since they readily induce hedonic effects, tolerance, and a withdrawal syndrome. The incidence of opiate abuse in the United Kingdom is not certainly known but was estimated as 20 000–30 000 in 1983 (Breckon 1983), rapidly increasing to 50 000 by 1985 (*The Listener* 1985). In the United States, the prevalence is probably over half a million (Jaffe 1980). It is of interest that long-term heavy opiate usage is not necessarily incompatible with apparently normal physical and mental health and long life (Brecher 1972) and, ex-heroin users have been maintained on high doses of methadone for over 10 years without ill-effects (Jaffe 1980).

However, the annual death rate among young abusers is several times higher than that of matched control groups; causes of death include infections resulting from unhygienic injection techniques, and overdoses and rections to impurities in illicit supplies of fluctuating potency (Jaffe 1980).

The hedonic effects of opiates in man, the reinforcing effects in animals, and the actions on opioid receptors in the limbic system have already been mentioned. Kornetsky *et al.* (1979) showed a close relationship between the abuse potential in man of various drugs and their ability to lower the threshold for intracranial self-stimulation in rats. Of the drugs studied, morphine and cocaine caused the maximum lowering of self-stimulation threshold; nalorphine, a partial agonist/antagonist, was intermediate, and the antagonist naloxone was neutral (Table 7.2). Nelson *et al.* (1981) found maximal dose-dependent increases in self-stimulation with morphine if the stimulating electrodes were placed in the locus coeruleus or lateral hypothalamus, but decreases if the electrodes were in the substantia nigra. Both effects were naloxone-reversible. These authors suggested that there are critical pathways for the reinforcing effects of morphine, possibly related to noradrenaline release in specific areas.

Pharmacodynamic tolerance develops rapidly to many of the effects of morphine and other opiates. In mice, a twenty-fold tolerance to the analgesic effects can be demonstrated within 3 days of regular morphine administration (Way *et al.* 1969). Naloxone can precipitate a withdrawal reaction from therapeutic doses given for only a few days in man. Tolerance develops readily to the respiratory depressant, sedative, and emetic effects, but is less marked for the constipating and meiotic effects. The question of how much tolerance develops to the hedonic effects is controversial. Many studies have

Table 7.2. Effects of drugs on intracranial self-stimulation (ICCS) thresholds of rats

Drug	Mean effect on ICCS Threshold*	
Morphine	−25%	(*n*=10)
Cocaine	−19%	(*n*=4)
Pentazocine	−10%	(*n*=4)
Phencyclidine	−10%	(*n*=4)
Nalorphine	−4%	(*n*=4)
Cyclazocine	−1%	(*n*=4)
Naloxone	+20%	(*n*=4)

* Mean difference from lowest threshold after saline.
Electrodes were implanted in median forebrain bundle—lateral hypothalamus area. Effects were independent of doses (morphine 2–8 mg/kg; cocaine 1–40 mg/kg; pentazocine (5–30 mg/kg; phencyclidine 0.5-5 mg/kg; nalorphine 4-16 mg/kg; cyclazocine 0.05-1.0 mg/kg; naloxone 1–4 mg/kg).
Reference: Kornetsky *et al.* 1979.

shown little tolerance to the effects of intracranial self-stimulation in animals (Kornetsky et al. 1979; Bush et al. 1976; Lorens 1976; Olds and Travis 1960; Pert and Hulsebus 1975). In man, it has been claimed that tolerance does develop to this effect and that the dose required to produce a 'rush' or 'high' must be continually escalated (Jaffe 1980). It is claimed that eventually many addicts continue to take opiates to avoid withdrawal effects rather than to receive rewarding effects. However, Kornetsky et al. (1979) quote evidence that dependent subjects still experience both a 'rush' and a sustained 'high' and that these effects are continued over the entire course of addiction, with no evidence of tolerance.

The mechanisms of opiate tolerance are not clear. Endogenous opioid systems are involved, since the development of tolerance is blocked if naloxone is administered concurrently with morphine (Way 1973) and potentiated by the administration of leucine enkephalin (Takemori et al. 1982). There is little evidence at present for changes in the affinity or density of opioid receptors after chronic administration of opioid agonists, although antagonists produce increases in receptor density (Herz et al. 1980b). However, tolerance to opioid agonists may involve changes at the effector part of the receptor system, rather than at the recognition site, since changes in the sensitivity of tissues to other neurotransmitters are induced by exposure to opiates. In particular, the sensitivity to serotonin and prostaglandins E1 and E2 is increased in the isolated guinea-pig ileum, a tissue rich in mu receptors (Herz et al. 1980). Furthermore, reduction in the functional activity of serotonin inhibits the development of tolerance while increase in serotonin synthesis (produced by loading with L-tryptophan) enhances the development of tolerance (Ho et al. 1975). Alterations in the activity of noradrenaline or acetylcholine do not affect the degree or rate of development of tolerance, although they affect the analgesic actions of opiates (Way 1978).

Modulation of adenylate cyclase activity and of levels of cyclic AMP in the brain has been proposed as a possible cellular mechanism for opiate tolerance and dependence West and Miller (1983). Opiates decrease basal intracellular concentrations of cyclic AMP and also inhibit the enhancement of cyclic AMP formation by prostaglandins and noradrenaline. Intravenous or intraventricular injection of cyclic AMP reverses morphine analgesia in tolerant and non-tolerant animals. In cultured neuroblastoma cells, opiates and opioids decease cyclic AMP formation acutely, but concentrations return to normal with continued administration, suggesting that the cells become tolerant. A rebound increase in cyclic AMP concentration occurs on sudden withdrawal or challenge with naloxone. Although these observations appear to constitute an attractive model for tolerance and dependence, the opioid receptors in these tumour cells are delta-receptors and it is not known whether mu-receptors are linked to adenylate cyclase.

A high degree of cross-tolerance develops between morphine, heroin and methadone, which act primarily on mu-receptors, but much less between these drugs and those such as ketazocine which act mainly on kappa-receptors. The degree of tolerance declines steadily after withdrawal and fatalities have occurred in addicts who have resumed their previous dosage after a period of abstinence.

Withdrawal syndrome (i) Clinical features. The character of the opiate withdrawal syndrome varies with individuals, drugs, dosage, duration of use, and other factors. Time of onset and intensity depends mainly on pharmacokinetic factors. Symptoms are almost immediate and severe if withdrawal is precipitated by naloxone, rapid in onset with quickly eliminated drugs such as pethidine, and delayed or less intense with slowly eliminated drugs such as methadone. However, the general features of the abstinence syndrome are similar for all opiates (Jaffe 1980).

Peak symptoms include those of widespread autonomic overactivity with increased glandular secretion, and cardiovascular and gastrointestinal symptoms. General central nervous system excitation is manifested by tremor, insomnia, restlessness, irritability, and dilated pupils. Psychological symptoms include intense anxiety, depression, and severe craving. Hallucinations are not a marked feature in comparison with alcohol, barbiturate, and benzodiazepine withdrawal, and convulsions are not usual. However, death can occur in debilitated subjects as a result of dehydration, acidosis, and cardiovascular collapse. Gross-symptoms recede in about 10 days, but are followed by a protracted abstinence syndrome with lethargy, inability to tolerate stress, hypochondriasis, depression, and continued craving—which may last several months. These effects contribute towards the high tendency to relapse in compulsive opiate users.

The neonatal withdrawal syndrome appears on the first day in the babies of heroin-dependent mothers, but may be delayed for several days in babies exposed to methadone *in utero*. It consists of irritability, high-pitched crying, hyperreflexia, increased sucking activity, and signs of autonomic overactivity. The signs are more severe after methadone than heroin (Zelsen *et al.* 1973).

(ii) Mechanisms. One of the mechanisms contributing to the withdrawal syndrome may be a deficiency of endogenous opioids resulting from chronic receptor activation by exogenous opiates. In rats, long-term morphine administration (1 month or more) decreased the concentration of methionine enkephalin and beta-endorphin in some pituitary, septal, and midbrain areas and in plasma (Herz *et al.* 1980; Herz 1981; Herz and Holt 1982). In human heroin addicts, Herz (1981) and Ho (1980) found reduced concentrations of beta-endorphin and methionine enkephalin in plasma and cerebrospinal fluid. In heroin addicts showing signs of withdrawal, Clement-Jones *et al.* (1979) found low concentrations of methionine enkephalin in the cerebrospinal fluid but elevated beta-endorphin levels in both blood and cerebrospinal fluid. In this context, it is interesting that acupuncture can alleviate acute symptoms in heroin withdrawal (Wen and Cheung 1973; Clement-Jones *et al.* 1979). This procedure was found to increase cerebrospinal fluid concentrations of methionine enkephalin. Relief of clinical symptoms occurred concurrently with this rise in four out of six patients; one patient who did not respond showed little change in methionine enkephalin concentration.

The rebound rise in noradrenergic activity which occurs on withdrawal from narcotics (and other central nervous system depressants) undoubtedly contributes to the anxiety and central nervous system hyperexcitability of the abstinence syndrome. Gold *et al.* (1978b, 1979a) suggested that noradrenergic activity in the locus coeruleus is particularly implicated and that this could be controlled with the alpha$_2$-adrenoceptor stimulant clonidine, which inhibits release of noradrenaline at this site. Clonidine (5 μg/kg) was effective in the management of heroin withdrawal and also suppressed narcotic withdrawal signs in animals (Lal and Fielding 1983). This effect was attributed to the fact that opiates inhibit locus coeruleus activity via an opioid mechanism while clonidine inhibits it via an adrenergic mechanism. Subsensitivity to opioid inhibition is thought to develop with tolerance during narcotic use, and on withdrawal endogenous opioids (which may also be reduced) are unable to suppress locus coeruleus activity. The activity, however, can still be suppressed by drugs that act on adrenergic receptors. Sicuteri (1981) reported a marked supersensitivity (in the smooth muscle of the hand dorsal vein) to dopamine and serotonin in the narcotic withdrawal syndrome, and in volunteers with a mild abstinence reaction induced by 3 days treatment with morphine. This peripheral supersensitivity was immediately abolished by a further dose of morphine. Antagonists of alpha$_1$- and beta-adrenoceptors and dopamine receptor antagonists have also been used in opiate withdrawal (Lal and Fielding 1983). The standard pharmacological treatment at present remains that of methadone substitution, although the success rate is not high (Menon *et al.* 1986). Withdrawal techniques are described by Jaffe (1980).

Other narcotic analgesics

A number of semisynthetic or synthetic opioids have actions which are similar to those of morphine and are presumably due to effects mainly on mu-receptors. Some of these are mentioned below and in Table 7.1.

Heroin

Heroin is diacetylmorphine. It is 1.5 times more potent than morphine as an analgesic. It is absorbed more rapidly from the gastrointestinal tract and enters the brain faster than morphine; hence it has a shorter onset of action. It is quickly metabolized, one of its metabolites being morphine, and has a shorter duration of action.

Pethidine

Pethidine is a synthetic compound structurally different from morphine although its actions and adverse effects are similar at equianalgesic doses. However, it does not constrict the pupil or depress cough reflexes. Its elimination half-life is 2–4 h and it has a rapid tissue distribution.

Methadone

Methadone is a synthetic substance which is structurally different from morphine but exerts similar effects. It reaches the brain in only small amounts, attaining a peak concentration within 1–2 h after oral administration, and causes less euphoria and drowsiness. Methadone is bound to protein in various tissues, including the brain, and may gradually accumulate during chronic administration. On cesation of treatment, it is slowly released from these tissues. The apparent elimination half-life after a single dose is about 15 h, but after chronic administration this rises to 22 h (Jaffe and Martin 1980). Methadone is mainly used in the management of withdrawal from other narcotics. Although it produces tolerance and dependence, management is easier and the abstinence syndrome is less intense.

Dextroprophoxyphene

Dextropropoxyphene is similar in structure to methadone but has less potent analgesic effects. In the United Kingdom it is commonly combined with paracetamol. Overdose of this preparation can cause respiratory depression, convulsions, and hypotension as well as paracetamol toxicity. In high doses it has euphoric effects, and dependence and abuse may occur (Wall *et al.* 1980).

Fentanyl

Fentanyl is a synthetic opioid which has an analgesic potency 80–100 times that of morphine. It is short acting, the peak effect lasting only 20–30 min due to rapid redistribution. The elimination half-life is 2–4 h. It is used with the neuroleptic droperidol to produce neuroleptanalgesia (Chapter 10), and also as a post-operative analgesic. High doses produce marked muscular rigidity which is naloxone-reversible and may be due to an action on dopaminergic transmission in the corpus striatum.

Mixed opioid agonists/antagonists

A group of synthetic opioids have mixed agonist/antagonist actions at various opioid receptors. Many of these have been developed in an effort to find a potent analgesic that does not produce respiratory depression or dependence and abuse. A singular property of some of these drugs is that small doses produce agonist effects (such as analgesia, respiratory depression or inhibition of gastrointestinal motility) but reversal of these effects occurs as dosage is increased and antagonistic actions develop (Fig. 7.1). The maximum agonist effect (efficacy) of these drugs is usually lower than that of pure agonists. Many of them have greater effects on delta-, kappa-, and sigma-receptors than morphine and thus have rather different pharmacological profiles; some have agonist effects on some types of opioid receptors but antagonist effects on others. Suitable doses of mixed agonists/ antagonists can reverse the toxic effects of agonists, but they can also precipitate withdrawal reactions and induce toxic effects of their own. Some produce pscyhotomimetic and dysphoric effects, thought to be mediated by sigma receptors. A few of these drugs are mentioned below. They have recently been reviewed by Rance (1983).

Nalorphine

Nalorphine appears to exert mainly antagonistic effects on mu-receptors but agonist effects on kappa- and sigma-receptors. It antagonizes the effects of morphine, heroin, methadone, and pethidine and has some analgesic and respiratory depressant effects of its own. However, it produces bizarre and terrifying hallucinations which are naloxone-reversible and thought to be due to actions on sigma receptors. Because of its dysphoric effects, it has little abuse potential.

Pentazocine

Pentazocine appears to have mainly antagonist actions at mu-receptors, but agonist effects at kappa- and sigma-receptors. It produces analgesia,

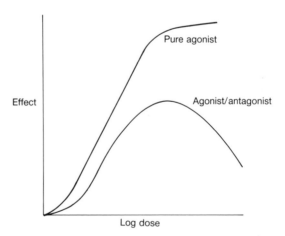

Fig. 7.1. Dose-response curve for a pure opioid agonist and a mixed agonist/ antagonist. For the agonist/antagonist, small doses produce agonist effects while reversal of these effects occurs as dosage is increased and antagonistic actions develop. The maximum agonist effect is usually lower than that of a pure agonist.

sedation, respiratory depression, and constipation at low doses, but the intensity of these effects does not increase progressively with increased dosage. Its efficacy is less than that of morphine, and it is less likely to cause nausea and vomiting. Unlike morphine, it has stimulant effects on the cardiovascular system, and can cause systemic and pulmonary hypertension. High doses produce naloxone-reversible dysphoric and psychotomimetic effects, but at therapeutic doses these are less marked than with nalorphine. Pentazocine appears to have less dependence-producing potential than morphine-like drugs; nevertheless, dependence and compulsive use does occur. *Butorphanol* and *nalbuphine* are similar to pentazocine, but have lower levels of agonist activity at sigma receptors and are hence less likely to produce dysphoria (Rance 1983).

Buprenorphine

Buprenorphine appears to act mainly on mu-receptors on which it has powerful agonist effects, but almost equivalent antagonist effects at higher doses. It has analgesic, sedative, respiratory depressant, emetic, and euphoric effects like morphine, but the actions are slower in onset and longer in duration, and do not continue to increase with increasing dosage. The respiratory depressant and other effects are not reversed by nalorphine and only partially by naloxone, probably because buprenorphine is not easily displaced from receptors. Buprenorphine can precipitate withdrawal reactions in narcotic addicts and can also alleviate withdrawal symptoms after narcotic abstinence. Dependence on buprenorphine occurs and its withdrawal after chronic use causes an abstinence syndrome after a delay of several days. However, its dependence potential is much less than that of morphine. *Propiram* is a partial mu-receptor agonist similar to buprenorphine (Rance 1983).

Opioid antagonists

A few synthetic drugs have almost pure antagonist actions at opioid receptors. None of these are completely selective for one type of receptor.

Naloxone

Naloxone is a relatively selective antagonist at mu-receptors but has some antagonist activity at delta-, kappa- and sigma sites. It has almost no intrinsic agonist activity and in low doses produces little discernible effect on normal subjects apart from subtle effects on subjective mood ratings (File and Silverstone 1981). In very high doses (2–4 mg/kg) morphine-like euphoria or dysphoria occurs (Cohen *et al.* 1981). Small doses can cause hyperalgesia in subjects under stress, aggravate some types of clinical pain, and prevent or reverse placebo analgesia and analgesia caused by acupuncture or transcutaneous electrical stimulation (Levine *et al.* 1978; Frid and Singer 1979; Skjelbred and Lokken 1983). These actions are thought to be due to antagonist effects on endogenous opioid systems which have been activated by pain, stress, or treatment. Naloxone reverses the actions of narcotic analgesics and opioid agonists/antagonists, although the reversal of buprenorphine effects is only partial. It exerts some antagonistic action on the central nervous system depressant effects of nitrous oxide, barbiturates, benzodiazepines and perhaps alcohol (Nuotto *et al.* 1983; Catley *et al.* 1981; Badawy and Evans 1981; Jeffcoate *et al.* 1979; Jeffreys *et al.* 1980). The effects of naloxone are very rapid in onset (within minutes), but the elimination half-life is only 20 min, much shorter than that of opiates. Thus, dosage must often be repeated in the treatment of narcotic overdose. Withdrawal reactions, which can be dangerous, are precipitated by naloxone in patients dependent on opiates or opioids. Longer acting analogues of naloxone, such as naltrexone and others, are in the process of development.

Endogenous opioids

Purified preparations or synthetic analogues of various endogenous opioids have potent analgesic effects when administered directly into the cerebrospinal fluid. Synthetic *beta-endorphin* (3 mg intrathecally) was found by Omaya *et al.* (1980) to induce profound analgesia, sedation, and euphoria lasting 22–74 h in 14 patients with intractable pain. Beta-endorphin (1 mg intrathecally) used for obstetric anaesthesia, provided complete relief of labour pains although patients remained alert (Omaya *et al.* 1982). *Enkephalins* injected intrathecally or into the cerebral ventricles in animals have analgesic effects which are weaker and shorter-lasting than those of beta-endorphin. Their actions can be prolonged by the addition of thiorphan, an inhibitor of enkephalinase A (Clement-Jones and Besser 1983). *Dynorphin* appears to be a potent analgesic (Goldstein *et al.* 1981; Wen, personal communication) and also produces behavioural effects (Katz 1980). Experience in the use of these substances in pain relief, narcotic withdrawal, or psychiatric states is still limited, but they all produce behavioural effects as well as analgesia, and Kosterlitz (1979) observes that all natural and synthetic opioids are liable to produce dependence.

Alcohol (Ethanol)

Alcohol has few therapeutic uses, but is the most widely used and clinically important drug of dependence. Like other such drugs, it exerts hedonic effects, induces tolerance, and can produce an abstinence syndrome on withdrawal. The incidence of alcoholic dependence (alcoholism) is about 5 per cent of the adult population in the United States and Western Europe (Rogers *et al.* 1981). The prevalence of alcoholism in a polulation is closely related to the overall level of alcohol consumption, which is in turn related to the cost of alcohol relative to average income (Hore and Ritson 1982; *Lancet*

1984a,b,c,d). In the United Kingdom, alcohol consumption doubled between 1950 and 1976, and is still increasing, and there are probably over a million alcoholics in Britain (Paton 1985). The heavy social and medical consequences of alcohol use are discussed by Glatt (1977), Madden (1979) and Jaffe (1980), among others.

Pharmacokinetics

Alcohol is readily absorbed from the gut, mainly in the small intestine. Fats and carbohydrates delay absorption, and large amounts of alcohol are absorbed relatively slowly. Small single doses start to appear in the plasma within 5 min, reaching a peak after 30 min to 2 h. There is considerable individual variation in rate of absorption, which may be more rapid in chronic drinkers. Alcohol is widely distributed and penetrates the cerebrospinal fluid and placental barrier.

Alcohol is 95 per cent metabolized in the liver, the rest being excreted unchanged in the breath, urine, and sweat. In the liver it is oxidized to acetaldehyde. The major pathway is by cytoplasmic alcohol dehydrogenase using nicotinamide adenine dinucleotide (NAD) as coenzyme. Some of the toxic effects of alcohol may be due to accumulation of lactate, beta-hydroxybutyrate, glutamate, malate, and alpha-glycerophosphate which require NAD for their metabolism (Rogers *et al.* 1981). This accumulation results in impaired gluconeogenesis, hypoglycaemia, and fatty infiltration of the liver. Associated nutritional deficiencies in alcoholics may add to the tissue damage. Acetaldehyde is further converted in the liver mitochondria to acetyl coenzyme A which enters the tricarboxylic acid cycle to produce 7 Kcal/g of alcohol. The rate of alcohol metabolism varies between individuals but is on average 10 ml/h. A modest increase in the rate of oxidation occurs in chronic alcoholics.

Chronic alcoholism is associated with reduced concentrations of cytosolic acetaldehyde dehydrogenase in the liver and erythrocytes (Thomas *et al.* 1982; Jenkins *et al.* 1982; Peters 1983; Agarwal *et al.* 1983). It is not clear whether a pre-existing deficiency of this enzyme predisposes to alcoholism or whether the deficiency is caused by heavy drinking. However, the observation that enzyme concentrations return to normal during abstinence suggests that excess consumption of alcohol impairs its own metabolism (Jenkins *et al.* 1982 1984; Agarwal 1983; Towell *et al.* 1983).

Other investigations have shown that acetaldehyde can condense *in vivo* with catecholamines to form tetrahydroisoquinolines, such as salsolinol, which have narcotic properties. Similarly, indole amines can condense with acetaldehyde to form tetrahydro-beta-carbolines (Blum *et al.* 1978). The importance of these metabolic conversions in the development of alcohol dependence is discussed below. It is possible that degradation products of these monoamine derived tetrahydroisoquinolines and beta-carbolines may contribute to brain and nerve degeneration in chronic alcoholism (Collins 1982).

Actions
Central nervous system

Acute effects Alcohol is a general central nervous system depressant, producing a dose-dependent decrease in the level of arousal in a manner similar to that of general anaesthetics. The most sensitive areas of the brain are polysynaptic structures such as the reticular activating system, so that impairment of consciousness occurs with small doses. This is manifested in deterioration of discrimination and judgement, concentration, attention, and psychomotor performance—a combination which may result in traffic accidents. The apparent stimulant effects of small doses are probably due to disinhibition. However, like other central nervous system depressants, small doses of alcohol may actually improve performance in some psychomotor tests, especially in anxious subjects (Chapter 2, Linnoila, 1974). Effects on sleep are similar to those of other hypnotics and consist of a decrease in REMS and SWS, with rebound effects often occuring the same night as blood alcohol concentrations fall. Alcohol also impairs learning and memory (Chapter 8).

The effect on mood is complex. Small doses produce mild euphoria and a pleasant sense of relaxation, similar to that seen with tranquillizing drugs. An increase of aggression is common with slightly higher doses. Emotions may be generally dulled, but sometimes there may be an increased sense of poignancy or sentimentality. Depression with self-pity occurs in some subjects; gay hilarity and fatuousness in others. Intoxication with alcohol sometimes gives rise to hallucinations. In animals alcohol appears to be definitely rewarding (Chapter 6).

Alcohol has analgesic effects: the ingestion of 60 ml of 95 per cent alcohol raises the pain threshold by 35–40 per cent without alteration of other sensory perceptions; the emotional reaction to pain is also dulled (Ritchie 1980). This rather specific analgesic action combined with euphoria is reminiscent of the effects of morphine.

As dosage is increased, ataxia, slurred speech, and eventually stupor, deep anaesthesia, and coma ensue. The respiratory response to carbon dioxide is depressed; at blood concentrations of 400 mg/l or more, respiratory depression may be lethal. Vasomotor and cardiac centres are also depressed. Alcohol exerts anticonvulsant effects in doses that cause general depression, but a period of hyperexcitability with increased liability to convulsions occurs during recovery and (in animals) may last 12 h after a single dose and several days after chronic administration (Ritchie 1980). The relationship between the acute central nervous system effects of alcohol and blood concentrations in

normal subjects and alcohol equivalents of various drinkers are shown in Fig.
7.2.

Chronic effects Chronic alcoholism, with associated vitamin deficiencies, may
lead to degenerative changes in brain cells. Wernicke's encephalopathy and
Korsakoff's psychosis, which are associated with memory defects, are
described in Chapter 9. These conditions respond partially to thiamine. They
appear to be more common in individuals who have a genetic abnormality
of the enzyme transketolase with reduced affinity for its coenzyme, thiamine
(Rogers *et al.* 1981). A significant loss of brain tissue, mainly from the white
matter of the cerebral hemispheres, was shown in a necropsy study of 22
chronic alcoholics (10 with Wernicke's encephalopathy and 14 with liver
disease; Harper *et al.* 1985). Peripheral neuropathy and retrobulbar neuritis
are also associated with thiamine deficiency in alcoholics, and a pellagra-like
state may occur due to nicotinic acid deficiency. Chronic alcoholism may
also lead to chronic cerebral degeneration with dementia and demyelinization
of the corpus callosum or central pontine areas. As already mentioned, toxic
metabolites as well as thiamine deficiency may contribute (Collins 1982).

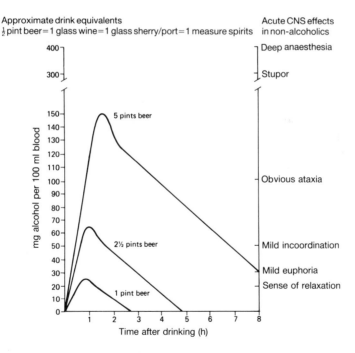

Fig. 7.2. Blood alcohol concentrations, acute central nervous system effects, and
approximate equivalents of various drinks. (Adapted from Laurence 1962, by kind
permission of Churchill Livingstone.)

Computed tomography (CT) techniques have shown that cerebral atrophy, as well as psychological impairment, is common in chronic alcoholics even in the absence of classical Wernicke–Korsakoff's syndrome. Lee *et al.* (1979) found evidence of cortical atrophy on CT scans in 49 per cent of a group of 37 young adult males and 59 per cent had intellectual impairment on psychometric testing. Several other studies reported similar results (*British Medical Journal* 1981). While one in 10 patients seen in alcoholic units have clinically obvious organic brain damage, over half of the remaining 90 per cent have brain shrinkage and specific cognitive defects with particular impairment of memory, abstract thinking, problem-solving, and psychomotor speed. However, Melgaard *et al.* (1986) found no correlation between severity of alcoholism, intellectual impairment, and cerebral atrophy. Nevertheless, minor brain damage with cognitive impairment may play a part in precipitating loss of drinking control and also in the high relapse rate of alcoholics who have undergone withdrawal. Psychological performance improves during a period of abstinence and even brain scan appearance can show slight slow improvement (*British Medical Journal* 1981). The mechanisms for minimal brain damage may be the same as those which produce Wernicke–Korsakoff psychosis; in addition, brain protein synthesis is reduced by chronic alcohol exposure in well-nourished animals (Ellingboe 1978), and this may contribute to psychomotor impairment, especially of memory functions.

Cardiovascular System

Acute cardiovascular effects of alcohol include skin vasodilatation with sweating which may lead to hypothermia. This effect is probably centrally induced and is accompanied by splanchnic vasoconstriction. Alcohol also increases myocardial excitability (Rogers *et al.* 1981) and chronic alcohol ingestion may produce hypertension in some subjects (Klatsky *et al.* 1977). However, in moderate daily amounts it may raise the concentration of high density lipoproteins and protect against coronary heart disease (Ritchie 1980). Chronic alcoholism combined with thiamine deficiency may lead to cardiac and skeletal myopathy (Hudgson 1984).

Gastrointestinal system

Low concentrations of alcohol increase gastric acid and mucus secretion. Higher concentrations decrease gastric secretions, are directly irritating to the mucosa, and may cause gastritis and peptic ulceration. Pancreatic secretions are increased and obstruction of the pancreatic duct may cause pancreatis. Fatty infiltration of the liver occurs on chronic ingestion and may lead to hepatic cirrhosis.

Urinary system

Alcoholic acts as a diuretic partly due to suppression of pituitary antidiuretic hormone secretion. Acidosis may result from increased excretion of ammonia ions and increased acidity of the urine. Hyperuricaemia also occurs and may precipitate gout.

Effects in pregnancy

Alcohol crosses the placenta and may damage the foetus. The foetal alcohol syndrome (Jones *et al.* 1974), consisting of maldevelopment particularly of the central nervous system, is common (up to 40 per cent incidence) in babies born to mothers who are chronic alcoholics. Risks associated with drinking in pregnancy are discussed by Ashton (1983b).

Endocrine effects

Various endocrine changes including hypoglycaemia, pseudo-Cushing's syndrome, and decreeased ACTH response to stress have been described.

Drug interactions

Alcohol potentiates the effects of other central nervous system depressants, mainly because of additive efects on arousal systems. It also increases the rate of absorption of benzodiazepines and can inhibit the metabolism of chloral, pentobarbitone, and meprobamate. It is a weak hepatic enzyme inducer and can increase the rate of metabolism of mepobramate, barbiturates, phenytoin, warfarin, and other drugs. Alcohol can enhance the hypoglycaemic effects of insulin and oral hypoglycaemic agents, and cause adverse reactions with some oral hypoglycaemic agents, metronidazole, and other agents, perhaps due to accumulation of acetaldehyde. It enhances the gastric irritant effects of drugs such as aspirin and non-steroidal anti-inflammatory agents. Interactions with opioid agonists and antagonists are described below.

A general review of alcohol and disease is given by Sherlock (1982). Whether or not there are 'safe' levels for chronic alcohol consumption is controversial and is discussed by the Royal College of Psychiatrists (1979), the Health Education Council (1983) and Anderson *et al.* (1984).

Mechanisms of action in central nervous system
Acute effects

Surprisingly little is known about the mode of action of alcohol in the central nervous system, a question reviewed by Littleton (1983), Myers (1978) and Richards (1980). The physical properties of alcohol, including its lipid solubility, are similar to those of general anaesthetics and it seems likely that they act in the same manner. These compounds all decrease synaptic transmission: they probably act both pre-synaptically, decreasing neurotransmitter release, and post-synaptically, affecting neurotransmitter receptors. There is evidence that the presynaptic action is due to inhibition of calcium influx through voltage-dependent channels in nerve terminals, thus preventing the rise in intracellular calcium which normally acts as a trigger for neurotransmitter release (Harris and Hood 1980). The effect on calcium may result from the partitioning of alcohol into membrane lipids or from binding onto membrane proteins (Franks and Lieb 1982).

The effects of alcohol on receptors, and on the release and turnover of individual neurotransmitters appear bewildering and confused at present; experimental results in animals are often complicated by changes due to tolerance. Carmichael and Israel (1975) showed that alcohol, in doses compatible with moderate to severe intoxication, reduces the release of at least six neurotransmitters from slices of rat cortex. These include, in order of their sensitivity to alcohol, acetylcholine, serotonin, dopamine, noradrenaline, glutamate, and GABA. *In vivo* experiments confirm that systemically administered alcohol causes a marked suppression of acetylcholine release from the cerebral cortex and reticular formation (Phillis and Jhamandas 1971; Erickson and Graham 1973), and this effect may partially explain its sedative actions.

However, *in vivo* alcohol, in moderate doses given acutely, increases the output of noradrenaline and adrenaline, raising the concentration of these catecholamines and their metabolites in the urine. This change is accompanied by alterations in turnover, with decrease in concentrations of catecholamines in the adrenal medulla and central nervous system (Ritchie 1980; Myers 1978). Mullin and Ferko (1983) reported that low doses of alcohol acutely stimulate dopamine synthesis, utilization and potassium-stimulated release in rats, while high doses inhibit dopamine utilization and release. Serotonin turnover and accumulation in the brain is also increased acutely by alcohol (Ellingboe 1978).

Alcohol, like benzodiazepines and barbiturates, may produce some of its depressant effects by enhancement of GABA activity. Nestoros (1980) found that locally applied or intravenous alcohol potentiated the inhibition of firing of single cortical neurones produced by iontophoretically applied pulses of GABA in the cat. This effect appeared to be due to an action on the post-synaptic membrane and it seems possible that GABA may interact at some site on the GABA receptor complex. Such a site is not the same as the benzodiazepine site, since alcohol does not bind to the benzodiazepine receptor. Acute administration of alcohol, however, increases the number of low affinity GABA binding sites and increases the binding of ^{3}H-diazepam (Ticku 1983).

Central opioid mechanisms appear to be involved in the acute effects of alcohol, and these interact with dopamine and probably GABA. For example, Barbaccia *et al.* (1981) found that acute alcohol administration induced a significant increase in striatal dopamine metabolism and turnover in selected strains of mice whose nigrostriatal dopaminergic fibres are rich in enkephalinergic receptors. Acute administration of alcohol to mice in moderate doses (which caused slight sedation) selectively increased methionine enkephalin concentrations in the corpus striatum and beta-endorphin concentrations selectively in the hypothalamus, in both cases by about 20 per cent (Schulz et al. 1980). It seems likely that effects on endogenous opioids as well as on catecholamines may account for the hedonic and perhaps analgesic effects of alcohol.

A further intriguing link between effects of alcohol and endogenous opioids is suggested by the possibility that acetaldehyde, the highly reactive metabolite of alcohol, may condense with catecholamines in the brain to form opioid-like alkaloids. The evidence is reviewed by Blum et al. (1978), Myers (1978a,b), and Collins (1982). Endogenous formation of tetrahydroisoquinoline and salsolinol from dopamine has been demonstrated in normal humans, in alcoholics, and in patients with Parkinsonism treated with L-dopa. Tetrahydroisoquinoline has also been detected in the brain of L-dopa treated rats exposed to alcohol and an orthomethylated derivative of salsolinol has been found in the corpus striatum of mice exposed to ethanol vapour. A similar isoquinoline alkaloid, tetrahydropapaveroline, is an intermediate in the biosynthesis of morphine in the opium poppy (papaver somniferum). Both tetrahydroisoquinoline and salsolinol have antinociceptive properties when injected intraventricularly in rats, with a potency similar to that of the enkephalins, and the effect is naloxone-reversible (Kemperman 1982). Isoquinoline alkaloids also potentiate morphine analgesia, increase ethanol-induced sleep time in mice, inhibit calcium binding to synaptic membranes, release endogenous stores of catechol amines, and some have hallucinogic properties (Kemperman 1982).

Furthermore, some studies have shown that naloxone can reverse alcohol-induced coma in man (MacKenzie 1979; Jeffereys et al. 1980; Lyon and Anthony 1982; Lancet 1982a). Jeffcoate et al. (1979) found that naloxone (0.4 mg) prevented impairment of performance by low blood concentrations of alcohol (40 mg/100 ml) in a four-choice serial reaction time test in non-alcoholic subjects. However, Bird et al. (1982) reported that the same dose of naloxone given before or after alcohol (blood alcohol concentrations 74–101 mg/100 ml), had no effect on the performance of 'social drinkers' in a battery of psychomotor tests which were impaired by alcohol (Bird et al. 1982). In animals, reversal of the acute effects of alcohol by opioid antagonists has been observed, but there is a significant genetically determined difference in the response (Kiianmaa et al. 1983). Thus, the isoquinoline hypothesis in human alcoholism remains controversial, but if true it would appear that 'when one imbibes alcohol a central opiate-like substance is, in essence, produced' (Blum et al. 1978, p. 119).

In addition, acetaldehyde can condense with indoleamines, such as serotonin, to form tetrahydro-beta-carbolines. These substances have been demonstrated in vivo both in the rat and in man and their concentration increases after the parenteral administration of aceteldehyde (Kemperman 1983). These beta-carbolines are striking inhibitors of serotonin uptake and also bind weakly to serotonin receptors, resulting in decreased serotonergic activity in the brain (Kemperman 1983). It is possible that this effect acutely contributes to the anxiolytic action of alcohol, like that of benzodiazepines (Gray 1981), and chronically to the associated depression and sleep disturbances (Kemperman 1983).

Tolerance and dependence

Behavioural and clinical aspects

Chronic alcohol consumption quickly leads to tolerance with profound adaptive changes in the body, especially in the central nervous system. The progression from tolerance, which occurs to some degree in regular drinkers, to dependence, with compulsive drinking behaviour and a severe withdrawal syndrome, is subtle and there is no clear dividing line. However, dependent subjects tend to consume larger amounts of alcohol within a given time, to drink faster and to report a stronger desire to continue drinking after a priming dose of alcohol than non-dependent drinkers (Wodak *et al.* 1983). Alcoholics tend to lose control over their drinking so that the behaviour becomes self-perpetuating. Some make repeated attempts at abstinence but then indulge in binge-drinking; others maintain a steady blood alcohol concentration by constant topping up. Eventually motivation becomes centred on alcohol and social disintegration occurs. In addition, periods of amnesia (alcoholic blackouts), disorders of affect (rage, depression, pathological jealousy), insomnia, hallucinations, and convulsions may occur in chronic alcoholics, probably as a combined result of alcohol intoxication and degenerative brain changes. A history of affective disorders (major depression, neurosis, and personality disorders) is more common in patients with alcoholic liver disease than in patients with non-alcoholic liver disease (Ewusi-Mensah *et al.* 1983), suggesting that some patients use alcohol, at least initially, as an antidepressant or tranquillizer.

Wodak *et al.* (1983) were impressed by the rarity of severe withdrawal symptoms in patients admitted for investigation of alcoholic liver disease. They estimated the degree of dependence by means of a questionnaire in 193 of these patients and found that only 18 per cent could be classified as being severely dependent, compared with 56 per cent of patients without overt liver disease who were attending an alcohol treatment unit. Severity of dependence was closely correlated with average daily alcohol intake in both groups. The authors suggest that subjects who become highly dependent on alcohol and drink large amounts develop behavioural symptoms relatively early and present for treatment, while those who are less dependent are able to sustain a more moderate consumption over many years and thus expose themselves to hepatic damage. Tolerance to the toxic effects of alcohol on other body systems clearly does not develop in parallel with tolerance to its central nervous system effects.

There appears to be considerable individual variation in susceptibility to alcohol dependence [which may be partly genetically determined (*British Medical Journal* 1980a)] and possibly also to alcohol-induced hepatic and neurological changes. These and other clinical aspects of of human alcohol dependence are reviewed by Cicero (1978) and Mello (1978).

Mechanisms of tolerance

Acute tolerance Some degree of pharmacokinetic tolerance occurs with repeated alcohol administration but pharmacodynamic tolerance is much more important. As previously noted (Chapter 6) *acute pharmacodynamic tolerance* to alcohol occurs extremely rapidly and can be demonstrated in man and animals during the time course of absorption and elimination of a single dose. Edwards *et al.* (1983) suggests that adaptations in noradrenergic receptor activity may be involved since the administration of a range of alpha$_1$- and alpha$_2$-adrenoceptor antagonists inhibited the development of acute tolerance (within 30 min of alcohol dosing) in mice. Dopamine receptor blockade with spiperone and general central nervous system depression with phenobarbitone did not affect tolerance.

Chronic tolerance Behavioural tolerance to alcohol in man may involve operant and classical conditioning and other forms of learning (Bierness and Vogel-Sprott 1984; Annear and Vogel-Sprott, 1985; Shapiro and Nathan 1986; Newlin 1986). Pharmacodynamic tolerance after subacute or chronic administration of alcohol appears to result from multiple complex adaptations involving both pre-synaptic and post-synaptic neurones and neurotransmitter metabolism. Many of the changes occuring during tolerance are opposite to those of the acute response to alcohol. These changes may include increased sensitivity of the calcium-dependent pre-synaptic release of acetylcholine (Littleton 1983); decreased post-synaptic GABA receptor density (Volicer and Biagiani 1982); decrease in central serotonergic activity (Kemperman 1983; Myers 1978a,b); complex changes in catecholaminergic activity (Myers 1978a,b; Mullin and Ferko 1983; Reggiani *et al.* 1980; Barbaccia *et al.* 1981); decrease of endogenous opioid concentrations (Schulz *et al.* 1980); and increased vasopressin release (Crabbe and Rigter 1980). In addition the formation of opioid-like alkaloids such as salsolinol may play a role in alcohol tolerance and dependence. Sjoquist *et al.* (1982) measured postmortem concentrations of salsolinol in the brains of intoxicated alcoholics, sober alcoholics (who had not drunk for several days), and control non-alcoholic drinkers. Salsolinol was present in all subjects: the concentrations were highest in intoxicated alcoholics and lowest in sober alcoholics in all brain regions examined (caudate nucleus, putamen, hippocampus, frontal cortex, and precentral gyrus). Salsolinol concentrations correlated with those of dopamine, suggesting endogenous formation from dopamine. The authors speculate: 'If endogenous salsolinol has a physiological role it could be that alcoholics drink to increase their abnormally low salsolinol brain levels' (Sjoquist *et al.* 1982, p. 676).

Cross-tolerance

Some cross-tolerance to other central nervous system depressants develops in alcohol-tolerant subjects. However, such cross-tolerance is only seen in relatively sober alcoholics: when blood alcohol concentrations are high, the effect of other depressants is additive (Jaffe 1980). Since the identification of opiate-like alkaloids in the central nervous system after alcohol ingestion, there has been much interest in the question of whether there is cross-tolerance between alcohol and opiates. If so, the dependence-producing effects of these classes of drugs might involve similar mechanisms. Several animal studies reviewed by Myers (1978a,b) support an alcohol-opiate link. For example, morphine suppresses alcohol consumption in alcohol-dependent rats, mice, and hamsters, and naltrexone, a long-acting opioid antagonist, increases alcohol consumption in these animals. Morphine-dependent rats undergoing withdrawal prefer alcohol mixtures to water, suggesting that alcohol suppresses the morphine-withdrawal syndrome. Mayer *et al.* (1983) reported cross-tolerance between alcohol and morphine to the hypothermic effects in rats and the inhibiting effects on the isolated guinea-pig ileum. In rats bred selectively for their sensitivity to alcohol, this sensitivity generalized to the effects of morphine. At the neuronal level, Berger *et al.* (1982) reported that naloxone antagonized the excitatory action of alcohol and salsolinol on hippocampal cells. On the other hand, Shearman and Herz (1983) found that rats trained to discriminate between saline and the narcotic analgesic fentanyl were not able to generalize this discrimination to alcohol, tetrahydropapaveroline, salsolinol, or 3-carboxysalsolinol, although they did generalize to morphine. Thus, the alcohol-opiate link cannot yet be regarded as firmly established.

Alcohol Withdrawal Syndrome

Clinical features

Abrupt withdrawal from alcohol in subjects who have developed a high degree of oppositional tolerance (Chapter 6) causes an abstinence syndrome which is generally similar to that seen on withdrawal of hypnotics, and has some features in common with the narcotic withdrawal syndrome. The severity of the syndrome may correlate poorly with the amount and duration of previous alcohol consumption since it depends partly on individual drinking patterns (Jaffe 1980). Withdrawal symptoms usually appear within 12–72 h of total alcohol abstinence, but in subjects tolerant to high blood alcohol concentrations, even a relative drop (e.g. from 300 to 100 mg/100 ml) can precipitate a withdrawal reaction. Chronic alcoholics who drink irregularly may experience withdrawal symptoms while continuing to drink.

In mild cases, the withdrawal syndrome consists of sleep disturbance, nausea, weakness, anxiety, and tremor lasting for less than a day. Such mild withdrawal symptoms may contribute to the hangover experienced after a drinking bout by individuals who are not chronic alcoholics. The classical syndrome in subjects with severe alcohol dependence (described by Jaffe 1980) starts similarly but proceeds to hyperreflexia, vomiting, abdominal cramps, and craving, followed by hallucinations. The intensity of this state increases to a peak within 24–48 h, and major convulsions may occur within the first 24 h, although they are less common than in barbiturate withdrawal. However, the EEG shows dysrhythmias and photic stimulation may reveal paroxysmal abnormalities and occasionally precipitate seizures (De Keyser *et al.* 1984). Sleep disturbance is also prominent, with rebound of REMS.

If the syndrome progresses, a phase of delirium tremens is entered. The patient becomes disorientated, agitated, and a prey to terrifying hallucinations. This stage occurs about the third day of total abstinence and may be accompanied by exhaustion and fatal cardiovascular collapse. However, the syndrome appears to be self-limiting and recovery from the acute withdrawal reaction can begin within 5–7 days without treatment. A protracted abstinence syndrome, as with opiates, follows alcohol withdrawal, with weakness, depression and continued craving, and is likely to lead to relapse.

A neonatal withdrawal syndrome occurs in the babies of chronic alcoholic mothers. This occurs within 48 h of birth and includes sleep disturbances, tremor, hyperreflexia, and feeding difficulties.

Mechanisms of withdrawal syndrome

In view of the complex mechanisms involved in alcohol tolerance, it is not possible to explain particular features of the withdrawal syndrome in terms of any one neurotransmitter. Central degenerative changes and vitamin deficiencies associated with chronic alcoholism further confuse the picture. One mechanism, common to the narcotic withdrawal syndrome, may be a deficiency in central endogenous opioid concentrations. As already mentioned, concentrations of methionine enkephalin and beta-endorphin are decreased by chronic alcohol administration in rats (Schulz *et al.* 1980). Such a deficiency might contribute to the craving and drug-seeking behaviour characteristic of early withdrawal. Added to this effect would be a sudden decrease in the formation from acetaldehyde and endogenous catecholamines of opioid-like tetrahydroisoquinolines such as salsolinol which are thought to be intrinsically rewarding. Collins *et al.* (1979) observed that the concentration of salsolinol dropped to control-levels within 2 or 3 days of abstinence in alcoholic patients.

The generalized central and autonomic overactivity is likely to result from unopposed tolerance to the alcohol-induced impairment of synaptic transmission, so that release of and response to several excitatory neurotransmitters including acetylcholine and catecholamines is increased. As in the withdrawal syndromes of other central nervous system depressants, clonidine and propranolol partially relieve some of the symptoms due to noradrenergic overactivity (Wilkins *et al.* 1983). Benzodiazepines and barbiturates are helpful in controlling convulsions and other withdrawal symptoms, probably because they counteract depressed GABA activity (Volicer and Biagioni 1982). Other drugs which show cross-tolerance with alcohol, such as chloral hydrate, paraldehyde, and chlormethiazole, as well as sodium valproate and lithium may give symptomatic relief. The management of alcohol withdrawal (including social and psychotherapeutic measures) are discussed by Jaffe (1980). The relapse rate after withdrawal is unfortunately high, probably less than 20–30 per cent of patients remaining permanently abstinent (Hore and Ritson 1982).

Nicotine

Nicotine, a plant alkaloid structurally related to acetylcholine, has properties which make it perhaps the most subtley addictive of all drugs. Taken as tobacco, it vies with alcohol for pride of place amongst recreationally used pharmacological agents. The prevalence of cigarette smoking in adults has declined to about 43 per cent in Britain over the last decade, but tobacco use is rising in underdeveloped countries (Capell 1978; Taha and Ball 1980). The psychopharmacology of smoking is reviewed by Ashton and Stepney (1982) and Mangan and Golding (1984).

Pharmacokinetics

When inhaled in cigarette smoke, nicotine is swiftly and efficiently absorbed from the lungs. It is also rapidly absorbed from the nasal mucosa when taken as snuff, but absorption from the buccal mucosa from chewing tobacco, nicotine-containing chewing gum, and the relatively alkaline smoke of cigars and pipe tobacco is slower. When swallowed, little nicotine reaches the bloodstream because it undergoes 'first pass' metabolism in the liver.

Once in the bloodstream, nicotine is quickly distributed throughout the body, reaching the brain in 7–8 s (Russell 1978a), where it is briefly concentrated (Larson and Silvette 1975; Schmiterlow *et al.* 1967). Inhaled puffs of cigarette smoke produce intermittent highly concentrated boli of nicotine in the blood (Russell 1978). This factor appears to be important in determining the actions of nicotine, since similar doses given more slowly do not produce the same effects in animals (Armitage *et al.* 1969).

Nicotine is metabolized to cotinine, nicotine-N-oxide and other products, mainly in the liver, and its elimination half-life is approximately 30–60 min. There is considerable interindividual variation in the rate of metabolism, and the rate is increased in chronic smokers. Due to hepatic enzyme induction, nicotine increases the rate of metabolism of several other drugs (Rogers *et al.* 1981). Nicotine and its metabolites are excreted by the kidney at a rate which depends on the pH of the urine and is greatest under acidic conditions (Feyerabend and Russell 1978).

Actions and mechanisms

Central nervous system

Biphasic effects The pharmacological actions of nicotine are mainly due to its ability to combine with nicotinic acetycholine receptors. Nicotine exerts a biphasic, dose-dependent stimulant/depressant action on these receptors at cholinergic synapses. The initial combination of nicotine with the receptor stimulates a response, but persistent occupation of the receptors and prolonged effects on the neuronal membrane may block further responses. The degree of stimulation versus block depends on the amount of nicotine present relative to the number of receptors available. In general, small doses of nicotine produce predominantly stimulant effects at synapses and larger doses produce mainly depressant effects. Lethal doses block synaptic transmission completely.

When puffs of cigarette smoke are intermittently inhaled, the time/dose relationship of nicotine reaching the brain can be such as to produce either stimulant or depressant effects. Thus, by varying factors such as size of puff and depth of inhalation, a smoker can obtain predominantly inhibitory or predominantly excitatory effects, or a mixture of both, from one cigarette. The ease with which nicotine can produce rapid, reversible, biphasic effects over a small dose range is probably a major factor determining the popularity of the smoking habit. These effects are exerted on many brain systems including those involved in arousal, reward, and learning and memory.

Effects on arousal Small doses of intravenous nicotine (0.005–0.01 mg/kg) or puffs of cigarette smoke introduced into the nostrils or lungs cause behavioural and EEG arousal in sleeping animals (Domino 1979; Hall 1970). These effects can be blocked by the centrally acting ganglion blocker, mecamylamine. Armitage *et al.* (1969) showed that electrocortical arousal produced by cigarette smoke or intravenous nicotine in anaesthetized cats was accompanied by increased output of acetylcholine from the cortex. Cigarette smoking in man also causes alerting effects on the EEG, producing low voltage, high frequency patterns and an increase in alpha wave frequency (Knott and Venables 1977; Murphree *et al.* 1967; Lambiase and Serra 1957; Mangan and Golding 1978). Cigarette smoking and intermittent intravenous shots of nicotine can also increase the magnitude of event-related slow cortical potentials and auditory evoked responses (Ashton *et al.* 1974, 1980). Smoking has been shown to improve performance in tasks requiring vigilance and sustained attention in man (Wesnes and Warburton 1978; Tarriere and Hartemann 1964).

Under certain conditions, however, smoking and nicotine may decrease the level of arousal. Armitage *et al.* (1969) showed that some doses could cause slowing of EEG activity and a fall in cortical acetylcholine output in the anaesthetized cat. Mangan and Golding (1978) demonstrated in human subjects that under conditions of mild stress, induced by white noise, smoking increased the amount of slow alpha-activity in the EEG. Ashton *et al.* (1980) found that the effect of nicotine on the slow cortical evoked potential (contingent negative variation) was dose-dependent, small doses causing a stimulant effect (increased magnitude) but larger doses producing a depressant effect (decreased magnitude). Performance in some tasks, such as complex reaction times in a driving simulator, may be increased or decreased by smoking (Ashton *et al.* 1972).

These and other experiments show that nicotine and cigarette smoking can both increase and decrease arousal, at least partly through effects on cholinergic arousal systems. There appears to be an interaction between dose, personality, and environment which determines which effect predominates. Smokers can manipulate their nicotine dosage to obtain the desired effect in particular circumstances (Ashton and Watson 1970; Ashton *et al.* 1974; 1980; Armitage *et al.* 1968). Smokers themselves report that the subjective effects of smoking can be either in the direction of relaxation or of stimulation, and there is considerable evidence (reviewed by Ashton and Stepney 1982) that smokers self-regulate their nicotine intake when smoking cigarettes of different strength.

Effects on reward systems Nicotine is reinforcing in animals: certain doses enhance intracranial self-stimulation and animals will self-administer nicotine orally, by injection, or by inhalation of cigarette smoke (Clark 1969; Deneau and Inoki 1967; Jarvik 1967; Ando and Yanagita 1981; Spealman and Goldberg 1982). In humans, smoking is reported to be pleasurable by nearly 90 per cent of chronic smokers, although it clearly does not produce a 'high' comparable with that of many other drugs of dependence. In addition it reduces pain and anxiety in stressful situations (Pomerleau *et al.* 1984). Hall and Turner (1972) demonstrated that nicotine and cigarette smoke increase the release of noradrenaline and dopamine from limbic areas and hypothalamus in animals; this may be the basis for its rewarding effects (Burn 1961). In addition, nicotine may interact with opioid reward systems (Karras and Kane 1980); smoking has been shown to increase plasma concentrations of beta-endorphin-beta-lipotrophin in man (Pomerleau *et al.* 1983).

It also seems likely that certain doses of nicotine may reduce activity in punishment systems, possibly by a depressant effect at cholinergic synapses, for example in the periventricular system. Such an effect would tend to allay unpleasant emotions such as anxiety, fear, frustration, and anger. Situations which give rise to these emotions have been shown to be those which increase the intensity of smoking in smokers. Schachter *et al.* (1977) noted an increase in the number of cigarettes smoked under a high anxiety condition induced by electric shocks, and Mangan and Golding (1978) found an increase in the number and 'strength' of puffs when smokers were stressed by white noise. A similar relationship between stress and smoking intensity has been shown in questionnaire studies (Emery *et al.* 1968; Thomas 1973). Nicotine has been shown to attenuate the disruptive effects of stress on performance in several animal tests (Hutchison and Emley 1973; Nelson 1978; Hall and Morrison 1973). Aggressive behaviour, in particular, appears to be modified by nicotine and smoking. Berntson *et al.* (1976) and Hutchison and Emley 1973) showed that nicotine decreased aggressive behaviour in animals, and in humans Heimstra (1973) found that subjects allowed to smoke during a 6 h vigilance task did not increase their ratings of aggression while smoking-deprived smokers and non-smokers did. Dunn (1978) reported that smoking prevented the disruption in performance caused by frustration in a complex perceptual motor task.

Effects on learning and memory Learning and memory are affected by the level of arousal and appear to involve particularly cholinergic pathways (Chapter 8). Nicotine and smoking have been shown to effect some learning and memory processes in animals and man. For example, Flood *et al.* (1978) reported that nicotine improved memory consolidation, and Alpern and Jackson (1978) observed complex dose-dependent biphasic effects of nicotine on various stages of the memory process in mice. Morrison and Armitage (1967) found that nicotine could increase the rate of learning of reward or avoidance tasks in rats, depending on the dose and time after injection. In man the effects of smoking on learning and memory are complex, dose-related and biphasic; in general smoking appears to improve selective attention and memory consolidation, while not affecting or slightly impairing initial learning (Andersson 1975; Mangan and Golding 1978 1983; Andersson and Hockey 1977; Wesnes and Warburton 1978; Williams 1980). In addition to effects on cholinergic and monoaminergic systems, nicotine may affect memory by an effect on arginine vasopressin, the plasma concentrations of which are increased by smoking in man (Pomerleau *et al.* 1983).

Effects on other systems

Nicotine exerts its characteristic dose-dependent biphasic effects on both sympathetic and parasympathetic components of the autonomic nervous system. The typical effects of smoking a cigarette include tachycardia, peripheral vasoconstriction, and a rise in blood pressure from central and peripheral sympathetic stimulation, but bradycardia and a fall in blood pressure can result from parasympathetic stimulation or sympathetic depression. Low doses stimulate respiration by stimulation of medullary respiratory centres, chemoreceptors in the carotid and aortic bodies, and sensory receptors in the respiratory tract, but large doses produce respiratory paralysis. Nausea and vomiting may result from stimulation of the medullary chemoreceptor trigger zone, and peripheral vagal and spinal reflex pathways. The usual effect on the gastrointestinal tract is an increase in tone and motor activity. Metabolic and endocrine effects of smoking include a rise in plasma triglycerides, and of cortisol, antidiuretic hormone, and growth hormone.

Adverse Effects
Acute toxicity
Acute nicotine poisoning, which may occur from exposure to nicotine-containing insecticide sprays, is marked by the rapid onset of salivation, nausea, vomiting, diarrhoea, tremor, sweating, and mental confusion. Cardiovascular and respiratory collapse ensue with paralysis of respiratory muscles, and this may be followed by terminal convulsions. The acutely fatal dose of nicotine for an adult is about 60 mg of the base; cigarettes deliver when smoked about 0.05–2.5 mg nicotine (Taylor 1980).

Tolerance, dependence, withdrawal effects
Some pharmacokinetic tolerance to nicotine develops in smokers, but pharmacodynamic tolerance is more important in determining smoking behaviour. Acute tolerance can readily be demonstrated in animal tissues: if a few equal doses of nicotine are applied in close succession, the later doses have less and less effect. This tachyphylaxis is probably due to persistent occupation of cholinergic receptors by nicotine, but its importance in human smoking is not known. Chronic pharmacodynamic tolerance develops unevenly in smokers, who become tolerant to the emetic and irritant effects of nicotine but still exhibit tachycardia, rise in blood pressure, peripheral vasoconstriction, and endocrine and metabolic responses to smoking. Some aspects of tolerance appear to decrease rapidly: in chronic smokers the first cigarette of the day elicits greater cardiovascular responses than later cigarettes, and many smokers say that they get the greatest hedonic effects from the first daily cigarette.

Gross escalation of dosage of nicotine dosage does not occur in smokers. Since the rewarding effects of nicotine are probably derived from a combination of stimulant and inhibitory actions, and most smokers seek both these effects, they may be forced into maintaining a medium dosage. Any substantial increase in dose would lead to a predominance of inhibitory (as well as unpleasant) effects and would simultaneously deprive the smoker of the stimulant effects. This fine balance between stimulant and inhibitory effects may constitute the root of the tobacco habit. Subjects can obtain mild hedonic effects from nicotine without the disruption of performance or after-effects that occur with other dependence-producing drugs. In fact, performance may be improved, as discussed above, and nicotine from ciga-rette smoke can be delivered in a controlled dosage to allow the subject to regulate his psychological comfort and performance in a way that is optimal in a range of environments (Ashton and Stepney 1982).

Cessation of smoking can give rise to a definite abstinence syndrome (Jaffe 1980; Brecher 1972; Hatsukami et al. 1984). In keeping with the biphasic effects of nicotine, this syndrome shows characteristics of the withdrawal reaction from both stimulant and depressant drugs. The severity and clinical picture of the syndrome varies greatly within individuals, and some smokers can give up with minimal withdrawal effects. The most consistent signs and symptoms, in addition to a craving for tobacco, are nausea, headache, constipation, diarrhoea, and increased appetite (Jaffe 1980). Drowsiness, fatigue, lethargy, depression, increased low frequency activity on the EEG, and decreased psychomotor performance occur in some subjects and are similar, though less intense, to withdrawal effects of stimulants such as amphetamine. A fall in heart rate and blood pressure and peripheral vaso-dilation may also occur. Just as common, and often coexistent with the above symptoms, are insomnia, vivid dreaming, anxiety, tremor, increased excretion of noradrenaline, irritability, and increased aggression. These effects are similar to the withdrawal syndrome from central nervous system depressants. The nicotine abstinence syndrome starts within 24 h of smoking cessation and some symptoms may persist for many weeks or months. The symptoms may be partially alleviated by nicotine chewing gum (Russell et al. 1980) but the relapse rate of smokers advised to stop smoking for health reasons or attending anti-smoking clinics is high, only about 10–30 per cent of such subjects being still abstinent after 1 year (British Thoracid Society Research Committee 1983; Raw 1978; Jarvis et al. 1982). It is possible that other substances in cigarette smoke apart from nicotine contribute both to the hedonic effects and the dependence.

Cocaine

Cocaine, an alkaloid present in the leaves of the cocoa plant, is a potent local anaesthetic and also has central nervous stimulant properties similar to those of amphetamine (Chapter 4). It has hedonic effects and is subject to abuse, a practice which fluctuates in popularity but is at present increasing in the United States and Europe (Jaffe 1980).

Pharmacokinetics

Cocaine is lipid soluble; it is readily absorbed from the skin and mucous membranes and enters the central nervous system. It is mainly degraded by plasma and hepatic esterases, and about 10 per cent is excreted unchanged by the kidney. After oral or nasal application, the plasma half-life is approximately one hour.

Actions

Local anaesthesia

Like other local anaesthetics, cocaine blocks nerve conduction when applied locally to nervous tissue. It prevents both the generation and conduction of nerve impulses by inhibiting the rapid influx of sodium ions through the neuronal membrane. The mechanism is thought to be displacement of calcium from sites on membrane phospholipids, causing configurational changes which constrict sodium channels (Rogers *et al.* 1981).

Central nervous system

Acute effects Cocaine, and all related local anasethetics, produce an initial central nervous stimulation followed by depression. The effect observed depends on dosage and rate of administration. With steadily increasing doses, restlessness proceeds to tremor and agitation, followed by convulsions and then central nervous system depression with death from respiratory failure. The ability to produce convulsions correlates with local anaesthetic potency among the various agents. Rapid administration, or very large doses applied locally, produce death from central nervous system depression with only transient or no signs of stimulation. However, cocaine appears to exert a particularly powerful stimulant effect on the cortex compared with other local anaesthetics (Ritchie and Greene 1981).

In small doses, cocaine has definite hedonic effects. Addicts describe a euphoria similar to that obtained from amphetamine, consisting of mood elevation, increased energy and alertness, loss of fatigue, a feeling of enhanced physical and mental capacity, and loss of desire for food. In laboratory situations, addicts cannot initially distinguish between the subjective effects of 8–10 mg cocaine or 10 mg dextamphetamine given intravenously. However, the effects of cocaine only last a few minutes after intravenous administration, while those of some amphetamines (e.g. methamphetamine) endure for hours. Other local anaesthetics also appear to be rewarding: subjects cannot distinguish between the euphoric effects of cocaine or lignocaine taken intranasally, and animals will self-administer both procaine and cocaine (Jaffe 1980)

The effects of small doses of cocaine on behaviour are also similar to those of amphetamine: at first the subject is garrulous, excited, and insomniac, but with increasing doses tremor, agitation and anxiety are prominent. Some individuals experience dysphoria even with small doses. Further dose increases may lead to vomiting, from stimulation of medullary vomiting centres, and convulsions before the depressant effects supervene.

Chronic effects Repeated use of large doses of cocaine produces a psychosis similar to that produced by large doses of amphetamine. The syndrome may be clinically indistinguishable from some forms of schizophrenia and typically includes paranoid ideation, thought disturbance, stereotyped movements, and hallucinations which may be visual, auditory, or tactile. Formication is a characteristic feature: a feeling of pricking or crawling under the skin which may lead to picking and excoriation and delusions of parasitosis (Jaffe 1980; Brecher 1972).

Sympathetic nervous system

Cocaine potentiates the responses of sympathetically innervated neurones to noradrenline, adrenaline, and sympathetic nerve stimulation, probably by blocking reuptake of catechol amines at adrenergic nerve endings. This action produces vasoconstriction and mydriasis, contributes to tachycardia, and may precipitate cardiac arrhythmia.

Cardiovascular system

Small doses of cocaine may produce bradycardia as a result of vagal stimulation, but larger doses cause tachycardia from central stimulation and peripheral actions at adrenergic nerve terminals. Rise in blood pressure occurs for similar reasons but large doses produce vasomotor collapse from central depression combined with direct toxic actions on the myocardium.

Body temperature

Cocaine produces hyperthermia probably as a combined result of increased body activity, vasoconstriction, and direct effects on central heat regulating centres.

Acute intoxication

Acute intoxication with cocaine (or amphetamine) produces a state of extreme agitation and a toxic psychosis, with the physical accompaniments of tachycardia, hypertension, cardiac arrhythmias, sweating, hyperpyrexia, and convulsions. Without treatment, death may occur from cardiovascular and respiratory collapse or from convulsions. Drug treatment includes chlorpromazine, which antagonizes the psychotic effects, hypertension and hyperpyrexia, and diazepam as an anticonvulsant. Chronic users may become tolerant to the cardiovascular and hyperthermic effects of both cocaine and amphetamine.

Mechanisms of action

The central stimulant effects of cocaine and other local anaesthetics are usually ascribed to depression of inhibitory pathways due to the local anaesthetic effects on neuronal membranes, i.e. they result from disinhibition rather than stimulation of neurones (Rogers *et al.* 1981). Ritchie and Greene (1981) review some of the evidence for this claim. For example, application of procaine to neurones in isolated slabs of cerebral cortex produces only a depressant effect on directly evoked cortical responses. Similarly, procaine causes only depression of monosynaptic and polysynaptic spinal reflexes. Thirdly, local anaesthetics can produce total anaesthesia when administered to animals after sub-anaesthetic doses of general anaesthetics. Fourthly, local anaesthetics can inhibit convulsions produced by electric shock or pentylenetetrazol.

On the other hand, cocaine and other local anaesthetics produce many stimulant actions which are indistinguishable from those of amphetamine, and there is cross-tolerance between at least some of the actions of cocaine, amphetamine, and other sympathomimetic agents (Leith and Barrett 1981). Amphetamine is known to act largely by releasing catecholamines from nerve endings, although it also has some direct stimulant action on noradrenergic receptors, some catecholamine reuptake blocking activity, and some monoamine oxidase inhibitory action. Sympathomimetic amines, when applied to isolated neurones, cause stimulation in some and inhibition in others. The close similarities between local anaesthetics and indirectly acting sympathomimetic amines suggests that they have some mechanisms of action in common. Of the local anaesthetics, only cocaine blocks the reuptake of catecholamines, and other drugs with this action, such as tricyclic antidepressants, are not reinforcing in animals and are not abused. Thus, reuptake block can be ruled out as a common mechanism of action. Monoamine oxidase inhibition can also be ruled out on several grounds, including the fact that monoamine oxidase inhibitors (except those with additional amphetamine-like actions) are not reinforcing in animals.

Both cocaine and amphetamine produce stereotyped behaviour in man and animals. This can be blocked in animals by dopamine receptor antagonists and by selective lesions in dopaminergic pathways in the corpus striatum. Thus, both drugs appear to enhance dopaminergic activity in parts of the brain. The euphoric effects in both cases also appear to involve dopamine. The reinforcing effects of cocaine and amphetamine in animals (both self-administration and enhanced intracranial self-stimulation) are blocked by the dopamine receptor antagonist pimozide and destruction of dopamine neurones in the nucleus accumbens attenuates dopamine self-administration in rats (Pettit *et al.* 1984). Some central effects of amphetamine are antagonized by inhibition of tyrosine hydroxylase, with consequent decrease in dopamine synthesis, suggesting that amphetamine acts by releasing newly formed dopamine, a possibility recently supported by Langer and Arbilla (1984). Inhibition of this enzyme does not attenuate the central effects of cocaine. However, depletion of central catecholamines with reserpine blocks the effects of cocaine but not those of amphetamine. It is difficult to avoid the conclusion that at least some of the actions of cocaine involve a fairly specific interaction with dopaminergic systems in addition to the local anaesthetic effects, which apply to all neurones. Such an interaction with dopaminergic systems may not involve a mechanism identical with that of amphetamine, but the final effect is similar. As in the case of amphetamine (Chapter 4) interactions with other monoamines, including noradrenaline and serotonin, may also occur with cocaine.

Tolerance, Abuse, Dependence

Acute tolerance to cocaine appears to occur in man, since the euphoric effects following intranasal use decay more quickly than plasma concentrations (Jaffe 1980). To maintain a euphoric state, cocaine addicts tend to take the drug every 30–40 min. Chronic tolerance to the convulsant and cardiorespiratory effects has been reported in man, but increased sensitivity to the sympathetic effects may also occur, and is attributed to catecholamine reuptake block (Ritchie and Greene 1981). Cross tolerance between cocaine and amphetamine has been reported for the anorectic effects (Jaffe 1980) and for the enhancement of intracranial self-stimulation in animals (Leith and Barrett 1981). The latter authors demonstrated that tolerance to chronic amphetamine was due to decreases in post-synaptic dopamine receptor density. The fact that the animals were then tolerant to cocaine, again suggests an action of this drug on dopaminergic systems, although it does not show whether such an action is pre- or post-synaptic. Changes in dopamine receptor density after chronic cocaine administration do not appear to have been systemically studied, but an increase in beta adrenoceptor binding has been reported (Creese and Sibley 1981).

Although the chewing of coca leaves, as practised by natives living high in the Andes, does not give rise to signs of tolerance or dependence, or any difficulties with withdrawal, the taking of cocaine in higher doses by 'snorting' or intravenous injection not only produces an intense 'high' , but can also give rise to compulsive drug-taking behaviour in some subjects. The pattern of drug use is similar for cocaine and amphetamine, and characteristically includes 'runs' of often repeated dosage for several days, followed by periods of abstinence. Animals self-administering these stimulants show similar cyclical patterns (Villarreal and Salazar 1981). Some individuals may use these drugs for months or years without developing a toxic psychosis, which may suddenly appear during the course of a single 'run'. Cocaine and amphetamine use is often combined with the taking of central nervous system depressant drugs, preferably opiates, which are used to combat the dysphoric and psychogenic effects of the stimulants.

Sudden cessation of cocaine after a 'run' of high dosage is followed by a deep sleep lasting 12–18 h or more. Upon awaking, a withdrawal syndrome of craving, lethargy, hunger, sleep disturbance with rebound of REMS, and depression appears and may run a protracted course. The symptoms are immediately alleviated by a further dose of the drug, thus reinstating the pattern. The withdrawal syndrome appears to be more marked with cocaine than with amphetamine, although it is clinically similar. Nevertheless, there is a population of cocaine users who only take an occasional 'snort' and not appear to become dependent, although they are often abusers of other drugs.

Phencyclidine

Phencyclidine was introduced as a general anaesthetic and is structurally related to the anaesthetic agent ketamine. It was used as an anaesthetic in man, but discarded because patients experienced delirium, vivid dreams, and hallucinations on emerging from anaesthesia. However, it became popular as a recreational drug (under the names Angel Dust, PCP, Peace Pill, and others), and by the 1970s it was one of the most commonly abused drugs in the United States. Phencyclidine, and analogues with similar properties, is easy to synthesize and many such agents are sold illicitly as 'street drugs' in America. Ketamine abuse has also been reported. At present the recreational use of such drugs is only sporadic in the United Kingdom, but may be increasing (*British Medical Journal* 1980b).

Pharmacokinetics

Phencyclidine is well absorbed from any route and may be sniffed, smoked, ingested, or injected. It is lipid soluble and widely distributed in the body, and enters the nervous system and cerebrospinal fluid. Hydroxylation occurs in the liver, and the metabolites are conjugated with glucuronic acid and excreted in the urine. There is considerable gastroenteric recirculation which prolongs the action of the drug. The elimination half-life is about 1–2 h after small doses, but up to 3 days after overdose (Jaffe 1980). The conjugates are detectable in the urine for 72 h to 1 week after exposure, depending on dosage (*British Medical Journal* 1980).

Actions

Central nervous system
Acute effects Phencyclidine has anaesthetic, analgesic, central nervous system stimulant and depressant actions, and is one of the most powerful psychotomimetic agents known (Jaffe 1980; *British Medical Journal* 1980b). In man,

small doses produce a sense and appearance of drunkeness with staggering gait, slurred speech, nystagmus, and numbness or complete analgesia of the fingers and toes. At this stage subjects describe a 'high' consisting of euphoria, sense of intoxication, increased response to external stimuli, and general excitement. Sweating, catatonic muscular rigidity, disturbances of body image, disorganized thoughts, restlessness, and anxiety may accompany the 'high'. Bizarre and sometimes aggressive behaviour and a schizophreniform psychosis may occur. There may be amnesia for the episode of intoxication. The typical 'high' from a single dose lasts 4-6 h and is followed by an extended 'coming down' period.

With increasing dosage, analgesia becomes marked and anaesthesia, drowsiness, stupor or coma and convulsions may follow. Anaesthesia and profound analgesia can coexist with normal pharyngeal and laryngeal reflexes. In some anaesthetic doses, a type of sensory isolation may occur (dissociative anaesthesia) in which the subject's eyes are wide open but he appears unresponsive to the environment. However, sensory impulses may reach to the cortex and be experienced in distorted form. Unlike most anaesthetics, phencyclidine stimulates respiratory and cardiovascular systems, and autonomic activity generally: tachycardia, hypertension, sweating, hypersalivation, fever, repetetive movements, and muscle rigidity on stimulation are described. The course of intoxication is prolonged, due to the slow elimination of the drug, and a schizophrenia-like psychosis can persist for several weeks after a single dose. 'Flashback' psychotic episodes may occur several weeks after cesation of phencyclidine use.

Complications of acute phencyclidine intoxication include adrenergic crises precipitating high output cardiac failure, cerebrovascular accidents, malignant hyperthermia, and status epilepticus. Acute rhabdomyolisis has been described, probably resulting from excessive isometric muscular contractions (*British Medical Journal* 1980b). However, the principle causes of death associated with phencyclidine are homicide or suicide. Death from respiratory arrest can occur when phencyclidine is taken with barbiturates.

The management of acute intoxication involves keeping the patient in quiet surroundings; external stimulation aggravates the already hyperexcited state. Fits and muscular rigidity respond to benzodiazepines and haloperidol is recommended for psychotic symptoms. Acidification of the urine and continuous gastric suction hastens elimination of the drug.

Chronic effects Phencyclidine is often abused chronically. About half the users claim to take the drug at least once a week. 'Runs' of drug-taking lasting 2-3 days are not uncommon and are followed by depression and disorientation upon wakening. Some take the drug regularly several times a day. It is sniffed (snorted), taken orally, or injected intravenously, but usually it is sprinkled on tobacco or cannabis and smoked as a cigarette. Polydrug abuse including phencyclidine is also common.

Chronic phencyclidine usage appears to produce an organic brain disorder with long-term neuropsychological damage. Chronic abusers become aggressive, suffer loss of recent memory, have dysphasic speech difficulties and difficulty in time estimation, develop personality disorders with anxiety and a psychosis indistinguishable from schizophrenia which can last 6 months to a year after stopping the drug. Drug tolerance and dependence can almost certainly develop, although the phenomenon has not been fully studied. Phencyclidine is reinforcing in animals and tolerance develops in some species. Monkeys apparently show no clear withdrawal syndrome, even months after chronic administration—possibly because of the slow elimination of the drug. However, craving has been reported in man and compulsive drug use certainly occurs. Some of the symptoms observed in chronic users may represent withdrawal effects.

Mechanisms of action

The mechanisms of action of phencyclidine are at present unknown: various possiblities are discussed by Henderson (1982). Changes in the concentration and turnover of monoamines in the brain have been observed *in vivo*. *In vitro* studies on peripheral tissues, brain slices, and synaptosomal preparations show that phencyclidine competetively inhibits the neuronal uptake of noradrenaline, dopamine, and serotonin at concentrations within the range that induces behavioural changes in animals. Higher concentrations directly increase release of monoamines (Ary and Komiskey 1982). Locally applied phencyclidine also depresses the firing rate of cerebellar Purkinje cells. This effect appears to be mediated by enhancement of activity in the inhibitory noradrenergic pathways from the locus coeruleus to the cerebellar Purkinje neurones, and is possibly due to inhibition of noradrenaline reuptake. This mechanism may explain the ataxia induced by phencyclidine, but whether a similar mechanism underlies the psychological effects is not clear, since other reuptake blockers, such as the tricyclic antidepressants, do not produce similar psychological effects. Other studies have shown that phencyclidine decreases the firing rate of locus coeruleus neurones, increases that of neurones in the substantia nigra and has no effect on dorsal raphe neurones.

Phencyclidine may have some effect at cholinergic synapses. It has muscarinic agonist actions on cardiac muscle and muscarinic antagonistic actions on guinea-pig ileum. It does not appear to have direct effects on nicotinic receptors, but inhibits acetylcholinesterase.

One mechanism which may be common to phencyclidine and some opioids is an interaction with the sigma opioid receptor (Chapter 5). Pert and Quirion (1983) report that radioactively labelled phencyclidine binds to specific receptors in the rat brain, and that it can be displaced by opioids acting on sigma receptors (such as cyclazocine, SKF-10047, pentazocine), but not by monoamine transmitters, neuropeptides, serotonin, LSD, other opioid agonists and antagonists, dopamine receptor agonists and antagonists, benzodiazepines, tetrahydrocannabinol, or local anaesthetics, and only by high concentrations of muscarinic and nicotonic receptor agonists and antagonists. Phencyclidine binding sites are concentrated in the frontal cortex, hippocampus and subiculum. In addition, Pert and Quirion (1983) found a good correlation between receptor affinity and behavioural potency in certain animal tests amongst a range of phencyclidine analogues. It was concluded that the phencyclidine receptor and the sigma opioid receptor are identical and that the psychomimetic effects of phencyclidine and opiates may be related. Greenberg and Segal (1986) suggest that phencyclidine may interact with mu- as well as with sigma- opioid receptors, since some of its behavioural effects (including ingestive behaviour) are similar to those of morphine-like opiates and are antagonised by low doses of naloxone.

However, phencyclidine shares many effects with a large number of psychotropic drugs, including general anaesthetics, alcohol, narcotics, hallucinogens, cocaine, and amphetamine and it is possible that it has several mechanisms of action. Some of the drugs with which phencyclidine has common actions have been linked to schizophrenia (Chapters 13, 14), and an understanding of the modes of action of these drugs might shed light on the neurochemical nature of this psychosis. EEG studies of phencyclidine in Rhesus monkeys syggest that the major sites of action are the limbic and hypothalamic-reticular systems, on which it has biphasic depressant and excitatory effects (Matsuzaki and Dowling 1985).

Organic solvents

The abuse of household and industrial organic solvents appoears to be have originated in the United States and Puerto Rico in the 1950s. It became widespread in the United States in the 1960s and in the United Kingdom in the 1970s, and the practice appears to be growing, not only in the western world but even in some Pacific islands (Daniels and Latcham 1984). Adolescents in relatively deprived social groups are mainly involved; boys somewhat outnumber girls, and glue sniffing has been reported in children as young as 8 years old (King et al. 1981). Some of the substances abused are shown in Table 7.3; they all have properties similar to those of alcohol and gaseous anaesthetics. Usually, the solvent vapour is inhaled by means of a variety of techniques designed to increase the available concentration (such as inhaling deeply from a bag or placing a plastic bag over the head), but occasionally they are ingested in liquid form.

Table 7.3. Some products used in solvent abuse

Antifreeze	Lighter fuel
Dry cleaning products	Nail varnish remover
Dyes	Oven cleaners
Hair lacquers	Paint and paint thinners
Industrial solvents	Petrol
Inks	Polystyrene glues and cements
	Bronchodilator inhalers
	for asthma

Some volatile substances present in abused products

acetone	hexane
amyl acetate	
amyl alcohol	isobutanol
	isopropanol
benzene	
butane	methane
n-butanol	methanol
n-butyl acetate	methylene chloride
	methyl ethyl ketone
Carbon tetrachloride	
Chloroform	perchlorethylene
	propane
1,4 dioxan	*i*-propyl acetate
1,2 dichlorethane	
ethane	styrene
ethanol	
ether	toluene
ethyl acetate	trichlorethane
ethylene chloride	trichlorethylene
	toluene
formaldehyde	
freons	xylene

References: Black 1982; Garriott and Petty 1980; Oliver and Watson 1977.

Pharmacokinetics

The pharmacokinetics of industrial solvents are described by Waldron (1981). They are readily absorbed though the lungs and reach variable concentrations in the blood, depending on the blood/air partition coefficient of individual substances. They are highly lipid soluble and widely distributed in the body, reaching highest concentrations in the nervous system and fat depots.

Actions

Central nervous system

Like general anaesthetics and alcohol, the organic solvents produce a dose-dependent central nervous system depression. Mild intoxication occurs within minutes of inhalation, lasting up to 30 min. However, with judicious repeated sniffing this state can be maintained for up to 12 h (Black 1982). There is an initial euphoria with apparent excitatory effects, probably due to disinhibition, followed, as dosage is increased, by confusion, perceptual distortion, hallucinations, and delusions. At this stage there may be marked aggressive and risk-taking behaviour. As central nervous system depression increases, ataxia, nystagmus, and dysathria become pronounced, followed by drowsiness and coma, and sometimes convulsions. On recovery there may be complete amnesia for the episode. Vomiting may occur at any stage and there is a risk of inhalational asphyxia.

Chronic solvent abuse produces organic damage in the nervous system, and the changes may sometimes be irreversible. Peripheral neuropathy has been described, especially with toluene, tichlorethylene, petrol containing lead, n hexane and methyl butyl ketone. The latter two substances are metabolized to 2,5 hexanedione which causes giant axonal neuropathy. Cerebral cortical atrophy may occur with toluene, petrol containing lead and probably others, and prolonged cerebellar dysfunction may occur with chronic toluene abuse. Optic atrophy has also been described (Black 1982; Waldron 1981; *Drugs Newsletter* 1981; King *et al.* 1981; *Lancet* 1982c) and delayed latencies of visual evoked potentials were noted by Cooper *et al.* (1985).

Psychological changes with chronic use include craving, apathy, impaired psychomotor performance, and possibly precipitation of schizophrenia (Daniels and Latcham 1984). Drug dependence definitely occurs and withdrawal symptoms probably contribute to continued use. Chronic solvent abusers have a variety of somatic and psychological complaints including headaches, photophobia, anxiety, irritability, tremor, sleep disturbance, hallucinations, anorexia, nausea vomiting, abdominal pain, fits, tinnitus, diplopia, and paraesthesiae (O'Connor 1984). These symptoms probably represent a mixture of toxic and withdrawal effects.

Liver

Chloroform and carbon tetrachloride and other dry-cleaning fluids are potent hepatotoxics, producing fatty infiltration of the liver and, in high doses, centrilobular necrosis. Trichlorethylene and related drugs can also cause liver damage but only at high concentrations. Some of the hepatotoxic efects may be due to the formation of free radicals during metabolism (Waldron 1981).

Kidney

Organic solvents which are hepatotoxic are also nephrotoxic, particularly carbon tetrachloride and chloroform. The main effects are on the proximal tubule, and result in polyuria, glycosuria, proteneinuria and, in massive doses, anuria and renal failure. Probably, renal metabolism to free radical intermediates is responsible for the damage, as in the liver (Waldron 1981).

Cardiovascular system

Solvent abusers sometimes die suddenly from cardiac arrhythmias. High concentrations of fluorocarbon propellants and halogenated hydrocarbon solvents have been particularly incriminated, and butane is also cardiotoxic (Black 1982). The mechanisms of action are discussed by Garriott and Petty (1980), and Waldron (1981).

Respiratory tract

Many organic solvents are irritant to the respiratory tract mucosa and can cause laryngeal spasm when sprayed directly into the mouth. Cough, increase in upper respiratory tract secretions, reddening of the conjunctiva, and a pustular rash around the mouth occur in chronic abusers. Inhalation of vomitus during intoxication can cause further respiratory complications, and aerosol residues in the lungs can cause asphyxiation.

Bone Marrow

Haematological complications appear to be rare. However benzene can produce aplastic anaemia and bone marrow suppression possibly by inhibition of DNA synthesis. Exposure to benzene has also been associated with an increased risk of leukaemia (Waldron 1982).

Pregnancy

Organic solvents readily cross the placenta and when taken in late pregnancy may cause neonatal depression. There is also a suspicion that they may have teratogenic effects (Ashton 1985).

Mortality

Between 1970 and 1981 there were 117 deaths in the United Kingdom associated with abuse of volatile substances (Black 1982). Causes of death include accidents or suicide during intoxication, asphyxiation, cardiac arrhythmia, and hepatic and renal failure.

Dependence, tolerance, withdrawal syndrome

Earlier reports suggested that physical dependence did not occur in solvent abusers (Glaser and Massengale 1962). Many adolescents appear to sniff organic solvents as part of a group activity and after a short period move on to some other activity. However, further experience indicates that drug dependence can occur and is not uncommon in 'solitary sniffers' who use solvents as adults use alcohol and regularly become intoxicated and euphoric (Herzberg and Wolkind 1983). Tolerance is evidenced by the observation that 'in the initial stages of inhalation, prior to habit formation, a few whiffs of the vapors will produce a "jag"... but chronic users often have to "take" the contents of as many as 5 tubes ... of cement in order to experience the desired results' (Glaser and Massengale 1962, p. 90). O'Connor (1982) describes several chronic abusers taking regular inhalations at least 4 days a week for a minimum of 3 h a day, with a history of abuse of at least 6 months. In cases of this sort, abrupt cessation of organic solvents undoubtedly gives rise to a withdrawal syndrome. This appears to be similar to the alcohol abstinence syndrome, although usually milder, and includes anxiety, tremor, hallucinations, sleep disturbances, and a variety of somatic and psychological symptoms.

The mechanisms of action on the brain and the central changes involved in tolerance and withdrawal have not been systematically studied for organic solvents. It seems likely, however, that they are fundamentally similar to those of alcohol. Methods of treatment and sociological factors in solvent abuse are discussed by O'Connor (1982, 1984); Lowenstein (1982), and Herzberg and Wolkind (1983).

Part III
Learning and memory

8

Learning and memory systems

Learning and memory can be viewed as a system for modifying behaviour as a result of experience. Both functionally and anatomically this system is inextricably bound up with the systems for arousal (Chapter 2), and for reward and punishment (Chapter 5). In the simplest terms, arousal supplies the necessary degree of alertness and attention while reward/punishment supplies motivation, and the degree of either attention or motivation affects the efficiency of learning and memory. The three systems operate in synchrony, utilizing the same neurotransmitters and modulators, and relaying in many of the same brain structures and pathways.

Each new experience to which an animal is exposed is interpreted in the light of previous memories. The brain does not merely act as a blank screen for recording facts; it translates and edits external or internal information on the basis of previously acquired information. Just as the brain exerts a control over its own sensory input, as described in Chapter 2, so it selects which experiences are laid down as a basis for future action and which are discarded or forgotten.

The process of learning involves physical as well as functional changes in the brain. Yet there is no separate structure for memory, which resides to some degree in every living cell. In the central nervous system, various structures make particular contributions to certain aspects of memory, and there is considerable localization of function for specialized forms of memory. Even so, multiple interconnections between many parts of the brain are involved, and the formation and retrieval of memories is probably possible through numerous alternative and simultaneously active pathways. There is no discrete location in the brain for any one memory; rather each memory is synthesized as a pattern of selective neural activity in many pathways and in many areas. Activity in these pathways is almost infinitely adaptable and learned behaviours can be altered or reversed by later experience. There is increasing evidence, discussed below, that the crucial neural alterations necessary for memory occur at synapses. The speed and efficiency of learning and memory and the capacity for information storage and retrieval are closely allied to, and may even constitute, the quality described as intelligence.

The general organization of learning and memory systems and some of the mechanisms thought to be involved are outlined in this chapter. The localization and biochemistry of memory in man is further explored in Chapter 9 in relation to clinical memory disorders, while some drugs which affect memory functions are described in Chapter 10.

Stages of learning and memory

Learning and memory are conventionally described as a continuum of stages: (1) *acquisition* or registration of information, (2) *ultra-short-term memory* (immediate memory), a transient form of retention by means of which information of transitory significance, such as a series of digits, is retained for a matter of seconds, (3) *short-term memory* (intermediate memory), a temporary form of retention which may last for minutes, hours or days and may be prolonged by 'rehearsal' —mental repetition of the data, (4) *long-term memory* a form of retention in which information, initially in short-term memory, is transferred to a more permanent store (*consolidation*) which may endure for decades or even a life-time. Finally (5) *retrieval* (recall), is a process whereby stored information is selectively made accessible as required. Whether or not these hypothetical stages of memory are really separate (and particularly whether long-term memories are stored or encoded in a different form from shorter-term memories) is controversial.

During learning, all the stages operate simultaneously. For example, new information, after initial registration, enters immediate or short-term memory; on the second and subsequent presentations, the information is added to that already entered in short-term memory, which is recalled as the information becomes familiar. Meanwhile, data relevant to the new information is retrieved from long-term memory, and finally the newly learned information, interpreted and edited in the light of previous experience, is itself consolidated and stored in long-term memory. Since learning depends on information storage, all types of learning are based on memory, and learning and memory can be viewed as parts of the same process. Some authors however, prefer to separate them (Zornetzer 1978).

Types of learning

Several types of learning have been described (Kupferman 1981). More complex types of learning may be based on these elementary forms, but the many processes of 'higher' learning, especially those involving language, are not fully understood.

Habituation

Habituation is the decrease in a behavioural response following repetition of an initially novel stimulus, such as diminution of the startle response to a repeated sound. 'Habituation ... is probably the most widespread of all forms of learning. Through habituation animals, including human beings, learn to ignore stimuli that have lost novelty or meaning ... Habituation is thought to be the first learning process to emerge in human infants and is commonly used to study the development of intellectual processes such as attention, perception and memory'. (Kandel 1979; p. 64) Failure of normal habituation may occur in certain mental diseases such as schizophrenia and after some psychotropic drugs such as LSD (Chapters 13 and 14).

Sensitization

Sensitization is a slightly more complex form of learning which consists of a prolonged enhancement of the response to a stimulus if it is preceded by a noxious or intense stimulus. 'Whereas habituation requires an animal to learn to ignore a particular stimulus because its consequences are trivial, sensitization requires the animal to learn to attend to a stimulus because it is accompanied by potentially painful or dangerous consequences' (Kandel 1979; p. 67). Clearly both types of learning are accompanied by changes in arousal. Sensitization has been described as a precursor form of classical Pavlovian conditioning; in both types of learning a response to one stimulus is enhanced as a result of activation by a different stimulus.

Operant conditioning

Operant conditioning, described by Thorndike (1911), represents a process of trial and error learning. For example, if a rat is placed in a cage containing a protruding lever it will, in its random activity, occasionally press the lever. If this action is rewarded by food or drink or punished by an electric foot-shock, the animal soon learns to associate the action with the outcome and to modify its behaviour accordingly. Thus, the frequency of lever pressing increases if the result is rewarding (reinforcement) and declines if the result is aversive (punishment). An interaction with reward and punishment systems is obviously necessary for this type of learning.

Classical conditioning

Classical conditioning was described by Pavlov (1927) who showed that if a neutral (conditional) stimulus such as the sound of a bell is repeatedly paired with a second (unconditional) stimulus, such as food on the tongue, the animal learns to associate the two stimuli and will respond to the first stimulus in anticipation of the second. Thus, the sound of the bell initially elicits little overt response although the presentation of the food evokes obvious responses including salivation. After conditioning, the bell alone evokes many of the responses, including salivation, originally elicited only by the food. A conditioned response also develops if the second stimulus is aversive.

In both operant and classical conditioning, the strength of the response is related to the probability of occurrence of reinforcement or punishment. If after conditioning the expected result no longer occurs, the response undergoes *extinction*, a form of relearning which terminates a response to a stimulus which is no longer relevant. However not every stimulus or response needs to be reinforced to maintain conditioning; the rate of extinction can be slowed by various systems of partial reinforcement. In operant conditioning, the highest rates of response are obtained when rewards only occur after a number of responses have been made. In both types of conditioning the time interval between the stimulus or operant response and the reinforcement is critical; in general the longer the delay the poorer the associative learning.

There is evidence (Siegal 1975, 1983) that operant and classical conditioning, both of which involve reward and punishment systems (Chapter 5), contribute to drug dependence and behavioural tolerance to drugs in man and animals (Chapters 6, 7).

Types of memory

The tremendous scope and complexity of memory defies classification. Some categories of memory which have been classified largely from clinical data in man and lesion experiments in animals are mentioned here. They do not, however, cover the full range and subtlety of memory or convey how a single word can conjure up a host of further associations—pictures, smells, events, emotions, and other phenomena—and also trigger off a variety of physical responses.

Short-term memory

Although there is no direct evidence, it has been widely accepted that immediate and short-term memory may depend on reverberatory neural circuits maintained by excitatory feedback connections, and that such memories are temporarily encoded in terms of the firing patterns of complex sets of neurones (Hebb 1949). Immediate memory has a limited capacity of five to ten items in man and is acoustically rather than semantically coded (Warrington 1981). At some stage more permanent changes (perhaps synaptic) are thought to occur, with the result that a selection of the information is preserved in a more lasting form.

Long-term memory

There is evidence that long-term memory involves several functionally and anatomically separate systems, which can be selectively impaired by localized damage to the brain (Warrington 1981; Oakley 1981; Ojemann 1983). This hierarchy of different types of memory has developed with the expansion of the brain and of more sophisticated forms of environmental adaptation in the course of evolution (Oakley 1981). In practice, however, the different types of memory function interdependently.

Association memory

Association memory is the form of memory involved in learning by operant or classical conditioning. It requires the formation of an association between two events (e.g. stimulus and reinforcement or conditional and unconditional stimuli). This type of memory appears primarily to involve subcortical structures. It survives total removal of the neocortex in mammals; it can still be demonstrated after removal of all brain tissue rostral to the thalamus in the rat; and is still present after severe reductions in neural mass in man (Oakley 1981). The major locus for the associative mechanism is thought to be in the brainstem reticular formation.

Event memory or representational memory

A second type of memory has been termed event memory (Warrington 1981) or representational memory (Oakley 1981). This type of memory forms a record of the individual's experiences. A major difference from association memory is that event memory includes the ability to retain a representation or image of a prior event in the absence of the original stimulus. In addition, event memory involves not only the storage of single events, but also their organization into a spatiotemporal map or template which allows an orientation of each event in relation to space and time. The existence of such a template also confers predictive ability; future events can be compared or matched with past events, allowing appropriate action to be taken in familiar or unfamiliar circumstances.

The capacity of event memory is very large; indeed for practical purposes it is almost infinite (Warrington 1981). However, it is relatively unstable and appears to undergo continuous modification, possibly as a result of interaction with previous and subsequent learning and memories (Piaget and Inhelder 1969; Kupferman 1978). For example, subjects asked to repeat a previously learned story tend to shorten and reconstruct it, making alterations from the original and emphasizing the most important points. Apparent forgetting may therefore be due to reinterpretation as well as to failure to register, store or retrieve information. The neurological substrates for event memory consist of diencephalic and temporal lobe structures, including the hippocampus, mammillary bodies, certain thalamic nuclei, and the frontal neocortex. In man, event memory may be selectively impaired in the amnesic syndrome (Chapter 9) in which there is damage to these structures. Memory for recent events is more vulnerable to disturbance than that for remote events.

Semantic memory or abstract memory

Semantic memory (Warrington 1981) or abstract memory (Oakley 1981) is memory for words, facts, and concepts, including numerical concepts. It represents a general store of information composed of facts abstracted from several specific instances. The items in the memory are context free and lacking in spatiotemporal identity, and the meaning of objects and events are preserved separately from memories of the specific incidents in which they occurred. Such memories appear to represent abstracts of a prototype for each item as a result of the entry of similar examples into storage (Oakley, 1981). Semantic memory has a very large, but probably limited capacity; it is extremely durable and relatively accessible. Thus, normal individuals have a large though limited vocabulary, and their visual and auditory memory of words and the meaning of words is immediate, almost permanent, and relatively unchanged by use. Semantic memory is associated primarily with the neocortex, particularly the occipital, parietal and temporal regions. Specialized cortical areas are involved in memory for language and are discussed further below and in Chapter 9.

Recognition memory

The ability to recognize places, people, objects, or events may involve semantic, event, and association memory systems. Conscious recognition of the *meaning* of sensory stimuli depends on semantic memory, and cortical lesions may result in 'psychic blindness' or agnosia. For example, destruction of the temporal cortex in the Rhesus monkey or man leads to inability to differentiate edible from inedible objects and loss of fear reactions to previously frightening visual stimuli (Oakley, 1981). Agnosia may be limited to one sensory modality: in visual agnosia an object is not recognized by sight but may be recognized by touch, while the opposite is true of tactile agnosia. In prosopagnosia in man (discussed by Damasio, 1985), there is inability to recognize by sight previously familiar faces, although faces as a category are recognized, and the familiar person may be recognized by voice. This agnosia results from bilateral lesions of occipitotemporal cortex. Prosopagnosia does not occur with unilateral lesions and it appears that each hemisphere can recognize faces via different strategies.

Despite the lack of conscious recognition, there is evidence that familiar faces are recognized at subcortical levels, since the faces of the subject himself, relatives, or friends generate greater autonomic responses than unfamiliar faces. This observation suggests that one level of recognition involves association memory. The lack of conscious recognition appears to be due to a failure of visual stimuli to activate other memories pertinent to the familiar face and suggests the existence of a template system for the individual recognition of faces. Such a template system or visuospatial map is an attribute of event memory, involving subcortical temporal lobe structures including the hippocampus. Failure of recognition of previously (and often) experienced faces, places, pictures, etc., occurs in the amnesic syndrome, associated with damage to these structures. Such stimuli never become familiar, however often they are repeated. Possibly such experiences are normally processed through event memory at each repetition, before being abstracted into semantic memory. The various aspects of recognition memory demonstrate the interdependence of the several categories of memory.

Motor memory

Motor memory is the ability to store and recall motor movements in temporal and spatial sequence. It appears to be subserved by a system located in the cerebellum (Marr, 1969; Young 1979; Iverson 1977; Anderson 1982).

Neural mechanisms of learning and memory

In the widest sense learning and memory are incorporated in every body cell. The coding of information in DNA constitutes a type of genetic memory which interacts with the environment to determine which of a range of possible characteristics are selected for expression. In the nervous system too, the basis of learning and memory appears to be a process of selection between a range of genetically possible patterns of neural activity, followed by amplification of the selected paths and shutting down of alternative paths (Young 1979; Mark 1978; Marr, 1969; Eccles, 1977; Changeux and Danchin, 1976; Edelman, 1978). It seems likely that many of the underlying changes occur at the synaptic level and involve most of the brain as well as the spinal cord and probably much of the peripheral nervous system. However, different parts of the brain make specific contributions to various aspects of learning and memory. The major advantage of learning and memory in the nervous system is that it is far more plastic and rapidly adaptable than genetic memory and can alter behaviour in response to short-term or unpredictable changes in the environment.

Synaptic plasticity

Several recent studies have shown that synapses are capable of undergoing both structural and functional modification in response to environmental alterations. These modifications result in changes of synaptic efficiency and may increase or decrease the likelihood of transmission of impulses, with consequent modulation of behaviour. In some cases such synaptic plasticity appears to be directly linked to learning and memory.

Learning in invertebrates

Habituation Some mechanisms of learning and memory have been elucidated for the sea hare *Aplysia californica* (Kandel 1978, 1979, 1983; Kandel and Schwartz 1982). This mollusc has a reflex for withdrawing its gill in response to stimulation of mechanoreceptors in the skin. The reflex involves mono-synaptic connections between skin sensory neurones and gill motoneurones, and exhibits habituation, sensitization, and a form of classical conditioning.

Short-term habituation, lasting a few hours, can be induced rapidly in a single training session of 10–15 tactile stimuli. It has been shown to be due to a progressive decline in amplitude of the synaptic potentials generated by the sensory terminals as the innocuous stimulus is repeated. The diminution of synaptic transmission is due to shutting down of calcium channels at the sensory nerve terminals with a consequent reduction of the amount of neurotransmitter released at the sensory-motor synapse. Eventually, insufficient transmitter is released to evoke an action potential in the motoneurones, and no withdrawal response is elicited.

Long-term habituation, lasting for weeks, can be induced over four training sessions of 10 stimuli each. In this case, similar but more profound changes in synaptic efficiency occur with disruption of the functional connections of many previously effective synapses. These results show that short-term and long-term habituation involve the same neuronal loci, and suggest that short-term and long-term memory share a common locus, the synapse, and differ only in the degree of functional change induced by learning.

Sensitization Sensitization of the gill withdrawal reflex can be elicited by a strong stimulus to the head of the animal. As with habituation, sensitization can last for hours or weeks, depending on the amount of training. In short-term sensitization, Kandel (1979) showed that noxious stimuli activate facilitatory interneurones which liberate serotonin at the terminals of the sensory neurones from the mechanoreceptors involved in the reflex. The serotonin increases the amount of 3′,5 cyclic AMP in the presynaptic sensory terminals. Through a series of steps, this increase leads to opening of calcium channels and an increased release of transmitter at the sensory-motor synapse. Consequently there is increased spike-propagation at the post-synaptic motoneurone and a greater reflex response occurs.

In long-term sensitization following noxious stimuli repeated over a few days, there is enhancement of the connections made by the sensory neurones on both the facilitatory interneurone and the motoneurones, with even further release of transmitter. In addition, the response becomes generalized to include increased escape locomotion and other defensive reflexes.

Classical Conditioning A form of classical conditioning can also be demonstrated in *Aplysia* (Kandel 1983). If an unconditional noxious stimulus producing sensitization is paired for a few days with a conditional stimulus (exposure to shrimp extract which normally produces no response), the animal learns to respond with all the signs of long-term sensitization to the conditional stimulus alone. The mechanism for this response has not been elucidated, but it is suggested that the unconditional stimulus increases the activity of the facilitatory interneurones. This type of associative learning also occurs in other invertebrates including the octopus (Young 1966) and appears similar to the classical conditioning demonstrated in dogs by Pavlov (1927).

These simple forms of learning thus involve (presynaptic) modulation of the strength of previously existing synaptic connections. What is known of the properties of neurones and synapses of higher animals, including the importance of calcium currents in synaptic transmission (Berridge 1981), suggests that similar processes may occur in more complex forms of learning. However, as discussed later, post-synaptic mechanisms may be of equal or greater importance in mammals.

Collateral sprouting in vertebrates

There is evidence in vertebrates for the growth of new synapses, for the activation of previously 'silent' synapses, and for change in the efficacy of existing synapses in the brain. For example, if kittens or newborn macaque monkeys are monocularly deprived by surgical closure of one eye during a critical period of their development, plastic changes occur in the connections to the visual cortex (Wiesel and Hubel 1963; Hubel and Wiesel 1977; Pettigrew 1978). The cortical columns which receive imput from the normal eye become enlarged at the expense of those receiving imput from the deprived eye, so that most of the neurones are activated only by the eye which has been open, instead of most neurones being binocularly activated, as in normal animals. This alteration may be due to synaptic competition, the input from the open eye displacing the synapses of the deprived eye terminals. These plastic changes do not occur if the noradrenergic neocortical projections of the locus coeruleus are destroyed by intraventricular injections of 6-hydroxydopamine, but a degree of cortical plasticity can be restored by localized perfusion with noradrenaline (Pettigrew, 1978). The mechanism of these catecholamine-induced effects is not known; some possibilities are discussed by Mayes (1983).

Such morphological and functional synaptic plasticity is not limited to the growing nervous system of immature animals, but also occurs in adults (Raisman 1969; Bjorkelund and Stenevi 1979). For example, Azmitia (1978) showed in the adult rat hippocampus that normal serotonergic fibres in the infracallosal bundle exhibited collateral sprouting in response to destruction of supracallosal serotonergic fibres. The new fibres reinnervated the denervated areas of the dorsal hippocampus and took over the function of the degenerated neurones. Tsukahara (1981) demonstrated similar collateral sprouting in the cat red nucleus following lesions of some of its connections. At present it appears that while several fibre systems have the potential to sprout, others for reasons which are not clear, do not.

Studies of structural plasticity in the brain of adult songbirds are reviewed by Bottjer and Arnold (1984). In the canary the size and weight of certain brain nuclei are directly related to the learning of song sequences: the greater the vocal virtuosity, the greater the volume of these song-control nuclei, demonstrating a correlation between the degree of learning and the amount of space devoted to it in the brain. The canary's song-control nuclei are influenced by testosterone and enlarge each spring in male birds, coincident with a rise in endogenous testosterone concentration and the onset of singing. Female birds do not normally sing and have small or absent song-related nuclei. However, these can be induced by treatment with testosterone in adults and with the development of song-control nuclei, female birds start to sing. Histological studies reveal that testosterone treatment in females increases the size of the dendritic field of the neurones in the song-related nuclei, presumably increasing the number of synaptic connections made. In addition, Paton and Nottebohm (1984) showed by radioactive labelling techniques that neurogenesis can occur in the song-control nuclei of adult canaries and that the newly generated neurones are incorporated into functional brain circuits.

Functional synaptic changes in vertebrates

More rapidly occurring functional synaptic changes, without collateral sprouting, have been demonstrated in the red nucleus in a cat preparation and shown to be associated with learning by classical conditioning (Tsukahara 1981; Fig. 8.1). Corticorubral fibres in the cerebral peduncle were stimulated electrically as the conditional stimulus, after section of the cerebral peduncle caudal to the red nucleus. This initially produced no behavioural response. Electrical stimulation of the forelimb skin, to produce flexion, was used as the unconditional stimulus. After 5 days of training in which the two stimuli were paired, the conditional stimuli alone produced forelimb flexion. This conditioned reflex also showed extinction in the classical manner. The neurological substrate of the conditioned change, which could last for several weeks, appeared to be a functional alteration in efficacy of the corticorubral synapses, since there was no evidence of axonal sprouting and no detectable change in transmission along any other of the pathways involved in the reflex.

Long-term potentiation Functional synaptic changes may also account for the phenomenon of long-term potentiation described in the rat and rabbit hippocampus (Bliss 1979; Bliss and Gardner-Medwin, 1973). Electrical stimulation of the perforant pathway to the hippocampus produces an extracellular post-synaptic potential or synaptic wave in the hippocampus. The amplitude of this synaptic wave remains constant if test shocks are given at intervals of 2–3 s, but if the test shocks are interrupted by brief trains of higher frequency conditioning shocks (10 Hz or more), a large increase in the amplitude of the synaptic wave develops (Fig. 8.2). The effect occurs within minutes of one 50 s burst of conditioning shocks, and after three or four such trains the

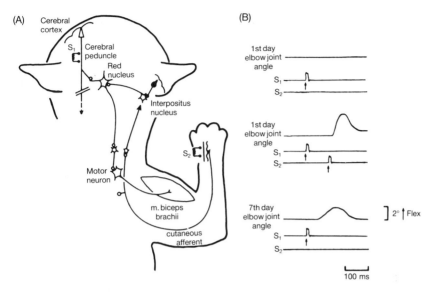

Fig. 8.1. Classical conditioning mediated by the red nucleus in the cat. (A) Arrangement of experimental preparation. (B) Record of elbow flexion on first and seventh day after conditioning. S_1, conditional stimulus (electrical stimulation of corticorubral fibres in the cerebral peduncle, after section caudal to the red nucleus). S_2, unconditional stimulus (electrical stimulation of forelimb skin). S_1 initially produced no elbow flexion, but after 5 days training in which S_1 and S_2 were paired, S_1 alone produced this response. (From Tsukahara 1981.)

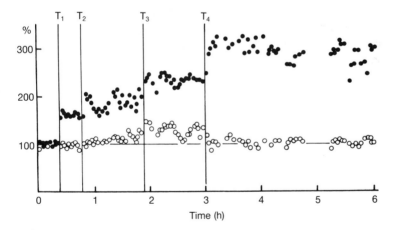

Fig.8.2. Long-term potentiation in the hippocampus. Stimulating and recording electrodes located bilaterally in the perforant path. Conditioning trains (15 Hz for 10 s) delivered to one side at times 1–4. Amplitude of synaptic wave evoked by a contant test shock (ordinate) plotted against time (abscissa). Open circles, control side; filled circles, conditioned side. (From Bliss 1979.)

synaptic wave can show a 300 per cent increase in amplitude which can last for days. This phenomenon has been shown in anaesthetised and awake rats and rabbits and in *in vitro* preparations of hippocampal slices. Possible links with memory and learning include the observation that senescent and malnourished rats are deficient in simple memory tasks, and also in the ability to sustain long-term potentiation and that the amplitude of the long-term potentiation is correlated with the speed of complex maze learning.

Both pre- and post-synaptic mechanisms may be involved in the genesis and maintenance of hippocampal long-term potentiation (Bliss and Dolphin 1982; Rawlins 1984). There appears to be an increased release of excitatory neurotransmitters including glutamate and aspartate. In addition, the phenomenon is extremely sensitive to calcium ion concentration. Long-term potentiation can be prevented from occurring in hippocampal slices by reducing the concentration of calcium in the batheing medium, and can be induced by increasing calcium ion concentration. These calcium-induced changes suggest a mechanism similar to that of sensitization in *Aplysia*. However, post-synaptic changes have also been observed in relation to long-term potentiation. These include an increase in the diameter of dendritic spines, an increase in the number of synapses and an increase in the density of glutamate receptors. In addition, there may be an increase in coupling mechanisms related to spike-generation in individual neurones. These changes are discussed further below.

Dendritic spines Several authors (cited by Crick 1982; Bliss 1979) have drawn attention to the possible importance of dendritic spines in synaptic plasticity. Dendritic spines are small projections from the dendrites of certain types of neurones (pyramidal cells and stellate cells; Peters *et al.* 1976; Fig. 8.3). Spiny cells are numerous in the cerebral and cerebellar cortex, accounting for about 90 per cent of neurones in the cerebral cortex, and each may have from 300 to 30 000 spines. The spines are synaptic sites and most of them are believed to be excitatory, accounting for the great majority of excitatory synapses in the cerebral cortex. In most neurones the dendritic spines are post-synaptic, and vesicles of neurotransmitter can be seen on the pre-synaptic terminals with which they make contact.

The function of dendritic spines is not known, but it has been suggested that alterations in their width or conformation might account for some types of synaptic plasticity (Crick 1982; Koch and Poggio 1983). Contraction of a spine would increase the width of its neck, reducing its electrical resistance and increasing the amplitude of a synaptic current being conducted into a dendrite and reaching the impulse-generating site of the nerve cell (the initial segment of the axon). Converse changes in electrical resistance would occur if the neck of the spine elongated and became narrower. Large variations in the size and shape of spines, seen on the same dendrite, have been observed

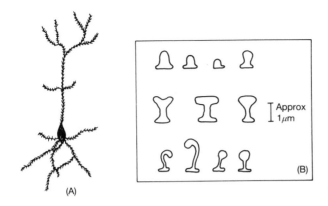

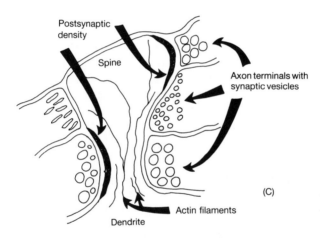

Fig. 8.3. Dendritic spines. (A) Pyramidal cell showing dendritic spines. (B) Observed variations in shape and form of dendritic spines. (C) Dendritic spine bearing synapses with axon terminals containing large, small, and elongated synaptic vesicles. (References: Crick 1982; Peters *et al.* 1976.)

(Peters *et al.* 1976; Fig. 8.3) and increases in the diameter of dendritic spines have been reported in the hippocampus after high frequency stimulation of the perforant pathway under conditions that give rise to long-term potentiation (Bliss 1979).

Matus *et al.* (1982), and Fifkova and Delay (1982) have demonstrated the presence of the contractile protein actin in dendritic spines in the rat cortex and hippocampus. They suggest that the actin is triggered to contract by the influx of calcium ions at the end of the action potential. The greater and more prolonged the amount of synaptic activity, the larger the calcium influx and the greater the conductance change caused by dendritic spine contraction. Very rapid changes in synaptic efficiency produced by muscle contraction might occur during short-term memory, while longer-lasting conductance changes produced by repeated synaptic activity could facilitate learning and consolidation of memory by ensuring preferential selection of the pathways involved on future repetitions of the same stimuli, at the expense of other possible pathways. In certain areas of the brain, patterns of activity unique to each event could be envisaged to be built up over time. Portions or segments of these patterns might gradually be strengthened by events, while portions would tend to fade through under-use as the dendritic spines slowly reverted to their uncontracted state. In this way, the patterns for each memory would constantly be edited and changed over the years.

Increased receptor density The properties of dendritic spines and the phenomenon of long-term potentiation have been linked in a biochemical hypothesis of memory (Fig. 8.4; Lynch and Baudry 1984; Siman *et al.* 1985). These authors propose that in certain pathways of the brain the release of the excitatory neurotransmitter glutamate, following brief bursts of high frequency neural activity, produces a transient elevation of calcium in (post-synaptic) dendritic spines. This ionic change activates a membrane-associated proteinase (calpain), which has been demonstrated to occur in neural membranes. The enzyme degrades a membrane protein, fodrin, which has also been identified as a substrate for calpain. Degradation of fodrin exposes glutamate receptors on the post-synaptic membrane of the dendritic spines. The increase in the number of active glutamate receptors increases the size of the postsynaptic potential. Repetition of the these events is followed by contraction of actin filaments in the neck of the dendritic spine causing structural changes and permanent exposure of glutamate receptors, with long-lasting synaptic potentiation.

Lynch and Baudry (1984) have demonstrated that calpain, which is sensitive to low concentrations of calcium, is present only in the cortex, striatum, and hippocampus and not in the brainstem. Furthermore, the activity of the enzyme is greatly reduced at temperatures below the body temperature of mammals. These observations suggest that the mechanism accounts for 'higher' forms of learning involving the telencephalon of mammals. In support of the hypothesis, increased glutamate binding has been demonstrated in the telencephalon after learning in rats and rabbits, and inhibition of calpain by leupeptin was shown to impair several forms of learning in these rodents.

Formation of new synapses In addition to increased efficiency in individual synapses, there is considerable evidence for the formation of new synapses during learning. Greenhough (1984) has shown that synaptic density is more than doubled after long-term potentiation in rat hippocampal slices. The

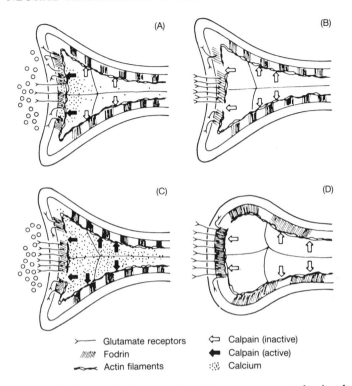

>— Glutamate receptors	⇦ Calpain (inactive)
///// Fodrin	◀ Calpain (active)
⌒ Actin filaments	⠋ Calcium

Fig. 8.4. Hypothetical synaptic changes subserving memory: a mechanism by which brief periods of high frequency activity produce long-lasting changes in synaptic efficacy. (A) Release of glutamate, following brief bursts of high frequency neural activity, causes a transient elevation of calcium in postsynaptic dendritic spines. This change activates the enzyme calpain which degrades fodrin, uncovering occluded glutamate receptors. (B) Calcium is removed from the spine, inactivating calpain. (C) Subsequent high frequency activity produces a larger influx of calcium because of the greater number of receptors. This stimulates fodrin throughout the spine causing widespread disruption of the fodrin network and leads to a configurational change in the dendritic spine. (D) Calcium is again eliminated, but the structural and receptor changes remain. (From Lynch and Baudry 1984.)

increase involved synapses onto axonal shafts and a specific type of dendritic spine synapse (sessile spines). Increases in synaptic density and in the frequency of dendritic spines were also observed in the occipital cortex of rats reared in complex, 'enriched' environments compared with litter mates reared singly or in groups in standard laboratory cages. The relationship of such changes to learning was demonstrated by experiments in which rats were exposed to maze training after total transection of the corpus callosum and eye occlusion arranged to direct visual input to one hemisphere. In these rats, increases in synaptic numbers were found in occipital cortical pyramidal neurones only in the hemisphere exposed to visual stimulation during maze training. Greenhough (1984) suggests that in young animals learning is dependent upon the establishment of synapses in preferred pathways, among a selection of potential connections, while in adults it is dependent on making new synaptic connections in already established pathways.

The relation of memory to 'intelligence' is discussed by Hendrickson (1983a,b) and current theories on the biological basis of intelligence are brought together by Eysenck (1983).

Localization of learning and memory functions

Reward and punishment systems

Although in cellular terms learning and memory are widely represented in the brain, different parts appear to be organised to contribute in different and specific ways. Young (1966, 1979) has described in the octopus brain separate pairs of lobes that signal reinforcement or punishment for vision and touch. The output from these lobes allows the animal to select either approach/attack or avoidance behaviour for the object seen or touched, and it can be conditioned to avoid objects if their presence is paired with a painful electrical shock. Removal of the lobe signalling punishment deprives the octopus of the ability to learn *not* to approach objects even when such behaviour results in painful shocks.

Reinforcement and punishment pathways in vertebrates (Chapter 5) are intimately concerned with learning and the selection of approach or avoidance behaviour. Rolls *et al.* (1981), in microelectrode recordings from single cells in the monkey hypothalamus, found certain neurones which responded only when a visual discrimination stimulus presented to the animal was associated with a food reward, not to stimuli associated with saline. The activity of such neurones was suggested to underlie stimulus-reinforcement associations. Routtenberg (1978) found that continuous electrical stimulation of some rewarding areas (median forebrain bundle, substantia nigra, frontal cortex) during learning in the rat disrupts subsequent recall, but if the animals are allowed to self-stimulate for reward after learning, their retention is improved. He suggests that 'when something is learned, activity in the brain-reward pathways facilitates the formation of memory' (Routtenberg 1978; p. 129).

In the reward/punishment system, a specific role for the amygdala in learning and memory has been suggested by several authors. For example, Kapp and Gallagher (1979) noted that tests associated with painful stimuli were readily remembered and in many species the possibility of receiving a repeat stimulus evoked a fear reaction leading to avoidance. The site of this memory system may be based in the amygdala and may involve an opioid mediation since retention of aversive stimuli in rats is influenced by opioid agonists and antagonists, injected into the amygdala. The authors suggested that an amygdaloid opioid system is involved in generating an emotional component to painful experiences, and may interact with the noradrenergic system of the locus coruleus with which it has anatomical connections. Kesner and Hardy (1983) suggest that the amygdala encodes, stores, and retrieves the hedonic qualities—rewarding or aversive—of all stimuli. In this function it interacts with the hippocampus, which at the same time encodes the environmental context of the same specific memory.

Arousal systems

The locus coeruleus (Mason 1979, 1980) and the amygdala (Douglas and Pribram 1966) may also be important in selective attention which, along with optimal activation of arousal systems, appears to be necessary for efficient learning and memory. In particular, lesions of the locus coeruleus in animals cause perseveration of inappropriate behaviour, increased distractibility and overinclusiveness of attention. Involvement of the locus coeruleus in arousal, anxiety, and reward systems is mentioned in Chapters 2, 3, and 5, respectively. The possible relationship of paradoxical sleep to memory is discussed in Chapter 2.

The hippocampus

Both the locus coeruleus and the amygdala have anatomical connections with the hippocampus which is widely believed to play a specific though complex role in memory functions, particularly in relation to event memory. It and the cerebral cortex are the only brain structures in animals known to exhibit long-term potentiation (described above), and many clinical studies indicate its importance in human memory.

It has been generally accepted since the clinical investigations of Scoville and Milner (1957) that bilateral surgical lesions involving the temporal lobes and hippocampus in man cause a characteristic amnesic syndrome with loss of memory for recent events, but preservation of immediate memory (normal digit span) and of remote memories. Similar memory impairment is seen in many other lesions involving damage to the hippocampus or its connections (Chapter 9). In addition, Penfield and Jasper (1954) observed that electrical stimulation of the temporal lobe in patients sometimes elicits complete memories similar to those which may occur spontaneously in temporal lobe epilepsy; these effects are thought to involve hippocampal activity.

As a result of these clinical observations, it has been suggested that a function of the hippocampus may be the tranfer of short-term memories into a permanently encoded or long-term store. However, such dramatic amnesic syndromes are not observed in animals with experimental bilateral hippocampal lesions and the question of whether the clinical findings are actually due to hippocampal damage or to disruption of neighbouring structures is in a state of flux at present (Horel 1978; Squire 1980). Even in human subjects it appears that the amnesia is not as complete as previously thought and that apparently forgotten events can be recalled if suitable clues are provided (Weiskrantz 1977, Chapter 9). Thus, the hippocampus may also be involved in the retrieval of memory.

Another function ascribed to the hippocampus is that of acting as a cognitive map (both spatial and temporal) of the environment (O'Keefe and Nadel 1978). Patients with hippocampal lesions are sometimes permanently lost even in their everyday surroundings, if these are different from their surroundings prior to the lesion, and animal studies show that certain hippocampal neurones discharge only when the animal is in a particular place in relation to the environment. The hippocampus of the dominant hemisphere appears to be concerned with visual environment features, and that of the non-dominant hemisphere with spatial features (Norton 1981). In this capacity the hippocampus may act as a type of match/mismatch or error evaluation system which compares present environmental stimuli with those previously experienced and allows alteration of response in accordance with environmental changes (O'Keefe and Nadel, 1978). Douglas (1967, 1975), and Douglas and Pribram (1966) stressed the inhibitory nature of the hippocampus which, in animals at least, appears to allow suppression of incorrect responses and hence selection of responses more appropriate to the circumstances. The importance of the postulated hippocampal behavioural inhibition system (Gray, 1982) in anxiety is discussed in Chapter 3. Rawlins (1984) attempts to reconcile the many postulated functions of the hippocampus by suggesting that it acts as a high capacity memory for all types of information which is then retained (by long-term potentiation) for a considerable time. This retention allows the association of items occurring at widely separated times and also allows comparison and evaluation of presently occurring events with a spatiotemporal representation of previous events.

Despite the probably important functions of the hippocampus in vertebrates it is perhaps noteworthy that a hippocampus is not essential for all types of learning and memory. The octopus can learn but has no hippocampus (Young 1966) and animals with extensive hippocampal lesions can form and use long-term memories (Rawlins, 1984).

Diencephalic structures
Memory defects similar to those produced by temporal lobe and hippocampal lesions also occurs after damage to diencephalic structures in man. Thus, the amnesic syndrome due to thiamine deficiency, tuberculous meningitis, some cerebral tumours, and surgical lesions has been associated with pathological changes in the inner portions of the dorsomedial, anteroventral and pulvinar nuclei of the thalamus and the mammillary bodies (Brierley 1977). It has been claimed that the amnesic syndrome can occur after bilateral destruction

of the mammillary bodies alone (Mair *et al.* 1979). These diencephalic structures are connected to the hippocampus via the fornix and other tracts and there is some evidence that they are directly involved in certain memory functions. Gaffan (1972) noted that lesions of the fornix disrupted recognition memory in the rat. More recently, microelectrode recordings of the activity in single neurones in the brain of the Rhesus monkey have shown that certain cells located in the far anterior and medial region of the thalamus respond to familiar but not to unfamiliar visual stimuli (Rolls *et al.* 1981). It is suggested that such cells might form the basis of recognition memory. In man, some lateral thalamic nuclei also seem to play an important part in modulating cortical language and spatial memory functions (Ojemann 1983).

The cerebral cortex
The cerebral cortex is not essential for some types of learning. Oakley (1979) has shown that associative learning, including classical and operant conditioning, can occur, and may even be shown more clearly, after removal of the whole neocortex in rats and rabbits, indicating that such forms of learning must involve subcortical structures. Indeed, learning of a sort can occur at all levels of the nervous system including the isolated spinal cord preparation which can show associative conditioning.

Lateralization
However, in humans the cerebral cortex is essential for the more complex forms of learning and memory involving abstract thought and language (Oakley 1981). It has long been known that there is considerable lateralization of function in the cortex. In the majority of individuals, the left hemisphere is specialized for language, logical analysis and deduction, the programming of refined manual movements, abstract and symbolic reasoning, and possibly an appreciation of temporal causality. The right hemisphere, on the other hand, is dominant and superior in spatial visualization, memory for and recognition of faces and other complex stimuli which are resistant to verbal description, musical appreciation, and possibly appreciation of physical principles and spatial organization. The left hemisphere is superior to the right in memory for temporal rhythm and pattern, while the right is superior in memory for non-verbalizable spatial patterns. In particular, the right hemisphere is able to represent the rich qualities of sensory and emotional experience and complex spatial relationships which defy description in terms of language (Sperry 1973, 1974, 1976; Beaumont 1983; Levy 1979; Ross 1984).

The advantages of such deduplication of cerebral function are discussed by Levy (1979) who concludes that the lateralization of function found in the human brain reflects a trend towards the optimally efficient use of neural space. The potential information capacity of the human brain is greatly increased by reduction in redundancy and the coexistence of mutually exclusive, but equally important mechanisms for understanding the environment. The lateralization of language function appears to be present soon after birth in humans (Woods 1983), and neuroanatomical asymmetries are present in human and non-human species (Geschwind and Levitsky, 1968; Sherman *et al.* 1982; Le May 1982). Aberrations of hemispheric and interhemispheric function may occur in depression (Chapter 11) and schizophrenia (Chapter 13).

Language Functions

Early information concerning cortical language functions came from clinical studies relating various defects of speech and memory to brain lesions at particular sites. From such studies, the critical sites in the dominant hemisphere for the comprehension and production of written and spoken language have been classically held to include (Lane and McLeod 1981; Fig. 8.5): Broca's area (the portion of the frontal lobe just anterior to the face, lip, tongue, and mouth area of the motor cortex), Wernicke's area (the posterior portion of the superior temporal gyrus), the connection between these two areas through the arcuate fasciculus, the interconnections between these areas and various parts of the cortex, and parts of the visual and auditory cortex. Damage to different sites in these systems is thought to account for various

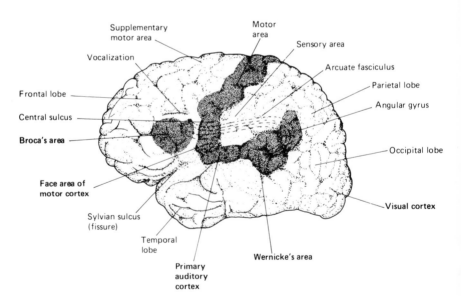

Fig. 8.5. Cortical areas classically associated with language functions. Areas concerned with language functions include Broca's area, Wernicke's area, their connections through the arcuate fasciculus, and parts of the visual and auditory cortex. (Reference: Kandel and Schwartz 1982.)

types of aphasia and alexia described in Chapter 9. However, it is always difficult in clinical studies to relate specific defects to particular areas of damage, and the traditional view may require revision.

More recently, brain electrical stimulation techniques in conscious subjects have allowed more detailed mapping of cortical language and memory functions (Ojemann 1983). Stimulation at certain discrete sites during a naming task evokes repeated errors, while at closely adjacent sites (0.5 cm or less) similar stimulation evokes no errors. Regions in which repeated naming errors occur on stimulation are often well outside the traditional Broca and Wernicke zones, and in many patients naming changes do not occur when the classical areas are stimulated. Yet areas where errors are evoked seem to be essential for language function, since cortical resections encroaching on these areas produce aphasia. Sites where naming errors were evoked by electrical stimulation in one subject are shown in Fig. 8.6. The location of these areas varies somewhat between individual subjects and between males and females, and is related to verbal ability.

Examination of other language functions by this technique revealed that stimulation at different sites produced errors of different types including naming, reading, short-term verbal memory, and phoneme (single speech

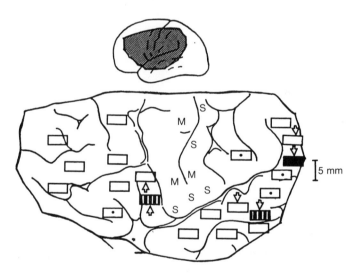

Fig. 8.6. Cortical sites in language-dominant hemisphere of one subject at which repeated naming errors were evoked by electrical stimulation. Open rectangles—no errors evoked; filled and striped rectangles, repeated errors; Single dot, single errors in multiple trials. Arrows identify adjacent sites separated by 5 mm or less. M,S, sites of evoked motor movements or sensations. Stimulation by trains of 60Hz stimuli of 2.5 s duration, biphasic pulses at 8 mA, delivered through bipolar electrodes 5 mm apart. (From Ojemann 1983.)

sound) identification. Not only different language functions, but the same function in different languages appears to be separately represented; thus, in the subject in Fig. 8.6, the naming of objects in English and in Greek was disrupted by stimulation at different sites. It is possible that the localization of these sites exhibits a degree of plasticity since they may change position after injury (Ojemann 1983).

From the results obtained with these techniques in several subjects, Ojemann (1983) concludes that language functions in the human cortex are organized in a mosaic of small areas subserving separate aspects: some sites are concerned with orofacial movements and identification of speech sounds; others relate only to syntactical aspects of language or only to word naming; yet other sites appear to subserve a short-term verbal memory system in which storage and retrieval of verbal memory can be separately interrupted by localized stimulation.

The cortical verbal memory system appears to be closely linked to a common memory and language system in the dominant lateral thalamus. From experiments in which thalamic sites were stimulated, Ojemann (1983) suggested that thalamo-cortical activating circuits select the cortical mosaics appropriate to the language task. A similar mechanism, modulating memory for spatial information processed in the opposite hemisphere, may be present in the non-dominant thalamus. The basal ganglia appear also to be involved in the processing of language. Lesions in this area may cause language disturbances which include not only articulatory difficulty but also fluent aphasia and impairment of auditory comprehension (DiMasio 1983). It is becoming increasingly clear that language is by no means a monopoly of the cerebral cortex.

The cerebellum

The cerebral cortex, hippocampus and locus coeruleus all send impulses to the cerebellum which is possibly the seat of motor learning in vertebrates (Marr 1969; Changeaux and Danchin 1976; Young 1979; Anderson 1982). The cerebellar Purkinje cells normally exert an inhibitory influence on muscle fibres, but this inhibition is opposed by afferents to the Purkinje cells from proprioceptors in the muscles. The learning of motor skills has been shown to be associated with selective changes in the firing of Purkinje cells, and it is suggested that proprioceptor activity from the particular muscle groups required for a motor task leads to adaptive changes in their cerebellar synapses (possibly in dendritic spines) which lessen the inhibitory discharge of the Purkinje cells and so increase the activity of the selected muscles. Due to the synaptic changes, the particular sequence of contractions will occur 'automatically' in the future (once initiated by cortical 'commands'). Motor learning usually involves a complex sequence of movements and the cerebellum may also function as a timing device by which the required strength and sequence of muscular contractions are learned. The cerebellum has also been implicated as a site of associative learning involving motor responses (Gellman and Miles 1985; Stein 1985).

Other brain sites undoubtedly make their own contributions to various aspects of learning and memory. In a sense, as many have claimed since Lashley's classic description ('In search of the engram', Lashley 1950) which revealed that memory could not be localized anywhere in the brain, learning and memory may be diffusely distributed throughout the nervous system. Nevertheless, it appears that a co-operative effort between closely inter-connected structures is also involved, with critical changes occurring perhaps in different localities for different facets of the process. The more complex the development of learning and memory the greater the degree of local-ization that appears to be required. If learning is essentially a selective process, then the higher and more localized levels of the nervous system may allow a more versatile selection of responses from a much larger repertoire of behavioural possibilities than are provided for by the more 'primitive' parts of the brain. Exactly how the selections are made and then communicated to the selected sites has yet to be unravelled. In particular, the process of recall remains the least understood and yet the most fundamental of all memory processes. The importance of the cytoarchitecture of the cortex in mammals and its organization into horizontally integrated columnar modules which act as processing and distributing units is discussed by Mountcastle (1978) and Gilbert (1985).

Pharmacology of learning and memory

Many drugs and physical agents affect learning and memory. Such treatments can be administered at different times in relation to the time of initial learning and by this means their effects on various stages of the memory process can sometimes be distinguished (Mondadori 1981; Mathies 1980; Zornetzer 1978). If a substance is administered before a learning trial (*pre-trial*), any subsequent changes in memory may be due to a direct effect on memory processing, but may also be due to indirect effects on other functions such as perception, vigilance, and motivation. If a treatment is administered soon after the learning trial (*post-trial*) it cannot affect the initial learning, and any effects in later retention tests are traditionally ascribed to an action on mem-ory processing. However, the memory is only susceptible to modulation for a short period after the learning, and this time depends on species, task, and type of treatment. Furthermore it is not usually clear whether any memory defects are due to specific interference with some encoding process, con-solidation, or retrieval. When treatment is deferred until before the test for retention (*pre-retest*), its effects may be limited to the retrieval processes, but these may also be indirectly affected by effects of the drug on other systems.

Thus, the study of drug effects on memory presents methodological problems and poses difficulties of interpretation. Other variables include the dose and route of administration of the drug and the type of memory test employed. Many drugs produce dose-dependent effects which may be central or peripheral and which vary with task complexity. There is also the problem of 'state-dependent learning'. Differences in performance may arise if learning and retention are not tested in same drug state (Mondadori 1981). Furthermore, changes in the functional condition of any single transmitter system in the brain almost certainly affects the function of other transmitter systems, and almost any functional change in the brain is likely to have consequences for learning and memory. In spite of these shortcomings, drug studies have provided some insights into the pharmacological aspects of memory.

Brain protein synthesis

The part played by brain protein synthesis in learning and memory has been the subject of a large number of animal studies (reviewed by Agranoff *et al.* 1978; Dunn 1980; Squire and Davis 1981; Mayes 1983). Learning-associated changes in RNA and various proteins, glycoproteins, and phosphoproteins have been demonstrated in several brain regions, including the hippocampus and forebrain. However, the results are difficult to interpret and have not always been reproducible. Dunn (1980) concluded that while the brain is almost certainly altered biochemically during learning, and some of the changes appear to be regionally, biochemically, and behaviourally specific, it is unlikely that any of the changes represent stored information. 'It is much more likely that they indicate the general cellular activation necessary for learning to occur' (Dunn 1980; p. 359).

Another experimental approach has been to administer agents which inhibit brain protein synthesis at different times before and after learning, and to measure any effects produced on subsequent performance in tasks requiring retention of the learning. Drugs which impair brain protein synthesis include puromycin, anisomysin, cycloheximide, and acetoxycycloheximide. Some of these agents also produce convulsions, and other convulsant drugs such as pentylenetetrazol, strychnine, and flurothyl, as well as electrically induced convulsions and cerebral anoxia (all of which also inhibit protein synthesis), have similar effects on memory. The general conclusion from work on a wide variety of animals using these agents is summarised by Squire and Davis (1981): 'When cerebral protein synthesis is inhibited by 90–95 per cent just before or after training in a simple task, initial learning is normal but amnesia develops gradually and is present within a few hours. When inhibition is established 30 min. or longer after training or just prior to retention testing, memory is not affected. The results have generally been taken to mean that brain protein synthesis during or shortly after training is required for the formation of long-term memory' (Squire and Davis 1981; p. 331).

However, this conclusion remains controversial since amnesia following brain protein synthesis inhibition can be reversed or protected against by a variety of agents. Behavioural manipulation such as 'reminders' can reverse the amnesia, and increasing training strength and several pharmacological agents can not only reverse the amnesia but also render the animals non-susceptible to amnesic treatment (Dunn 1980). These agents include stimulants such as caffeine and nicotine, sympathomimetic drugs such as amphetamine, and alpha- and beta- adrenoreceptor stimulants, monoamine oxidase inhibitors, and various hormones and polypeptides [ACTH, vasopressin, melanocyte-stimulating hormone release-inhibiting factor (MIF), enkephalin, cortisol, corticosterone, dexamethasone]. Although these drugs protect against or reverse the effects of amnesic agents on memory (and often enhance performance in the absence of amnesic treatment), they do not significantly decrease the inhibitory action of amnesic agents on brain protein synthesis, according to a number of studies (cited by Dunn 1980). Hence, it cannot be concluded that protein synthesis is essential for the formation of long-term memory. At present it seems unlikely that long-term memories are stored in the form of some specially encoded protein or nucleic acid macromolecules as suggested in some models (Levitt and Goedel 1975), but it is possible that protein synthesis is generally involved in the establishment of permanent synaptic changes related to memory. These may include the synthesis of the proteolytic enzyme, calpain, (Lynch and Baudry 1984) and the protein actin (Crick 1982) in dendritic spines, increased dendritic branching (Greenough 1984), and other plastic neuronal changes (Mayes 1983). Such processes may be facilitated in animals by the administration of RNA precursors such as orotic acid which has been shown to improve retention in young and old rats (Ruthrich et al. 1983).

It seems clear that protein synthesis is not required for short-term memory since initial learning can occur normally despite amnesic treatment and occurs too quickly to allow time for de novo protein synthesis (Agranoff et al. 1978). It may be that short-term memory results from rapidly occurring synaptic changes (such as alterations in the contacts made by dendritic spines) and that protein synthesis is only one of several steps which establish persisting patterns of neuronal connectivity in certain synapses reflecting long-term memory, a process which may be modulated by other neurotransmitters and neurohormones (Squire and Davis 1981).

Acetylcholine

Several authors (Deutsch 1971; Drachman 1978; Squire and Davis 1981) have put forward the view that it is in cholinergic synapses that specific alterations related to memory occur. Other agents such as biogenic amines and polypeptides act as modulators which can influence the development, maintenance and expression of memory but are not themselves essential. Animal work (Deutsch 1971) has shown that drugs which affect cholinergic synaptic transmission can impair, facilitate or have no effect on retention, depending on the age of the memory at the time of treatment. For example, the same dose of an anticholinesterase (physostigmine, diiso-propylfluorophosphate: DFP) injected intracerebrally in rats had no effect on performance if administered 1–4 days after learning a task, impaired performance if given 7 days after learning, and improved memory if injected 21 days after learning, at a time when untreated animals exhibited forgetting. Opposite, time-related effects occurred with anticholinergic drugs such as scopolamine. Furthermore, the effects of cholinergic drugs depend on the efficiency of the original learning. Stanes et al. (1976) divided rats into slow learners and fast learners and found that physostigmine given 4 days after learning improved memory in slow learners, but impaired memory in fast learners. Dose-effects were also apparent and the direction of effects on memory of different doses depended on the age of the memory.

These results were interpreted to mean that memory storage involves changes in the efficiency of transmission which develop over time at certain cholinergic synapses. Deutsch (1971) suggested that, in the appetitive and aversive tasks which he studied in rats, there was a gradual increase in efficacy of cholinergic transmission which continued for several days after learning until it reached an optimal level at about 2 weeks, and thereafter a gradual decline in efficacy during the course of forgetting (Fig. 8.7). During the initial period, when cholinergic activity was rising, anticholinesterases were assumed to raise the synaptic concentration of acetylcholine above the optimal level and cause synaptic blockade, thus impairing performance. During the period of forgetting, however, when cholinergic activity was declining, the effect of anticholinesterases would be to improve synaptic efficacy and thus enhance memory. A similar interpretation is possible for fast and slow-learning rats (Stanes et al. 1976) if it is assumed that slow learners take longer to reach optimal levels of synaptic efficacy. By the same reasoning, different doses of drugs affecting cholinergic transmission will be required to produce a given effect at different times after learning.

Deutsch (1971) suggests that these learning-related changes in cholinergic synaptic efficacy are not due to alterations in the amount of acetycholine released pre-synaptically, but to variation in the sensitivity of post-synaptic membrane, because responsiveness to carbachol, a cholinergic receptor agon-ist, is greatly increased 7 days after learning. It is conceivable that an increase in the number of synapses made by dendritic spines could account for such a change in post-synaptic sensitivity.

The idea that learning is subserved by gradual synaptic changes whose

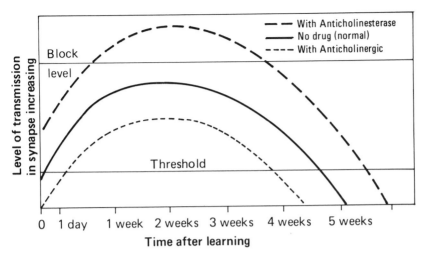

Fig. 8.7. Hypothetical effects of cholinergic and anticholinergic drugs on transmission in cholinergic synapses subserving memory functions. It is suggested that training causes a gradual increase in efficacy of cholinergic transmission which reaches an optimal level after about 2 weeks and then declines. Anticholinesterases initially increase the synaptic concentration of acetylcholine above the optimal level while anticholinergic drugs reduce it to suboptimal levels. Later, when cholinergic activity is declining anticholinesterases improve synaptic efficacy. (From Deutsch 1971.)

time-course is related to the duration of the memory and that cholinergic synapses are involved is supported by some observations on human subjects. In normal young subjects, a series of studies (cited by Squire and Davis 1981) showed that cholinergic drugs (infusion of arecoline or physostigmine and oral choline) in suitable doses can improve word recall, while larger doses of physostigmine can impair cognitive function. Drachman (1978) found that central cholinergic blockade with scopolamine did not affect immediate memory (digit span) but seriously affected the ability to store new information (serial order of digits and free recall of words) and also impaired retrieval of old information as well as lowering general cognitive performance. The impairment induced by scopolamine was reversed by physostigmine, in doses which had no effect on memory or cognitive function when given alone, but not by the general stimulant amphetamine.

The memory and cognitive deficits produced by scopolamine closely resemble those which develop in normal elderly subjects, suggesting that the cognitive disorders or normal ageing may result from a relatively specific dysfunction of cholinergic transmission. This raises the possibility that cholinergic drugs might improve cognitive function in the aged, and Drachman (1978) noted a trend toward improvement in memory storage and IQ function in 13 normal elderly patients following a small subcutaneous dose of physostigmine (0.8 mg). It has been suggested that the commonest form of senile dementia, Alzheimer's disease, might in its early stages result from selective loss of cholinergic neurones (Chapter 10).

Anatomical sites in which cholinergic pathways may be involved in memory and other cognitive functions include the cortex and the limbic system, particularly the septal-hippocampal structures and pathways. However, cholinergic systems, whether they are specific sites of memory or not, undoubtedly interact crucially with other systems, such as those involving monoamines.

Monoamines (Noradrenaline, dopamine, serotonin)

Pharmacological studies in animals and man suggest that monoamines play some role in learning and memory. In general, agonists of monoaminergic systems improve while antagonists interfere with learning and memory. However, the literature is confusing and it appears that the involvement of monoaminergic systems is much less specific than that of cholinergic systems.

Many authors (cited by Squire and Davis 1981; Mayes 1983) have studied the effects of altering central monoaminergic activity in animals. Post-trial intraventricular and localized intracerebral injections of noradrenaline and isoprenaline have been reported to improve retention and partially to reverse memory deficits induced by various adrenergic antagonists in rats, while beta-adenergic and dopaminergic receptor antagonists impair acquisition and retention. As mentioned above, adrenergic agonists also reverse the amnesic effects of brain protein synthesis inhibitors. In humans, systemically administered (pre-trial) amphetamine and methylphenidate can improve learning and memory in normal subjects, especially in boring or fatiguing tasks, and in learning-disabled children, healthy aged subjects and depressed patients (Squire and Davis 1981). A major effect of amphetamine appears to be on the acquisition of information and the effect is biphasic, resulting either in facilitation or in disruption, depending on dosage and the state of arousal of the subject (Zornetzer 1978).

However, in other studies, acute manipulation of brain monoamines had no effect on learning and memory in a range of tasks. Chronic depletion of forebrain monoamines with reserpine and 6-hydroxydopamine in rats did not affect learning and memory in a reliable way (Palfai et al., 1978). Similarly, lesions of the locus coeruleus, which reduce cortical and hippocampal noradrenaline concentration by 60–80 per cent, and lesions of the substantia nigra, reducing striatal dopamine concentrations by 95 per cent, do not appear to affect retention in several studies cited by Squire and Davies (1981).

Nevertheless, catecholamines may modulate memory processes by both peripheral and central effects. Squire and Davis (1981) draw attention to observations that disruption of memory occurs in animals after combined lesions of the dorsal adrenergic bundle and adrenalectomy, but not after either treatment alone. In addition, intraperitoneal amphetamine can facilitate post-training retention, but this effect is blocked by adrenal demedullation. Phentolamine, an alpha-adrenergic antagonist which does not cross the blood-brain barrier can block the retrograde amnesia induced in rats by the alpha-adrenergic agonist clonidine (Gozzani and Izquierdo, 1976).

Peripheral effects may be due to changes in blood flow or blood pressure in the central nervous system or to other reflex changes resulting from peripheral sympathetic activity. With regard to central effects, Kety (1970) proposes that the extremely diffuse projections of the adrenergic neurones of the locus coeruleus make them ideally suited to reinforce significant information associated with arousal or stress at individual synapses. The importance of the locus coeruleus in arousal and sleep, selective attention, and motivation has already been noted. Dopaminergic projections are also widely distributed in the limbic system and forebrain and are involved in arousal and reward systems. Possibly the locus coeruleus also plays a more direct role in memory through its effects on cortical plasticity (Pettigrew, 1978). Zornetzer (cited by Izquierdo, 1984) observed that electrical or chemical stimulation of the locus coeruleus over a period of months prevented the normal decline of memory in senescent rats and that there was a significant correlation between cell counts in the locus coeruleus and some types of avoidance learning in rats.

Information concerning the part played by serotonin in memory is confusing (Mondadori 1981). Post-trial injection of serotonin into the hippocampus inhibits the retention of some learning tasks, and the administration of serotonin precursors depresses performance in active avoidance responses. However, serotonin reuptake inhibitors (zimelidine and alaprocate) administered 24 h after training facilitate memory retention of an inhibitory avoidance task in mice (Altman *et al.* 1984). Serotonin depletion appears to facilitate learning and memory in some tests but to inhibit them in others. Raphe lesions which lower the serotonin content of the forebrain may facilitate memory. Amnesic treatment with electroconvulsive shocks and CO_2-anoxia influence brain serotonin turnover, and the extent of the amnesia appears to be related to the serotonin content of the hippocampus. On the whole, the evidence at present points to a general permissive rather than a specific role for monoamines in learning and memory. They may act indirectly as modulators and in this general role they appear to interact closely with polypeptide hormones and neuromodulators.

Amino acid neurotransmitters

There is little information concerning the role of GABA in learning and memory, although it would be expected to exert at least an indirect influence through its effects on arousal (Chapter 2). Conflicting results have been reported (Mondadori 1981). Thus, pre-trial injection of GABA into the lateral ventricle exerts a dose-related, time-dependent facilitating effect on the learning of a dark-light discrimination task in rats. Pre-trial blockade of GABA by picrotoxin has been reported to improve learning in some studies but to impair memory in others. Benzodiazepines have amnesic effects which are thought to be due to enhancement of GABA activity (Chapter 4). Information on the role of excitatory amino acid transmitters such as aspartate and glutamate is also lacking, in spite of their postulated importance in hippocampal long-term potentiation (Lynch and Baudrey 1984).

Neuropeptides

Increasing evidence points to the involvement of pituitary hormones and polypeptide neuromodulators in learning and memory. Of the 20 or more biologically active peptides present in the mammalian nervous system, ACTH, ACTH fragments, oxytocin, vasopressin, and opioid peptides have been most studied in this respect.

ACTH

Removal of the anterior lobe of the pituitary interferes with the acquisition of conditioned avoidance behaviour in rats (Rigter and van Riezen 1978). This behaviour can be restored by ACTH and by ACTH fragments 1-10, 1-13 (alpha- MSH), and 4-10 (de Wied 1974; de Wied and Gispen 1977). The action is presumably due to a central effect, since ACTH fragments are devoid of adrenocorticotrophic properties. In intact rats, ACTH and ACTH 4-10 can stimulate acquisition in certain learning situations and, when given just prior to testing, can also delay the extinction of conditioned avoidance behaviour, sexually motivated behaviour and approach behaviours (Dunn 1980). Furthermore, as already mentioned, ACTH and ACTH fragments, when administered immediately before retention testing, can reverse the effects of amnesic agents including carbon dioxide, electroconvulsion, and drugs (Meyer and Beattie 1977). However, ACTH does not appear to be indispensable for memory since total hypophysectomy does not prevent an animal from learning new responses (Rigter and van Riezen 1978).

In humans, the effects of ACTH on memory appear to be small, though perhaps subtle. In normal subjects, intravenous infusion of ACTH fragments have been reported to delay habituation, improve performance in some memory tests (Benton Visual Retention Test, Wechsler Memory Test) and to enhance selective attention (Rigter and van Riezen 1978; Ashton *et al.* 1976).

Vasopressin

Removal of the posterior lobe of the pituitary does not impair the acquisition of conditioned avoidance behaviour in rats; instead, it causes premature extinction of avoidance behaviour, suggesting a defect in consolidation or retrieval of memory. This abnormality can be reversed by lysine vasopressin and also by the fragment desglycinamide lysine vasopressin, which is devoid of endocrine and autonomic activity (Rigter and van Riezen 1978; Crabbe and Rigter 1980). Thus, the effect appears to be mediated by a central action. The situation is, however, complicated by the fact that both ACTH and alpha- MSH also reverse the extinction deficit following posterior pituitary lobectomy, while lysine vasopressin also reverses the acquisition deficit associated with anterior pituitary lobectomy (de Wied 1969). Nevertheless, there are clear differences between the behavioural effects of anterior and posterior pituitary hormones. The effect of ACTH and ACTH fragments is short-lived and cessation of treatment results in rapid loss of effect. By contrast, the effects of lysine vasopressin are long-lasting, persisting over seven days after cessation of a week's treatment in an avoidance acquisition test (Bohus *et al.* 1973; Fig. 8.8).

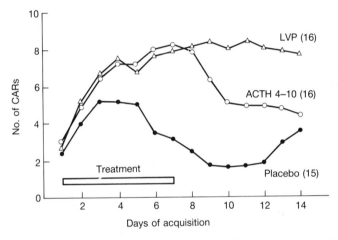

Fig. 8.8. The effect of ACTH 4–10 and lysine vasopressin on memory in rats. ACTH 4-10 (20 g/day) and lysine vasopressin (LVP)(1 g/day) administered subcutaneously for 7 days. Numbers of animals (male hypophysectomised rats) in parentheses. CAR's, = correct responses in shuttlebox conditioned avoidance task. (From Bohus *et al.* 1973, by kind permission of S. Karger AG, Basel.)

In intact rats, both arginine and lysine vasopressin produce a prolonged delay in extinction of various avoidance behaviours, persisting after discontinuation of treatment, and improve active and passive avoidance behaviour, especially if given immediately after the learning trial (Kovacs *et al.* 1982). Lesions of the rostral septal region and the anterodorsal hippocampus prevent the effects of vasopressin on the extinction of active avoidance behaviour. Injection of minute amounts of arginine vasopressin into the dorsal septal area, hippocampal dentate gyrus or midbrain dorsal raphe nucleus facilitates passive avoidance behaviour, while injection of anti-vasopressin serum into the same areas impairs passive avoidance behaviour.

In addition, vasopressin, like ACTH, can attenuate or reverse the effects of amnesic treatments in rats and mice (Kovacs *et al.* 1982; Rigter and van Riezen 1978). Microinjection of arginine vasopressin into the amygdala can partially reverse the amnesia produced by pentylenetetrazol, but injections of vasopressin into the dorsal septal area and dorsal raphe nucleus are ineffective. Kovacs *et al.* (1982) suggest that certain limbic areas are specifically sensitive to vasopressin and that different areas are concerned with different aspects of memory, particularly consolidation and retrieval. Muhlethaler *et al.* (1982) observed that low concentrations (10^{-8}–10^{-6m}) of vasopressin increase the rate of firing of neurones in the CA1 area of rat hippocampal slices and conclude that vasopressin can act as a transmitter or modulator in the mesolimbic hippocampus.

However, it is controversial whether vasopressin has direct effects on particular memory processes or whether its effects are secondary to general actions on arousal or to peripheral autonomic effects. The question has recently been debated by Gash and Thomas (1983, 1984) and de Wied (1984a,b). Some investigations have found that vasopressin has dose-dependent, biphasic effects on memory which are influenced by the strain of rats used and their state of arousal (Hamburger *et al.* 1985). Gash and Thomas (1984) conclude: 'while the thesis that vasopressin directly modulates memory processes is becoming increasingly untenable, evidence is mounting that vasopressin has direct visceral (autonomic) effects which may indirectly influence other behaviours, perhaps by modulating emotional-motivational (arousal) and temperamental factors subserving the specific responses from which higher cognitive functions (like 'memory') are inferred' (Gash and Thomas 1984; p. 198). The use of recently developed selective vasopressin agonists and antagonists (Manning and Sawyer 1984) may help to clarify the issue.

A few double blind placebo controlled studies on a small number of subjects suggest that vasopressin may be involved in human memory. Lysine vasopressin and desmopressin (*l* -desamine-8-D-arginine vasopressin) administered as nasal spray for several days or weeks have been reported to improve memory processes as well as concentration, attention and motor performance in normal subjects, both young and elderly and in patients with depression (Weingartner *et al.* 1981; Legros *et al.* 1978; Gold *et al.* 1979). The global improvement suggests that any effect on memory is secondary to changes in arousal. Clinical studies are described further in Chapter 10.

Oxytocin

The other posterior pituitary neuropeptide, oxytocin, appears to have effects which are opposite to those of vasopressin. Oxytocin facilitates rather than delays extinction of active avoidance behaviour and attenuates rather than enhances passive avoidance behaviour in rats (Kovacs *et al.* 1982). Bohus and others (1978) suggest that oxytocin might be a naturally occuring amnesic polypeptide. In the clinical field, oxytocin is used in obstetrics and is also normally released during labour. Possibly its amnesic effects play a physiological role during labour and delivery, isolating the mother from external stimuli (Ferrier *et al.* 1980). The same authors studied the effect of oxytocin nasal spray on cognitive functions in six normal male and female subjects and reported that it reduced memory recall. However, information on the importance of this neurohormone on memory processes is sparse.

Opioid peptides

The opioid peptides may also participate in a neurohumoral system which induces forgetting rather than remembering. The evidence for such a function has mostly been obtained from investigations in rats and is reviewed by Izquierdo (1982a). The intraperitoneal or intraventricular injection immediately after training of small doses of beta-endorphin causes retrograde amnesia for avoidance tasks and for habituation learning. This effect is competetively reversed by naloxone. The effective dose of beta-endorphin is extremely small, much smaller than that required to produce analgesia and similar to the amount released endogenously from the brain during training (5–25 ng per rat). Beta-endorphin does not, however, affect acquisition of avoidance or habituation learning even in doses that produce full amnesia. Subanalgesic doses of morphine, methionine enkephalin, leucine enkephalin, and des-tyr-metenkephalin also produce naloxone-reversible retrograde amnesia.

Naloxone administered immediately post-training by contrast causes retrograde memory facilitation for a wide variety of tasks. This facilitation is independent of the response required and of the presence or absence of pain associated with training. It is prevented by beta-adrenergic or dopaminergic receptor antagonists and potentiated by concurrent administration of nicotine or *d* -amphetamine. Izquierdo, (1982a) suggested that naloxone acts by releasing central beta-adrenergic and dopaminergic systems from inhibition by endogenous opioids. Naloxone also completely blocks the amnesia induced by post-training electroconvulsive shock, a procedure which is accompanied by a massive release of beta-endorphin and methionine enkephalin from the hypothalamus and amygdala from the rat brain. Presumably, the amnesia results, at least partly, from the release of opioid peptides, the actions of which can be prevented by naloxone (Izquierdo 1982a). From a study of the relative potency of memory enhancement of various opioid antagonists, it appears that mu-opioid receptors are preferentially involved in opioid memory systems (Izquierdo 1983).

The fact that opioid agonists and antagonists affect memory when administered post-training confirms the view that the memory of an event continues to be modified after learning; perhaps the consequences of an event determine whether it, or which part of it, is remembered and which forgotten (Gold and McGaugh 1975). The presence of a polypeptide-mediated amnesic system in the brain might improve learning efficiency by allowing useless or obsolete information, or responses that have become inappropriate, to be economically discarded. Under many conditions this system would be independent of pain.

In man, narcotic analgesics (Chapter 7) induce forgetfulness, but this effect may be related to their sedative action. However, it seems possible from human experience that there might be a connection between opiate or opioid analgesia and the quick forgetting of pain. It is said that the pain of childbirth or of torture is rapidly forgotten. Those who have suffered pain 'may remember very vividly all the circumstances surrounding, or pertaining to, their painful experience, but can never actually revive the pain itself' (Izquierdo 1982a, p. 457). Kapp and Gallagher (1979) suggest that an opioid-mediated system in the amygdala is involved in attenuating the pain and fear of unpleasant experiences. There is remarkably little information on the effects of naloxone in human memory (Chapter 10).

Several authors (Dunn 1980; Squire and Davis 1981; Meyer and Beattie 1977) have remarked on the general similarity of the effects on memory of the catechol amines and the pituitary polypeptides which enhance retention or retrieval. Like the catechol amines, the neuropeptides appear to be modulators rather than prerequisites of the memory process. Indeed the close connections between polypeptide and catecholaminergic systems suggest that they function together: for example ACTH may stimulate the release of dopamine and noradrenaline, and vasopressin also affects catecholamine metabolism (Dunn 1980) and is found in high concentration in the locus coeruleus (Rossor *et al.* 1980). There is now abundant evidence that many central neurones liberate and respond to both polypeptides and catechol amines (Lundberg and Hokfelt 1985).

The opioid amnesic system also interacts with catecholamine systems: for example, Kapp and Gallagher (1979) cited evidence for an opiate-noradrenaline interaction between the amygdala and the locus coeruleus. Many polypeptides, including the endorphins, produce long-lasting synaptic changes. Such effects may modulate memory and other processes by reinforcing or inhibiting the shorter-acting synaptic changes induced by catecholamine and other neurotransmitters, thus underlining or erasing the effects of experience.

Peripheral mechanisms may also be involved in catecholamine-neuropeptide interactions. Izquierdo (1982b) points out that both the memory-enhancing effect of vasopressin and the amnesic effect of methionine enkephalin, when administered intraperitoneally after training, are attenuated by adrenal medullectomy and reinstated by the systemic administration of adrenaline in rats, and suggests that these neuropeptides require the presence of peripheral adrenaline to be effective.

In summary, pharmacological studies suggest the presence of multiple overlapping back-up systems controlling learning and memory, similar to those described for pain modulation (Chapter 5) and appetite control (Chapter 11). These systems probably involve both peripheral and central functions, both generalised and localised processes, and both specific and modulatory neurotransmitters which simultaneously co-ordinate memory, arousal, and reinforcement systems. The detailed mechanisms of how memory is stored or recalled remain obscure but at present some fundamental requirements in vertebrates appear to be a mechanism for synaptic plasticity, possibly provided by dendritic spines, the presence of cholinergic synapses, and, for higher functions such as language, a considerable degree of specialization in localized cortical-subcortical structures. Clinical findings in patients with memory disorders, described in the next chapter, in general support these conclusions and give further information on how memory systems might work.

9

Disorders of memory

Clinically occurring memory disorders are difficult to classify on the basis of the hypothetical stages of memory discussed in Chapter 8. Since pathological processes extend over time and are rarely limited to particular pathways or structures, any resulting memory loss is usually mixed. Certain conditions, however, give rise to characteristic memory disturbances, sometimes global, sometimes relatively discrete, sometimes associated with a limited anatomical involvement, and sometimes showing a fairly specific biochemical disruption. These clinical disorders provide a window through which to study the organisation and dynamics of memory functions in man.

Non-specific memory impairment

Since memory functions are widely distributed in the brain, memory disturbance forms part of the clinical picture in many pathological states. These include acute conditions with alterations of consciousness, due to a variety of diseases or drugs, and chronic or progressive conditions involving brain damage secondary to vascular, infective, neoplastic, traumatic, metabolic and other causes. Memory may also be impaired in psychiatric disorders and in epilepsy. Such memory disturbances are usually non-specific, involving several stages of memory, albeit to varying degrees, and are overshadowed by other clinical features. Much less commonly, relatively selective memory loss occurs and memory disturbance forms the primary or major clinical symptom.

Impairment of immediate memory

Warrington (1981) described a rare syndrome characterized by a relatively selective loss of immediate memory with inability to repeat strings of digits or words. One such patient had a digit and letter span of only one to two items (normal: five to nine items), although he had no aphasia, could converse without difficulty, and performed well in a variety of verbal learning tasks. He could remember stimulus items normally if they were presented visually rather than acoustically. Other patients have been described with similar immediate memory defects, and it appears that the critical site for a lesion to produce this type of impairment is the left inferior parietal lobe of the brain (Fig. 9.1).

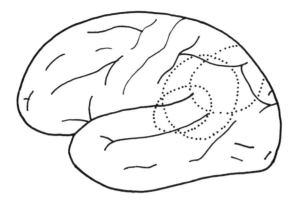

Fig. 9.1. Sites of lesions causing selective impairment of auditory-verbal immediate memory in three patients. (From Warrington 1981.)

Impairment of semantic memory

Occasionally cerebral lesions lead to selective impairment of semantic memory: some forms of aphasia and alexia may be regarded as disorders of semantic memory, an amnesia for words or their meanings. The critical sites in the dominant hemisphere for the comprehension and production of written and spoken language have been described in Chapter 8 (Fig. 8.5). Different types of aphasia may result from damage at several of these sites, but since lesions are rarely discretely localized, most clinically occuring aphasias are mixed. They are usually classified functionally (Walton 1977; Lane and McLeod 1981; Geschwind 1975).

Nominal aphasia (anomic or amnesic aphasia) results from lesions in or near the angular gyrus of the dominant hemisphere interrupting the connection between Wernicke's area and the rest of the brain, and may occur with lesions at other sites (Ojemann 1983); it is also seen in non-focal widespread disease of the brain. The dominant feature is an inability to name objects, although comprehension is not greatly affected and the patient can usually describe objects by paraphrasing. Articulation of words is unimpaired and patients can repeat names supplied by the examiner, only to forget them rapidly. Reading and writing are similarly impaired and acalculia (difficulty in carrying out calculations) may be present. Limited forms of nominal aphasia may be encountered rarely. Warrington (1981) described two patients in whom the semantic deficit was category-specific: in one, comprehension of concrete words (blacksmith, macaroni) was much more impaired than that of abstract words (soul, opinion), while in the other the reverse was true. These patients showed no apparent general intellectual deficit, no amnesia for events, and were not disorientated in time or place. Studies of further patients with similar disorders led Warrington (1981) to conclude that the critical lesion for this type of semantic defect was in the temporo-occipital region of the brain and that memories for concrete and abstract word meanings are represented in structurally separate pathways.

Other forms of aphasia are not conventionally considered as memory disorders but are included here since they involve semantic memory systems (Ojemann 1983). In *Broca's aphasia* (*expressive or motor aphasia*), usually ascribed to damage to Broca's area, comprehension of speech and writing is normal but the patient is unable to translate speech into articulate sounds (non-fluent aphasia), or to write normally. The brain damage involves the dominant hemisphere and there is nearly always a crossed hemiplegia. In *Wernicke's aphasia* (*sensory or receptive aphasia*), ascribed to lesions involving Wernicke's area, comprehension of spoken and written language is impaired, but the patient can articulate words normally, although his conversation makes little sense (fluent aphasia). There is usually no hemiplegia. Occasionally cortical insufficiency or anoxia gives rise to the *syndrome of isolated speech area*, in which a lesion is thought to occupy a C-shaped configuration which spares Broca's area, Wernicke's area, and their interconnections, but destroys the cortex and underlying white matter which surround the region. The most striking clinical feature is an almost total lack of comprehension but normal repetition and no dysarthia. *Conduction aphasia* (*syntactical aphasia, central aphasia of Goldstein*) is usually ascribed to lesions which disrupt the connection between Broca's and Wernicke's areas, just above the Sylvian fissure. Comprehension of spoken and written language is intact, but speech and writing, though fluent, are severely impaired. *Global or total aphasia*, with impairment of both comprehension and production of speech and writing, results from damage to the dominant frontal and temporal lobes.

Impairment of recognition memory

Various agnosias, inability to recognize complex stimuli although perception is intact, appear to represent disorders of recognition memory. Such disorders may be associated with aphasias or with global amnesia, but occasionally occur as isolated defects, and may be limited to one sensory modality. The commonest form is *visual agnosia* in which faces or objects, or pictures of them, are not recognized by sight. Damasio (1985) reviews recent findings in prosopagnosia, impaired recognition of previously familiar faces. Such patients also have difficulty in differentiating specific objects within a class, such as recognizing their own car, clothes, dog, or specific foods. The lesions in this case are bilateral and involve the mesial occipitotemporal region. The physiological basis of the defect appears to be a failure of visual stimuli to activate the host of memories pertinent to those stimuli. A similar type of dysfunction appears to underlie *auditory agnosia* (amusia), failure to recognize musical tunes, caused by temporo-sphenoidal lobe lesions, and *tactile agnosia*, inability to recognize an object placed in the hand, resulting from perietal lobe lesions.

Impairment of motor memory

Apraxia, the inability to perform a learned act or purposive movement in the absence of motor paralysis, sensory loss or ataxia, is sometimes clinically associated with aphasia. Some forms of apraxia may represent an amnesia for motor learning. Dressing apraxia may reflect a defect of spatial under-standing and can occur after lesions of the non-dominant hemisphere. Right hemisphere lesions can also cause anosognosia, a tendency to neglect the left side of the body (Chapter 2). Left and right dissociation occurs after lesions of the corpus callosum.

However, most aspects of motor learning and memory appear to be func-tionally and anatomically separate from both semantic and event memory. Thus, motor learning is often preserved in patients with semantic memory defects and in the amnesic syndrome described below. It seems likely that the neural substrates for motor learning lie outside the brain sites damaged in these cases, possibly in the cerebellum (Marr 1969; Young 1979; Iverson 1977).

Impairment of event memory

Selective impairment of event memory can result from diverse pathological causes discussed below. The anatomical feature common to all these disorders is damage within the diencephalon involving the mammillary bodies and certain thalamic nuclei or in the interconnected temporal lobes involving the hippocampal formation (Brierley 1977). The importance of these structures in the organisation of memory has been discussed in Chapter 8. Their dys-function may give rise to the amnesic syndrome first described by Korsakoff in 1887 (cited in Zangwill 1977).

Memory loss in the amnesic syndrome has been intensively studied (Milner 1970; Scoville and Milner 1957; Mair *et al.* 1979; Iverson 1977; Zangwill 1977; Warrington 1981). The impairment is most marked for recent events, both verbal and non-verbal, and typically patients forget new names, new faces, and new places, although they retain memories of distant events. In new surroundings, they cannot remember the geography for long enough to find their way around. In a sense, such patients exist in a timeless void, permanently lost among strangers. Occasionally, if the lesion is focal or unilateral, impairment of recent memory may be limited to one sensory modality, one half of the body, or to the function of one cerebral hemisphere (Ross 1982).

In addition to the anterograde amnesia, the inability to retain the memory of events since the onset of the lesion, there is a variable degree of retrograde amnesia or inability to recall events that occurred prior to the illness. The retrograde amnesia may extend backwards for several years but if recovery occurs may shrink up to the time of onset of the memory disturbance. Spontaneous recovery of memory for events which occurred during the period of anterograde amnesia apparently does not occur (Ross 1982).

Despite the severe restriction of event memory, in the purest form of the amnesic syndrome, attention, immediate recall, language (semantic memory), perception, performance in various types of intelligence tests and motor learning and memory are all normal (Ross 1982; Warrington 1981). An example of relatively undiminished intelligence coupled with severe memory deficit is illustrated by the noted patient H.M. who had undergone bilateral surgical removal of the medial temporal cortex, amygdala, hippocampus and associated connections (Milner 1970; Iverson 1977).

'Consider, for example, H.M's response to the direction to remember the numbers "584". In the absence of distraction he was able to retain this for about 15 minutes, apparently by working out elaborate mnemonic schemes. .....when asked how he had been able to retain the number for so long, he replied: "Its easy. You just remember 8. You see 5, 8 and 4 add to 17. You remember 8, subtract it from 17 and it leaves 9. Divide 9 in half and you get 5 and 4 and there you are: 584. Easy". A minute or so later, H.M. was unable to recall either the number 584 or any of the associated complex train of thoughts; in fact he did not know that he had been given a number to remember because, in the meantime, the examiner had introduced a new topic.' (Iverson 1977, p. 137).

Much investigation, reviewed by Piercy (1977), has been directed to the question of which stage or stages of memory are impaired in the amnesic syndrome. Immediate memory appears to be intact, although unduly sensitive to interference. Several possibilities have been suggested to explain the impairment of event memory: (a) a defect of consolidation, (b) inadequate encoding of information at the time it is entered into store, and (c) failure of retrieval of information. The fact that the retrograde amnesia can shrink suggests a defect of retrieval with normal storage, at least in those cases in which shrinkage occurs. However, if a general defect of retrieval is postulated it is hard to explain how amnesic patients are often able to recall remote memories with little difficulty, although exhibiting retrograde and anterograde amnesia. Possibly remote and recent memories are recalled through different pathways, and those for remote memory escape damage in the amnesic syndrome.

Nevertheless, careful testing suggests that neither the retrograde amnesia when present, nor the anterograde amnesia, are so absolute as they appear. In both cases some investigators have shown that learning can be considerably improved by cued recall techniques (Warrington 1981; Warrington and Weis-krantz 1970). Word fragments, initial letters of a word, and category information can be used as clues by amnesic patients suggesting that they can encode and consolidate information, both pictorial and verbal, and that their difficulty is one of access to the stored material.

It is possible that these results could also be explained in other terms such as a failure to encode material in a form that is accessible for normal retrieval, limitation of capacity of event memory systems, or an abnormality of forgetting rather than of remembering. The question is far from solved and Piercy (1977) points out that attempts to explain the memory defect are in any case based on hypothetical and controversial ideas of memory. The picture may be further complicated by the fact that patients who have been investigated are not homogeneous either in aetiology or localization of brain damage. For example, the amnesic syndrome can follow lesions of either the mammillary bodies and certain thalamic nuclei, or of the temporal lobes and hippocampal formation, but memory performance has rarely been compared in patients with lesions limited to one or other of these locations. Memory loss may be partial rather than absolute and may affect more than one subfunction (e.g. both consolidation and retrieval). These questions are discussed further at the end of this chapter.

Closer investigation of the various causes of disturbance of event memory, and particularly correlations of the memory defects with the localisaton of the associated lesions, has shed some light on the way memory systems are organized in the brain. Some types of the amnesic syndrome present particular features, such as the confabulation so typical in the alcoholic amnesic syndrome, or particular temporal patterns, as seen in some closed head injuries, and both the site and extent of the brain damage as well as the quantity and possibly quality of the memory defect varies from case to case.

Thiamine deficiency

Of the original patients on whom Korsokoff based his description of the amnesic syndrome, a number were alcoholics, and the Korsakoff syndrome is still most commonly seen in chronic alcoholics (Whitty *et al.* 1977). The amnesia probably results from brain damage caused by the associated dietary thiamine deficiency; a similar syndrome is sometimes seen in other thiamine-deficient states (Handler and Perkin 1983) and can be induced in animals by thiamine deficient diets (Brierley 1977). The psychological abnormalities are not limited to memory defects, although loss of recent memory is prominent and retrograde amnesia is usual. A striking feature is a facile and expansive confabulation, a tendency to fill in memory gaps with improvized and often implausible explanations, and a marked lack of insight into the disability, both intellectual and physical.

Studies which have attempted to correlate the psychological features with neurological damage in chronic thiamine deficiency have been reviewed by Brierley (1977) and by Mair *et al.* (1979). The presence of amnesia appears to be related to bilateral damage to diencephalic structures, and the important foci of such lesions appear to include the inner portions of the dorsomedial, anteroventral, and pulvinar nuclei of the thalamus, the mammillary bodies, and the terminal portions of the fornix. Damage to the hippocampus, septal region, cortex, brainstem or cerebellum does not appear to be a constant feature, although changes here may account for associated cognitive and physical symptoms seen in individual cases. The pathological processes include demyelinization and neuronal loss in some areas, and proliferation of microglia and fibrous astrocytes. The mammillary bodies are almost invariably markedly affected. The precise mechanism by which thiamine deficiency induces the acute or chronic changes is not known.

Brain surgery

Neurosurgical procedures have been used for the removal of tumours and for the relief of epilepsy, Parkinson's disease, and chronic psychiatric states. Patients undergoing such operations have pre-existing brain damage or dys-function, but some have developed postoperatively particular memory deficits clearly related to the surgical intervention and not to the original disease. The induction of memory disorders by removal or section of known brain structures has provided strong evidence for the critical participation of temporal lobe sites in certain memory functions in man.

Scoville and Milner (1957) reported the appearance of the typical amnesic syndrome in patients following bilateral removal of the anterior two-thirds of the hippocampus and hippocampal gyrus along with the uncus and amyg-dala. The memory defect was permanent and was confined to loss of memory for recent events with some retrograde amnesia, but no deterioration in personality, intelligence, or previously learned motor skills. Similar results have sometimes followed unilateral surgical lesions of this type, but in such cases there is probably pre-existing bilateral brain disease (Whitty *et al.* 1977; Iverson 1977; Brierley 1977). These results have been confirmed by others and have led to the conclusion that temporal lobe structures are involved in the registration of recent memory. Brierley (1977) pointed out that the inner portions of the temporal lobes, the hippocampus, and hippocampal gyrus seem to be essential for normal memorizing and there is proportionality between the amount of hippocampal formation removed at operation and the severity of the ensuing memory defect.

Severe defects of recent memory probably result only from bilateral tem-poral lobe damage. However, unilateral temporal lobe damage is not entirely without effects on memory. Patients with left temporal lobectomies show disruption of performance in verbal-auditory recent memory tasks, while in patients with right temporal lobectomies visual-spatial and non-verbal auditory recent memory tasks is impaired (Ross 1982). Localization of function of verbal and non-verbal recent memory between the hemispheres is also confirmed by the differential results of unilateral left and right electroconvulsive therapy and by brain stimulation experiments, discussed below.

Less consistent memory defects follow operations on other brain areas. Operations on the frontal lobes rarely produce permanent memory deficits, although defects in retention and marked distractibility occur in the immediate post-operative period, along with a patchy retrograde amnesia (Whitty *et al.* 1977). Transient difficulty in remembering the temporal sequence of events has been observed after limited ablations of the anterior cingulate cortex. Operations on the thalamus produce various memory disorders depending on the site affected, but interference with the anterior thalamic nuclei may cause gross and permanent defects of recent memory. Surgical interference with the fornix has produced variable results; it seems likely that bilateral section of the fornix does not produce memory loss unless there is coincident damage to periventricular structures (Whitty *et al.* 1977; Brierley 1977).

Cerebral tumours

Cerebral tumours usually cause generalized effects, including a rise of intracranial pressure and interference with blood supply, and memory changes form only part of a widespread disturbance of consciousness. Occasionally, however, a characteristic and florid confabulatory amnesic syndrome occurs with localized tumours, in the absence of generalized mental disturbance or evidence of pre-existing alcoholism. Whitty *et al.* (1977) and Brierley (1977) have reviewed the evidence suggesting that localized damage to particular brain structures is the cause of amnesia in these cases. The tumours usually involve deep midline diencephalic structures in the region of the hypothalamus and third ventricle either by neoplastic changes or by compression. Craniopharyngiomas are commonly associated with memory loss and removal of the tumour or removal of fluid from it can restore normal memory, suggesting that the amnesia is due to pressure on structures on the floor of the third ventricle. The amnesic syndrome has been described in patients with secondary neoplastic deposits confined to the mammillary bodies. Temporal lobe tumours are sometimes associated with selective memory impairment, depending on whether the tumour is situated on the dominant or non-dominant side.

Frontal lobe tumours have also been reported to cause amnesia, especially if they are bilateral and involve the corpus callosum. However, in these cases there is also a defect of motivation and attention which seriously interferes with memory testing. Tumours of the cerebral hemisphere may produce different types of impairment depending on their location, including a variety of aphasias when certain areas of the dominant hemisphere are affected and loss of memory for motor skills when the right parietal area is involved.

Intracranial infections

In herpes encephalitis, tissue necrosis and haemorrhage, with intranuclear inclusion bodies in nerve cells and glia, chiefly affect limbic structures: the uncus, amygdaloid nucleus, hippocampus, hippocampal and cingulate gyri, post-orbital regions, and sometimes the fornices and mammillary bodies (Whitty *et al.* 1977; Brierley 1977). The pathological changes are so discrete that the term 'limbic encephalitis' has been applied to this condition. A marked impairment of recent memory with the features of the amnesic syndrome including confabulation is found in such cases. The syndrome is not common as a major defect in other forms of encephalitis, in which the pathological changes in the brain are more widespread.

The amnesic syndrome can also occur in tubercular meningitis. Following an early confusional stage, a phase may develop showing all the features of the amnesic syndrome, with retrograde and anterograde amnesia and confabulation but preservation of immediate and remote memory and general intelligence. Pathological studies in patients dying at stage have revealed an inflammatory process with exudation largely limited to the more anterior basal cisterns of the brain and directly involving the floor of the third ventricle (Whitty *et al.* 1977). Other forms of meningitis are not associated with particular memory defects or such localized brain changes. Occasionally cerebral abcesses involving limbic system structures can cause the amnesic syndrome.

Vascular disorders and hypoxia

Vascular disorders can precipitate the amnesic syndrome in acute or chronic form (Whitty *et al.* 1977). Transient disturbance of recent memory, probably secondary to localized cerebral ischaemia, can occur in migraine, hypertensive encephalopathy, thromboangitis obliterans, and systemic lupus erythematosus. It has been suggested that in this case the amnesia is due to vertebral-basilar artery spasm with consequent ischaemia in the brainstem reticular formation, mammillary bodies, and hippocampal formation.

More permanent amnesia results from destruction of cerebral brain tissue following vascular lesions. Typical features of the amnesic syndrome, with or without confabulation, develop and, depending on the site and extent of the lesion, may be combined with general intellectual impairment, and physical signs and symptoms. Following sudden vascular catastrophes, such as strokes, memory loss is sudden, although it may have been preceded by transient ischaemic attacks, and some recovery may occur. Steady progress of central arteriosclerotic disease may produce the gradually increasing impairment of arteriosclerotic dementia. This usually begins at about the age of 60 or 70 with progressive, but stepwise intellectual deterioration in which impairment of recent memory is often an early and at first isolated sign. The clinical picture differs little from other dementias of old age, but post-mortem studies show multiple small cerebral infarcts. The amnesic syndrome can also follow severe hypoxia from any cause (Brierly 1977; Iverson 1977; Whitty *et al.* 1977).

Where post-mortem examinations have been related to the amnesic symptomatology, the results indicate that loss of recent memory occurs after bilateral damage to the medial temporal lobes, and usually involves the uncinate gyrus, hippocampus and sometimes the mammillary bodies and fornix (Brierley 1977). Localized vascular lesions may give rise to fractional disorders of recent memory; for example, Ross (1982) described two patients with posterior cerebral artery lesions causing infarction in the inferior occipital lobes and inferior-posterior, but not medial temporal lobes, bilaterally. These patients had recent memory disorders limited to the visual system.

Head injury

The typical results of a moderate to severe closed head injury are: a period of loss of consciousness, a period of behavioural confusion, a post-traumatic anterograde amnesia extending forwards in time from the first two events, and a retrograde amnesia extending backwards in time from the loss of consciousness (Whitty and Zangwill 1977). The duration of the post-traumatic amnesia correlates well with the severity of the injury. During this period the patient may behave apparently normally yet later have no recollection of events. Sometimes confabulation, delusions, or automatism occur during post-traumatic amnesia. The duration of the retrograde amnesia is usually much shorter than the post-traumatic amnesia, but its length is also roughly proportional to the severity of the injury; it may last from a few seconds to months. Usually the retrograde amnesia shrinks as recovery occurs, but the return of memory is often patchy and does not necessarily occur in chronological order. A residual memory defect of some degree is probably common in spite of otherwise full recovery, although it may be difficult to detect. There may be some degree of impairment of recent memory and also 'islands of amnesia' well outside the period of retrograde amnesia. These residual effects may last for months or even permanently after severe injuries, and may be difficult to differentiate from post-traumatic neurosis.

The anatomical basis of post-concussional amnesia is usually difficult to establish and the site of injury differs with the location and direction of the blow to the head. However, Whitty and Zangwill (1977) point out that in the common injury to the front of the head, the frontal and temporal lobes as well as the brainstem are especially liable to damage. The amnesic syndrome may also follow penetrating injuries of the temporal lobes, and bilateral diencephalic or hippocampal injuries.

Epilepsy

Transient amnesia forms an integral part of many types of epileptic attacks. In generalized tonic-clonic seizures (grand mal epilepsy), memory is usually lost during the convulsion. After the attack, a period of mental clouding is common and in this post-convulsive confusional stage outbursts of aggressive or destructive behaviour may occur, of which the patient later has no recollection. A period of retrograde amnesia may also occur. The memory disturbance probably results from the general impairment of consciousness and it does not appear to be an essential clinical feature since, rarely, memory persists even during the attack (Whitty *et al.* 1977). Memory may be generally impaired in epileptics by antiepileptic drug treatment (Trimble and Thompson 1981).

Absence seizures, (petit mal), originating subcortically and characterized by three per second spike and wave activity on the EEG, are also accompanied by short memory gaps during the periods of inattention, and by brief periods of retrograde amnesia. However, there does not seem to be clear temporal relationship between the EEG spike and wave activity and behaviour, since EEG changes may precede or follow behavioural changes. Occasionally, generalized EEG discharges may occur without obvious motor manifestations although registration of events and subsequent memory is disturbed. There is some evidence that thalamic structures are involved in the propagation of such discharges, although they are probably not the source of activity. This possibility provides a link between petit mal and temporal lobe epilepsy since the thalamus and hippocampus are anatomically connected via the fornix, mammillothalamic tract, and septal pathways (Whitty *et al.* 1977).

Disturbances of memory is a characteristic feature of temporal lobe epilepsy. The aura preceding the attack may include feelings of intensified familiarity with the surroundings or situation (deja vu) or feelings of strangeness and unfamiliarity. There may also be confusion, with difficulty in recalling words, and a variety of epigastric gustatory or olfactory sensations accompanied by salivation and lip-smacking. Manifestations of the subsequent seizure are variable and may consist only of a dazed look, confused behaviour, automatic repetition of an inappropriate motor sequence, a period of aggressiveness, or a prolonged fugue. Amnesia for the period of the seizure is the rule, and the amnesia typically has an abrupt onset and ending.

Study of temporal lobe epilepsy has been of particular value in localizing some of the sites involved in memory. Much evidence (reviewed by Brierley 1977) has shown that the attacks result from epileptic discharges originating in the medial temporal lobe. EEG recordings during attacks have shown spontaneous epileptic discharges in the medial and inferior temporal regions in most cases. Furthermore, electrical stimulation of these areas, especially around the amygdala and deep in the uncus, can reproduce both the automatism and the amnesia. Electrical stimulation of the medial aspect of the temporal lobe in unanaesthetized subjects can also reproduce the premonitory auras of epileptic attacks. Stimulation of the lateral aspects of the temporal lobes in cases where these are already the site of epileptic discharge can give rize to false recollections or 'experimental hallucinations'. These memories are often the same as those which occur in the spontaneous epileptic attacks (Penfield and Perot 1963). Similar 'stereotyped memories' have been induced by stimulation through implanted electrodes and the same memories can be evoked on several occasions by repeated stimulation (Bickford *et al.* 1958). Thus both amnesia and memories can be evoked by localized electrical stimulation in discrete temporal lobe areas.

Patients with temporal lobe epilepsy have been reported to show a preponderance of particular personality traints, characterized essentially by high 'psychoticism' (Bear *et al.* 1982). Temporal lobe activity probably contributes to personality chacteristics but brain damage and anticonvulsant drugs may also produce abnormal behaviour (Reynolds 1983). Frank psychosis, clinically indistinguishable from schizophrenia (Chapter 13), may also occur in temporal lobe epilepsy (Trimble 1981) and temporal lobe surgery sometimes induces psychosis (Polkey 1983).

Electroconvulsive therapy

A reversible memory deficit invariably follows electroconvulsive therapy; the impairment is very similar to that following a closed head injury or an epileptic convulsion. The clinical features, reviewed by Williams (1977), consist of a retrograde amnesia, a confused phase following the convulsion, and a period of anterograde amnesia similar to post-traumatic amnesia. The retrograde amnesia usually shrinks rapidly until it occupies only a few seconds, although there may be patches of amnesia which extend further back in time. During the anterograde amnesia, the main impairment is memory for recent events and is similar to the amnesic syndrome from other causes; this phase typically lasts about 4–6 h. There may be some residual memory defect persisting for some weeks. These effects are believed to be mainly due to the convulsion itself, and to be little affected by medication or by the nature of the illness (usually depression; see Chapter 11).

In general, the memory defects appear to be proportional to the strength and duration of electrical stimulation and to the duration of the seizure. They can, however, be considerably modified if unilateral rather than bilateral electroconvulsive therapy is employed (Williams 1977; Iversen 1977; Ross 1982). Unilateral electroconvulsive therapy applied to the dominant hemisphere produces a limited memory defect, mainly affecting performance in verbal recent memory tests. When the shock is applied only to the non-dominant hemisphere, the resulting memory impairment is even less marked and affects performance predominantly in non-verbal recent memory tests. The therapeutic effects of unilateral convulsive therapy appear to be only slightly, if at all, inferior to the bilateral treatment (Green 1978).

The amnesic effect of electroconvulsive therapy is probably due to disruption of temporal lobe activity: the electrodes are normally applied over the temporal lobe; they cause local electrical charges as well as generalized activity; and the hippocampus has a very low threshold for electrically induced convulsions. Furthermore, electrical stimulation of the temporal lobe in conscious patients, when followed by an epileptic after-discharge, seriously impairs memory for recent events (Iverson 1977). Electroconvulsive therapy given through electrodes placed over the frontal lobes appears to cause less memory impairment but also less antidepressant effect (Williams 1977).

Senile and presenile dementias
Alzheimer-type dementia

Progressive deterioration of intellectual activity leading to dementia is common with advancing years but not inevitable (Davison 1982). Its occurrence is a major problem in modern societies with ageing populations and has stimulated much recent research into age-related dementias. Historically, the term Alzheimer's disease was applied to a type of progressive dementia starting between the ages of 45 and 65, while the term senile dementia was used for a similar condition commencing at the age of 65 and over. Because of the close clinical and pathological similarities, however, Alzheimer's disease (or Alzheimer-type dementia) is now used by many authors to describe both the senile and presenile forms (Gottfries 1980; Corkin 1981; Rossor 1982). Alzheimer's disease is the commonest of the presenile dementias and it accounts for over 50 per cent of elderly patients diagnosed clincally as demented. About half a million people in Britain and over two million in the United States are affected (Corkin 1981; Wiesnieski and Iqbal 1980; Bousefield 1982). Other dementias in old age include those caused by vascular disease which account for 15 per cent, mixed forms which account for 22 per cent, and a small group of rarer disorders (Besson 1983).

Clinical features Alzheimer's disease, which is more prevalent among women than men, begins insidiously and is characterized by marked deficits in many cognitive functions, including memory, language, and complex sensorimotor and perceptual capacities. Typically the first symptom is loss of memory for recent events, and often there is especial difficulty in recalling names and words, a disability soon merging into an amnesic dysphasia, although memory for remote events may be relatively unimpaired. Memory loss is more prominent in Alzheimer's disease than in most other dementias. Ultimately generalized intellectual impairment and disorientation develops, social behaviour degenerates, and there may be associated disorders of affect, agitation, sleep disturbances, poor appetite, decreased sexual activity and unsteadiness of gait.

Morphological changes Since memory disruption is prominent, and Alzheimer's disease is more common than most other causes of the amnesic syndrome, the histological and neurochemical changes found in the brain post-mortem are of particular interest as a source of information on the neural substrates of memory. Morphological changes consist of diffuse neocortical degeneration which is most marked in the temporal, parietal, and occipital lobes, but also involves the posterior cingulate gyrus, amygdala, hippocampus, hypothalamus, some midbrain and brainstem structures (Corkin 1981), and olfactory nucleus (Averback 1983). Ball *et al.* (1985) stress the importance of degenerative changes in the hippocampus as a factor in the memory defects. There is also marked neuronal loss (up to 76 per cent; Tagliavini and Pilleri 1983) in the basal nucleus of Meynert, situated in the basal forebrain (Whitehouse *et al.* 1982), and sometimes in other nuclei including the nucleus of the diagonal band of Broca, the medial septal nucleus, and the locus coeruleus (Davison 1982). However, the anterior cingulate gyrus, caudate nucleus, thalamus, and mammillary bodies are only minimally affected.

Several distinctive pathological changes have been described (Fig. 9.2): (1) senile (neuritic) plaques, in which deposits of extracellular amyloid-like material are surrounded by abnormal unmyelinated neuronal processes; (2) neurofibrillary tangles, consisting of intracellular bundles of filaments in the cytoplasm surrounding cell nuclei; (3) progressive deterioration of the dendrites of pyramidal cells in the cortex and hippocampus and of dentate granule cells; (4) the development of vacuoles in the cytoplasm of hippocampal pyramidal cells, especially in areas CA1–3 (Wiesnieski and Iqbal 1980); (5) intraneuronal accumulation of the pigment lipofuscin in the parietal cortex and especially in the inferior olivary nucleus (Dowson 1982). These changes occur bilaterally in the brain but are not necessarily symmetrical. Inclusion bodies have also been found in adrenal medullary cells (Averback 1983). The importance and pathogenesis of some of these changes are discussed by Wiesnieski and Iqbal (1980), Dowson (1982), and Selkoe (1982). More detailed cytological changes are discussed further below.

Biochemical changes Accompanying these morphological changes, distinct neurochemical abnormalities have been found in post-mortem specimens. Compared with age-matched non-demented control subjects, there is significant impairment of cholinergic function in the brain in Alzheimer's disease, as indicated by a 50 per cent or more decrease in the activity of the enzyme choline acetyltransferase (CAT), which is involved in the synthesis of ace-

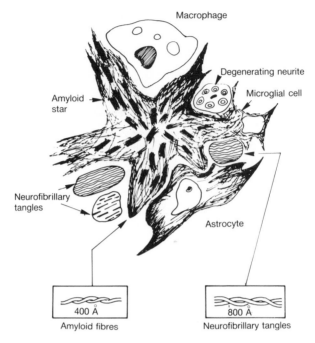

Fig. 9.2. Diagram of pathological features in the brain in Alzheimer-type dementia. Diagram shows various elements of a neuritic (senile) plaque, consisting of a central amyloid star containing paired helical fibres of amyloid-like material, surrounded by degenerating neurites with neurofibrillary tangles containing intracellular bundles of paired helical filaments, and by macrophages, fibrous astrocytes, and microglial cells. (Adapted from Wiesnieski and Iqbal 1980.)

tylcholine and is a specific marker for cholinergic neurones. In addition, acetylcholinesterase activity and acetylcholine synthesis are reduced significantly in biopsy samples *in vitro* . The areas of the brain involved include most of the cortex, especially the frontal and temporal lobes, the hippocampus, amygdala, and in some cases caudate nucleus and putamen. These post-mortem changes have been confirmed in many studies reviewed by Deakin (1983), Besson (1983), Rossor (1982), Coyle (1983a,b), Bowen and Davison (1984), Corkin, (1981) and Gottfries (1980). Acetylcholinesterase activity is also reduced in the cerebrospinal fluid during life (Appleyard *et al.* 1983; Arendt *et al.* 1984).

The cerebral cortex contains few intrinsic cholinergic neurones, and the CAT deficit reflects impairment of ascending cholinergic projections which mainly arize from the basal nucleus of Meynert, the medial septal nucleus, and the diagonal band of Broca (Fig. 9.3; Coyle *et al.* 1983a,b). There is no evidence, however, that post-synaptic muscarinic receptors in the cortex are affected (Corkin 1981; Caulfield *et al.* 1982). A close correlation exists

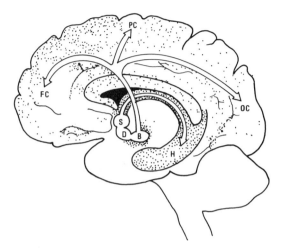

Fig. 9.3. Diagram of brain showing origin of ascending cholinergic projections from the basal nucleus of Meynert, the diagonal band of Broca, and the medial septal nucleus. B, basal nucleus of Meynert; D, diagonal band of Broca; S, medial septal nucleus; FC, frontal cortex; PC, parietal cortex; OC, occipital cortex; H, hippocampal formation. (Adapted from Coyle *et al.* 1983b).

between the degree of intellectual deterioration in patients with Alzheimer's disease and the decrease in CAT activity found post-mortem. This correlation strengthens the suggestion that cholinergic systems are important for learning and memory (Chapter 8) and also suggests that mental function in Alzheimer's disease might be improved by cholinergic agents (Corkin 1981; Chapter 10). It is of interest in view of the proposed important of dendritic spines in memory (Chapter 8) that widespread dendritic degeneration occurs in Alzheimer's disease.

Although there appears to be a relatively selective degeneration of cholinergic projections in some cases of Alzheimer's disease, monoaminergic systems may also be affected. There are decreases in brain concentrations of the enzymes tyrosine hydroxylase and dopamine decarboxylase and of the neurotransmitters dopamine, noradrenaline, and serotonin and their metabolites, and an increase in monoamine oxidase activity. These changes are seen in normal ageing but the sum of damage in the different systems seems to be greater in Alzheimer's disease (Gottfries 1980). However, Corkin (1981) pointed out that catecholamine deficiences might indicate the concomitant presence of Parkinson's disease or might be secondary to cholinergic loss. Nevertheless, the locus coeruleus has an important population of noradrenergic neurones which send projections to the cortex, and Bondareff *et al.* (1983) found cell numbers in this nucleus to be reduced by nearly 80 per cent in some patients with severe and early Alzheimer's disease. Reduction in cell numbers may also occur in the raphe nuclei (serotonergic) and substantia nigra (dopaminergic) (Besson 1983). Recent work indicates in addition that there are also large reductions in the concentration of the polypeptide somatostatin in the temporal cortex and perhaps of other polypeptides but not cholecystokinin, vasoactive intestinal polypeptide or vasopressin (Zeisel *et al*. 1981; Selkoe 1982). Reduced concentrations of GABA have been noted in cortical areas, hippocampus and amygdala (Deakin 1983; Rossor 1982; Rossor *et al*. 1984) and glutamate concentration may also be reduced. Harrison (1986) suggests that initially corticocortical and corticofugal pathways are selectively affected, and that the disease process extends retrogradely, involving the many neurotransmitters utilized in these pathways.

It may be that the cognitive impairments seen in Alzheimer's disease result from defects in many transmitters or modulator systems; the degree of mental deterioration correlates not only with decrease in CAT activity, but also with the numbers of neuritic plaques and neurofibrillary tangles. Total cerebral blood flow is also reduced and variations in regional blood flow correlate with the type of intellectual impairment (Ingvar 1982). Memory disturbance is associated with low flow in temporal regions, disorientation with low flow in parieto-occipital regions, and speech disturbance with low flow in the dominant hemisphere which is most marked anteriorly in motor aphasia and posteriorly in sensory aphasia.

Relationship to age and to normal ageing It has been suggested that Alzheimer's disease is not a single entity but appears in two distinct forms with either early (middle-age) or late (old-age) onset (Bondareff 1983; Rossor *et al*. 1984). Although the clinical picture and general pathology are similar, the early onset type is characterized by much greater and more widespread neuronal and neurotransmitter loss. The late onset form consists of a relatively pure cholinergic deficit confined to the temporal lobe and hippocampus and a reduction in somatostatin concentration in the temporal cortex. Other authors (Anderson and Hubbard 1981; Wilcock and Esiri 1983) argue that the basic mechanism for both types is the same and that generalized severe changes are less likely to be seen in older patients because they die before such changes develop.

The relation of Alzheimer's disease to normal ageing has also been debated. Most of the morphological and neurochemical changes that have been described in Alzheimer's disease also occur in non-demented elderly subjects (Selkoe 1982; Perry and Perry 1982; Gottfries 1980; Corkin 1981). There is progressive loss of neurones, particularly in the cortex, from adulthood onwards, and even in normal individuals a steady accumulation of neuritic plaques, neurofibrillary tangles, and lipofuscin deposits begins in about the fifth decade. At the same time there is a fall in cholinergic function which, unlike Alzheimer's disease, includes loss of cholinergic receptors in brain tissue (Gottfries 1980), and a fall in monoaminergic activity. There is a substantial neuronal loss in the locus coeruleus, although major cell losses in the basal nucleus of Meynert may be confined to Alzheimer's dementia (Tagliavini and Pilleri 1983). All these changes in normal ageing occur without gross loss of cognitive function or memory, although most people past middle age admit to some deterioration of learning ability and memory, and the elderly are more susceptible to mental disruption from central depressant drugs (Chapter 4). These findings suggest that Alzheimer's disease reflects an acceleration of the normal ageing process. It is interesting that age-related brain atrophy occurs at an earlier age in females than males (Hubbard and Anderson 1983), perhaps explaining the higher incidence of senile dementia in women. However, Rossor et al. (1984) do not accept the view that Alzheimer's disease and ageing reflect the same process. The neurotransmitter changes they found in 54 aged subjects were confined to relatively moderate reductions in cholinergic and GABA-ergic systems in limited brain areas. The losses of noradrenaline and somatostatin seen in Alzheimer's disease were not found to be a feature of normal ageing.

Nevertheless, the distinction between normal human brain ageing and Alzheimer's disease seems to be essentially quantitative, Alzheimer's disease being characterized by the greater density and wider distribution of the changes. Thus, it is possible that knowledge of the molecular pathogenesis of Alzheimer's disease might shed light on the mechanisms of neuronal ageing in general.

Molecular pathogenesis Much interest has focussed on the molecular structure of neurofibrillary tangles, amyloid-like deposits and lipofuscin deposits (Selkoe 1982; Wiesnieski and Iqbal 1980). Neurofibrillary tangles (Fig. 9.2) consist of pairs of helically wound filaments which resemble normal neurofilaments except for their helical conformation. The nature of the filamental proteins has not been identified with certainty; they appear to be unusual, highly insoluble, protein polymers bound together by covalent bonds. The amyloid-like deposits consist of rigid fibrils which, like the tangles, are very insoluble and resistant to proteolytic digestion. High concentrations of aluminimum and silica (present as aluminimum silicate) have been found in the centre of senile plaques and also in neurofibrillary tangles (Candy et al. 1984, 1985, 1986; Perry and Perry, 1985). These salts have the staining properties of amyloid, a fibrillary structure, and form rigid, self-replicating crystals. Lipofuscin granules may be derived from mitochondria, lysosymes, or both by a process of autophagocytosis. They include lipoids, proteins, cations, and acid hydrolysis-resistant residues. The lipid moiety contains oxidized polymers of polyunsaturated fatty acids, and it is possible that the production of these results in the formation of lipid/free radical molecules which can, through a series of reactions, disrupt lipoidal structures, and also cross-link and damage proteins or nucleic acids. Thus, the development of tangles, plaques, and lipofuscin in the brain may lead to an accumulation of rigid, insoluble intra- and extracellular deposits and could be the cause, rather than the result of progressive neuronal degeneration and death (Selkoe 1982).

Aetiology What initiates the changes is still conjectural. It is possible that the paired helical filaments result from faulty assembly of normal brain constituents (Wiesnieski and Iqbal 1980). Faulty protein assembly may occur generally in old age due to an accumulation of errors (Hayflick 1979), and dementia may result when neuronal loss reaches a critical level of distribution. Genetic or environmental factors may render some individuals more vulnerable to cell loss. A genetic link is suggested by observations that the incidence of Alzheimer's disease is increased among the relatives of patients (Heston and Mastri 1977) and that most patients with Down's syndrome who survive to the age of 40 develop dementia with histological changes resembling those of Alzheimer's disease (Selkoe 1982; Rossor 1982; Besson 1983).

Alternatively, cell loss may be precipitated or aggravated by certain viruses. Neuritic plaques can be induced in mice by the scrapie agent. Although this agent has not yet been isolated, it causes a disease in sheep which has an incubation period of 5–15 years, suggesting a slow virus. In Creutzfeld–Jacob disease and Kuru there are similar pathological changes in the brain; these diseases cause dementia in humans, are thought to be caused by slow viruses, and can be transmitted from humans to experimental animals. Paired helical filaments are also found in post-encephalitic Parkinson's disease and in some cases of subacute sclerosing panencephalitis caused by a measles-like virus (Wiesnieski and Iqbal 1980). It has also been suggested that reactivation of latent herpes may lead to its transport into the brain (Bowen and Davison 1984). However, it has not yet been possible to transmit Alzheimer's disease from humans to animals and a viral aetiology remains unproved.

A primary increase in the permeability of the blood-brain barrier, allowing the penetration of environmental toxins such as aluminium has been proposed as a possible aetiological factor (Banks and Kastin 1983). Aluminium is concentrated in plaques and neurofibrillary tangles (Candy *et al.* 1984 1985) and it is possible that aluminium absorption is increased in certain conditions. For example, typical plaques and tangles occurred in amyotrophic lateral sclerosis associated with calcium deficiency in a population in Guam (Garruto *et al.* 1984). Other suggested aetiologies included an autoimmune response (Davison 1982) and trauma. Pearce (1984a,b) noted excessive senile plaques and neurofibrillary tangles in the cortex of subjects who had been boxers, and attributed this change to repeated brain trauma during life. It seems likely that Alzheimer type dementia could result from any one, or a combination, of several causes.

Other presenile dementias

Other presenile dementias, which are rare compared with Alzheimer's disease, are reviewed by Gottfries (1980), Small and Jarvik (1982), and Rossor (1982).

Pick's disease, is clinically similar to Alzheimer's disease, but the histology of the brain is quite different, consisting of a localized cerebral atrophy in the frontal lobe. The aetiology is unknown. Creutzfeld–Jacob disease may be induced by a virus in genetically susceptible individuals (Oppenheimer 1985), and neuritic plaques can be found in the brain. Huntingdon's chorea is a hereditary disease in which progressive choreiform movements dominate the clinical picture but dementia is an almost invariable accompaniment. Pathological features (Bird 1978; Spokes 1981) include severe degeneration in the neostriatum with loss of interneurones, and generalized cortical shrinkage and thinning, particularly of the deeper layers. Biochemical analysis shows a marked loss of GABA, and of glutamic acid decarboxylase in the caudate nucleus and substantia nigra, loss of choline acetyltransferase in the caudate nucleus, and of substance P and tyrosine hydroxyclase in the substantia nigra. There also appears to be a selective depletion of angiotensin-converting enzyme and of enkephalin in the basal ganglia. On the other hand there are significant increases in dopamine and noradrenaline concentrations. It is suggested that the movement disorder results from dopaminergic and possibly adrenergic overactivity due to degeneration of GABA-ergic, cholinergic, and possibly other neurones in the basal ganglia. The neurochemical changes which account for the dementia have not been defined.

A proportion of patients with Parkinson's disease develop dementia; estimates vary from 20–40 per cent (Small and Jarvik 1982) to 3–15 per cent (Lees 1985). The main lesion accounting for the muscular disorder is degeneration of dopamine-containing cells in the substantia nigra. The changes underlying the dementia are not known, but the mesolimbic dopaminergic system, the serotonergic system, and the noradrenergic projection from the locus coeruleus may all be affected, and there may be a reduction in cortical CAT activity (Rossor 1982). These changes suggest a degree of overlap between Parkinson's disease and Alzheimer's disease.

Application of clinical studies to memory mechanisms in man

The theoretical basis of learning and memory (discussed in Chapter 8) is largely derived from experimental work on associative memory in animals, and it is generally agreed from this work that many basic memory functions are widely distributed in the brain. In man, memory functions are vastly more complex because of their close association with language, both verbal and numerate, and with the human capability for abstract thought. A study of clinically occuring memory disorders might thus be expected to provide an opportunity for testing the applicability of animal work to human memory. Clinical studies have indeed allowed some tentative conclusions to be drawn with regard to the organization of memory in man, but in general the information is limited to *where* memory occurs rather than *how* it occurs.

Clinical investigations clearly confirm the considerable degree of localization of memory functions in the human brain. This specialization has presumably arisen in the course of its evolutionary development (Oakley 1981). Thus, as mentioned in Chapter 8, the neocortex is the main neural substrate for semantic memory; limbic structures including the hippocampus are the main substrates for event memory (including spatial and temporal orientation); subcortical structures are concerned in association memory, and the cerebellum probably subserves motor memory. For this reason, gross defects in event memory, for example, are compatible with apparently normal semantic memory (although new words cannot be learned), and vice versa. Localization of memory function also appears to exist within the main structures, and discrete lesions can lead to very discrete memory defects. A semantic memory deficit, for example, may be limited to recall of auditorally but not visually presented words or digits, or involve only abstract or only concrete word meanings (Warrington 1981). Similarly, event memory deficits may affect only recent memory, leaving long-term event memory unimpaired; within recent event memory, impairment may be limited to a single sensory modality (Ross 1982). Specific memory defects result from localised lesions, and the same lesion produces the same defect in different subjects. Conversely, the same memory can be evoked repeatedly by stimulation of the same brain area. Thus, the 'hard-wiring' of established memories appears to be both relatively discrete and relatively fixed.

These observations may seem to suggest that different types of memory are 'stored' in particular places in the brain. However, the fact that a certain type of memory is lost after a localized lesion does not necessarily mean that the memory itself was housed at this site. It seems more likely that such lesions interrupt pathways that are critical either for the formation or recall of the memory. Each particular subjective memory, may, like each emotion, be conjured temporarily into existence as a three-dimensional pattern of neural activity involving many synapses, which are often congruent with those activated by other memories. (It is doubtful whether a memory exists as an entity at all, except during the times of learning or recall when the particular pattern is actually being used). Certain synapses may be crucial for the establishment or recall of specific components of memory, and dysfunction at these synapses could result in different types of amnesia. For example, the neural activity stimulated by an event may need to be referred through circuits in the temporal lobes in order to activate patterns which include an association with geographical or time location. If these circuits are lacking due to a lesion, the full memory pattern cannot be formed, and the patient will be lost in time and space.

Each memory pattern is envisaged to be honed into shape by synaptic modulations occurring during learning, so that once activity is triggered by a familiar stimulus it will tend to follow preferential pathways. The patterns initiated by a single memory would tend to spread like ripples in a pond as associated memory patterns are in turn sparked into activity. Thus a subject with nominal aphasia can still describe the attributes of an object even if he cannot name it. The ability to use memories, especially once they are well established, and to alter behaviour because of them, undoubtedly involves widespread interconnections between many brain areas, and it is likely that many different possible pathways can be utilized both in the process of learning and in the execution of a learned behaviour. Because of this redundancy, selective memory loss is compatible with normal performance in many tests of intelligence. Yet the total capacity of the brain to store or recall information, with all its associated nuances, must be reduced by memory loss. Hence intelligence in the widest sense—global intelligence or maximal intellectual performance—must be correspondingly impaired.

Interpretation of the often confusing and conflicting results of investigations in amnesic syndromes has been beset by major difficulties. First, the memory tests employed in man, mainly designed to test aspects of semantic or event memory, are not comparable with those used in animals, which mainly test associative memory. Second, the memory tests have been based on hypothetical ideas of memory and it has often been assumed that memory deficits are absolute and that they are limited to one supposed subfunction of memory (e.g. encoding, consolidation, or retrieval). Yet these processes may not be separable and several of them may be partially affected to varying degrees in different patients with disease of different severity or aetiology.

With regard to the biochemical basis of human memory, clinical studies have so far yielded limited information. Investigations of patients with Alzheimer's disease conform with other evidence indicating that cholinergic connections are of importance, at least in event memory. However, they do not rule out the possibility that other neurotransmitters are involved, since the post-mortem changes are diffuse, and patients do not usually die when the intellectual disability is limited to the amnesic syndrome. Cerebral blood flow studies have yielded interesting information demonstrating the localised nature of changes in cerebral metabolic activity associated with different types of memory loss in Alzheimer's disease. As to the nature of the synaptic changes postulated to underlie memory, degeneration of both dendritic spines and microtubular structures occurs in Alzheimer's disease, but other major pathological changes, including large-scale neuronal loss, occur in addition. Thus, it has not been possible to pinpoint the cellular mechanisms of memory loss.

Pharmacological treatments aimed at restoring deficient neurotransmitters or stimulating neuronal metabolism in the central nervous system are considered in the next chapter.

10

Drugs and memory

Increasing interest has focused recently on the possibility of pharmacological treatment for memory disorders. Drugs, of course, cannot be expected to replace degenerated neurones, but they might theoretically improve the function of surviving neurones in chronic diseases, hasten neuronal recovery in acute conditions, and perhaps prevent further neuronal damage in both. Possible approaches include non-specific central nervous system stimulation, replacement of depleted neurotransmitters or neuromodulators, improvement of brain oxidation by increasing cerebral blood flow or stimulating neuronal metabolism, administration of putative memory modulators, or inhibition of endogenous amnesic systems. Such measures may not necessarily have specific effects on memory, since the same transmitters and metabolic processes are utilized in many brain activities, but improvement of memory may occur along with general improvement in mental efficiency. Clinical results so far have not been encouraging, but with greater experience and better patient selection, pharmacotherapy may find a useful if limited place in the management of memory disorders.

In other circumstances it may be advantageous to facilitate forgetting by means of drugs. For example, the use of benzodiazepines or anticholinergic drugs as premedication before surgery may not only calm the patient but also forestall the laying down of unpleasant memories. The combination of opiate narcotics with neuroleptics to induce neuroleptanalgesia, a state of drowsy numbness, also has uses in surgery.

Drugs for improving memory

Central nervous system stimulants

Central nervous system stimulants such as amphetamine and caffeine can improve performance of normal subjects in certain tasks, particularly in the presence of fatigue or boredom. However it is doubtful that such drugs can contribute much to the treatment of memory disorders. In general, they do not appear to have direct effects on memory, although they may influence it by affecting arousal and attention. Because of the inverted U-shaped relationship between performance and arousal, the effects of stimulant drugs depend on initial state, task variables, and dosage.

In normal subjects, *d*-amphetamine can enhance, impair, or have no effect on paired-associate learning (Zornetzer 1978). Methyl-phenidate over a range of doses has been reported to impair performance in memory tasks by disrupting attention during learning (Squire and Davis 1981), but to facilitate the learning of a pictorial paired-associate task in hyperactive children (Shea 1982). Facilitation of word-list recall has been observed after d-amphetamine in depressed patients (20 mg) and in normal children (0.5 mg/kg; Squire and Davis 1981). Pemoline and other central nervous sysem stimulants reviewed by Ban (1978) have also been claimed to increase general performance, although not specifically memory, in fatigued or elderly subjects, and to reverse the sedative effects of central nervous system depressants.

Cholinergic agents

The possibility that loss of central cholinergic activity may underlie the cognitive and memory impairments of Alzheimer type dementia (Chapter 9) suggests a therapeutic potential for cholinergic agents in these conditions. The rationale for such treatment is strengthened by the probability that the cholinergic abnormality is presynaptic in origin, with little evidence of involvement of post-synaptic muscarinic receptors (Corkin 1981). Furthermore, the memory defects produced by anticholinergic agents are similar to those which develop in old age and can be reversed by physostigmine (Drachman 1978; Chapter 8). A parallel between dopamine replacement in Parkinson's disease and acetylcholine replacement in Alzheimer's disease is immediately suggested.

However, the results available suggest only limited therapeutic benefit from cholinergic agents and at present drugs do not appear to provide a dramatic treatment for dementia. This conclusion is not altogether surprising in view of the neuropathological and neurochemical heterogeneity of clinical populations with dementia (Zeisel *et al.* 1981). Treatment, if it is to be effective, must probably be started early in the disease and continued for long periods, perhaps for life. Dosage may also be critical, since the effects of cholinergic drugs on memory are biphasic (Stanes *et al.* 1976; Corkin 1981). Coyle *et al.* (1983b) point out that functional deficits caused by degeneration of the cholinergic system, which is normally phasically active, with rapid neuronal discharge rates conveying spatially and temporally coded information (Chapter 8), may not be amenable to pharmacological correction.

Trials with several cholinergic agents including acetylcholine precursors (lecithin and choline), the anticholinesterase physostigmine, and the muscarinic cholinergic agonist arecoline have been reported, although these drugs have not been fully assessed in large scale, well designed, long-term trials (Squire and Davis 1981; Zeisel *et al.* 1981). Dietary supplements of choline and lecithin increase the synthesis and concentration of acetylcholine in the rat brain, and may possibly do so in humans. Corkin (1981) reviewed 11 studies in which either choline (doses in the range of 10–20 g choline chloride or equivalent daily) or lecithin (doses in the range of 30–100 g 20 per cent phosphatidyl choline daily) were administered for periods of 2 weeks to 3 months to patients with Alzheimer dementia. No overall changes were seen although individual patients showed improvement in some memory tests. Levy *et al.* (1983) reported the preliminary results of a double blind trial of a preparation containing 90 per cent phosphatydyl choline (25 g daily) in 52 patients with early Alzheimer dementia. A significant improvement in a test of general cognitive function and in a paired associate learning test was found in patients taking the drugs for 6 months. Pomara and Stanley (1982) raise the possibility that long-term treatment with cholinergic precursors might lead to acetylcholine muscarinic receptor desensitization and eventually produce the opposite effect from that intended. In addition, non-selective stimulation of cholinergic transmission might theoretically cause unwanted effects by enhancing transmission in pyramidal and extrapyramidal systems (Davies 1983). Cholinergic muscarinic agonists selective for receptors in cortical and hippocampal regions or drugs which selectively enhance the sensitivity of these receptors would represent a much-needed therapeutic advance.

Physostigmine has been used in some trials in dementia, but it may produce adverse effects and has a short half-life and a narrow effective dose range (Castleden 1984). However, enhanced performance in some memory tests, including verbal recall, has been reported in patients given 0.5 mg or less of physostigmine by intravenous infusion.

Combination therapy with lecithin and physostigmine (3 patients), and lecithin and tetrehydroaminoacridine, an oral anticholinesterase (10 patients), has been given in short trials with apparent improvement in long-term recall of words (Corkin 1981). Davies (1983) also reports some response in selected patients to physostigmine and lecithin. Possibly such drug combinations merit further long-term studies. A combination of choline with piracetam or hydergine derivatives, which may increase septohippocampal release or utilisation of acetylcholine, has also been suggested as a possibility for future investigation (Corkin 1981; Zeisel 1981; Davies 1983).

Drugs which increase cerebral blood flow or enhance cellular metabolism in the brain

In cerebral arteriosclerosis, which occurs to some degree in about 30 per cent of patients with senile dementia, cerebral blood flow is reduced and areas of brain tissue are hypoxic (Scott 1979). Several drugs have been tested for their ability to relieve cerebral hypoxia in animals. It was found, however, that many of the drugs, although vasodilators, also stimulated cerebral metabolism. This action is probably more important than vasodilatation since cerebral vascular tone depends largely on local factors and sclerotic blood vessels in anoxic areas are likely to be already maximally dilated. Vasodilatation in other blood vessels may therefore increase cerebral blood flow through normal areas without affecting, or even at the expense of, hypoxic areas. Recent efforts have therefore been directed towards developing drugs which increase neuronal oxidative activity, in the hope of improving neural function both in cerebrovascular disease and Alzheimer's disease.

Papaverine

Papaverine produces vasodilatation by a direct action on arterial smooth muscle. It may also have some dopamine receptor blocking activity and may inhibit phosphodiesterase, resulting in raised tissue concentrations of cyclic AMP, which may stimulate neuronal metabolism (Scott 1979). It is rapidly inactivated in the body, but sustained release preparations are available.

Papaverine reduces the symptoms of cerebral ischaemia due to arterial spasm. Its effects in arteriosclerotic dementia or other dementias of old age are controversial. Nevertheless some trials have reported favourable results. Branconnier and Cole (1977) reported that performance compared with placebo was improved in geriatric outpatients given 300 mg papaverine hydrochloride daily for 2 months, and Culebras (1976) found that papaverine had a stimulating effect on EEG activity compared with placebo in elderly patients with dementia associated with diffuse cerebrovascular disease. Other placebo controlled trials showing generally favourable results with papaverine in various dementias are cited by Ban (1978). Not surprisingly, beneficial effects when they occur are modest and are not restricted to memory functions. Similarly, procaine may have beneficial effects on mood, but there is little evidence that it improves cognitive function in senile dementia (Reisberg *et al.* 1981).

Cyclandelate

Cyclandelate has pharmacological properties similar to papaverine but is a more potent vasodilator. In doses of 800–1600 mg daily it has been shown to improve the general performance of patients with impaired mental abilities (Ban 1978). Improvement is, however, small although Scott (1979) suggested that it may prevent the steady decline in mental performance which usually occurs over time in senile dementias.

Dihydrogenated ergot alkaloids

Co-dergocrine mesylate (Hydergine) is a mixture of dihydrogenated derivatives of the constitutent alkaloids of ergotoxine. These substances block adrenergic receptors and act as partial agonists/antagonists at dopaminergic and serotonergic sites (Castleden 1984). They may increase the microcirculation in the brain but their major action appears to be on neurone metabolism. Co-dergocrine is reported to inhibit the action of Na/K ATPase, adenylate cyclase, and phosphodiesterase in brain cells, thus decreasing the breakdown of ATP and cyclic AMP, improving the energy balance of the cell, and enhancing cyclic AMP-mediated effects (Meier-Ruge *et al.* 1975). These changes are thought to account for an 'activating' effect on the EEG observed in hypoxic rats and elderly patients. Cerebral oxygen consumption is also reported to be increased by hydergine in patients with cerebrovascular disease (Sandoz 1977).

Castleden (1984) discussed the pharmacokinetics of co-dergocrine which appears to be poorly absorbed from the gut and has a bioavailability of only 5-12.5 per cent when taken by mouth in single doses. Little is known about the effects of chronic dosing or about its penetration into the central nervous system in normal subjects or in patients with dementia. Several placebo controlled double blind with dihydrogenated ergot alkaloids studies have shown significant improvement in general and cognitive functioning, including memory functions, in cerebrovascular disorders in geriatric patients (Thibault 1974; Rao and Norris 1972; Ditch *et al.* 1971; and others reviewed by Castleden 1984; Reisberg *et al.* 1981). Although co-dergocrine treatment was associated with improvement in certain memory items tested, such as 'recognition memory' and 'forgetfulness' , it was clear that the beneficial effect of the drug was on global cognitive and affective functioning and not specific for memory. Burian (1974) reported a dramatic improvement in general intellectual and motor function after 90 days treatment with hydergine in a 62-year-old patient shown by brain biopsy to have Alzheimer's disease. The effects of hydergine do not become evident for several weeks and improvement when it occurs continues for at least 3 months; life-long treatment may be required.

Naftidrofuryl

Naftidrofuryl is a vasodilator with sympatholytic and local anaesthetic properties; it is also said to stimulate brain metabolism (Scott 1979). The drug is well absorbed from the gastrointestinal tract, but undergoes first pass hepatic metabolism so that its bioavailability is only 24 per cent. The elimination half-life is only about 40 m, but some of the metabolites may be pharmacologically active, and there is some evidence that the drug penetrates into the central nervous system (Castleden 1984). It has been used in a number of small studies in patients with mixed dementias and may be modestly effective in improving cognitive performance in some patients (Brodie 1977; Castleden 1984).

Other vasodilators

Several other vasodilator drugs which also stimulate cell metabolism have been used in cerebrovascular disease. These include isoxsuprine, vincamine, nicergoline and cinnarizine. Some studies have suggested that they are of therapeutic value and these are reviewed by Scott (1977) and Ban (1978).

Piracetam

The term nootropic was applied to the compound piracetam which was claimed to be the first of a new class of drugs that enhance learning and memory by a selective effect on brain integrative mechanisms in the telencephalon, without altering neuronal excitability or neurotransmitter activity (Giurgea 1976). A synthetic compound, piracetam (2-oxo-pyrrolidine acetamide) can be regarded as a cyclic derivative of GABA. Its mechanism of action has been investigated in normal, hypoxic, and aged rats. It is reported to increase the turnover of ATP in brain cells by increasing both the rate of synthesis from ADP and the rate of utilization, as shown by an increased rate of incorporation of ^{32}P into phospholipids and nucleic acids, although not all studies agree (Scott 1979). Electron microscopy studies have shown that the drug prevents polysomial damage induced by hypoxia in the rat brain and other organs (Giurgea 1976). This action is presumed to increase the energy available to neurones for macromolecular synthesis and membrane polarization, thus enhancing neuronal efficiency, especially when this is impaired by hypoxia and other noxious influences to which telencephalic structures are specially sensitive.

Later studies have suggested that piracetam is not without effects on neurotransmitter activity. Rago et al. (1981) found that it increased the concentration of dopamine metabolites, but not the dopamine content, in the rat striatum and suggested that it increased dopamine turnover. Corkin (1981) and Zeisel (1981) suggest that it may increase acetylcholine release in the septum and hippocampus. The implications of its structural similarity to GABA in relation to possible effects on GABA-ergic systems is not known.

Piracetam is well absorbed by mouth, enters the brain and cerebrospinal fluid, has a plasma half-life of 4.5 h in man, is eliminated 98 per cent unchanged by the kidney and appears to be remarkably non-toxic (Giurgea 1976).

Effects in animals The effects in animals have been reviewed by Giurgea (1976). Piracetam was initially found to be effective in blocking the central nystagmus induced by electrical stimulation of the lateral geniculate body, and also peripheral rotatory nystagmus in rabbits. It exerted no demonstrable actions on reticular and limbic formations, caused no disturbances of sleep or wakefulness, had no effect on pain or aggression, and did not alter sensory perception in several animal species even in high doses (10 g/kg/day in dogs).

However, piracetam exerted a marked protective action against the damaging effects of cerebral hypoxia in brain function. For example, hypoxia induced in rabbits by nitrogen inhalation causes a flattening of the EEG trace, progressing to electrical silence. Intravenous administration of piracetam delayed the appearance of electrical silence and markedly accelerated the recovery of the EEG to a normal pattern when the animal was allowed to breathe air. The effect was not due to a stimulating action in the respiratory centre, since it also occurred in curarized animals under artificial respiration.

The protective effect of piracetam against anoxia, to which the neocortex is particularly sensitive, along with its apparent lack of effect on reticular or rhinencephalic structures, suggested a telencephalic site of action and led to investigation of its effects on learning and memory. In normal rats, daily treatment with piracetam, administered before testing, increased the speed of learning and decreased the number of errors made in swimming out of a cold water maze, compared with placebo, and also improved acquisition of learning in a number of other tests. In addition, it was highly protective against the deleterious effects of electroconvulsive shocks, hypoxia, old age, and alcohol intoxication on learning acquisition in the water maze and other tasks.

The effect of piracetam on consolidation or retrieval of memory was investigated in a number of tests in which amnesic procedures were administered after training sessions in rats. In several tests, including operant conditioning and passive avoidance conditioning, piracetam protected against the amnesic effects of hypoxia, electroconvulsive shocks, and the protein synthesis inhibitor 8-azaguanine. It was concluded that the drug affects both acquisition and consolidation or retrieval of memory. Further behavioural investigations (Sara et al. 1979) led to the conclusion that piracetam facilitated retrieval of memory without impairing extinction in normal rats.

The hypothesis that these effects were due to an action on the cortical association areas was examined in a study of the drug's effects on cortical evoked potentials in rats. In curarized animals under artificial respiration, the cortico-cortical potential, evoked by stimulating the median suprasylvan gyrus, an area of 'association' cortex, and recorded from the same site on the contralateral hemisphere (transcallosal response), was greatly increased following intravenous piracetam (2–100 mg/kg). By contrast, cortical potentials evoked by stimulation of the thalamus or the sciatic nerve and recorded from the contralateral sigmoid gyrus were not facilitated. A large range of psychotropic drugs were also tested in this model but none showed the selectivity of piracetam in facilitating only the transcallosal response. It was concluded that piracetam exerted its effects, unlike other psychotropic drugs, by an action exclusively on the association areas of the cortex. The ability of piracetam to enhance interhemispheric transfer of memory was confirmed in behavioural tests in rats (Buresova and Bures 1976). It was suggested that the blocking effect on piracetam on central and peripheral nystagmus was due to facilitation of cortical control over subcortical structures involved in nystagmus.

Effects in man Piracetam appears to cause little if any disruption of normal brain function in man. Oswald and Lewis (cited by Giurgea 1976) showed that it had no detectable effects on sleep stages, and no changes in excitability thresholds, reflex activities, or psychodysleptic phenomena have been recorded during piracetam treatment. It has been claimed that a dose of more than 20 g per day produces virtually no toxic effects, although rarely, aggressiveness, slight psychomotor agitation, and insomnia, have been reported.

Antinystagmus activity for nystagmus produced by rotation or calorically has been reported (Giurgea 1976), as well as protection against brain hypoxia in normal subjects. Lagergren and Levander (1974) investigated the effects of piracetam on psychomotor performance (critical flicker fusion, reaction time, and visual acuity) in volunteers fitted with a cardiac pacemaker and made artifically hypoxic by means of controlled reduction of heart rate from 70 to 45 beats per min. The subjects received 1 week of treatment each with placebo and piracetam (4.8 g daily) in a double blind cross-over trial. Piracetam had little effect on performance at normal heart rate, but significantly lessened the deterioration in performance caused by hypoxia when the heart rate fell to 45 beats per min.

Dimond and Bronwers (1976) reported that piracetam enhanced verbal memory in 16 healthy young university students who took the drug for 3 weeks. There was no effect compared with placebo on remembering lists of words after 1 week, but significant improvement in recall after 2 weeks. Dimond (cited in Giurgea 1976) also reported that piracetam improved dichotic listening in normal subjects, a finding consistent with the possibility that the drug facilitates interhemispheric transfer of information in humans.

Piracetam has also been investigated in a number of clinical trials in patients with impaired mental function of mixed aetiology (Giurgea 1976; Dimond and Bronwers 1976; Scott 1979; Castleden 1984). It has been reported to produce variable degrees of improvement in general mental function in cerebrovascular disease, post-concussional syndrome, senile and presenile dementia, chronic and acute alcoholism, and alcohol withdrawal syndromes, to shorten the duration of coma following drug intoxication, and to hasten recovery after neurosurgery (Richardson and Bereen 1977). As a treatment for senile dementia, piracetam has received little support, eight out of 13 studies reviewed by McDonald (1982) showing no difference between drug and placebo. However, trials with a combination of piracetam and choline in Alzheimer's dementia may be worth pursuing (Castleden 1984).

On the whole, clinical results with this drug have been disappointing in spite of its promising pharmacological profile in animals. However, it may prove of some use in hastening brain recovery after acute hypoxia as in neonatal asphyxia (Giurgea 1976), near-drowning, drug intoxications, carbon monoxide poisoning, trauma, neurosurgery, and cerebral vascular accidents. It has also been claimed to have antipsychotic effects in schizophrenia (Kabes et al. 1979), in which there may be abnormalities in interhemispheric transfer (Green 1978, Chapter 13). The possibilities of improving mental function in normal subjects opens up another uncharted field.

Etiracetam, Aniracetam, Pramiracetam

Three compounds closely related to piracetam: pramiracetam, etiracetam, and aniracetam have been introduced more recently. Their properties are very similar to those of piracetam (Cumin *et al.* 1982; Sara 1980; Murray and Fibiger 1986). There have been few clinical studies but preliminary data indicate that aniracetam is well tolerated in man and that it may improve EEG activity in cerebrovascular unsufficiency (Cumin *et al.* 1982).

Vasopressin

In spite of the demonstrable effects of vasopressin on memory in animals and the suggestion that it may be involved in human memory (Chapter 8), the use of vasopressin or its synthetic analogues for treatment of memory disorders in man has met with variable success. Vasopressin is usually administered by nasal catheter or as a nasal spray in doses of about 16 IU daily, and treatment must usually be continued for some weeks before a measurable response occurs.

In alcoholic and post-traumatic amnesia, no improvement after vasopressin or desmopressin was found by Blake *et al.* (1978), Jenkins *et al.* (1979) or Koch-Henrikson and Neilson (1981). However, occasional reports have noted improvement after vasopressin in learning ability in the alcoholic amnesic syndrome (Le Boeuf *et al.* 1978) and partial reversal of retrograde amnesia due to head injury (Oliveros *et al.* 1978) or electroconvulsive therapy (Weingartner *et al.* 1981). Vasopressin has also been reported to improve learning and memory in patients with primary affective disorders (Gold *et al.* 1979; Weingartner *et al.* 1981). Improvement in cognitive function was independent of changes in mood, although mood also improved in some patients. Kovacs *et al.* (1982) claim that memory defects occurring in diabetes insipidus, in which there is a lack of endogenous posterior pituitary hormones, can be reversed with vasopressin or its derivatives. Vasopressin does not appear to be a hopeful treatment for Alzheimer dementia since brain vasopressin levels are usually normal, but it is possible that somatostatin might be beneficial since selective depletion of this neuropeptide has been reported (Coyle *et al.* 1983b).

Opioid antagonists

Considering the probable importance of opioid peptides in a physiological amnesic system and the proven effects of naloxone on memory in animals (Chapter 8), it is perhaps surprising that there is little published data on the effects of opioid antagonists on memory in man. Naloxone does not appear to improve memory in normal subjects (Volavka *et al.* 1979; File and Silverstone 1981; Wolkowitz and Tinklenberg 1983). Reisberg *et al.* (1983) conducted a double blind, placebo controlled, multiple dose (single intravenous injections of 1.5 or 10 mg) trial of naloxone in seven patients with Alzheimer's dementia.

They noted significant improvement in tests of digit span and recall as well as in general cognitive function. In isolated cases, naloxone has been reported to reverse neurological defects associated with cerebral ischaemic attacks. Baskin and Hosobuchi (1981) described two patients with cerebral ischaemia who received intravenous infusions of naloxone or saline. Naloxone restored consciousness and reversed hemiplegia in both patients. The effect was short-lived, since naloxone has a brief duration of action, but was repeatable on several occasions. Bousigue *et al.* (1982) reported a similar effect of naloxone in a patient with a cerebral ischaemic attack and suggested on the basis of EEG findings that naloxone may stimulate the reticular formation and motor pathways.

Drugs for forgetting

A number of clinically used drugs can produce adverse effects on memory (Whitty et al. 1977; McClelland 1985; Libiger and Ban 1981). Acute toxic confusional states may result from overdose or idiosyncratic reactions. The main defect is usually one of acquisition with persisting amnesia for the period of confusion. Chronic intoxication with central nervous system depressants such as barbiturates, benzodiazepines and other hypnotics and sedatives, antiepileptic drugs, alcohol, and narcotic analgesics produces impairment of concentration and memory, and sometimes disorientation, particularly in the elderly. However, in certain doses both alcohol (Parker *et al.* 1981) and benzodiazepines (Liljequist *et al.* 1978) may improve recall while impairing acquisition.

The amnesic effects of certain drugs can sometimes be put to clinical use as preoperative medication or during minor surgical procedures.

Benzodiazepines

The amnesic effects of intravenous diazepam (10 and 20 mg), flunitrazepam (1 and 2 mg) and lorazepam (4 mg) given preoperatively to healthy females undergoing minor gynaecological operations were assessed against a saline control by George and Dundee (1977). All the drugs produced an anterograde amnesia as tested by recognition of cards shown to the patients at various times after drug administration. There was no retrograde amnesia. The amnesia was accompanied by sedation, although the patients were rousable, and the sedation far outlasted the amnesic effects. No adverse effects were noted and this study confirmed other reports that the benzodiazepines are effective amnesic agents for minor operations. Webberly and Cuschieri (1982) note that the amnesic effect of diazepam is valuable in ensuring future compliance with repeat gastrointestinal endoscopy, especially in patients with high neuroticism personality traits.

Several authors have tested the effects of orally administered benzo-

diazepines on memory in healthy adults. Jones *et al.* (1978 1979) compared
the effects of single doses of diazepam (5 mg) and nitrazepam (5 mg) with
those of hyoscine (0.3 mg) and placebo. They found that the benzodiazepines
and hyoscine impaired short term memory (recall of serial order of digits)
but not recall of word lists. Liljequist *et al.* (1978) compared the effects of
diazepam (10 mg) given as a single dose or daily for 14 days, chlorpromazine
(25 mg) given singly or daily for 4 days, and placebo on several tests of
memory in normal young subjects. They found, using a paired-association
learning task, that diazepam impaired acquisition but slightly facilitated
recall while chlorpromazine had no effect. Ghoneim *et al.* (1981) studied a
group of normal subjects during 3 weeks medication with diazepam (0.2
mg/kg daily) and also noted impairment of acquisition, but not of recall.
Their evidence suggested the development of partial tolerance to the memory
decrement after 3 weeks, and complete recovery of memory occurred by 1
week after drug withdrawal.

Although the general effect of benzodiazepines on memory thus appears
to be limited to a deficit in acquisition which has been attributed to an
impairment of encoding, similar to that produced by anticholinergic agents
(Caine *et al.* 1981), not all subjects show this response. Desai *et al.* (1983)
found that in normal subjects with high state anxiety oral diazepam (5 mg)
improved short term memory, while impairing it in subjects with low state
anxiety. This result is not surprising considering the known interactions of
psychotropic drugs with starting state and personalty. It seems likely that
the effects of benzodiazepines on memory result from general central nervous
system depression, due to enhancement of GABA activity (Chapter 4), rather
than from any specific efects on memory mechanisms. The degree to which
benzodiazepines affect different aspects of memory (acquisition, retention,
recall) is probably dose-related, and it appears from the data of Liljequist *et
al.* (1978) and Ghonheim *et al.* (1981) that acquisition is impaired at lower
doses than retrieval.

Anticholinergic drugs

Atropine and scopolamine primarily block the actions of acetylcholine at
muscarinic receptors, although at high doses they may have some nicotinic
receptor blocking action as well. Both muscarinic and nicotinic receptors
appear to be involved in cholinergic transmission at cortical and subcortical
levels in the brain. While the depressant effects of atropine and scopolamine
are usually ascribed to central muscarinic blockade, stimulant effects may
result from other actions. The drugs cause an increase in acetylcholine turnover which may result in the activation of nicotinic receptors in the brain
(Weiner 1980a). The mixed stimulant/depressant effects of these drugs
depend on dose and on individual susceptibility. Since cholinergic systems
are involved both in arousal (Chapter 2) and memory (Chapter 8), amnesic

effects of anticholinergic drugs could result from disruption of either or both
of these systems.

In the clinical setting, therapeutic doses of scopolamine (0.6 mg) usually
produce drowsiness, euphoria, amnesia, fatigue, and dreamless sleep with
decreased REM activity (Weiner 1980a). This action is useful when scopolamine is employed for preanaesthetic medication or as an adjunct to anaesthetic agents. However, some patients respond to the same doses with
excitement, restlessness, hallucinations, and delirium. The excitatory effects
are most common in patients with severe pain, occur regularly with high
doses, and are also seen with high doses of atropine.

Several investigators have compared the effects of scopolamine (0.8 mg
IM, 1 mg SC), methscopolamine, a peripherally acting muscarinic blocker
(0.5 mg IM, 1 mg SC), and normal saline on the performance of normal
subjects in multiple memory tests (Caine et al. 1981; Drachman 1978). From
both studies, it appeared that the effects of scopolamine on memory were not
global and not due simply to non-specific central nervous system depression,
although the subjects were drowsy. Scopolamine impaired initial memory
acquisition and retrieval, but even at these doses there was no decrement in
immediate memory and no decrease of attention or initial signal detection in
an auditory vigilance task. Caine et al. (1981) suggest that the amnesic effect
of scopolamine was on definable neuropsychological processes, especially
encoding of new information and retrieval of well-learned old information.
Drachman (1978) showed that the pattern of memory deficits of normal
young subjects given scopolamine was similar to that shown by normal,
undrugged, elderly subjects. The effect of scopolamine was presumed to be
mediated via cholinergic mechanisms since it was reversed by physostigmine,
but not by the stimulant drug amphetamine.

Neuroleptanalgesia and dissociative anaesthesia

Neuroleptic drugs themselves rarely cause impairment of memory (Whitty
et al. 1977); they produce a state of quiescence with indifference to the
surroundings and reduction of anxiety, while consciousness and the ability
to obey commands is maintained (Chapter 14). However, they potentiate the
effects of other central nervous system depressants (Marshall and Wollman
1980) and when a neuroleptic such as droperidol is combined with a potent
narcotic analgesic such as fentanyl, a state of neuroleptanalgesia supervenes.
During this state, a number of minor surgical procedures can be
accomplished without discomfort to the patient. Neuroleptanalgesia can be
converted to neuroleptanaesthesia by the administration of 65 per cent
nitrous oxide in oxygen (Marshall and Wollman 1980). The amnesic effect
of the narcotic presumably results from a combination of general central
nervous system depression and activation of opioid amnesic systems.

Some arylcycloalkylamines induce a state of dissociative anaesthesia. The state is characterized by sedation, immobility, amnesia, marked analgesia, and a strong feeling of detachment similar to neuroleptanalgesia (Marshall and Wollman 1980). Phencyclidine (Chapter 7) has been used for this purpose but readily gives rise to dysphoria, hallucinations, and psychological complications, possibly due to an action on opioid sigma receptors. These effects are much less common with ketamine hydrochloride which can be administered intravenously as an anaesthetic induction agent. A feeling of depersonalization occurs within 15 s, followed shortly by unconsciousness which lasts 10–15 min after a single dose. Analgesia persists for some 40 minutes and amnesia may last for 1–2 h. Full recovery after multiple dosage takes several hours and about 50 per cent of patients over 30 years of age experience unpleasant dreams, hallucinations, delirium, or excitement, during the recovery period. 'Flashbacks' with disagreeable psychological symptoms may occur days or weeks later. However, in younger adults and children these adverse psychological experiences are not nearly so common. Ketamine is thought to act on the cortex and limbic system (Marshall and Wollman 1980) and has some pharmacological effects in common with LSD (Chapter 14).

Future prospects

While the use of drugs for forgetting, as described above, has reached a considerable degree of sophistication, the use of drugs to improve memory remains problematic. Despite intense interest in the pharmacology of memory over the past few years (Chapters 8 and 9), and considerable advances in understanding, it appears that the subject has hardly reached the stage of direct clinical application to memory disorders. From experience to date, it seems unlikely that drugs which influence neurotransmitter or modulator function (cholinergic drugs, vasopressin, naloxone) will have major effects in clinical conditions—although possibly the development of drugs with specific sites of action in the brain is worth striving for. Drugs which improve cerebral oxygenation and stimulate neuronal metabolism may be of more value in dementias and other amnesic syndromes if used early enough, but again specificity in site of action is so far lacking. The greatest hope for the future would seem to lie in drugs which stimulate neuronal plasticity, and such drugs are still in their infancy. Early information on the biological actions or nerve growth factor is reviewed by Greene (1984). Since adult neurones are capable of increasing their dendritic arborizations and are hormone-responsive, at least in animals (Chapter 8), it might be possible (perhaps with a combination of nerve growth factor and hormones) to encourage surviving neurones to take over the functions of degenerated neurones in human dementias.

Part IV
Depression and mania

11
Depression and mania: clinical features and brain mechanisms

In previous chapters, brain systems for arousal and sleep, reward and punishment, and learning and memory have been considered. It is clear, from the clinical manifestations and observed physiological changes, that all of these systems are involved in depression and mania, but the central feature is an alteration of affect. Although alterations in affect may occur in organic brain disease, no structural abnormality has been found which could account for affective disorders in general. These conditions thus appear to result from some, usually reversible, functional disorder in the brain systems controlling emotional tone. Present evidence, discussed in this chapter, points to a dysfunction of the limbic system, particularly in pathways subserving reward and punishment. Depression and mania can thus be viewed as disorders of reward and punishment systems, with features in common with drug dependence and chronic pain syndromes (Chapter 6). Because of the integrated nature of brain systems, such disorders have secondary effects on arousal and sleep and on cognitive, autonomic and endocrine function.

All brain systems utilize similar multiple neurotransmitter and modulator mechanisms and their neurones run in overlapping and interconnected pathways. Hence, attempts to incriminate any one chemical or any one brain location in affective disorders have not been successful. Furthermore, within any one functional system there are often redundant subsystems having similar effects, but utilizing a different series of transmitters. Such back-up systems have been described for pain modulation (Chapter 5) and exist for other vital processes. Malfunction at various different sites can therefore bring about similar behavioural effects. The clinical, neurophysiological and biochemical evidence discussed below all suggests that both the syndrome of affective disorders and the symptoms of depression or elation may be triggered by several aetiological factors acting through a final common path in the limbic system, but the ultimate mechanisms remain elusive.

Classification

A great deal of energy has been used in attempts to classify affective disorders, and the problems are still 'sufficient to keep armies of psychiatrists disputing happily for years' (Paykel 1983; p. 155S). Classification is difficult because depressive states are heterogeneous and the symptoms may merge with the symptom clusters of anxiety, schizophrenia, personality disorders, and even with normality. Thus, neither classifications based on possible aetiology nor those based on clinical manifestations are at present satisfactory. Classification is discussed by Hamilton (1979), Roth and Barnes (1981), Gelder *et al.* (1983), and Paykel (1983).

For clinical purposes, a division of depressive states into endogenous (psychotic) and neurotic (reactive) groups is widely used. Endogenous depression may be subdivided into bipolar and unipolar types. In bipolar depression there are episodes of mania, while in the unipolar type only depressive episodes occur. These divisions have to some extent characteristic symptoms and clinical course, but there is considerable overlap between all groups. The clinical assessment of depression is discussed by Lader (1981). The difficult distinction between the *symptoms* of depression and elation, which are experienced normally and seen in many illnesses, and the *syndromes* of affective disorders is discussed by Gelder *et al.* (1983).

Symptoms of depression

Psychological symptoms

The symptoms of depression encompass a whole gamut of emotional states, of which sadness and misery as normally experienced form only a part, and stand somewhere in the middle of the range. At one extreme there may be a feeling of hopelessness and despair, inability to experience pleasure or to envisage it in the future, and an attitude of apathy. At another extreme there may be intense anxiety, fear, agitation, irritability, and sometimes specific phobias. Yet another dimension of depression is characterized by feelings of guilt and unworthiness, feelings of deserved punishment, delusions, hallucinations of accusatory voices, obsessional ruminations, and hypochondriasis. There is considerable overlap in the clinical presentation of these symptoms and almost any combination may exist in individual patients. The symptoms may be present in any degree of severity. They may be so mild as to be within the range of normal experience or so severe as to suggest a major psychosis.

Behaviour

The behaviour and appearance of the depressed patient varies according to the symptoms. Facial expression, posture, and movement are expressive of misery. Apathetic patients show psychomotor retardation: they walk and react slowly and take little interest in their surroundings. Thoughts are slowed and response to speech is noticeably delayed. On the other hand, agitated patients cannot remain still: they may be continually wringing their hands, pacing up and down, and repetitively expressing their fears. Suicidal behaviour is not uncommon in patients who are not too anergic to undertake it; 11–17 per cent of patients with severe depressive disorders eventually commit suicide (Gelder *et al.* 1983).

Somatic symptoms

A wide range of somatic symptoms may be present. Complaints of disturbed sleep are common: early morning waking is characteristic, but frequent awakenings during the night and delay in falling asleep may also occur. Typically, the psychological changes of depression are worst in the morning, coinciding with early waking, and mood may improve during the day. However, patients with anxiety may feel worst at the end of the day, coinciding with difficulty in falling asleep. Other patients sleep excessively, but still wake feeling unrefreshed and pessimistic. Loss of appetite and weight are common and are associated with poor sleep; in patients with excessive sleep, however, there may be increased eating and weight gain. Constipation, loss of libido, amenorrhoea, lethargy, impaired memory and concentration, and generalized aches and pains are all frequent symptoms.

Hypochondriacal preoccupation and sometimes bizarre somatic delusions are prominent in some patients. However, physical disease may coexist with depression. As previously discussed (Chapter 6), disease, especially chronic pain, can cause depression, and depression can aggravate chronic pain. Sometimes the presenting symptoms are purely physical, and in such masked depression alteration of mood may not be apparent and may even be hidden beneath a smiling exterior.

Symptoms and signs of mania

The symptoms and signs of mania are of variable severity, but are generally characterized by elevation of mood, hyperactivity, and self-important ideas. The mood may be predominantly one of euphoria or elation, but is typically labile and interspersed with irritability, episodes of anger, and brief periods of depression. Expansive ideas are common but insight and judgement are impaired so that extravagant and impractical projects are recklessly undertaken. Grandiose or sometimes persecutory delusions, and hallucinations, may occur.

The behaviour reflects the changes in mood. The patient is hyperactive; he starts many activities, but often leaves them unfinished. He may become exhausted and present a dishevelled appearance. He sleeps little and may talk incessantly. Speech is rapid and may become incoherent, reflecting flight of ideas. Appetite and libido are increased, and social behaviour may be uninhibited. Rarely, a manic stupour may occur in which the patient is mute and immobile but his facial expression is one of elation.

Relation to other psychiatric disorders

The difference between anxiety syndromes and neurotic depression is based clinically on the relative severity of the anxiety and depressive symptoms and the order in which they appear (Gelder *et al*. 1983). It is said that the course and response to treatment differs between the two groups, but a distinction is probably artificial; in practice borderline cases are usually treated with both antidepressant and anxiolytic drugs. Similar difficulties arise when phobic or obsessive symptoms are mixed with anxiety/depression. In the same way, the distinction between some manifestations of schizophrenia and depression or mania is so blurred that patients who have equal proportions of schizophrenic and depressive or manic symptoms are classed as having a schizoaffective disorder. The overlap between depression and chronic pain syndromes has been discussed in Chapter 6. Depression may also be a prominent feature of organic brain disease and may follow the use of various drugs, as described below.

Peripheral and central indices of affective disorders

Some of the symptoms of affective disorders are accompanied by measurable changes in peripheral autonomic and central activity. In the periphery, there is some evidence of reduced electrodermal responsivity in depressed patients, especially in those categorized as endogenous or retarded (Christie *et al*. 1980). Resting forearm blood flow and heart rate appear to be higher in patients with agitated compared with endogenous depression, but there is little evidence for a consistent deviation from normal levels (Christie *et al*. 1980). However, some patients with agitated depression have abnormally high concentrations of plasma noradrenaline (Siever *et al*. 1983). There is no direct relationship between blood pressure and plasma noradrenaline concentration in these patients and it has been suggested that subsensitivity of peripheral alpha-adrenergic receptors develops in the face of prolonged sympathetic overactivity.

Sleep studies

Electroencephalographic studies have revealed marked abnormalities in the sleep profiles of depressed patients consistent with their symptoms of sleep disturbance (Christie *et al*. 1980; Perris 1980). Characteristically, patients with depression show reduction in Stage 4 sleep, fragmentation of the sleep pattern, multiple awakenings, and decreased total sleep time. A fairly consistent feature is a shortened latency to the first REMS episode and increased REMS density (Coble *et al*. 1976; Kupfer and Foster 1972). Several longitudinal studies indicate that REMS correlates inversely with the severity of depressive symptoms, the greatest amount of REMS and the shortest REMS latency occurring when the symptoms are worst (Schulz *et al*. 1978). These observations suggest that selective REMS deprivation might be of therapeutic value in depression. Awakening at the start of REMS episodes has been reported to improve endogenous depression, but is not a practicable procedure for wide application (*British Medical Journal* 1975). Several antidepressant drugs reduce REMS, but this effect does not always coincide with clinical improvement.

Paroxysmal features including slow focal spikes and small sharp spikes have also been observed in the sleeping EEG in depressive disorders. Similar changes in sleep profiles occur in mania.

Waking EEG studies

Studies of the waking EEG in affective disorders have given confusing results. Overall there seems to be no consistent difference in alpha frequency or power between manic or depressed patients and normal subjects. Beta activity has been found to be increased in both mania and depression. Paroxysmal and other abnormal EEG patterns appear to be more common in manic-depressives than in normal subjects. Some investigations (Perris 1980) have shown that the mean integrated amplitude of the EEG is reduced during depressive episodes, with lower values and decreased variability in the dominant hemisphere. After recovery, mean integrated EEG amplitude increases and the interhemispheric difference disappears. Further studies by Perris (1980), analysed by complex computerized techniques, suggest that the lateralization of EEG activity may differ between depressed patients with high or low anxiety and that different distributions of activity in temporal and occipital lobes may occur.

Cortical evoked potentials in depression are reviewed by Shagass *et al.* (1978). In general, the amplitude of the later components of the auditory, visual, and somatosensory evoked potentials are decreased, and their latency prolonged, and in some patients the changes disappear on recovery (Ashton, unpublished observations). However, conflicting results have also been reported since the responses vary with the intensity of the stimulus (Buchsbaum *et al.* 1971), and also depend upon which components are measured. Perris (1980) has reported interhemispheric differences in evoked potential amplitudes during depression with diminution of the difference on recovery. The magnitude of the slow cortical potential, the contingent negative variation, may also be reduced and its negativity prolonged during depression (Shagass *et al.* 1978) although again there are conflicting findings.

Cerebral blood flow

Measurements of cerebral blood flow with xenon-133 inhalation (Mathew *et al.* 1980) revealed greatly reduced values for grey-matter blood flow in depressed patients compared with age-matched controls. There was a significant inverse correlation between the degree of depression and the reduction in blood flow. No interhemispheric differences were found, but the decrease in blood flow was most marked in frontal regions. These studies suggest that there is a reduction in neuronal metabolism in depression and are consistent with the findings of decreased mean integrated EEG amplitude, decreased amplitude of cortical evoked responses, slowed psychomotor responses (Weckowicz *et al.* 1978), and cognitive dysfunction.

Incidence and clinical course

Depressive symptoms are reported by 13–20 per cent of the population, but are not necessarily part of a depressive affective disorder. Using strict diagnostic criteria (Gelder *et al.* 1983), the prevalence of bipolar depressive disorder is less than 1 per cent, with a mean age of onset of about 30 years. Females outnumber males by about 1.3 to 2:1. Unipolar depressive syndromes (including endogenous and neurotic depression) are more common, with a prevalence of about 3 per cent in males and 5–9 per cent in females. The preponderance in females may be partly due to a higher rate of recognition, but may also reflect genetic factors. The peak age of onset in females is between 35–40 years, while in males the prevalence increases with increasing age.

Genetic factors

The prevalence of affective disorders is greater in the relatives of depressed patients than in the general population. Parents, siblings and children of affected patients have a morbid risk of 10–15 per cent, several times greater than the general population. Twin studies have shown high rates of concordance (nearly 70 per cent) for manic-depressive psychosis in monozygotic twins, whether reared together or apart, and for dizygotic twins (23 per cent). Adoption studies have also provided strong evidence for genetic factors in the aetiology of depression. Bipolar disorders appear to be more common in the relatives of bipolar probands, but both bipolar and unipolar disorders occur in the families of unipolar probands. There is also some evidence of a greater than normal incidence of other psychiatric disorders, including schizophrenia, alcoholism, and personality disorders, in the families of patients with depressive syndromes. In addition, the families of probands with schizophrenia have an increased incidence of affective disorders.

At present, it seems clear that genetic factors are important in determining the incidence of affective disorders, but the mode of inheritance is not understood and no specific genetic markers have been found. Furthermore, most genetic studies have been concerned only with patients with severe disorders. The frequency of depressive symptoms (as opposed to frank illness) and of depressive personality traits in patients who later develop depressive illness or in their families is not known. It has been suggested that subjects with cyclothymic personality types might be prone to bipolar depression; those with high anxiety or obsessional traits to neurotic and endogenous unipolar depression (Shaw *et al.* 1982; Gelder *et al.* 1983). However, there is no evidence from prospective studies concerning premorbid personality in depressive disorders. Nor is it clear whether personality and illness are manifestations of the same processes.

Both unipolar and bipolar depressions follow a self-limiting, but recurrent course. Manic episodes, if untreated, usually last several months, sometimes years. Eventual recovery nearly always occurs, but recurrence of manic or depressive episodes is frequent. The course of unipolar depressive illness is variable: the usual duration of individual episodes is 6–12 months, but they may last from a few days to a few years. Most of the younger patients recover, but again there is a tendency to relapse. Even with modern treatment, up to 50 per cent of patients with unipolar depression have a further episode, although 95 per cent recover from the first episode. The effect of various drugs on relapse rates is discussed further in Chapter 12 and is reviewed by Freeman (1984) There appears to be a seasonal variation in the incidence of depressive episodes, with peak occurrences in March/April and September/October.

Factors causing depressive and manic symptoms

For purposes of clinical classification, psychiatrists have usually taken pains to separate the symptom of depression, which may occur in many conditions, from the syndrome of depressive disorder, in which depression of mood is usually a central feature. However, in attempts to understand the aetiology of depressive syndromes, it seems important to inquire into any factors which can give rise to the symptom of depression. As mentioned before, the symptoms of affective disorders merge at one end with normal emotions and at the other with psychiatric disorders. Even among the depressive syndromes, the symptoms are so variable, both in range and severity, as to suggest a heterogeneous group of disorders. It seems that there is nothing unique about either the quality or the degree of depression experienced as part of a depressive disorder. The mechanisms by which this emotion is generated, although perhaps triggered in different ways, are likely to be the same wherever it is found. The same considerations apply to the symptom of elation and the syndrome of manic states.

Organic Disease

Organic brain damage can give rise to disorders of affect. In dementia (chronic organic brain syndrome), depression can be marked although memory and cognitive impairment may also be prominent. Neoplastic, vascular, or infective brain lesions, especially of the frontal lobe, may cause expansive and uninhibited behaviour which can be difficult to distinguish from mania. Brain damage secondary to alcoholism may also give rise to depression and other affective disorders. Depression commonly occurs in the course of the Parkinsonian syndrome, and manic, depressive, or schizophreniform features may be associated with temporal lobe epilepsy.

Viral infections, particularly infectious mononucleosis, infectious hepatitis, and influenza, and some chronic bacterial infections such as brucellosis can give rise to prolonged depression. Chronic pain, neoplastic disease, and terminal illness can also (not surprisingly) cause depression.

Various endocrine abnormalities are associated with change in mood. Cushing's disease may be accompanied by either depression or by periods of elation, while Addison's disease, hyperparathyroidism, acromegaly, and hypopituitarism are associated with depression. Depression is common in the puerperium and may be severe enough to be classed as a puerperial depressive psychosis; depression may occur in the post-menopausal period and symptoms of depression may occur as part of the premenstrual tension syndrome. Endocrine abnormalities occuring in the affective disorders are discussed below.

Drugs

Several classes of drugs can cause depression. Many of these decrease the activity of monoaminergic systems in the brain. For example, reserpine, which depletes nerve terminals of monoamines, can cause a depressive reaction so severe that it leads to suicide, and such a reaction is more common in patients with a history of depressive disorder. Other antihypertensive drugs which interfere with neuronal release or storage of monoamines, such as guanethidine, debrisoquine, methyldopa and clonidine, can also cause depression. Monoamine receptor blockers, including beta-adrenergic receptor antagonists and neuroleptics, can have similar affects. Depression may also result from chronic use of central nervous system depressants, including alcohol, barbiturates, benzodiazepines, narcotics, and anticonvulsants, all of which decrease central catecholaminergic activity.

Depression is likewise a prominent symptom in drug withdrawal reactions, particularly from drugs with central nervous system stimulant effects, such as amphetamines, cocaine, and nicotine. In this case, drug withdrawal probably exposes catecholaminergic underactivity which has developed as the result of pharmacodynamic tolerance. Other drugs causing depression are reviewed by McClelland (1973a,b; 1985, 1986) and Tyrer (1981).

Other drugs can produce elation, euphoria, and in high doses manic states. Many of these drugs have central nervous system stimulant actions and increase activity in catecholaminergic systems in the brain. Thus, amphetamines, cocaine, laevo-dopa, tricyclic antidepressants, and monoamine oxidase inhibitors in high doses can all produce manic reactions. In patients in the depressive phase of a bipolar affective disorder, antidepressants may produce a rapid switch to the manic phase. Euphoric reactions also sometimes occur after small, disinhibiting, doses of alcohol, benzodiazepines, barbiturates, phencyclidine, and organic solvents. Manic states with hallucinations and delirium can occur as part of the withdrawal reactions from central nervous system depressants, probably reflecting central catecholaminergic overactivity due to drug tolerance.

The observed effects of many of the above drugs, which can induce mania or depression in normal subjects, and relieve or aggravate clinically occurring mania or depression, have formed the cornerstone of the various monoaminergic theories of affective disorders discussed below.

Environmental factors

Life events Depressive disorders often follow distressing life events. Of these, maternal deprivation in childhood has been suggested to be a predisposing factor to affective illness in later life. Death or departure of a parent, however, appears also to be non-specifically related to psychoneurosis, antisocial personality, and alcoholism (Paykel 1981). An excess of stressful or threatening life events, including loss or separation by death, has been shown in several studies to have occurred in the months before the onset of a depressive or manic disorder or a suicide attempt. However, a similar excess of events may precede the onset of neurosis, schizophrenia, cancer, and psychosomatic disorders, and only 10 per cent of people who experience loss develop a depressive syndrome (Paykel 1974). Thus, stress and bereavement appear to be non-specific factors in the aetiology of depression.

Animal separation studies There have been a number of studies of the affective responses to separation in monkeys and apes. Hinde (1977) noted that separation of an infant macaque monkey from its mother may cause a syndrome of despair which bears some resemblance to human depression. An initial stage of agitated activity is followed by depressed locomotor and play activity, and a generally depressed demeanour. This behaviour sometimes persisted for up to a month when the mother was returned after only a few days separation. Examination of the brain of infants during the early separation period showed an elevation of hypothalamic serotonin concentration, but no changes in other monoamines. It was also observed that the disturbance of behaviour was attenuated by anxiolytic drugs such as diazepam and chlorpromazine. These observations suggest that anxiety rather than depression was the major response to separation. Moreover, infants from a variety of other primate species do not show despair behaviour on separation (Everitt and Keverne 1979). The reaction displayed depends upon the social organization of the species. Thus, animal studies suggest that separation may also be a non-specific factor which may cause psychiatric disturbance, but not necessarily depression.

Peer separation has also been studied in monkeys, but this experience does not appear to provide a model for human depression. The reactions observed depend upon the strength of attachment of the separated individuals and the availability of substitutes in the new environment. However, in some primate societies, loss of social rank is sometimes associated with behaviour patterns seen in human depression. These include decreased locomotor activity, isolation from the group, suspension of sexual activity, cessation of eating, and death from inanition or infection. Changes in endocrine activity include elevated concentrations of cortisol and prolactin, low testosterone concentrations in males, and depression of luteinizing hormone and oestrogen responses in females (Everitt and Keverne 1979). Similar endocrine profiles are sometimes seen in human depression and human symptoms such as loss of self-esteem and feelings of rejection may be reminiscent of the role of a socially subordinate monkey.

The relevance of such animal studies to the symptom or syndrome of human depression is clearly limited, but Everitt and Keverne (1979) conclude that irreparable loss of important bonds, either social or connected with activities of personal importance (work, art, religion, etc.) may be fundamental.

Coping mechanisms Mills (1977), among others, has argued that depressive disorders may represent the breakdown of 'coping mechanisms' after periods of prolonged stress or repeated adverse events, the final event acting as a non-specific 'last straw' which eventually precipitates the illness. The sequence envisaged (Fig. 11.1) is that stressful events raise the general level of arousal. If the event is successfully coped with, the arousal level falls again. Moderate levels of arousal associated with successful coping are normally rewarding: in fact lack of a sufficient number of arousing events leads to dissatisfaction and boredom. However, if such events are particularly severe or come in quick succession, the demands of coping require a further rise in arousal level, which may need to be maintained. At this stage, because the arousal does not return to baseline, a sleep disturbance appears. Further environmental demands may lead to levels of arousal which are above the optimum for performance; such levels, instead of being rewarding, become unpleasant. Eventually, the capacity of arousal systems is exhausted and further coping responses become impossible. At this stage, coping ability declines, sleep disturbance continues, and the psychological and somatic symptoms of a depressive disorder are precipitated. Mills (1977) suggests that subjects particularly prone to such coping failure are those with an innately poor coping ability (inadequate personality), those who experience a chance succession of severe environmental challenges, and those who generate too many challenges for themselves by aiming at impossible goals.

This model, although perhaps describing a series of events which could lead to neurotic depression, seems to apply equally to the development of anxiety neurosis. It does not appear to account for some forms of endogenous

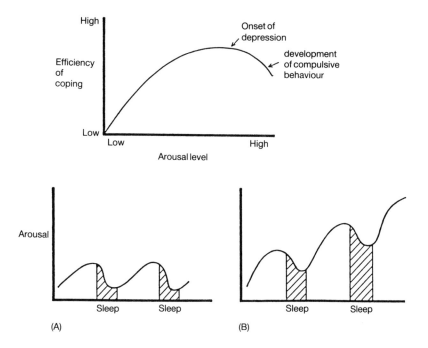

Fig. 11.1. Hypothetical relationship between arousal levels and coping mechanisms in the precipitation of depression. (From Mills 1977, by kind permission of the author.)

Top figure: biphasic relation between arousal and coping efficiency
A. normal pattern of arousal and sleep.
B. progressive elevation of arousal level under stress.
For fuller explanation see text.

depression in which the onset is apparently unrelated to life-events and in which the clinical picture of retardation and general slowness, with evidence of decreased neuronal metabolism in the brain (e.g., decreased cerebral blood flow; Mathew *et al.* 1980), is difficult to reconcile with a high general level of arousal. However, different individuals may have different patterns of response to stress, and some may fail to respond with increased arousal. In others, an anergic picture may reflect exhaustion of arousal systems and perhaps tolerance to excitatory neurotransmitters and endogenous opioids released during prolonged stress. Such a possibility was considered in relation to chronic pain syndrome (Chapter 6). Furthermore, as discussed below, different types of stress, whether real or perceived, may engender different responses.

A biochemical basis for the coping theory of depression has been proposed by Mills (1977), and this has received some support from animal work reviewed by Anisman *et al.* (1981). Acute stress increases the synthesis and utilization of noradrenaline in man (Chapter 3) and animals, and to a lesser extent that of dopamine and serotonin. The output of acetylcholine and of endogenous opioids (Chapter 6) is also increased. These changes are associated with increased arousal and escape or aggressive behaviour. However, if the stress is prolonged, repetitive, or severe, the rate of utilization of neurotransmitters may exceed the rate of synthesis so that temporary depletion occurs. Depletion of noradrenaline, dopamine, and serotonin has been shown to occur in a variety of brain regions in animals after exposure to severe or prolonged stress (Anisman *et al.* 1982), and may possibly be related to human depression.

Learned helplessness If animals are placed in a situation in which pain and stress are inescapable, for instance by being harnessed and subjected to electric shocks, a further reaction develops. During the stress, an initial period of hyperactivity and struggling is replaced by a state of immobility during which the animal apparently gives up all attempts to cope. In this situation central depletion of monoamines occurs much more readily than if the stress is escapable: this depletion is compatible with the more severe nature of the stress. However, if the animal is later exposed to an avoidable stress, it no longer tries to escape, exhibiting instead a severe deficit in escape avoidance behaviour. Such a response was described in dogs by Seligman (1975) and gave rise to the 'learned helplessness' theory of depression. The phenomenon has been observed in several animal species, and such animals display a behaviour bearing some resemblance to human depression, including reduced voluntary activity and decreased food intake. It was suggested that depression is a learned behaviour which develops when reward or punishment is perceived as no longer being contingent on the actions or responses of the animal.

However, Anisman *et al.* (1981) argued that learned helplessness behaviour depends not so much on cognitive functions involving learning and memory as on the biochemical responses to severe stress. Learned helplessness behaviour is accentuated by pharmacological manipulations which further deplete central monoamines or block monoamine receptors, and attenuated by drugs which prevent amine depletion or increase monoaminergic activity including a variety of antidepressant drugs (Kametani *et al.* 1983). Thus, depression and the consequent failure of coping is held to reflect an inability to sustain adequate concentrations of central monoamines, either because the stress is uncontrollable and severe or because of some deficiency in the adaptive process to stress.

This model seems to have some relevance to human depression, since drugs which deplete central monoamines or block their receptors induce depression in humans, while most drugs which act as antidepressants increase central monoaminergic activity. In addition some depressed patients (though not all) appear to have reduced brain concentrations of certain monoamines. However, the model suggests a continuum of states, as stress is increased, from anxiety to anxiety/depression to retarded depression which does not fully explain the rather separate clinical presentations of anxiety states, neurotic depression, and retarded depression nor the interrelationships between depression, mania and schizophrenia. No doubt this scheme is an oversimplification which does not take into account all the dimensions of affective states.

The validity of animal models of depression is assessed by Willner (1984) who concludes that those most relevant to human depression are intracranial self-stimulation (Chapter 5), chronic stress, and learned helplessness models in rats, and the primate separation model.

Cognitive factors

Gloomy and pessimistic thoughts (depressive cognitions) are characteristic of depessive disorders. Patients lose confidence and self-esteem and evaluate themselves as failures. They feel guilty, blame themselves unreasonably, and may dwell on unhappy past events. For the future, they see no hope, and there seems little point in continuing to live. By contrast, the thoughts in manic disorders are full of optimism with high hopes for the future and an exaggerated sense of self-confidence.

It has been questioned whether the thoughts are secondary to a primary disorders of mood, or whether a disorder of cognition is the primary, or at least an aggravating or perpetuating, factor. Beck (1967) suggested that people who habitually adopt certain ways of thinking are vulnerable to depression when faced with minor problems. To some extent, cognitive factors are also involved in psychoanalytic theories: some forms of depression are viewed as resulting from loss of a loved object, combined with inwardly turned hostility expressed as self-reproach (Gelder *et al.* 1983). The learned helplessness theory of Seligman (1975) also stresses the importance of cognitive factors.

All these theories imply that depression could be alleviated by educating patients to develop more successful cognitive strategies. In animals, pre-training has been shown to arrest the development of learned helplessness behaviour, but in humans educational, psychoanalytic, and psychotherapeutic approaches, although sometimes helpful, are far from uniformly successful (*Lancet* 1984c; Docherty and Parloff 1984). Nor is there any evidence that particular cognitive strategies are present before the onset of depression or that they are more frequent in those that develop depression than in those who do not (Gelder *et al.* 1983). The rapid, rationally uninfluenced, switches between mania and depression, accompanied (and sometimes preceded) by demonstrable somatic and biochemical changes, seen in bipolar affective disorders provide strong evidence for the primacy of emotional rather than cognitive factors. All recent investigations point to the primary involvement of limbic rather than cortical pathways in depressive disorders. Nevertheless, depression (or elation) as a symptom can undoubtedly be perpetuated or inhibited by cortical activity. An interesting view of the interplay between prevailing mood and rational evaluation is presented by Pollitt (1982).

Brain mechanisms in affective disorders

Adaptive value of depression

Since systems in the brain are capable of producing depression in man and behaviours resembling depression in animals, it may be pertinent to consider the adaptive role, if any, of depression in animal behaviour. Of all the emotions, depression seems the most difficult to understand. Anxiety, fear, excitement, rage, or aggression are clearly protective, and useful for escape and for defence of self, territory, or food supply. Pleasure of all kinds, love, affection, and hope, and certain displeasures including disappointment, disgust, and hate, are all important for positive or negative reinforcement and for motivation towards actions promoting individual or group survival. However, severe depression, with its associated inactivity, lack of motivation, and failure of coping seems maladaptive.

Nevertheless, under certain adverse circumstances a depressive reaction might be an economic strategy for an individual or his closely related group. In a situation in which extreme adversity is inescapable and irremediable, or in which an important loss is apparently irreplaceable, a shut-down of brain motivation systems and a state of inactivity may conserve energy until conditions improve. If there is no abatement, continuance of such behaviour may lead to death, yet this event not only protects the individual from further suffering, but also conserves food supplies and social energies of the group to which he belongs. As previously mentioned, in some animal societies, (Everitt and Keverne 1979), loss of social status and falling rank in a group appears to constitute a severe disruption of socially important bonds for certain individuals; these show marked inhibition of social, aggressive, and sexual behaviour, withdrawal from the group, refusal of food, and occasionally death. A similar picture is seen in some types of human depression, and it is possible that suicide in depressive disorders represents an echo of such self-destructive behaviour. Normal humans subjected to extreme inescapable adversity, such as imprisonment or torture, may manifest the same reactions.

More commonly occurring adverse circumstances, such as loss of a child or close relation, may also lead to a depressive emotional reaction. In animal separation studies, there is normally an initial stage of anxiety as well as obvious distress. Such combined arousing and aversive stimuli may produce goal-seeking behaviour, such as searching, which may clearly have an adaptive function. If the loss is irretrievable, adaptation or recovery usually occurs in both animals and man. Possibly the initial state of anxiety and distress is similar to that of anxiety/depression (reactive or neurotic depression) in humans.

Less severe situations produce milder symptoms and signs of depression. It appears that the clinical syndrome of depression, like that of anxiety (Chapter 4), represents an extreme range of activity in normally adaptive systems, and that the psychophysiological differences between normal depression and depressive disorders are quantitative rather than qualitative. Psychoevolutionary aspects of depression are discussed by Gilbert (1984).

Brain systems in affective disorders
Reward and punishment systems

The salient feature of depression is unhappiness, or absence of pleasure; that of mania, at least in its early stages, is elation and increased drive or motivation. Therefore, the brain systems most likely to be primarily involved in both the symptoms and the syndromes of affective disorder are those for pleasure (reward) and punishment. As discussed in Chapter 5, evidence for the existence of such systems rests largely upon intracranial self-stimulation experiments in animals, but rewarding and aversive brain sites appear also to be present in man. These systems are thought to be important in generating both the behavioural and emotional aspects of motivation, reinforcement or avoidance, and gratification. They are located in various interconnected limbic structures, have many interconnections with the cerebral cortex, and with endocrine and autonomic centres, and themselves form part of the limbic and reticular formation arousal systems. Like all functional systems of the brain, they utilize a number of different neurotransmitters, including catecholamines, serotonin, acetylcholine, and endogenous opioids. In addition, a number of separate brain sites may be involved in different aspects of reward and punishment. Perturbation in reward and punishment pathways, induced by stimulation, ablation, pharmacological manipulation, or organic dizease, are known to cause widespread effects on arousal, endocrine, and autonomic activity, and on behaviour.

It is generally agreed that these systems are responsible for mood, although the details of how the infinitely graded nuances of normal mood are achieved remain obscure. Primary dysfunction in reward and/or punishment systems could theoretically account for most of the changes found in affective disorders. Involvement of any particular limbic structure or pathway has not been demonstrated in such disorders. However, this is not surprising since affect is likely to be a reflection complex patterns of functional interplay between many neuronal structures and their transmitters, any part of which could be subject to malfunction.

Endogenous depression Patients with endogenous depression often report a lack of capacity for enjoyment; they seem to be singularly unresponsive to reward. Sometimes they seem unresponsive to punishment as well, describing an emotional anaesthesia or inability to feel either pleasure or pain. Such patients may have high thresholds for externally induced pain. They are lacking in drive or motivation, and their behaviour is apathetic and aimless. Such a picture suggests underactivity of the whole reward and punishment mechanism. Other patients experience strong feelings of punishment and guilt, complain of pain or develop a chronic pain syndrome, suggesting absolute or relative overactivity of certain punishment systems.

Stein (1968), Olds (1977), and others have suggested a biochemical basis for these symptoms. Depletion of catecholamines, blockade of catecholamine receptors, or destruction of catecholamine neurones at limbic sites all disrupt intracranial self-stimulation in animals, implying that these treatments decrease the reinforcing value of stimulation. Conversely, drugs which raise the central availability of catecholamines reverse these effects and enhance self-stimulation, implying that they increase its reinforcement value. Among the latter drugs are the clinically used antidepressants, tricyclic agents, and monoamine oxidase inhibitors, especially if used with amphetamine, which releases catecholamines. The inference of these findings is that depression is accompanied by a fall in catecholaminergic activity in reward systems, with perhaps relative overactivity in antagonistic punishment systems. Mania would be a reflection of the reverse process.

This hypothesis is consistent with the catecholamine theory of depression, discussed below, and also with the fact that drugs such as cocaine and amphetamine, which raise central catecholamine activity, cause elation, while depression is a marked feature of their withdrawal syndromes. Changes in catecholamine activity in reward and punishment pathways could result from a number of different mechanisms including alterations not only in catecholamine concentrations, but also in receptor sensitivity, and the model need not apply to all forms of depression, some of which may involve other transmitters (such as serotonin and endogenous opioids) utilized by the same systems.

Neurotic depression In neurotic depression, feelings of anxiety, fear, and of overwhelming catastrophe are commonly mingled with those of guilt and misery. The patient is tremulous and overactive, although productive behaviour is inhibited. This clinical picture suggests high levels of activity not only in punishment systems but also in those arousal systems (Chapter 3) which control affect and behaviour in threatening situations.

The anatomical pathways are probably similar or overlapping, and systems which generate anxiety no doubt also function as part of the reward and punishment system. Serotonergic connections appear to be of particular importance. Evidence has been given in Chapter 5 that a serotonergic pathway arising from the dorsal raphe nuclei acts antagonistically to noradrenergic reward pathways in the median forebrain bundle. Drugs which decrease serotonergic activity here enhance intracranial self-stimulation in animals, while serotonergic drugs suppress it. In addition, there is evidence, discussed in Chapter 3, that increased serotonergic activity in septo-hippocampal pathways (the behavioural inhibition system; Gray 1981a, 1982) is associated with increased anxiety and fear, while anxiolytic drugs decrease serotonergic activity here. Thus, increased activity in these serotonergic systems would simultaneously engender anxiety and antagonize reward.

Neurotic depression could arise when aversive serotonergic activity exceeds (rewarding) noradrenergic activity in these pathways, and be exacerbated if, as postulated by Mills (1977) and Anisman et al. (1981), prolonged or severe anxiety leads to exhaustion of catecholamine systems. The relative balance of activity between serotonergic and catecholaminergic activity in different reward and punishment pathways may determine which type of depression is manifested, and also contribute to the premorbid personality type of the individual (Gray 1982). At present there are no clear hypotheses concerning the role in depression of other neurotransmitters or modulators involved in reward and punishment pathways (for example, acetylcholine and endogenous opioids) but these too may colour the clinical picture.

Arousal systems

The fact that sleep disturbance almost always occurs in affective disorders suggests that arousal systems are closely involved. The usual pattern is a reduction in SWS and total sleep time with an increase in REMS, suggesting increased activity in arousal systems. However, hypersomnia can also occur in depression. In patients with endogenous depression, retardation, apathy, slow psychomotor performance, reduced and late evoked potential responses, and diminished cerebral blood flow all suggest decreased activity in central arousal systems. In some patients, there is evidence of reduced central monoamine metabolism, while reduced electrodermal responsivity suggest decreased activity in autonomic arousal systems. Thus, in many patients there is evidence of decreased arousal, in spite of sleep disturbance. There is also evidence of a shift or inversion of the normal clinical sleep/wake pattern in depression (Mellerup and Rafaelson 1979). On the other hand, patients with neurotic depression may be obviously hyperaroused and hyperactive, and may have raised blood concentrations of noradrenaline. Manic patients are also hyperaroused though irritable or elated rather than anxious.

The lack of a consistent pattern of activity in arousal systems in depression suggests that any changes are secondary to the emotional state. However, as discussed above, a prolonged or intense increase in arousal as a result of external or internal stress may be an important precipitating or aggravating factor. In discussing the role of stress in the aetiology of depression, Willner (1984) stated: 'Increasingly, theories of depresssion emphasize multi-dimensional causality, with stress as only one among several aetiological factors; in these theories, the underactivity of a central reward pathway has been proposed as a "final common path" to which the diverse precipitants lead' (Willner 1984, p. 11).

Cognitive systems

It has been claimed that depression is primarily a cognitive disorder which may develop as a result of learning (Seligman 1975) or of particular ways of thinking (Beck 1967). Certainly, cognitive dysfunction may occur in many patients with depression, as evidenced by the presence of delusions, hal-lucinations, rumination on pessimistic thoughts, and difficulty in learning and memory. However, the brain systems for rational thought, learning, and memory appear to have developed to evaluate rather than to generate emotions, and ablation or stimulation of large parts of the cortex is not associated with particular changes in mood. In fact, changes in mood, are much more likely to occur when subcortical structures are involved. Hence, it seems likely that the cognitive changes seen in depression (reflecting cortical dysfunction) are secondary to emotional changes resulting from subcortical (limbic) dysfunction.

Nevertheless, because of the close anatomical and functional connections between the cortex and the limbic system, cognitive factors may well play a part in maintaining or aggravating depression. The connections between the frontal, especially prefrontal, cortical regions and subcortical circuits in the limbic system have for many years been believed to be particularly implicated, and this belief has formed the basis for psychosurgery aimed at disconnecting these brain regions.

Hemispheric dysfunction

A number of observations reviewed by Flor-Henry (1979) suggest that there may be a disturbance of cerebral laterality in mania and depression. In psychosis associated with temporal lobe epilepsy, there is a trend for schizo-phrenia to be more common when the epilepsy involves the dominant lobe and for manic-depressive psychosis to occur more commonly when it involves the non-dominant lobe. Isolated cases have been described in which changes in motor laterality have occurred during transitions between mania and depression in patients with bipolar disorders (not associated with temporal lobe epilepsy). For example, Flor-Henry (1979; p. 4) cited a case of a woman who was '100 per cent sinistral during a manic episode, becoming 100 per cent dextral when asymptomatic' . Another patient with unipolar depression was ambidextrous when well, but repeatedly lost the manual skill of his left hand when depressed.

Studies of handedness in patients with affective disorders reveal a small, but significant excess of left-handedness compared with the general population, and a greater incidence of right-left confusion. The excess of sinistrality is mainly accounted for by patients with bipolar depression or schizoaffective psychosis. It is possible that bipolar depression is a separate clinical entity among the depressions, which is related to schizophrenia and particularly associated with disturbances in laterality. This might help to account for the relative rarity of bipolar depression (which has an incidence similar to that of schizophrenia) and the clinical similarities between mania and schizophrenia. Both may represent pathological alterations in the dominant hemisphere. Lateral dysfunction and handedness in schizophrenia is discussed in Chapter 13.

Some studies of electrodermal and EEG activity and of cerebral blood flow suggest shifts of laterality in depression (Tucker 1981; Wexler 1980; Benedittis and Gonda 1985) but on the whole the results do not show a consistent pattern. Although the picture is much less clear-cut than that of schizophrenia, it is possible that in some cases of depression the dysfunction is predominantly related to the right hemisphere, while in mania the left hemisphere is mainly affected.

Neurotransmitters in affective disorders

Catecholamines

The idea that specific alterations in central neurotransmitter activity might cause depression or mania was stimulated by the discovery of antidepressant drugs and the finding that they exerted profound effects on the function of certain transmitter systems. Early ideas were centred around the catecholamines, and the catecholamine hypothesis of affective disorders (Schildkraut, 1965; Bunney and Davis, 1965) proposed that 'some, if not all, depressions are associated with an absolute or relative deficiency of catecholamines, particularly norepinephrine, at functionally important adrenergic sites in the brain, whereas manias might be associated with excess of catecholamines' (Schildkraut, 1978, p. 1223). The original hypothesis proposed that an absolute or relative deficiency of noradrenaline at receptors could result from a number of different mechanisms, including decreased synthesis, impairment of binding or storage, increased release and deamination, or decreased receptor sensitivity. It was not claimed that such changes occurred in all types of depression, which was recognized to be a heterogeneous group of disorders.

The theory was consistent with what was then known about the actions of several types of drugs. For example, many antidepressant drugs increase the availability of catecholamines at receptor sites. Acute effects of the tricyclic and related antidepressants include blockade of presynaptic reuptake of catecholamines, while monoamine oxidase inhibitors decrease their deamination with the result that increased amounts are available for release (Chapter 12). Drugs such as amphetamine, which release catecholamines, have a temporary antidepressant effect and also cause euphoria in normal subjects. Amphetamine, antidepressant drugs, and dopaminergic agents precipitate mania. Conversely, drugs which reduce central catecholaminergic activity by depletion, interference with release, synthesis, storage, or receptor blockade can cause or aggravate depression, and also alleviate mania. The ability of a drug to reverse the effects resulting from monoamine depletion by reserpine in animals is a good predictor of antidepressant activity.

Thus, an impressive body of pharmacological evidence appeared to support the theory (Fig. 11.2). The theory is also consistent with results obtained from intracranial self-stimulation experiments which strongly suggest an important role of catecholamines in reinforcement and reward (Chapter 5). Clinical investigations were therefore undertaken of catecholamine activity in patients with affective disorders. These have been reviewed by Schildkraut (1973a,b, 1978), Schaffer et al. (1981), van Praag (1980b, 1982), Green and Costain (1979), Berger and Barchas (1977), among others.

Noradrenaline No consistent changes in plasma concentration of noradrenaline or its precursor tyrosine have been noted in depressed patients and no changes in brain concentrations have been found in post-mortem studies of depressed suicides (Bourne *et al.* 1968; Pare *et al.* 1969). Enzyme studies including investigations of monoamine oxidase activity in plasma and platelets and of cyclic AMP concentrations in urine and cerebrospinal fluid, have given inconclusive results (Berger and Barchas 1977). However, several studies have indicated changes in noradrenaline metabolism in some affective disorders.

(i) Noradrenaline metabolites. 3-methoxy-4-hydroxyphenylglycol (MHPG) or its sulphate conjugate is a major metabolite of brain noradrenaline and it has been estimated that 50–80 per cent of this substance found in human urine is derived from the brain rather than peripheral tissues (Schildkraut 1978; Goodwin *et al.* 1978). A number of studies have shown that the urinary concentration of MHPG is relatively low during depressive episodes and higher during manic or hypomanic phases in bipolar depressive disorders. In spite of a few negative findings, the weight of evidence indicates that urinary MHPG does vary with clinical state in bipolar disorders. Decreased urinary MHPG concentration has also been reported in schizophrenia-related depression and in schizoaffective disorders. In unipolar endogenous depression, urinary MHPG concentrations may also be reduced compared with controls, but the concentration does not appear to be related to clinical state (Joseph *et al.* 1985). Schildkraut (1978) suggested that patients

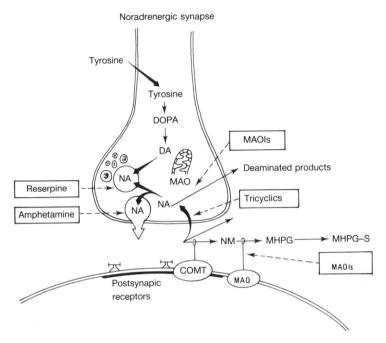

Fig. 11.2 Diagram of central noradrenergic synapse illustrating sites of action
of antidepressant drugs

NA noradrenaline; MAO monoamine oxidase; COMT catechol-0-methyl-
transferase; NM normetanephrine; MHPG 3-methoxy-4-hydroxyphenol-
glycol. Tricyclic antidepressants inhibit the reuptake of released NA; monoamine
oxidase inhibitors (MAOIs) inhibit the deamination of NA; amphetamine increases
the release of NA. Reserpine (which can cause depression) depletes NA storage sites.
For fuller explanation, see text. (Modified from Cooper *et al.* 1978, by kind permission
of Oxford University Press, New York.)

with abnormally high or low urinary MHPG concentrations may constitute
a biologically distinct subgroup of depressive disorders. It may be relevant
that in animals stimulation of the locus coeruleus produces a marked increase
in plasma MHPG concentration (Crawley *et al.* 1979).

Some investigations have suggested that depressed patients with low pre-
treatment urinary MHPG concentrations respond more favourably than
those with higher concentrations to drugs which have potent noradrenaline
reuptake blocking activity, such as desipramine, imipramine and maprotiline
(Maas *et al.* 1972; Beckman and Goodwin 1975; Rosenbaum *et al.* 1980;
Schatzberg *et al.* 1981). However, Veith *et al.* (1983) found that low urinary
MHPG concentration did not differentiate desipramine from amitriptyline
responders.

Scatton *et al.* (1986) reported that plasma concentrations of 3,4-hydroxyphenylethyleneglycol (DOPEG) and its sulphated metabolite were also decreased in drug-free patients with major depression compared with controls. The concentration of DOPEG was not related to the degree of clinically rated depression and did not differ between unipolar and bipolar patients. The results were interpreted as evidence of a general reduction in central noradrenergic activity in depression.

Dopamine The relation of dopaminergic activity to depression is relatively unexplored. No consistent changes in brain dopamine concentrations have been found in post-mortem studies in depressive suicides. However, van Praag (1980b) noted that there is an increased incidence of depression in Parkinson's disease and that drugs which increase dopaminergic activity such as amphetamine and direct dopamine agonists can produce euphoria or hypomania. Dopamine is also probably an important neurotransmitter in brain reward systems (Chapter 5).

(ii) Homovanillic acid (HVA). This metabolite of dopamine is present in cerebrospinal fluid and it is generally agreed that its presence reflects brain dopamine metabolism and that it may originate mainly from the caudate nucleus (Green and Costain 1979). Several investigations have shown that the concentration of HVA is reduced in the lumbar cerebrospinal fluid in both unipolar and bipolar depression, and some but not all have reported raised concentrations in mania (Schildkraut 1978). After blockade of HVA efflux from lumbar cerebrospinal fluid with probenecid, the accumulation of this metabolite in some depressed patients was less than in controls, indicating decreased dopamine turnover in the patients, and one study but not others, reported increased HVA accumulation in manic patients. Van Praag (1980b, 1982) suggests that alterations of dopamine metabolism in depressive disorders are related to motor components rather than mood, and that low concentrations of HVA in the cerebrospinal fluid are most likely to be found in patients with clinical signs of retardation.

(ii) Antidepressant drugs. Most of the tricyclic and related drugs block the reuptake of dopamine to a much lesser extent than that of noradrenaline and serotonin. However, nomifensine inhibits the reuptake of noradrenaline and dopamine equally and this drug has been shown to be clinically effective, especially in patients with low concentrations of cerebrospinal fluid HVA (van Praag 1982). Monoamine oxidase inhibitors impair the deamination of dopamine as well as noradrenaline and serotonin, and dopamine receptor agonists such as piribedil may be clinically effective in depressed patients with low cerebrospinal fluid HVA concentrations (Post 1978). Dopamine receptor antagonists such as phenothiazines and pimozide are effective in mania.

(iii) Catecholamine precursors. The administration of L-dopa, which probably raises brain concentrations of dopamine, has been found to produce improvement in some patients with depression, especially if given in high doses and combined with a peripheral dopamine decarboxylase inhibitor (Goodwin et al. 1970). However, the main effect appears to be a stimulation of motor activity and initiative rather than mood (van Praag 1980b). Exogenous tyrosine also leads to increased dopamine and noradrenaline synthesis in man; this precursor may have antidepressant effects (van Praag 1982).

Serotonin

A sister hypothesis to the catecholamine theory of depression is the indoleamine theory which suggests that, in some types of depression at least, there is serotonergic underactivity and that the therapeutic actions of antidepressant treatments are due to reversal of this deficiency. Serotonin metabolism in affective disorders is reviewed by Berger and Barchas (1977) van Praag (1980a 1982), Murphy et al. (1978), Green and Costain (1979), and Goodwin and Post (1983).

Post-mortem studies

Several post-mortem studies have shown decreased concentrations of serotonin or its metabolite 5-hydroxy-indoleacetic acid (5-HIAA) in the hindbrain or raphe nuclei in depressed patients or suicides compared with controls (Bourne et al. 1968; Lloyd et al. 1974; Birkmayer and Reiderer 1975). Such results are difficult to interpret since the changes may have occurred after death or have resulted from terminal anoxia and metabolic disturbance or from antidepressants or other drugs (Gelder et al. 1983; Owen et al. 1983). In addition, other studies, reviewed by Murphy et al. (1978), have reported no significant abnormalities in the concentration of serotonin or its metabolites in post-mortem brains of depressed patients.

Cerebrospinal fluid Asberg et al. (1976) found a bimodal distribution of 5-HIAA concentration in the lumbar cerebrospinal fluid of endogenously depressed patients, of whom 29 per cent had lower than control concentrations while the others had normal concentrations. There was little difference in the clinical features between the two groups, but it was suggested that low 5-HIAA concentrations are correlated with higher levels of anxiety, impulsive behaviour, aggression, and a greater risk of suicide (Banki 1977; Traskman et al. 1981; Goodwin and Post 1983). Bridges et al. (1976) reported lower values of both 5-HIAA and of the serotonin precursor tryptophan in the ventricular cerebrospinal fluid of patients with endogenous depression undergoing psychosurgery compared to patients with other psychiatric or neurological disorders. Terenius (1980) noted reduced concentrations of both 5-HIAA and endogenous opioids in a subgroup of patients with chronic pain syndrome, and Sternbach (1981) suggested that low serotonergic activity might underlie the triad of chronic pain, sleep disturbance, and depression.

These results are all suggestive of altered serotonin metabolism in a proportion of patients with endogenous depression. These patients appear to constitute a different group from those with altered catecholamine metabolism, since there is an inverse correlation between cerebrospinal fluid 5-HIAA and urinary MHPG (Goodwin et al. 1978). However, a number of negative reports with respect to 5-HIAA have also appeared (summarized by Murphy et al. 1978). Furthermore, low cerebrospinald fluid 5-HIAA concentrations appear to persist after clinical recovery in some depressed patients (Coppen 1972), a finding which may cast a doubt on the aetiological role of serotonin in depressed mood. In mania, normal or low rather than raised 5-HIAA values have been found in cerebrospinal fluid (Gelder et al. 1983).

Serotonergic precursors The amino acid tryptophan is a precursor of serotonin and the plasma concentration of free tryptophan correlates with brain tryptophan concentration, which in turn largely determines the rate of brain serotonin synthesis (van Praag 1980a). Plasma concentrations of free tryptophan have been reported to be lower than normal in a subgroup of patients with endogenous depression (Moller et al. 1976; Coppen and Wood 1978), and a correlation between reduced plasma-free tryptophan concentration and depressed mood was found in the first week after parturition by Stein et al. (1976) and Handley et al. (1977). Again, however, others have found no difference in plasma-free tryptophan concentrations between depressed and normal subjects (Murphy et al. 1978).

Several investigators have argued that if serotonin activity is diminished in depressed patients, loading with serotonin precursors might have a therapeutic effect. Some success has been achieved with 5-hydroxytryptophan (5-HTP), the immediate precursor of serotonin (van Praag 1982). However, 5-HTP enhances the synthesis of noradrenaline and dopamine as well as serotonin. Tryptophan, the immediate precursor of 5-HTP, enhances only serotonin synthesis, and the results with this substance in depression have been less encouraging. Some authors have found it to be as effective as imipramine or amitriptyline (Coppen, et al. 1972; Jensen et al. 1975) and to potentiate the therapeutic effects of clomipramine and electroconvulsive therapy (Murphy et al. 1978), while others have found it ineffective (Carroll et al. 1970; Murphy et al. 1974). It appears that and therapeutic effects of precursors are confined to the subgroup of patients with low concentrations of cerebrospinal fluid 5-HIAA (van Praag 1982).

Antidepressant drugs Many antidepressant drugs increase the availability of both catecholamine and serotonin at receptor sites (Chapter 12). However, selective serotonin reuptake inhibitors such as zimelidine have proved effective in depression and it has been claimed that a low concentration of cerebrospinal fluid 5-HIAA is predictive of response to antidepressants with predominantly serotonergic effects, (van Praag 1982; Goodwin *et al.* 1978). However, Montgomery (1982) found no difference in response to zimelidine and maprotiline (a predominantly adrenergic reuptake blocker) among patients with high or low cerebrospinal fluid concentrations of 5-HIAA.

Present status of classical monoamine theories of affective disorders

On the whole, the vast amount of research devoted to investigating the various classical monoamine theories of affective disorders has so far yielded inconclusive and somewhat tentative results. It does appear that there are certain biochemically definable subgroups: (1) a group with bipolar endogenous depression with disordered central catecholamine activity, and (2) a group with unipolar and bipolar endogenous depression with reduced brain serotonin activity. These groups may respond preferentially to treatments which specifically affect catecholaminergic or serotonergic function, respectively.

However, no coherent picture of any biochemical changes underlying the whole range of affective disorders has emerged, and little new information on the part played by monoamines in the control of mood generally. Such a result is not necessarily surprising. If, as seems likely, moods reflect *patterns* of activity in different, but overlapping subcortical and cortical pathways, each utilizing several of a number of different transmitters, gross alterations of monoamine metabolites in remote body compartments such as cerebrospinal fluid and urine would not be expected except in the most severe disorders. Even where alterations in monoamine metabolism have been observed, it is not clear whether such changes are causative or whether they merely reflect the secondary consequences of some primary aetiological factor. Nor is there any evidence concerning which parts of the brain might be involved, since alterations in metabolite concentrations do not necessarily reflect transmitter activity at receptor sites.

Yet the findings in affective disorders may represent the 'first word on the cerebral substrates of depression' (van Praag 1982, p. 1263) and several authors have discussed their possible significance in terms of neurotransmitter effects on mood and behaviour in man (*Medical Research Council Brain Metabolism Unit* 1972). The results relating to catecholamines in affective disorders are in general consistent with what is known about their function in reward pathways and arousal systems (Chapters 2 and 5). The results relating to serotonin metabolism in affective disorders seem somewhat paradoxical since serotonin appears to be a transmitter in punishment rather than reward pathways. Furthermore, cerebrospinal fluid levels of 5-HIAA remain low after clinical improvement. Van Praag (1982) suggests that cerebrospinal fluid concentrations of 5-HIAA do not correlate directly with mood, but that reduced central serotonergic activity is a predisposing factor which increases the risk of developing depression when the subject is exposed to stress.

Receptor sensitivity in affective disorders

The classical monoamine theories of depression were based largely on the observed acute biochemical effects of antidepressant drugs at monoaminergic synapses. A serious drawback of such theories has always been that drug effects at synapses develop rapidly, within hours or days, while the clinical effects take several weeks to develop (Iverson and Mackay 1979; Oswald *et al.* 1972), necessitating prolonged use of the drugs. This therapeutic time-lag does not seem to be explicable on pharmacokinetic grounds (Peet and Coppen 1979).

This and other discrepancies have led to the idea that the therapeutic effects of antidepressants are not due to acute changes in *transmitter concentration* but to changes in *receptor sensitivity* which occur secondarily over a longer time-course, in response to the chronic presence of the drugs in the body. As a corollary, alteration of receptor sensitivity might be an aetiological factor in depression, a possibility which would account for the lack of alteration of transmitter or transmitter metabolite concentration in most patients.

That changes in receptor sensitivity might be important in affective disorders was suggested in the original monoamine hypothesis (Schildkraut 1965). Recent technological advances have led to a much greater understanding of monoamine receptors and have added a new dimension to the investigation of the monoamine hypothesis of affective disorders. New techniques include receptor binding assays, single unit neurophysiological recording, measurement of brain adenylate cyclase activity, and behavioural methods involving pharmacological manipulation of monoaminergic receptors. In particular, two properties of receptors; their plasticity and their multiplicity have assumed increasing importance from such studies.

Receptor plasticity

As discussed in Chapter 6 (Fig. 6.2), receptors for neurotransmitters are dynamic structures which undergo adaptive changes in response to chronic alterations of agonist supply. Decreased neurotransmitter concentration results after a time in an increase in sensitivity of the specific receptors, while increased exposure to the neurotransmitter leads to a compensatory decrease

in receptor sensitivity. A characteristic of these changes, especially with therapeutic doses of drugs, is that they tend to develop over a slow time course,
of the order of weeks rather than hours or days. Since many antidepressants
increase agonist supply at monoaminergic synapses, they might be expected
to cause secondary changes in receptor sensitivity when chronically
administered.

Receptor multiplicity

It is becoming increasingly clear that there are several different receptors for
each neurotransmitter. In the case of adrenergic receptors (Fig. 11.3), several
different types of post-synaptic receptors (alpha$_1$, beta$_1$, and beta$_2$) have been
recognized for some time (Ahlquist 1948; Lands *et al.* 1967). These receptors
mediate the various responses to adrenergic stimulation. Their differing tissue
distributions and pharmacological profiles are well known, and post-synaptic
alpha- and beta-agonists and antagonists are widely used in medicine.

There is now evidence [reviewed by Langer, (1977, 1980) and Tepper *et al.*
(1985), although recently questioned by Kalsner and Quillan (1984) and
Laduron (1984)], for the existence, in addition, of adrenergic autoreceptors
whose function is to modulate the release of neurotransmitter. Pre-synaptic

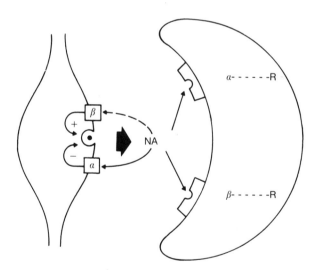

Fig. 11.3 Pre-synaptic and post-synaptic receptors for noradrenaline. (NA - noradrenaline.) Pre-synaptic alpha receptors mediate a negative feedback system for noradrenaline release under most physiological conditions; pre-synaptic beta receptors
mediate a positive feedback system for noradrenaline release when the concentration
of neurotransmitter in the synaptic cleft is low. Alpha and beta post-synaptic receptors
mediate different responses to adrenergic stimulation. (From Langer 1977)

alpha- receptors (alpha$_2$) appear to operate a local negative feedback system for noradrenaline release at the nerve terminal. They are stimulated by noradrenaline when the synaptic concentration reaches a certain threshold level, and the effect of stimulation is a decrease in noradrenaline release. Presynaptic beta- receptors operate a positive feedback system. They are stimulated at low concentrations of noradrenaline and the effect of stimulation is an increase in transmitter release. However, under physiological conditions the major local regulatory mechanism for noradrenaline release by nerve stimulation is probably mediated by alpha$_2$-receptors (Langer, 1977). In addition, somatodendritic autoreceptors, stimulated by release of transmitter from recurrent axon collaterals and/or dendro-dentritic synapses, reduce the firing rate, and thus, transmitter release from the neurone as a whole (Tepper *et al.* 1985).

Alpha$_2$-receptors have a different pharmacological profile from alpha$_1$-receptors, and a variety of agonists and antagonists with differing degrees of specificity for the two types of receptor are known (Table 11.1; Langer *et al.* 1980). Although alpha$_2$-receptors are situated presynaptically in the peripheral nervous system, they also exist at other sites. For example, they are present in platelets and in fat cells, and are located post-synaptically at some sites in the central nervous sysem. The alpha$_2$-receptors mediating cardiovascular depression in the medulla are postsynaptic, and alpha$_2$-somatodentritic autoreceptors mediate inhibition in the locus coeruleus. The effects of both pre- and post-synaptic beta receptors are mediated by stimulation of adenylate cyclase, while those of both pre- and post-synaptic alpha-receptors involve calcium gating mechanisms and probably other

Table 11.1. Relative order of potency of alpha$_1$ and alpha$_2$ adrenoceptor agonists and antagonists

Agonists	Receptors	Antagonists
Clonidine	more potent at alpha$_2$	Rauwolscine
Tramazoline	↑	Yohimbine
Alpha-CH3-noradrenaline		Piperoxan
Oxymetazoline		Dihydroergocryptine
Naphazoline		Tolazoline
Adrenaline		Mianserin
Noradrenaline	alpha$_1$=alpha^1	Phentolamine
Phenylephrine		Phenoxybenzamine
Methoxamine	↓	WB 4101
		Prazosin
	more potent at alpha$_2$	

Reference: Langer *et al.* 1980.

mechanisms in addition (Berridge 1981; Langer 1977; Barnes 1981; Tepper *et al.* 1985). In addition to the pre-synaptic noradrenergic autoreceptors through which noradrenaline modulates its own release, a whole mosaic of receptors for other substances appear to be present on pre-synaptic adrenergic nerve terminals, all of which can also modulate noradrenaline release (Langer 1977, 1980; Fig. 11.4).

Multiple receptor subtypes, both pre- and post-synaptic, also exist for other neurotransmitters (Langer 1980). Presynaptic alpha$_2$-receptors modulate adrenaline release in the central nervous system. The receptors for acetylcholine include muscarinic and nicotinic receptors. For dopamine, post-synaptic DA-1 and DA-2 receptors and pre-synaptic and soma-dendritic autoreceptors are recognized (Chapter 13). Serotonin receptors are discussed below.

The presence of multiple post-synaptic receptors which mediate different tissue responses, and of autoreceptors, which modulate release, thus appears to be a generalized phenomenon applicable to most neurotransmitters. Most of these receptors have been demonstrated in the central nervous system.

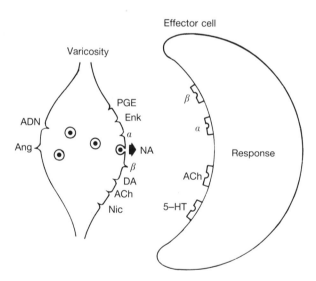

Fig. 11.4 Multiple pre-synaptic receptors on adrenergic nerve terminals. Schematic representation of pre-synaptic receptors at a noradrenergic synapse in the peripheral nervous system. Pre-synaptic receptors for PGE (prostaglandins of the E series), Enk (enkephalin), DA (dopamine), ACh (acetylcholine, muscarinic), ADN (adenosine) and alpha adrenergic receptors all inhibit NA (noradrenaline) release, while those for Nic (acetylcholine, nicotinic), Ang (angiotensin II) and beta adrenergic receptors enhance NA release. (From Langer 1977)

All types exhibit plasticity and chronic administration of several types of antidepressant drugs has been shown to cause changes in receptor sensitivity. Since such changes occur in both pre- and post-synaptic receptors, the effects of long-term dosage with antidepressant drugs are complex.

Receptor modulation by antidepressant drugs

Chronic administration of antidepressant drugs has been shown to cause secondary changes in adrenergic, serotonergic, and dopaminergic receptors.

Pre-synaptic-(alpha₂) adrenergic receptors Results from biochemical and physiological studies in animals and man (reviewed by Charney *et al.* 1981b; Langer *et al.* 1980) indicate that certain antidepressants when administered chronically cause down-regulation of adrenergic alpha₂-receptors, resulting in a secondary increase in the amount of noradrenaline release on nerve stimulation. The mechanism is probably a decrease in receptor density following the sustained rise in synaptic noradrenaline concentration caused by the drugs. For example, Crews and Smith (1978) found that chronic (twice daily doses for 3 weeks) but not acute (twice daily doses for 1 day) administration of desimpramine to rats enhanced the stimulation-induced release of radioactively labelled noradrenaline from left atrial strips. These results were thought to be due to a gradually developing subsensitivity of alpha₂-receptors which no longer inhibited noradrenaline release, and the authors suggested that this mechanism would explain the delay in the onset of clinical effects of the antidepressants. Chronic desipramine treatment has also been shown to decrease metabolic and endocrine response to the alpha₂-stimulant clonidine in the rat brain (Sugrue 1980; Eriksson *et al.* 1982). Chronic treatment with imipramine, nortriptyline, and amitryptyline similarly reduces the behavioural responses of rats to clonidine (Zebrowska-Lupin 1980; Green *et al.* 1982; Davis and Monkes 1982). Amitriptyline and several monoamine oxidase inhibitors decrease alpha₂-receptor binding in the rat brain (Cohen *et al.* 1982; Sugrue 1981; Smith *et al.* 1981). Alpha₂-receptor sensitivity in the locus coeruleus is also down-regulated by chronic treatment with some antidepressants. Desipramine decreases the responsiveness of the cells to the inhibitory effects of alpha₂-stimulation by clonidine, while mianserin stimulates the firing of cells in this (rewarding) brain area, presumably because of its alpha₂-blocking effect (Svenssen 1980; Svensson *et al.* 1981). However, one recent behavioural study in rats suggests that chronic imipramine treatment decreases locus coeruleus activity in rats (Mason and Engel 1983).

In man, Charney *et al.* (1981b) showed that long-term treatment with desipramine attenuated the effects of clonidine on MHPG excretion and blood pressure in depressed patients, indicating that alpha₂-receptors became subsensitive. Garcia-Sevilla *et al.* (1981) reported that chronic treatment of depressed patients with antidepressants produced a significant fall in the numbers of platelet alpha$_2$-receptors. In this study, platelet alpha$_2$-receptor density was significantly higher in depressed patients than in normal controls. Metz *et al.* (1983) also reported that platelet alpha$_2$-receptor density was higher in post-puerperal women developing symptoms of post-natal depression than in post-puerperal women without depression and normal controls.

These studies suggest not only that antidepressant drug effects might be mediated by the development of alpha$_2$-receptor subsensitivity, but also that alpha$_2$-receptor supersensitivity (increased alpha$_2$-density), perhaps induced by stress or other factors, might be a cause of depression. A critical site might be in central reward pathways such as the locus coeruleus, but it is not yet clear whether platelet alpha$_2$-receptor density mirrors that in the central nervous system. In rats, Campbell and Durcan (1982) showed that strains which were genetically susceptible to 'learned helplessness' had a greater density of alpha$_2$-adrenoceptors in the brainstem (though not in the fore-brain) than genetically more stable rats. Stress, caused by immobilization, significantly increased alpha$_2$-receptor density in the brainstem, and also increased beta-receptor density, but decreased alpha$_1$-receptor density, in the vulnerable animals; no marked changes were seen in the stable group.

The ability of some tricyclic antidepressants and monoamine oxidase inhibitors to down-regulate alpha$_2$-receptors does not appear to be shared by all antidepressants (Charney *et al.* 1981a). Some atypical antidepressants may, however, affect these receptors in different ways. For example, mianserin has been shown to exert an alpha$_2$-blocking action. Fludder and Leonard (1979) reported that chronic administration of mianserin to rats antagonized the behavioural effects of clonidine and produced metabolic changes in the brain similar to those of the alpha$_2$-antagonist yohimbine.

Post-synaptic (alpha$_1$) adrenergic receptors Evidence of adaptive changes in post-synaptic alpha$_1$-receptor sensitivity after chronic antidepressant treatment is conflicting. Binding studies have shown either no effect or a slight increase in alpha$_1$-receptor density after tricyclic drugs monoamine oxidase inhibitors or electroconvulsive treatment (Creese and Sibley 1981; Hu *et al.* 1981). Chronic treatment with the monoamine oxidase inhibitor clorgyline has been reported to cause a decrease in alpha$_1$-receptor binding (Cohen *et al.* 1982). However, Charney *et al.* (1981a,b) give evidence for enhanced physiological sensitivity of alpha$_1$-receptors in two brain areas (facial motor nucleus and dorsal lateral geniculate nucleus) after long-term treatment with several tricyclic drugs and iprindole. Increased sensitivity to noradrenaline has also been observed in the amygdala, an area whose adrenergic receptors appear to have neither alpha or beta properties.

Beta adrenergic receptors A large number of studies have shown that chronic (but not acute) administration of a variety of antidepressant agents results in down-regulation of beta-adrenergic receptors in the brain (Vetulani and Sulser 1975; Sulser *et al.* 1978; Sulser 1981; Wolfe *et al.* 1978; Sugrue 1980, 1981; Cohen *et al.* 1982; Creese and Sibley 1981; Mishra *et al.* 1983). Such an effect has been demonstrated with non-specific monoamine reuptake blockers, serotonin reuptake blockers, atypical antidepressants, including iprindole and mianserin, monoamine oxidase inhibitors, and after repeated electroconvulsive therapy (Sulser 1981; Table 11.2). Decreased beta-receptor density has been demonstrated in binding studies and/or functional subsensitivity by reductions in noradrenaline receptor coupled adenylate cyclase activity in the rat limbic forebrain. The effects seem to be largely due to changes in post-synaptic beta-receptors, although they may follow or be a consequence of pre-synaptic effects.

Table 11.2. Antidepressant treatments which cause beta-adrenergic subsensitivity in the brain

Treatments	Subsensitivity to noradrenaline or isoprenaline	Reduction in beta-receptor density
Non-selective reuptake blockers		
clomipramine	++	+
imipramine	++	+
amitriptyline	++	+
Predominantly noradrenaline reuptake blockers		
desipramine	++	+
nisoxetine	++	+
Selective serotonin reuptake blockers		
zimelidine	++	+
Atypical antidepressants		
iprindole	++	+
mianserin	++	+
Monoamine oxidase inhibitors		
pargyline	++	+
nialamide	++	+
tranylcypromine	++	+
Electroconvulsive treatment	++	+

Source: Sulser 1981.

These findings have led to the suggestion that the therapeutic actions of antidepressants are due to the delayed development of post-synaptic beta-receptor subsensitivity and that depression might be caused by hyper-sensitivity of post-synaptic beta receptors. Such a suggestion would appear to be the opposite of that proposed in the original monoamine hypothesis of depression. However, it may be supported by the report that the anti-depressant effect of the beta-adrenergic stimulant salbutamol had an anti-depressant effect which coincided with the delayed development of beta-adrenoceptor subsensitivity as measured by the plasma cyclic AMP response to intravenous salbutamol (Lerer *et al.* 1981). Previous inves-tigations, in which salbutamol was reported to have a rapid antidepressant effect, did not study receptor sensitivity (Widlocher *et al.* 1977; Simon *et al.* 1978; Lecrubier *et al.* 1980).

Down-regulation of beta-receptors by antidepressants does not appear to occur in all systems in humans. Thompson *et al.* (1983a,b) point out that the secretion of melanotonin is controlled by post-synaptic beta-receptors terminating in the pineal gland. Melanotonin secretion is blocked by the beta adrenoceptor blocker propranolol, but 3 weeks treatment with desipramine in six patients with depression and three normal subjects caused an increase in mean plasma melanotonin concentrations. Thus, imipramine does not appear to cause down-regulation of beta receptors at this site in man.

Synaptic stability The physiological significance of these varying effects of long-term antidepressant treatment on different adrenergic receptors is not clear. Many of the effects seem to be opposite: for example alpha$_2$-receptor subsensitivity would tend to increase noradrenergic transmission while post-synaptic beta-receptor subsensitivity would decrease the effects of nor-adrenaline. However, several authors have suggested that antidepressant drugs may increase the stability of noradrenergic synaptic transmission by pro-ducing effects which tend to cancel out but which limit the capacity for maladaptive positive or negative alterations in transmission (Maas 1979; Svensson and Usdin 1978; Willner and Montgomery 1980). Such an action might explain not only the normalizing effects of the drugs over a wide range of symptoms in depressive disorders, but also their relative lack of effect in normal subjects (Harrison-Read 1981). This idea suggests that instability of synaptic control rather than primary changes in receptor or transmitter activity, determines the onset of affective disorders. Synaptic instability might also account for the recurrent nature of the illness and the sudden switches that can occur between depression and mania.

Dopamine receptors There is relatively little information concerning the sen-sitivity of dopamine receptors in affective disorders. However, chronic treat-ment with imipramine, amitriptyline, and the atypical antidepressant iprindole induces subsensitivity of dopamine autoreceptors in the substantia nigra in rats (Antelman and Chiodo 1981). Similar effects were found after repeated electroconvulsive treatment. These autoreceptors, like alpha$_2$-adrenoceptors, may operate a negative feedback system for neurotransmitter release (Fig. 13.1). Dopamine autoreceptor subsensitivity occurring as a result of treatment in human depression would therefore increase dopamine release, an effect consistent with the catecholamine hypothesis. This effect might also explain the fact that antidepressant drug treatment can precipitate mania in bipolar disorders (Bunney 1978). Conversely, chronic treatment with neuroleptics, which are effective in mania, induces dopamine auto-receptor supersensitivity, tending to reduce dopamine release. The activity of post-synaptic dopamine receptors in affective disorders or after anti-depressant treatment does not appear to have been systematically inves-tigated, but binding studies suggest that chronic imipramine treatment modifies the density of post-synaptic dopamine receptors (Creese and Sibley 1981). Dopamine receptors are described in Chapter 13.

Serotonin receptors Catecholaminergic systems normally interact closely with serotonergic systems in the central nervous system. Most antidepressant drugs affect both systems and there is evidence that both may be involved in affective disorders. For these reasons, much attention has recently been paid to serotonin receptor activity in depression.

It is now possible to differentiate at least four types of recognition sites, or receptors, for serotonin at central serotonergic synapses (Langer and Briley 1981; Hamon *et al.* 1980; Peroutka *et al.* 1981; Fig. 11.5). These include two types of post-synaptic receptors: 5-HT-1 receptors, which are linked to adenylate cyclase and can be selectively labelled with tritiated serotonin, and 5-HT-2 receptors, which may be related to certain behavioural responses in animals (head twitch) and are selectively labelled with tritiated spiroperidol. Presynaptic autoreceptors, which operate a negative feedback control over stimulation-evoked serotonin release, have also been identified. Finally, there is a neuronal uptake site for serotonin linked to the active transport of transmitter into the nerve endings. This site is selectively labelled by tritiated imipramine; it is not a receptor in the classical sense, but has similar proper-ties in that it includes a serotonin recognition site, a coupling mechanism linked to the active transport of transmitter across the membrane, and it is inhibited by specific antagonists.

Langer and his associates (Langer and Briley 1981; Langer *et al.* 1980; Langer 1984) have proposed that this neuronal serotonin uptake site (high affinity imipramine binding site) is the locus of action at which tricyclic antidepressant drugs exert their clinical effects and that it may be closely linked to the pathogenesis of depression. The site is asymmetrically dis-

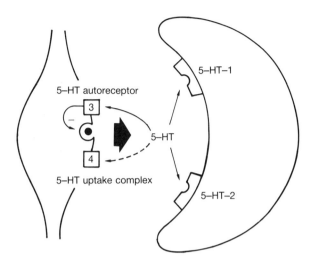

Fig. 11.5 Pre-synaptic and post-synaptic receptors for serotonin. (5-HT - serotonin.) Post-synaptic receptors include serotonin-1 (5-HT-1) and serotonin 2 (5-HT-2) receptors which mediate different responses. Pre-synaptic autoreceptors (3) operate a negative feedback control system for serotonin release. A neuronal uptake site (4) appears to be linked to the active transport of transmitter into the nerve endings. (Reference: Langer and Briley 1981)

tributed in the rat and human brain; the highest concentrations are found in the hypothalamus and amygdala, and the distribution parallels that of endogenous serotonin. It is also present in human platelets which are thought to represent a peripheral model for serotonergic neurones. Many tricyclic antidepressants bind with high affinity to this site (Table 11.3) and their affinity correlates significantly with clinically effective dosage. Some other monoamine uptake blockers also display moderate affinity, but the affinity of atypical antidepressants is low. Long-term treatment with tricyclic drugs decreases the density of high affinity imipramine binding sites in the brain of rats. Similar changes are produced by repeated electroconvulsive treatment and REM sleep deprivation. However, in human depression the density of these binding sites seems to be already low and is little influenced by antidepressant treatment. Several authors have reported reduced platelet imipramine binding in patients with untreated reactive and endogenous depression (Tuomisto *et al.* 1979; Langer and Briley 1981), and Stanley *et al.* (1982) found a reduction in imipramine binding in the frontal cortex of suicide victims. In clinical studies there was no correlation between receptor density and the severity of depressive symptoms and little change in receptor density after antidepressant treatment and clinical improvement. Langer and

Table 11.3. Inhibition of ^{3}H-imipiramine binding in rat cortex by antidepressants

Drug	IC$_{50}$ (nM)*
Tricyclic antidepressants	
imipramine	7
desipramine	18
protriptyline	20
clomipramine	25
amitriptyline	25
doxepin	300
Atypical antidepressants	
iprindole	5 500
viloxazine	11 500
mianserin	20 000
Monoamine uptake blockers	
fluoxetine	200
nisoxetine	200
quipazine	700
cocaine	900
amphetamine	>100 000
Monoamine oxidase inhibitor	
pargyline	>100 000

* IC$_{50}$, concentration of drug required to inhibit 50 per cent of the specific ^{3}H-imipramine binding, measured at 5 nM ^{3}H-imipramine. (Reference: Langer *et al.* 1980.)

Briley (1981) suggest that a decreased density of serotonin reuptake sites may be a genetic marker of vulnerability to depression, rather than a direct cause or reflection of depressed mood. This proposition would be in line with the findings of low cerebrospinal and brain concentrations of 5-HIAA in some depressed patients and their relatives, and the observations that cerebospinal fluid 5-HIAA concentrations do not always change with antidepressant treatment or clinical recovery.

Binding studies also suggest abnormalities in density of 5-HT-2 receptors in depression. Stanley and Mann (1983, 1984) found a 44 per cent increase in the density of these receptors in the brains of suicide victims. The increase in 5HT-2 receptor density was apparent in the frontal cortex, had a similar distribution to the (decreased) serotonin reuptake sites found previously in the same brains (Stanley *et al.* 1982) and was not thought to result from previous drug treatment. It is possible that the increase in 5-HT-2 receptor density may reflect post-synaptic supersensitivity developing as a result of decreased serotonin uptake and low serotonin turnover in depression.

Chronic treatment with several antidepressant drugs, including tricyclics, monoamine oxidase inhibitors and iprindole, has been shown to cause a reduction in density of 5-HT-2 receptors in animals in some studies (Charney et al. 1981a), but an increase in others (Green et al. 1983).

Investigations of 5-HT-1 receptors in binding studies have not shown consistent changes in man (Stanley and Mann 1984), but Savage et al. (1980) found a decrease in 5-HT-1 binding in the rat cerebral cortex after chronic administration of monoamine oxidase inhibitors, and Fuxe et al. (1981) report decreased 5-HT-1 binding after chronic zimelidine treatment in rodents.

Receptor binding studies thus suggest that a low density of neuronal serotonin uptake sites and a high density of post-synaptic 5-HT-2 receptor sites is associated with untreated depression, and that chronic antidepressant drug treatment may reduce 5-HT-2 and 5-HT-1 receptor density. Results from physiological and behavioural investigations, however, are somewhat confusing, partly because it has not always been clear which type of receptors are mediating responses. Several studies (Charney et al. 1981a; Svensson 1980; Svensson et al. 1981; Montigny and Aghajanian 1978; Green et al. 1983; Blier et al. 1984) have examined the physiological sensitivity of central neurones in animals to serotonin after long-term antidepressant treatment with a variety of drugs. These have shown enhanced sensitivity to serotonin in post-synaptic neurones in several brain areas, findings which seem to be at variance with binding studies showing reduced post-synaptic receptor density.

Many of the apparent inconsistencies in the various receptor sensitivity studies may be resolved by the findings of several recent investigations. With regard to serotonin receptors, Ogren et al. (1983) and Fuxe et al. (1983) showed that the observed changes in sensitivity after chronic antidepressant treatment depend on the area of the brain studied, the behavioural response measured, and the type and dose of agonist used to elicit physiological responses. These investigators were able to demonstrate both supersensitivity and subsensitivity of various serotonergically-mediated responses in rats after tricyclic antidepressants depending on the dose used. Similarly, binding studies showed marked regional differences in the alteration of density of 5-HT-1, 5-HT-2, and 5-HT reuptake binding sites induced by chronic antidepressant treatment. Such treatment could cause up- or down-regulation of receptors depending on the area analysed, and different antidepressants could cause different changes in the same areas.

A second recent illuminating observation is the discovery that down-regulation of beta-adrenergic receptors requires both a noradrenergic and a serotonergic input, and probably steroid and other hormones as well (Sulser et al. 1983; Barbaccia et al. 1983; Racagni and Brunello 1984). Similarly, both dopamine and noradrenaline are involved in changes of $alpha_2$ and dopamine autoreceptor sensitivity (Goldstein *et al.* 1983). It is likely that there are complex receptor–receptor interactions in local brain circuits, and adaptive receptor changes probably involve co-modulation by several different transmitters.

In the light of these findings, it may be vain to search for effects on particular transmitters or particular receptor adaptations to explain the antidepressant effects of the various drugs. The several effects on monoamine transmitter and receptor activity often have opposing actions: for instance, the combination of alpha$_2$- and beta-adrenergic subsensitivity would tend to cancel out. It seems more likely that the delayed therapeutic effects of antidepressant drugs result from the establishment, by a number of opposing actions, of greater overall stability at synapses for several monoamine transmitters, and/or from alteration of the balance between several neurotransmitter systems to a more optimal functional state. In addition, Ogren *et al.* (1983) observe that in some response systems, chronic antidepressant treatment appears to alter the signal-to-noise ratio, thus changing the gain to the receptor system. Such a change, possibly modulated through receptor–receptor interactions, may increase the efficiency of synaptic transmission through certain critical brain pathways.

Endogenous opioids in affective disorders

Although considerable knowledge has accumulated concerning the role of endogenous peptide systems in pain modulation (Chapter 5), much less is known of their actions in modulating emotion. Endogenous opioids are distributed in limbic structures; they are important in reward systems, along with catecholamines (with which they are co-released), and one of their most prominent clinical effects is an action on behaviour and mood. Panksepp (1981) proposed a role of opioid systems in mediating social reward rather than reward in general. He drew attention to some similarities between narcotic dependence and social attachments or bonding, and between the narcotic withdrawal syndrome and the behaviour induced by separation or loss in animals (Table 11.4), and suggested that the neurochemical underpinnings of the two conditions may be similar.

The similarity between the narcotic withdrawal syndrome and chronic pain syndromes has already been pointed out (Chapter 6), and the features of chronic pain syndromes described by Sternbach (1981; Table 6.3) are almost identical to those attributed to drug or social withdrawal by Panksepp (1981; Table 11.4). Chronic pain syndromes are in turn related to depression. The commonality between loss, pain, and depression were underlined by Panksepp who stated: 'From an evolutionary perspective, it is reasonable that social affect (panic, loneliness, comfort, and joy) might have arisen from brain systems which modulate pain.... The imprint of this evolutionary progression remains embedded within human and animal language. The

Table 11.4. Similarities between narcotic addiction and social dependence

Narcotic addiction	Social dependence
Psychological dependence	Love
Tolerance	Estrangement
Withdrawal syndrome	Loss of a loved one
psychological distress	loneliness
lachrymation	crying
anorexia	loss of appetite
depression	despondency
insomnia	sleeplessness
aggressiveness	irritability

Reference: Panksepp 1981.

semantics of social loss are the semantics of pain. It hurts to lose a loved one and we cry. Social separation makes young animals more sensitive to pain and they cry'. (Panksepp 1981, pp.170–1).

Stein (1978; Chapter 5) suggested that endogenous opioids in brain reward systems are important in signalling gratification on attaining an objective after goal-directed behaviour. Lack of a sense of gratification is a characteristic of some types of depression: activities which used to produce pleasure no longer do so. A similar incapacity may apparently be induced by giving naloxone to young animals, when they hurry to regain social contact but appear to gain little comfort from the contact (Bolles and Fanselow 1982). These and other observations all suggest that human depressions may be characterized by underactivity of endogenous opioid systems in limbic reward pathways. However, the evidence for this suggestion is extremely limited.

Very few direct measurements have been made of endogenous opioids in depression or mania. Pickar et al. (1980) reported a single case study of a patient with bipolar depression in whom daily estimations of plasma opioid activity were made during repeated manic and depressive episodes. Plasma opioid activity was measured as beta-endorphin-like radioreceptor activity assayed against beta-endorphin on rat brain membranes. Significantly higher levels of such activity were observed during two manic phases than during two intervening depressive phases, and there was no overlap between mania and depression values. There was a highly significant inverse correlation between clinical ratings for severity of depression and plasma opioid activity. Lindstrom et al. (1978) also reported greater opioid activity in the cerebrospinal fluid of bipolar patients during mania than during depression. Newnham et al. (1983) found reduced plasma concentrations of beta-endorphin in patients with post-partum depressive symptoms.

322 DEPRESSION AND MANIA

Apparently contradictory findings were reported by Terenius (1977) and von Knorring *et al.* (1978) who found low concentrations of endorphin-like activity in the cerebrospinal fluid of manic patients and high levels in patients with depression. In patients with chronic pain, those with psychogenic pain had normal concentrations of cerebrospinal fluid endorphin-like activity, as well as normal concentrations of 5-HIAA, while those with pain of organic origin had low concentrations of endorphin-like activity and low concentrations of 5-HIAA (Almay *et al.* 1980).

There have been few trials of opioid agonists or antagonists in the treatment of affective disorders. Terenius (1977) reported inconclusive results with naloxone in depression, but pointed out that this drug is very short-acting. No evidence for a therapeutic effect of intravenous beta-endorphin in depression has been found in double-blind studies (Clement-Jones and Besser 1983). In mania, some clinical studies have found beneficial effects of naloxone, but these effects were not confirmed in other studies. One double-blind study, but not others, have reported reduction of mania following intravenous injection of beta-endorphin (Koob and Bloom 1983).

Information on the relation between endogenous opioid activity and mood in affective disorders, and on the possible therapeutic benefits of opioid agonists and antagonists is thus sparse. In view of the complexity of endogenous opioid systems, their interactions with other neurotransmitter systems and their co-secretion by the same cells (Chapters 5 and 6) it is unlikely that any simple relationship exists. In contrast, there is considerable evidence that endocrine functions involving opioids and other endogenous polypeptides are disturbed in affective disorders.

Endocrine changes in affective disorders
A close relationship between depression and endocrine function is suggested by the fact that depression is a symptom of several endocrine disorders, and that patients with affective disorders often have evidence of endocrine dysfunction. Many endocrine disorders result from disturbance of hypothalmamic-pituitary function. The hypothalamus is part of the limbic system and is involved in mood control; furthermore, hypothalamic centres are partly controlled by monoamine systems postulated to be disturbed in affective disorders. In addition, the release of many anterior pituitary hormones is sleep-dependent and shows marked diurnal rhythmicity. Disorders of sleep and of circadian rhythm are prominent in depression (reviewed by Mellerup and Rafaelson 1979). These and other arguments have stimulated many investigations of endocrine function, particularly hypothalamic-pituitary relationships, in depression (see Sachar 1982, for a review). Although various endocrine abnormalities have been found, it is still not known what part (if any) is played in the control of mood by the plethora of neuroendocrine chemicals secreted by the body.

Hypothalamic-pituitary-adrenal axis

Of the endocrine changes in affective disorders, those of the hypothalamic-pituitary axis have been most widely investigated. The systemic concentration of cortisol is determined by a complex control system (Fig. 11.6) and represents the final outcome of at least four processes: (1) the effects of monoaminergic and cholinergic influences on the hypothalamic release of corticotropin-releasing factor, (2) the effects of corticotropin-releasing factor on the anterior pituitary release of ACTH, (3) the effects of ACTH on the release of cortisol by the adrenals, and (4) feedback affects of adrenal cortisol on pituitary ACTH release.

In about 50 per cent of patients with moderate to severe depression, the concentration of cortisol is raised above normal values in cerebrospinal fluid, plasma, and urine (Gelder *et al.* 1983; Calloway 1982). In addition, there is a change in the diurnal pattern of cortisol secretion: in depression plasma cortisol concentration remains high in the afternoon and evening and during

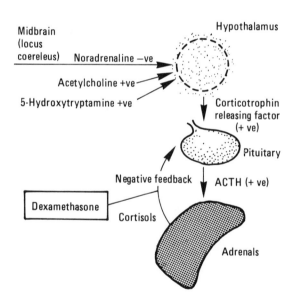

Fig. 11.6 The hypothalamic-pituitary-adrenal axis in the control of cortisol secretion. The systemic concentration of cortisol secretion is controlled by (1) monoaminergic and cholinergic influences on the hypothalamic release of corticotrophin releasing factor, (2) the effects of this factor on the anterior pituitary release of ACTH, (3) the effect of ACTH on adrenal release of cortisol, and (4) feedback effects of cortisol on pituitary ACTH release. The synthetic steroid dexamethasone normally suppresses release of ACTH and cortisol, but cortisol suppression is reduced in a proportion of patients with depression. (From Calloway 1982)

sleep, while in normal subjects there is a peak in cortisol concentration in the morning with declining concentrations later in the day and low levels at night. The raised cortisol secretion in depression is not thought to be the direct result of stress, which does not alter the diurnal pattern.

Dexamethasone suppression test In addition, 20-40 per cent of depressed patients do not show the normal suppression of cortisol secretion induced by administration of the synthetic steroid dexamethasone given at night. This lack of response forms the basis of the dexamethasone suppression test (DST) (Carroll *et al.* 1981; Fig. 11.6). This test has been held to have some diagnostic and possibly prognostic utility in depression, but it is not specific since non-suppression of cortisol secretion also occurs in 5-10 per cent of normal subjects, abstaining alcoholics, and patients with neuroses and senile dementias. Furthermore, the test does not appear to differentiate between endogenous and neurotic depression (Calloway *et al.* 1984a). Mellsop *et al.* (1985) suggest that the degree of non-suppression by dexamethasone reflects the degree of stress or distress experienced by a patient and does not relate to a specific disgnosis.

The mechanism of non-suppression of the DST in depression is not known, but is has been suggested that it is due either to excessive cholinergic or insufficient noradrenergic influence on the hypothalamus (see Fig. 11.6). If noradrenergic underactivity is responsible (a possibility consistent with the catecholamine theory of depression), it might be expected that non-suppressors would be most responsive to antidepressant drugs which selectively increase noradrenergic activity. A number of studies addressed to this possibility are mentioned by Amsterdam *et al.* (1983), but the results are conflicting and many of the investigations inadequate. The DST may, however, have an application in predicting relapse of depression on withdrawal of medication. In most patients, the DST returns to normal on clinical recovery. A few patients continue to show dexamethasone resistance in spite of clinical recovery, and Goldberg (1980a,b) found in a small series that all of such patients relapsed on cessation of drug treatment.

It remains puzzling that plasma cortisol concentrations in some depressed patients are in the same range as those found in Cushing's disease, yet depressed patients show no signs of hypercortisolism. Brain cortisol concentrations may be paradoxically decreased in depressed suicide victims, suggesting perhaps a decrease in tissue cortisol binding in depression (Carroll 1978). According to this author: 'The evidence for a primary limbic-hypothalamic neuroendocrine disturbance in endogenous depression is compelling. It is strengthened by the observation that all of the neuroendocrine abnormalities in endogenous depression occur in diencephalic Cushing's disease, in which a high incidence of depression is noted also' (Carroll 1978; p. 494).

Thyroid hormones

Circulating concentrations of thyroxine (tri- and tetraiodothyronine) are normal in depression, but in about 40 per cent of depressed patients the anterior pituitary release of thyroid stimulating hormone (thyrotropin, TSH) in response to an intravenous injection of synthetic thryotropin releasing hormone (TRH) is depressed (Carroll 1978; *British Medical Journal* 1973; Calloway *et al.* 1984b). The release of TSH is under inhibitory dopaminergic control and release is increased by dopaminergic receptor blockers such as chlorpromazine and, in hypothyroid subjects, by metoclopramide (Scanlon *et al.* 1977). There is no information relating cerebrospinal fluid concentration of the dopamine metabolite HVA to the TSH response in depression.

A blunted TSH response is also seen in patients on chronic glucocorticoid treatment and in Cushing's disease, and it has been suggested that the TSH responses are related to the high cortisol concentration. However, there appears to be no relation in depressed patients between TSH response and plasma cortisol concentration or the presence or absence of non-suppression in the dexamethasone suppression test (Calloway 1982). The TSH response may be used to predict response to treatment. Kierkegaard (1981) found that patients whose TRH response tended to return to normal after treatment remained well for 6 months while those in whom the TRH response remained blunted relapsed within 4 months.

Following earlier observations that triiodothyronine potentiated the anti-depressant effect of tricyclic drugs in female patients, Prange *et al.* (1972) compared the effect of a single intravenous infusion of TRH (600 g) with that of saline in 10 depressed euthyroid women with blunted TRH responses. They found a significant antidepressant effect lasting for over 3 days. Other workers reported similar results within intravenous TRH, but later trials using oral TRH showed no benefit in various types of depression (Prange *et al.* 1978; Mountjoy *et al.* 1974). The latter investigators commented that continuous oral use of TRH (40 mg daily) produced no signs of hyperthyroidism in depressed patients in spite of the fact that plasma TSH measurements showed that the medication was absorbed.

Growth hormone

Basal fasting plasma growth hormone concentration is normal in patients with depression. However, the response to stimulation of growth hormone release by insulin hypoglycaemia, L-dopa, and amphetamine is deficient in some patients (Carroll 1978). These procedures involve suprapituitary mechanisms and a poor response in depressed patients suggests a limbic-hypothalamic dysfunction. The regulation of growth hormone release is complex, but there is evidence that stimulation of release involves alpha-adrenergic, dopaminergic, and serotonergic systems, while inhibition of release involves beta-adrenergic systems and the polypeptide somatostatin.

Defective catecholaminergic activity in depression might be an explanation of the reduced growth hormone response since insulin hypoglycaemia, L-dopa, and amphetamine all exert their actions via catecholamines. It is not clear whether growth hormone responses differ between different types of depression (Langer and Sacher 1977; Mendlewicz *et al.* 1977; Carroll 1978), but some studies have found that bipolar patients with low urinary MHPG concentrations have the lowest growth hormone response to insulin hypoglycaemia. Diet and menopausal status effect the results, and the greatest growth hormone depression occurs in post-menopausal females (Mendlewicz *et al.* 1977).

Prolactin There is some evidence that prolactin secretion is slightly increased in depressive disorders, although results are conflicting (Carroll 1978; Calloway 1982; van Praag 1980b; Mendlowitz *et al.* 1980). Prolactin secretion undergoes diurnal rhythmic changes: it is released in a pulsatile fashion with a nocturnal rise which is dependent upon sleep (*Lancet* 1979a,b). Morning concentrations of prolactin have been reported to be increased in patients with bipolar depression. Prolactin secretion, like that of TRH is under inhibitory dopaminergic control and is suppressed by L-dopa and increased by dopamine receptor blockers. The suppression by L-dopa is more marked in bipolar depression, possibly implying dopaminergic dysfunction in these patients.

Investigations of the effects of antidepressant drugs on plasma prolactin concentrations in man have given confusing results (Carroll 1978; Meltzer *et al.* 1978). Spater *et al.* (1977) reported a doubling of prolactin concentration, without significiant changes in plasma cortisol, in depressed patients treated for 3 weeks with monoamine oxidase inhibitors while tricyclic antidepressants have been found in various investigations to elevate, decrease or have no effect on plasma prolactin concentration.

Sex hormones Many observations suggest a close relationship between sex hormones and affective disorders. Depression is twice as common in women as men, and women are most vulnerable between puberty and the age of 45 (*British Medical Journal* 1977). Affective disorders are associated with the puerperium, the menstrual cycle, the use of oral contraceptives, and perhaps with the menopause. Women with depression not uncommonly develop amenorrhoea, and in both sexes reduction of libido is a prominent symptom. Testosterone, as well as oestrogens, has marked behavioural effects (Tiwary 1974). In addition, the secretion of sex hormones exhibits pronounced circadian rhythmicity and there is evidence from sleep and biochemical studies for an upset in circadian rhythms in depression (Mellerup and Rafaelson 1979). Yet direct information relating sex hormone abnormalities to affective disorders is meagre. Plasma testosterone, oestrogen, and progesterone concentrations are within the normal range in most patients with depression (Calloway 1982).

Post-partum affective psychosis may be associated with the dramatic fall in circulating oestrogen levels that occurs at this time. This fall is normally accompanied by a decrease in peripheral alpha$_2$-receptor density. Metz *et al.* (1983) found that the decline in platelet alpha$_2$-receptors was significantly less in women developing 'maternity blues' after parturition than in controls. If these changes occur in the brain, central alpha$_2$-receptor hypersensitivity, with decreased noradrenaline release, may contribute to puerperal depression. Plasma concentrations of beta-endorphin also fall rapidly after delivery and another suggestion is that 'maternity blues' may represent endogenous opioid withdrawal symptoms (Newnham *et al.* 1983). No correlation was found between depressive symptoms and plasma beta-endorphin concentration, or with its rate of fall, but plasma concentrations may not reflect central opioid activity (Swyer 1985).

In relation to puerperal manic symptoms, Cookson (1982) cited evidence from animal studies that chronic treatment with oestradiol leads to an increase in dopamine receptor density in the striatum, and suggested that puerperal mania might be due to supersensitivity of dopamine receptors exposed by the sudden fall in oestrogen secretion. In support of this idea, the condition responds to dopamine receptor antagonists such as pimozide. The response to chlorpromazine is better, perhaps because receptors for other monoamines are also supersensitive.

Women with premenstrual tension syndromes have higher plasma prolactin concentrations that controls throughout the menstrual cycle. The cyclic decrease of oestrogen and progesterone concentrations, combined with high prolactin concentration, is thought to contribute to the affective symptoms (Carroll 1978). Cyclic changes in platelet alpha$_2$-receptor density also occurs, alpha$_2$-density being highest during the premenstruum (Grahame-Smith 1985), and this change may be more directly related to mood. Dalton (1964) found that the day of admission to hospital among women entering for depression was closely related to the menstrual cycle, 60 per cent being admitted on the 12 days of the month around ovulation, premenstruation, or during menstruation, and only 40 per cent on the other 16 days of the month.

The use of oestrogen/progesterone oral contraceptives is sometimes associated with effects on mood, and the frequency of depression as an adverse effect attributed to such use has been estimated to be between 2 and 30 per cent (Madsen 1974). Grahame-Smith (1985) reports that platelet alpha$_2$ density increases during the cycle of 21 days that the combined contraceptive pill is taken but decreases during the 7 days when it is stopped. Oestrogen/progesterone combinations also decrease the secretion of both luteinizing and follicle-stimulating hormones. It is not known how these alterations are related to mood but Whalley *et al.* (1985) report that plasma luteinizing hormone was significantly increased in drug-free young men with mania compared with controls.

Appetite and weight Disturbances in appetite and weight are common in affective disorders. Anorexia and weight loss is often associated with depression, but overeating and weight gain can occur. These changes, combined with endocrine and sleep abnormalities, suggest hypothalamic dysfunction. Somewhat similar changes are seen in anorexia nervosa, in which there is also evidence of hypothalamic-pituitary malfunction and which may be a type of phobic disorder which merges with the affective disorders.

The central control of appetite, reviewed by Morley and Levine (1983) (Fig. 11.7), involves a cascade of overlapping regulatory systems located in hypothalamic structures. These integrate information received from multiple sensory inputs describing the mileau interieur and maintain nutritional homeostasis by activating or suppressing food-seeking behaviour. Among several interconnected areas involved, a centre in the ventromedial hypothalamus has been termed the satiety centre. This is associated with a serotonergic pathway from the raphe nuclei of the pontine midbrain area and

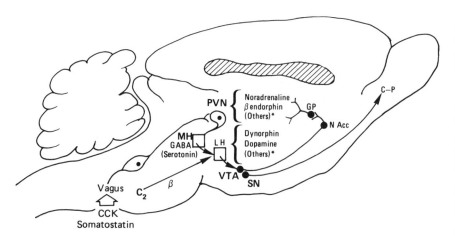

Fig. 11.7 Schematic representation of factors involved in the central control of appetite

PVN—paraventricular nucleus; MH—medial hypothalamus; LH-lateral hypothalamus; VTA—ventral tegmental area; SN—substantia nigra; N Acc—nucleus accumbens; C-P—caudate putamen; GP—globus pallidus; CCK—cholecystokinin; norepinephrine—noradrenaline.
*other transmitters in the PVN may include neurotensin, cHis-Pro-cyclo-histidyl-proline diketopiperazine, corticotropin-releasing factor and bombesin; in the LH they may include corticotropin-releasing factor, prostaglandins, calcitonin, bombesin, and GABA. (Modified from Morley and Levine 1983)

an adrenergic pathway, the ventral adrenergic bundle. Activity in the serotonergic pathway suppresses feeding, while activation of the (alpha) noradrenergic pathway antagonizes the serotonergic effect and stimulates feeding.
An area in the ventro-lateral hypothalamus is associated with the initiation
of feeding and has been termed the feeding centre. This area is associated with
the dopaminergic nigrostriatal tract, activation of which promotes feeding
behaviour. A beta-adrenergic pathway may inhibit the feeding centre, causing
satiety, and this may be the site of action of the anorectic effect of drugs such
as amphetamine. These serotonergic, noradrenergic, and dopaminergic pathways also form a part of the reward and punishment systems, and there is an
undoubted relationship between food and mood. GABA is also involved in
this complex regulating system. This neurotransmitter has a dual effect on
appetite: it can increase food intake by inhibiting serotonergic activity in the
satiety centre and decrease food intake by inhibiting dopaminergic activity in
the feeding centre.

In addition to the monoamines, several polypeptide neurotransmitters
and modulators are involved in appetite control. Morley and Levine (1983)
propose that endogenous opioids provide a tonic driving influence on
appetite. This food drive effect appears to operate through kappa opioid
receptors whose endogenous ligand is dynorphin (Chapter 5). Stress-induced
eating may result from activation of opioid systems. The opioid system
interacts with the dopaminergic system activating the contralateral hypothalamic feeding centre. Opioid binding sites are present on dopaminergic
terminals of the nigrostriatal pathways. Dopaminergic blockade inhibits
dynorphin-induced feeding and naloxone blocks dopamine-induced feeding.

Other non-opioid polypeptides appear, on the other hand, to inhibit
feeding. Calcitonin, cholecystokinin, bombesin, neurotensin and
thyrotropin-releasing hormone all suppress appetite. Corticotropin-releasing
factor (CRF), released during stress, also suppresses feeding behaviour. It is
possible that increased release of CRF in anorexia nervosa and in depression,
in which there is evidence of overactive or non-suppressible hypothalamic-
pituitary-adrenal function, accounts fot the loss of appetite in these
conditions. It is noteworthy that stress can produce either overeating by
activating endogenous opioid systems or anorexia through increased release
of CRF. Which reaction is manifestated presumably depends on the type of
stress and the constitutional balance of limbic-hypothalamic activity. The
elaborate organization of appetite control systems is reminiscent of the several redundant overlapping back-up systems modulating nociception (Chapter 5). In relation to depression, upsets of either monoamine or endogenous
peptide systems in limbic areas could result in either increase or decrease of
appetite and weight.

As well as those described above, other endocrine and metabolic changes,
including alterations in melatonin and in salt and water balance, have been

described in affective disorders; posterior pituitary hormones, involved in both sleep and memory (Chapter 8), do not appear to have been fully investigated. However, as in the case of the monoamine neurotransmitters, no particular endocrine pattern seems to characterize all cases of depression or mania. It is possible that the endocrine changes represent instability of control mechanisms, especially in the hypothalamus, rather than changes in the activity of any particular hormone. This instability could conceivably be secondary to instability of monoamine and/or polypeptide synaptic control as previously described, but as yet there is no information on this point.

12
Drugs used in depresson and mania

The development of antidepressant drugs in the last 30 years has greatly altered the management and considerably improved the prognosis of affective disorders. However, drug treatment is neither fully effective nor curative. Perhaps 80–90 per cent of patients with depression respond to antidepressant drugs, but 30–50 per cent also respond to placebo. About 80 per cent of patients with mania respond to lithium carbonate, and manic episodes can be further controlled with antipsychotic drugs. Nevertheless, the relapse rate of affective disorders is still of the order of 20 per cent after 6 months and 30–50 per cent after 1 or 2 years, even with maintenance drug treatment.

In this chapter, the main drugs used in affective disorders are described. Many drugs produce euphoria in normal subjects (Chapter 7) and some of these, at least temporarily, lighten mood in depressed patients. However, a characteristic of antidepressant drugs is that they have little effect on mood in normal subjects, yet restore normal mood in patients with clinical depression. Similarly, some drugs which are effective in mania (lithium, carbamazepine) have no discernible effects on mood in normal subjects. These drugs are thus essentially mood normalizers rather than euphoriants or mood-depressants. Most of them, even when effective, take some weeks to exert their therapeutic actions and there remains a core of patients who appear to be refractory to drug treatment. For these reasons, alternative measures, such as electro-convulsive therapy for depression, remain important for the treatment of affective disorders when rapid action is required and for drug non-responders.

As discussed in Chapter 11, some evidence suggests that affective disorders are characterized by instability of synaptic control mechanisms in multiple neurotransmitter pathways in the limbic system. The clinical course of these syndromes indicates that such instability is reversible and has a tendency to right itself. The possibility is suggested in this chapter that an action common to the diverse treatments effective in affective disorders is the restoration of synaptic stability and efficiency, and a consequent hastening of the intrinsic tendency towards remission.

Tricyclic antidepressants

Imipramine was the first tricyclic antidepressant to be introduced and has been followed by many others with similar chemical structure. The general characteristics of the drugs are discussed together here. Some of the properties of these and related drugs are shown in Table 12.1.

Pharmacokinetics

The pharmacokinetics of tricyclic antidepressants are reviewed by Peet and Coppen (1979), Rogers *et al.* (1981), and Bickel (1980). They are all well absorbed from the gut, widely distributed in the body, and concentrated in the brain, especially in limbic areas, basal ganglia, and cortex. They undergo extensive hepatic metabolism and some of the metabolites are pharmacologically active. Rates of metabolism are influenced by genetic and environmental factors and there are marked differences in steady state plasma concentrations between individuals on the same dose. In general there is little correlation between steady-state plasma concentration and clinical effect, despite evidence of a 'therapeutic window' for some tricyclic antidepressants (Asberg *et al.* 1971; Peet and Coppen 1979; Grahame-Smith and Orr 1978; Amsterdam *et al.* 1980; Montgomery 1980; Norman and Burrows 1983).

Biochemical actions

The biochemical actions of the tricyclic antidepressants have been reviewed by Sulser and Mobley (1980), Langer and Karobath (1980), Nielson (1980), Iverson and Mackay (1979), and Ghose (1980) among others.

Reuptake inhibition at monoaminergic synapses

A biochemical action common to all tricyclic antidepressants is inhibition of the high affinity, energy-dependent uptake of monoamines into cytoplasmic stores within the presynaptic membrane. This uptake (Uptake 1) is a saturable, stereochemically selective process which involves a Na/K-dependent carrier system and requires energy and Na/K-stimulated ATPase. Inhibition of this system by tricyclic antidepressants is competetive. It has been shown to occur *in vitro* and *in vivo* , both in peripheral tissues and in the brain in animals, and in peripheral tissues in man (Ghose 1980). Since this reuptake system normally terminates monoaminergic transmitter activity on synaptic neurones following nerve-stimulated release, the effect of its inhibition by tricyclic antidepressants is to prolong the actions of monoamines released at synapses, and to enhance their stimulation of pre- and post-synaptic receptors (Fig. 11.2). Among the tricyclic antidepressants, secondary amines have more potent effects on the uptake of noradrenaline, while tertiary amines are more potent in blocking the reuptake of serotonin (see Table 12.1). The reuptake of dopamine is much less affected by these drugs than that of noradrenaline and serotonin though all inhibit it to some degree.

Monoamine uptake block explains many of the pharmacological actions

Table 12.1. Pharmacological properties of some antidepressant drugs

Antidepressant drugs	Type	Plasma elimination half-life (h)	Noradrenaline uptake inhibition	Serotonin uptake inhibition	Anticholinergic effects	Sedative effects
Tricyclic compounds						
imipramine[1]	tertiary amine	4–18	++	+++	++	++
amitriptyline[2]	tertiary amine	10–25	+	+++	+++	++
clomipramine	tertiary amine	16–20	+	+++	++	++
nortriptyline	secondary amine	13–93	+++	+	++	○
desipramine	secondary amine	12–61	+++	○	+	○
protriptyline	secondary amine	54–198	+++	++	++	○
doxepin[3]	tertiary amine	8–25	+	+	+++	++
dothiepin						
Related compounds						
viloxazine (bicyclic)	secondary amine	2–5	+++	○	○	○
maprotiline (bridged tricyclic)	secondary amine	27–58	+++	+	+	+
mianserin[4]	tertiary amine	8–19	○	○	○	○
Unrelated compounds						
trazodone[4] (triazololpyridine)		4	○	+	○	++

1. Metabolized to desipramine.
2. Metabolized to nortriptyline.
3. Metabolized to desmethyldoxepin (beta half-life 33–81 h).
4. Inhibits presynaptic alpha$_2$ receptors.
Pharmacological activity: ○ = none; + = slight + + = moderate; + + + = marked.
References: Rogers *et al.* 1981; Amsterdam *et al.* 1980.

of the tricyclic antidepressants, and it has been widely accepted that it underlies their antidepressant effect. This possibility provided the main impetus
for the monoamine hypothesis of affective disorders (Chapter 11). Both
tricyclic antidepressants and monoamine oxidase in inhibitors (see below)
increase the availability of active monoamines at receptor sites and reverse
the biochemical, physiological, and behavioural effects of reserpine, a drug
which depletes monoamine stores at nerve terminals, causes behavioural
depression in animals, and can precipitate a depressive syndrome in man.
Reserpine-reversal by antidepressant drugs does not occur in rats whose
brains have been selectively depleted of catecholamines with 6-hydroxy-
dopamine (Sulser and Mobley 1980).

However, several of the newer, clinically effective, antidepressants are
neither reuptake blockers nor monoamine oxidase inhibitors; thus, such an
action does not appear to be a prerequisite for an antidepressant effect. In
addition, inhibition of monoamine uptake can be demonstrated within
minutes of the administration of tricyclic antidepresants while the clinical
antidepressant effect takes weeks to develop (Fig. 12.1). It has recently
become apparent that, with chronic administration, the initial reuptake
blocking effect gives rise to a number of secondary effects, both on monoamine synthesis and turnover, and on receptor sensitivity. At present, the long-
term effects on receptor sensitivity appear to have the most clinical relevance.

Other effects on monoamine systems

Animal studies indicate that the increased synaptic concentration of noradrenaline and serotonin, induced acutely by the tricyclic antidepressants,

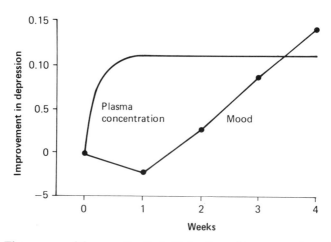

Fig. 12.1. Time course of therapeutic effect of tricyclic antidepressant drugs. Improvement in depression is considerably delayed compared with attainment of maximum
plasma concentration (and biochemical effects). (From Oswald *et al.* 1972.)

inhibits the synthesis of the respective monoamines through negative feed-back mechanisms, resulting in decreased cerebral turnover of noradrenaline or serotonin. Thus, tertiary amines have been observed to depress the firing of serotonergic raphe neurones (Koe 1983) while secondary amines depress the firing of noradrenergic locus coeruleus neurones (Sulser and Mobley 1980). The concentrations of metabolites of these transmitters in body fluids may fall after tricyclic antidepressant administration (Langer and Karobath 1980).

The effect of iontophoretically applied imipramine and desipramine on single cortical neurones of the cat has been studied by Bradshaw *et al.* (1974). When briefly applied, the drugs did not affect the spontaneous firing rate of the neurones, but both potentiation and antagonism of the responses of these neurones to noradrenaline and serotonin were observed. The direction of response depended on the concentration of the antidepressant drug, a lower concentration causing potentiation and a higher concentration causing antag-onism of response to either of the monoamines. Some cells were excited by noradrenaline or serotonin while others were inhibited; both types of response were potentiated or antagonized by the antidepressants, depending on dose. The authors suggested that the potentiation of response to mono-amines by imipramine and desipramine was at least partially due to monoamine reuptake blockade, and the antagonism to a (possibly post-synaptic) receptor blocking action. Similar dual effects on the response of neurones to acetylcholine were observed (Bevan *et al.* 1975). Bradshaw *et al.* (1974) raised the interesting possibility that a given concentration of antidepressant may have differential effects on different systems, potentiating the effects of one transmitter while, at the same dose, antagonizing those of another. In this way, the balance of activity between different neuronal systems might be altered, an effect which might be related to the therapeutic actions of these drugs in depression.

Monoamine receptor modulation with chronic administration

Chronic administration of tricyclic antidepressants leads to changes in the sensitivity of a number of receptors for monoamines. These changes are not apparent when only the acute biochemical effects are studied. They may represent, at least partially, a homeostatic response to the initial monoamine uptake blocking action of the drugs. Receptor adaptations to long-term antidepressant medication have been discussed Chapter 11. In general, it appears that tricyclic antidepressants, both secondary and tertiary amines, a number of non-tricyclic antidepressant drugs, and perhaps various other treatments for depression including lithium and electroconvulsive therapy, can produce some or all of the following changes in monoamine receptor activity in the brain:

(i) Down-regulation of presynaptic (alpha$_2$) adrenergic receptors has been demonstrated by biochemical and physiological studies in animals and man (Charney *et al.* 1981a,b; Langer *et al.* 1980) after imipramine, desipramine, nortriptyline, amitriptyline, and monoamine oxidase inhibitors. Binding studies in human platelets have produced conflicting results, probably because of differences in technique (Lenox *et al.* 1983; Pritchard *et al.* 1983), but some studies have reported a fall in platelet alpha$_2$ receptor binding (Garcia-Sevilla *et al.* 1981).

(ii) Down-regulation of post-synaptic beta-adrenergic receptors has been shown in binding, biochemical, and physiological investigations after tricyclic antidepressants and a large number of other antidepressant drugs and treatments (Sulser 1981; Creese and Sibley 1981; Table 11.2, Chapter 11).

(iii) For post-synaptic alpha$_1$-receptors, the evidence is conflicting: increases, decreases, and no change after antidepressant treatment have all been reported (Creese and Sibley 1981; Cohen *et al.* 1982; Charney *et al.* 1981a).

(iv) Down-regulation of dopamine autoreceptors has been shown to occur in animals after treatment with tricyclic antidepressants (Antelman and Chiodo 1981). There is little information in man and there have been few investigations of post-synaptic dopamine receptor density after antidepressants.

(v) Decreased density of serotonin reuptake sites (high affinity imipramine binding sites) has been demonstrated in the rat brain after tricyclic antidepressants (Langer and Briley 1981).

(vi) Studies of post-synaptic serotonin receptors (5-HT-1 and 5-HT-2) have given conflicting results. On the whole binding studies have suggested down-regulation (Rudeberg 1983) while some behavioural and physiological studies have suggested up-regulation after tricyclic and other antidepressant treatments (Charney *et al.* 1981a) and after mianserin (Blier *et al.* 1984).

As discussed in Chapter 11, the effects of chronic antidepressant treatment on receptor sensitivity may vary in different parts of the brain, and adaptive receptor changes probably involve co-modulation by several different neurotransmitters (Ogren *et al.* 1983; Fuxe *et al.* 1983; Sulser *et al.* 1983; Barbaccia *et al.* 1983; Goldstein *et al.* 1983). It seems likely that the therapeutic effects of chronic tricyclic antidepressant treatment stem from complex adaptive changes which ultimately result in greater synaptic efficiency and stability in several neurotransmitter systems.

Effects on other neurotransmitter systems

The tricyclic antidepressants are structurally related to the phenothiazines, and share with them both anticholinergic and antihistaminic effects. The anticholinergic effects may be due to a blocking action at muscarinic cholinergic receptors. Bevan *et al.* (1975) studied the effects of tricyclic antidepressants on the response of single cortical neurones to acetylcholine. As with the monoamines, both a potentiation and an antagonism of the cholinergic response was noted, depending on antidepressant concentration. Antagonism of response to acetylcholine was observed at higher doses and was ascribed to blockade of cholinergic muscarinic receptors. Potentiation of response was observed at lower doses of antidepressants, and also occurred with atropine; it was suggested that this effect was due to blockade of masked inhibitory cholinergic receptors. The anticholinergic effects of tricyclic antidepressants do not correlate with their antidepressant effects, and many of the newer antidepressants are almost devoid of anticholinergic activity. Cholinergic blockade may, however, give rise to adverse effects.

Antihistaminic effects are attributed to blockade of histamine H-2 receptors in the brain; they can also be demonstrated on peripheral tissues such as the guinea-pig ileum. There is no relationship between antihistaminic potency and antidepressant effect.

Effects on mood and behaviour

In most normal subjects, the tricyclic antidepressants have virtually no euphoriant or mood-elevating properties. Most of them induce at first a sense of fatigue and sleepiness, lightheadedness, and clumsiness, accompanied by anticholinergic symptoms such as dry mouth and blurred vision. These effects are usually perceived as unpleasant, and produce psychological discomfort and anxiety. Continued administration for several days leads to impairment of cognition with difficulty in concentration and logical thought, and a decline in psychomotor performance (Baldessarini 1980).

By contrast, about 70 per cent of patients with depression respond to the tricyclic antidepressants, after a delay of some weeks, with elevation or normalization of mood. The effect is usually one of dulling of depressive ideation rather than one of euphoric stimulation. Behaviour is correspondingly normalized with increased social interaction and cognitive and motor function. However, in patients with bipolar depression, the drugs may precipitate a sudden switch towards excitement, euphoria, and mania (Fig. 12.2). Such a switch may also be precipitated by L-dopa, monoamine oxidase inhibitors, amphetamine and ephedrine, even in patients receiving therapeutic doses of lithium (Bunney 1978).

Tricyclic antidepressants are sometimes effective in allaying the signs and symptoms of anxiety neuroses, including agoraphobia and obsessive/compulsive neuroses. Monoamine oxidase inhibitors have similar actions in these disorders. Certain tricyclic agents appear to have anxiolytic actions in addition to their antidepressant properties. These include imipramine, amitriptyline, dothiepin, and doxepin (Rogers *et al.* 1981), but it is not clear whether anxiolytic, antidepressant, and sedative effects are really separable— not whether anxiety is really separable from depression (Chapter 11).

In normal animals, the behavioural effects of the tricyclic antidepressants are usually those of mild central nervous system depression. Spontaneous

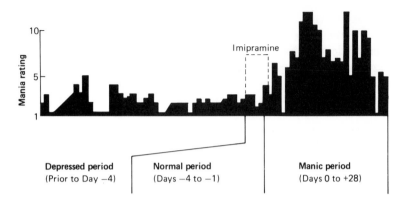

Fig. 12.2. Precipitation of mania by imipramine in a patient with bipolar depression. (Adapted from Bunney 1978, by kind permission of Raven Press, New York.)

motor activity is reduced, although the animals may show increased excitability (Nielsen 1980). Acquisition and peformance in conditional avoidance tasks is impaired (Baldessarini 1980). Muricidal behaviour is selectively blocked in rats, an action shared by amphetamine, neuroleptics, and some antihistamines. The tricyclic antidepressants exert little effect, when given alone, on intracranial self-stimulation behaviour, but potentiate the enhancing effect of amphetamine. They reserve the behavioural and physiological effect of reserpine and inhibit the development of 'depressive' behaviour in several animal models of depression, including behavioural despair in rodents, learned helplessness in dogs and rodents, separation distress in primates and abnormal behaviour in bulbectomized rats (Willner 1984).

Thus, the tricyclic antidepressants exert beneficial or therapeutic effects on mood and behaviour only in special circumstances. In animal models these circumstances are normally related to particular forms of stress. In man, the relationship to stress is less clear. The question of how the drugs influence thought patterns and ideation is obscure, even if it is accepted that they act by affecting synaptic transmission in the various ways discussed in previous sections. The question also arises of whether there is a critical point at which a previously normal person becomes depressed in the sense that he will respond to antidepressant drugs. Is it a matter of the severity of depression induced by external or internal stress, or is there a phase shift when limbic synaptic control mechanisms become unstable so that certain thought processes are no longer constrained or readily reversible? Yet the process is potentially reversible: a considerable proportion of patients with depression respond to placebo and most eventually remit without treatment. The antidepressant drugs appear to trigger or catalyse whatever processes are required for spontaneous remission.

Therapeutic efficacy of tricyclic antidepressants

Tricyclic antidepressants undoubtedly improve the prognosis in depression, but the degree to which they do this has been difficult to estimate. The drugs terminate attacks of depression in 60–80 per cent depending on the selection criteria for treatment (Amsterdam *et al.* 1980; Asberg and Sjoquist 1981; Lader 1982b) although their effects may not be apparent for several weeks. About 46 per cent of patients with acute depression and 16 per cent of those with chronic disorders respond to placebo but most randomly assigned, double blind, placebo-controlled trials show that tricyclic antidepressants are more effective than placebo (Berger 1977). No particular tricyclic drug appears to have greater overall therapeutic efficacy, although the incidence and severity of adverse effects varies between drugs. Tricyclic agents have become the standard drugs against which new antidepressant drugs are compared for efficacy.

Continued administration of tricyclic antidepressants also reduces the likelihood of recurrence of depressive episodes. About 30–50 per cent of depressed patients relapse in 6 months after treatment with electroconvulsive therapy alone, while the relapse rate after 6 months of drug treatment is 10–20 per cent (Rogers *et al.* 1981). Three large collaborative studies cited by Berger (1977) have confirmed the finding that continued (6 months) tricyclic depressants treatment reduces the relapse rate compared with short-term treatment (6 weeks).

Reasons for failure of therapeutic response are discussed by Amsterdam *et al.* (1980) and Kessler (1978). They include non-compliance, inappropriate dosage, and selective response to a particular tricyclic drug. Several reports suggest that the response is better in endogenous than in neurotic depression but others, reviewed by Amsterdam *et al.* (1980), give evidence that the drugs can be effective in both groups. There remains a core of depressed patients who do not respond to tricyclic antidepressants. These non-responders are clinically heterogeneous and there is no indication that their depression reflects a different aetiology from that of responders. Practical aspects of the treatment of depressive disorders with tricyclic drugs, including selection of patients, prediction of clinical response, choice of drug, and duration of treatment are discussed by Coppen and Peet (1979), Paykel (1979a,b), Berger (1977), and Kessler (1978).

Effects on sleep

Tricyclic antidepressants have pronounced effects on sleep (Kay *et al.* 1976; Hartmann 1976; Gaillard 1979). In depressive illness, Stage 4 sleep is decreased, REMS is increased, and there are frequent awakenings. This pattern is reversed by tricyclic antidepressant drugs which increase Stage 4 sleep, markedly decrease REMS, and decrease the number of nocturnal awakenings (Fig. 12.3). The effects on sleep commence soon after the start

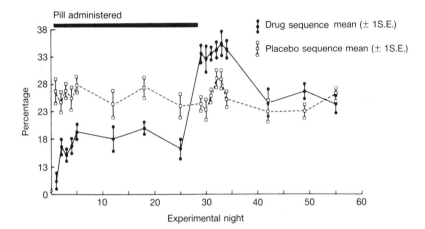

Fig. 12.3. Effect of amitriptyline on REMS percentage. Open symbols and dotted line, placebo; filled symbols and solid line, amitriptyline. $n = 10$. (From Hartmann 1976, by kind permission of John Wiley & Sons Inc., New York.)

of drug therapy and there is no temporal relationship with clinical recovery, despite reports that REMS deprivation without drugs may be of therapeutic value in depression (*British Medical Journal* 1975). The same effects on sleep are exerted by the drugs in normal subjects. A rebound of REMS occurs on cessation of antidepressant drug therapy.

The effects of tricyclic antidepressants on sleep are probably related to their actions on monoamine and endocrine function. As discussed in Chapter 2, serotonergic mechanisms in arousal and sleep systems probably actively promote SWS and inhibit arousal systems, and may in addition inhibit REMS. These serotonergic effects would all be enhanced by the serotonin uptake blocking effect of the tricyclic antidepressants. On this reasoning, sleep disturbance would be expected to be most marked in depressed patients with evidence of low serotonergic activity (decreased 5-HIAA cerebrospinal fluid concentrations) and the sleep of these patients would be most improved by tricyclic agents with patient serotonin reuptake blocking effects. Tertiary amines, which preferentially inhibit serotonin uptake, do have more marked sedative effects than secondary amines. However there do not appear to be any systematic studies of the relationships between sleep disturbance, cerebrospinal fluid 5-HIAA concentration, and the sleep response to tricyclic agents in depressed patients.

The role of catecholaminergic systems in sleep is less clear. In general, they appear to have effects on sleep which are opposite to those of serotonergic systems, promoting arousal and decreasing SWS and REMS. Tricyclic antidepressants which block catecholamine uptake may encourage activation of anergic patients and although they may normalize sleep patterns in these patients, they are less potent sedatives than the tertiary amines. Increased adrenergic and cholinergic activity in hypothalamic/pituitary systems induced by tricyclic antidepressants may tend to restore diurnal rhythmicity and endocrine secretion patterns during sleep, which are disturbed in depression. Cholinergic activity in sleep and arousal systems is thought to induce or facilitate REMS. Anticholinergic actions of tricyclic antidepressants may add to the REMS-reducing effects.

Effects on EEG

The effects of tricyclic antidepressants on the EEG are reviewed by Itil and Soldatos (1980), Gogolek (1980), Lader and Bhanji (1980), Fink (1975), Itil (1975). Quantitative analysis using digital computer methods has shown that the drugs produce a characteristic EEG profile which is common to all antidepressants, regardless of their chemical structure or supposed mechanism of action (Fig. 2.9). The ability to induce this profile is a predictor of antidepressant activity in newly developed drugs prior to clinical trial. The typical EEG changes after acute administration of a tricyclic antidepressant consist of an increase both in very slow and in fast activity, with a decrease in alpha activity. These effects are apparent within 3 h of oral dosage and occur in normal subjects and depressed patients. The drugs thus, appear to have a dual action consisting of activation of both central stimulant and central inhibitory processes.

On chronic administration in depressed patients, the effects are more variable and depend on dose and on the characteristics of the EEG prior to treatment. In general, slow wave activity is increased and alpha activity is more marked; increase in fast activity in the beta range persists. The total power of the EEG, which is reduced in untreated depression (Chapter 11) is usually increased. However, there is a tendency towards desynchronization and pre-existing paroxysmal abnormalities may be increased. These effects are dose-related and are accentuated by photic stimulation. The tricyclic antidepressants have anticonvulsant effects at low doses but are convulsant at high doses; epileptiform convulsions may occur in predisposed subjects and in overdose.

The effects on cortical evoked potentials are variable and depend on the strength of stimulus and the individual, but in some cases the amplitude of the late components of the auditory, visual, and somatosensory evoked potentials and the magnitude of the contingent negative variation are increased in treated depressed patients when clinical improvement occurs (Ashton unpublished observations; Lader and Bhanji 1980).

Adverse effects

Anticholinergic effects

Many of the tricyclic antidepressants have anticholinergic effects due to blockade of cholinergic (muscarinic) receptors (Table 12.1). Some tolerance appears appears to develop and the symptoms tend to recede as treatment continues.

Cardiovascular effects

Tachycardia and postural hypotension can occur. Cardiac arrhythmia may be provoked and cause sudden death. The effect may be related to peripheral monoamine reuptake blockade resulting in high concentrations of noradrenaline in cardiac tissues. Direct quinidine-like cardiac depressant effects may account for the development of myocardial infarction and congestive cardiac failure in some elderly subjects.

Central nervous system effects

Some of the tricyclic antidepressants, particularly those with anxiolytic effects may produce drowsiness or excessive sedation (Table 12.1). Others have stimulant effects and may cause restlessness or insomnia. Occasionally the drugs may precipitate mania in patients with bipolar disorders, acute psychosis in patients with a history a schizophrenia, or a toxic confusional psychosis in the elderly.

Acute overdose

Self-poisoning with antidepressant drugs is common. Each year there are over 100 000 cases of antidepressant overdose in the United Kingdom with about 400 deaths (Lader 1982b). A dose about 10 times the therapeutic dose can be lethal (Kessler 1978). The clinical picture includes a combination of central nervous system and cardiovascular toxic effects due to anticholinergic actions and increased adrenergic activity.

Drug interactions

A number of drugs which are highly protein-bound can displace tricyclic antidepressants from plasma protein binding sites (Baldessarini 1980). Several drugs affect their rate of metabolism, (Peet and Coppen 1979; Rogers *et al.* 1981). Hepatic enzyme inducers, particularly barbiturates (Chapter 4), increase the rate of metabolism and lower steady-state plasma concentrations, while neuroleptics inhibit the metabolism of some tricyclics leading to a rise in plasma concentration (Vandel *et al.* 1979).

Several drugs interact with tricyclic antidepressants at their sites of action. Monoamine oxidase inhibitors potentiate the increase of monoaminergic activity at synapses and the use of the two types of drugs together can precipitate excitement and hyperpyrexia. Rarely, this combination can also cause convulsions and coma, and the use of tricyclic antidepressants with monoamine oxidase inhibitors is generally contraindicated (Baldessarini 1980). Sympathomimetic amines may produce similar potentiation and give rise to a hypertensive reaction. On the other hand, the effects of certain antihypertensive drugs may be reversed. Drugs with anticholinergic effects, including anti-Parkinsonism drugs, may potentiate the central and peripheral anticholinergic effects of tricyclic antidepressants and at toxic concentrations produce a syndrome of hyperpyrexia, agitation and convulsions. Sedative/ hypnotic drugs, including alcohol, have additive effects with sedative tricyclic antidepressants.

Miscellaneous adverse effects

Tricyclic antidepressants can cause an increase in appetite with carbohydrate craving and a marked gain in weight. Blood sugar concentration may fall, particularly in diabetics. Amenorrhoea and menstrual irregularities may occur in women. Haemotological changes and allergic reactions are sometimes seen.

Effects in pregnancy

There is little evidence that tricyclic antidepressants are teratogenic, but several cases have been reported in which their use in late pregnancy caused undesirable effects in the neonate (Ostergaard and Pedersen 1982; Cowe et al. 1982; Webster 1973). Central nervous system depression, respiratory acidosis, cyanosis, hypothermia, tremor, hyper- and hypotonia, and urinary retention have been attributed to anticholinergic actions, and convulsions have been attributed to withdrawal effects. During lactation, maternal administration of amitriptyline, nortriptyline, imipramine, and mianserin appears to be compatible with breast feeding, since very small quantities are found in breast milk and none in the breast-feeding infant (Ashton 1985b; *Drug and Therapeutics Bulletin* 1983; Brixen-Rasmusson et al. 1982).

Withdrawal syndrome

Tolerance develops to the anticholinergic effects of the tricyclic antidepressants and a number of adaptive changes result from the monoamine uptake inhibition, as discussed above. Acute withdrawal effects, consisting of malaise, chills, coryza, muscular aches, nausea, and vomiting have been described after sudden cessation of imipramine (Baldessarini 1980; Berger 1977).

Tyrer (1984) studied patients with depressive anxiety and phobic neuroses who were withdrawn from maintenance treatment with tricyclic antidepressants or the monoamine oxidase inhibitor phenelzine. Some patients had no significant symptoms during a 4-week period after withdrawal; some were judged to have a relapse of the previous depression, but some developed new anxiety symptoms and perceptual disturbances which possibly represented true withdrawal phenomena. The incidence of this reaction was about 30 per cent with both types of drug, but symptoms were much milder on withdrawal from tricyclic antidepressants than from phenelzine. The occurrence of this reaction was related to duration of drug use and the authors suggested that it was unlikely to occur if the drugs had been used for less than 9 months. Similar symptoms on sudden tricyclic antidepressant withdrawal have been reported by Bialos *et al.* (1982) and Charney *et al.* (1982) and attributed to noradrenergic hyperactivity. The patients studied by Tyrer (1984) all had neurotic depression and the withdrawal symptoms were similar to benzodiazepine withdrawal symptoms (Chapter 4). In a study of 52 patients with neurotic depression who had taken therapeutic doses of doxepin for several years, Ayd (1986) reported that some patients experienced withdrawal symptoms after abrupt drug discontinuation or during 'drug holidays'. Symptoms included anxiety, irritability, restlessness, insomnia, nightmares, and gastrointestinal complaints. Symptoms emerged during the first two weeks after drug withdrawal and subsided during the next two weeks. There was no craving for the drug. It seems likely that the withdrawal syndrome of tricyclic antidepressants is related to the anxiolytic or sedative effects of the drugs.

Antidepressant withdrawal symptoms in which depression is a marked feature are difficult to distinguish from a relapse of the depressive disorder but careful studies of antidepressant withdrawal symptoms from patients after treatment of endogenous depression would be interesting. Since tricyclic antidepressants do not cause euphoria in most depressed patients, an amphetamine-like withdrawal syndrome or drug dependence would seem to be unlikely. Unlike amphetamine, tricyclic antidepressants are not self-administered by animals, although they can support intracranial self stimulation in certain circumstances (Chapter 11).

Individual properties of tricyclic antidepressants

The pharmacological properties and clinical effects of the many tricyclic antidepressants are broadly similar; differences between them relate mainly to their pharmacokinetics, their relative potency in blocking serotonin or noradrenaline reuptake, and the presence of central stimulant or depressant effects. However, *iprindole* should be mentioned for its slightly different profile of activity. This drug is a tricyclic agent, but has an indole nucleus and a cyclo-octane ring. It inhibits noradrenaline uptake in the brain, but has little effect in the peripheral nervous system. It has less anticholinergic and antihistaminic activity than other tricyclics and few adverse effects. It has little sedative effect. *Doxepin*, *dibenzapin* , and *dothiepin* appear to have anxiolytic effects and have been used in anxiety states (Chapter 3). They are sedative and may produce drowsiness. Adverse effects are similar to those of the other tricyclics, but the incidence and severity of these has been shown to be less with dothiepin which appears to be suitable for use in the elderly (Khan 1981; Dahl *et al.* 1981). *Lofepramine* is claimed to be relatively free from adverse effects (Dorman 1985). Individual properties of tricyclic antidepressant drugs are reviewed by Mindham (1982) and Dorman (1985).

New generation antidepressants

Following the apparent therapeutic success of the classical tricyclic antidepressants, a new generation of drugs was developed with the hope of finding agents with increased antidepressant potency, a more rapid onset of action, and fewer adverse effects. In spite of their diverse chemical structures, most of these new drugs have very similar therapeutic effects to the original tricyclics, including a delayed onset of action. On the other hand many have fewer adverse effects and are safer in overdose. These newer antidepressants are reviewed by Lader (1982b), and Barnes and Bridges (1982).

Maptrotiline

Maprotiline is a bridged tricyclic, only slightly different in chemical structure from other tricyclics. It has a beta half-life of 27–58 h and is a relatively selective inhibitor of noradrenaline uptake. It has sedative properties and its adverse and toxic effects are similar to those of imipramine (Knudsen and Heath 1984).

Mianserin

Mianserin has a tetracyclic structure. Its plasma beta half-life is 7.7–19.2 h and, because it is highly protein bound, only small amounts cross the placenta (Rogers *et al.* 1981). This drug appears to have a different biochemical action from the tricyclic antidepressants since it has no effect on monoamine uptake, no sympathomimetic activity, and no significant anticholinergic effects. It does not reverse the effects of reserpine in animal tests. There is some evidence, however, that it blocks presynaptic alpha$_2$ adrenoceptors, thus, inhibiting the negative feedback on noradrenaline release and increasing noradrenaline turnover (Fludder and Leonard 1979). It also decreases the density of postsynaptic serotonin (5-HT-2) receptors (Rudeberg 1983). The clinical profile of mianserin is similar to that of amitriptyline in depression. It also has anxiolytic, sedative, and antihistaminic effects. Apart from sedation, adverse effects are rare, and the virtual lack of cardiotoxic and anticholinergic effects make this drug suitable for the elderly and relatively safe in overdose.

Trazodone

Trazodone is a triazolopyridine derivative with a structure unrelated to other antidepressants. It has an elimination half-life of about 4 h. Its biochemical actions are complex. It inhibits neuronal serotonin uptake but blocks central serotonin receptors. At the same time, it blocks presynaptic alpha$_2$-adrenoceptors, having six times the affinity of mianserin for these receptors. Trazodone does not show the usual properties of antidepressants in animal tests; for example, it does not reverse the effects of reserpine or potentiate catecholamines and it has some properties which resemble those of anxiolytics. The clinical effects are similar to those of sedative tricyclic antidepressants. It appears to be effective in endogenous and neurotic depression, and in anxiety. It has been suggested that the anxiolytic effects result from blockade of central serotonergic receptors and the antidepressant effects from a combination of alpha$_2$-receptor antagonism and noradrenaline releasing effects (Peroutka and Snyder 1979). Adverse effects from trazodone appear to be minimal: there are no anticholinergic effects and little cardiotoxicity, but sedation may occur.

Other new antidepressants

A number of other compounds have been developed as new antidepressants. *Oxaprotaline* (Delini-Stula *et al.* 1983, Oxaprotaline Study Group 1983), and *nisoxetine* (Lemberger *et al.* 1983) are relatively selective noradrenaline reuptake blockers; *fluoxetine* (Lemberger *et al.* 1980) and *fluoxamine* (Wakelin 1983) are fairly specific serotonin reuptake blockers; *bupropion* (Miller and Stern 1983) is a potent inhibitor of dopamine uptake but appears to be free of amphetamine-like effects (Hamilton *et al.* 1983); while *diclofensine* (Burkard *et al.* 1983) inhibits the uptake of all three monoamines to an equal extent. All these drugs appear to have similar therapeutic efficacy to the tricyclic antidepressants with a similar delayed onset of action, but fewer adverse effects.

Monoamine oxidase inhibitors

The monoamine oxidase inhibitors were introduced as antidepressants in the 1950s at about the same time as the tricyclic compounds, but they were soon superseded by the tricyclics which had a wider therapeutic range and less severe adverse effects. Monoamine oxidase inhibitors are now used for certain subgroups of patients with depressive or anxiety disorders, including some which do not respond to tricyclic antidepressants. The drugs most often used clinically are the hydrazine derivates *phenelzine* and *isocarboxazid* and the non-hydrazine *tranylcypromine*. Another non-hydrazine, pargyline, has been used as an antihypertensive agent. The selective hydrazine monoamine oxidase-A inhibitor, *clorgyline*, has been introduced as an antidepressant more recently, while a selective monoamine oxidase-B inhibitor, deprenyl, is used in Parkinson's disease. The monoamine oxidase inhibitors are reviewed by Kline and Cooper (1980), and Tyrer (1982).

Pharmacokinetics

The monoamine oxidase inhibitors are all lipid soluble compounds which are rapidly absorbed after oral administration and widely distributed in body tissues including the brain. The metabolism of these drugs is poorly understood because it has been difficult to isolate the various metabolites. They are extensively metabolized in the liver into inactive compounds, by routes which probably include acetylation, oxidation, and oxidative deamination. The part played by acetylation in the inactivation of these drugs has been much discussed because the ability to acetylate foreign substances varies widely between individuals and may be related to the therapeutic and toxic effects of the monoamine oxidase inhibitors (Johnstone and Marsh 1973; Evans *et al.* 1965; Davidson *et al.* 1978). Paykel *et al.* (1982) followed the effect of phenelzine over 6 weeks in a double-blind controlled study. It was found that slow acetylators showed significantly more improvement with phenelzine than with placebo after 2 weeks, but fast acetylators showed a similar level of improvement after 6 weeks. The importance of acetylator status in the response to monoamine oxidase inhibitors is still debated.

Biochemical actions

Monoamine oxidase inhibition

As their name implies, the monoamine oxidase inhibitors inhibit the enzyme monoamine oxidase in brain and peripheral tissues. The hydrazines produce irreversible inhibition while that produced by non-hydrazines is slowly reversible. Monoamine oxidase exists in at least two forms in the body, MAO-A and MAO-B. These forms have different substrate specificities. The preferred substrate for MAO-A is serotonin, but it also deaminates noradrenaline and dopamine. The preferred substrate for MAO-B is benzylamine (Kline and Cooper 1980). Tyramine and tryptamine are substrates for both types. MAO-A is thought to be more relevant to the activity of antidepressant drugs. Most monoamine oxidase inhibitors with antidepressant properties inhibit both MAO-A and MAO-B, but the more recently introduced clorgyline is specific for MAO-A. New, selective, reversible monoamine oxidate inhibitors are in the process of experimental development and study (Benedetti and Dostert, 1985).

At monoaminergic nerve terminals, MAO-A appears to control the amount of transmitter which is held in synaptic storage vesicles. A stabilizing system seems to exist whereby the quantity of transmitter stored at these sites is kept roughly constant, any excess being deaminated by the enzyme and returned to the metabolic pool. Thus, the activity of monoamine oxidase determines the quantity of monoamine released into the synaptic cleft by a nerve impulse and the consequence of monoamine oxidase inhibition is an increase in the concentration of monoamine transmitter available to act on synaptic receptors following nerve stimulation (Fig. 11.2). This effect leads to enhancement of activity of serotonin, noradrenaline and dopamine, both centrally and peripherally. The effect persists for some weeks after the elimination of the drug from the body, because of the irreversible or only slowly reversible nature of the enzyme inhibition.

Monoamine oxidase inhibitors also have some catecholamine uptake blocking activity which adds to their effects (Kline and Cooper 1980). The non-hydrazine derivatives are similar in structure to amphetamine and have additional amphetamine-like effects including dopamine release.

In animal tests, monoamine oxidase inhibitors, like many other antidepressants, reverse the behavioural and physiological effects of reserpine, increase brain concentrations of monoamines, enhance intracranial self-stimulation, inhibit the development of learned helplessness and behavioural despair, and normalize the behaviour of bulbectomized rats.

Receptor modulation

On chronic administration, the monoamine oxidase inhibitors produce alterations in receptor sensitivity similar to those which have been observed with many of the tricyclic antidepressants. Thus, a reduction in $alpha_2$-adrenoceptor binding has been shown in the rat brain (Cohen et al. 1982; Sugrue 1981); decreased $alpha_1$-adrenoceptor binding was also found after chronic clorgyline administration by Cohen et al. (1982), but has not been shown in all studies (Creese and Sibley 1981). Down-regulation of beta-adrenoceptors has been shown in binding and biochemical investigations (Sulser 1981; Sulser et al. 1983; Sugrue 1981). Serotonin reuptake binding sites do not appear to be affected, but down-regulation of serotonin 5-HT-2 receptors (Charney et al. 1981a) and 5-HT-1 receptors (Savage et al. 1980) has been demonstrated in binding studies in the rat brain. The relevance of these findings to antidepressant effects are doubtful since similar adaptive receptor changes occur with pargyline which in clinical trials has little if any antidepressant effect (Tyrer 1982).

Relationship of biochemical effects to antidepressant action

It is not clear whether the inhibition of monoamine oxidase is responsible for the antidepressant effects of the monoamine oxidase inhibitors. At the time of the original catecholamine theory of affective disorders (Schildkraut 1965), it seemed likely that this was their main mechanism of action. However, major doubts are cast on this hypothesis by the fact that monoamine oxidase inhibition can be demonstrated in man (at least in peripheral tissues) within days of administration of the drugs, while the clinical effects may be delayed for 6 weeks or more, and the degree of monoamine oxidase inhibition does not correlate with the extent of clinical response.

On the other hand, peripheral monoamine oxidase activity (which is usually measured in man as MAO-B activity in platelets) may not correspond to MAO-A activity in the brain. It does appear that at least 80 per cent inhibition of platelet enzyme activity is necessary before a clinical response is obtained, suggesting some relationship. In addition, pharmacokinetic factors such as acetylator status may delay or prevent the attainment of adequate drug concentrations in the brain. Furthermore the offset of antidepressant effects on discontinuation of monoamine oxidase inhibitors has repeatedly been shown to occur after a period of weeks, a time that coincides with the resynthesis of endogenous monoamine oxidase (Tyrer 1982).

A further difficulty is the doubtful efficacy of monoamine oxidase inhibitors in many depressive disorders. The drugs were originally regarded more as 'psychic energizers' than antidepressants. Much of their effect on mood may be due to amphetamine-like actions resulting from enhancement of catecholaminergic activity following monoaminergic inhibition, or from dopamine release. Non-hydrazine monoamine oxidase inhibitors do have some amphetamine-like mood elevating effects with a relatively rapid onset of action. Furthermore, monoamine oxidase inhibitors can, like amphetamine, precipitate mania or a schizophreniform psychosis, and can aggravate the psychotic symptoms in schizophrenia. It might be expected that the drugs would elevate mood in patients with endogenous depression, especially those with severe disorders and psychomotor retardation. This type of depression responds better than neurotic depression to tricyclic antidepressants. However, the response of patients with severe endogenous depression to monoamine oxidase inhibitors is poor, although it is possible that adequate dosage had not been given (Tyrer 1982).

Yet certain types of neurotic depression, which are little affected by tricyclic antidepressants, appear to respond to monoamine oxidase inhibitors. These include disorders in which there is a strong anxiety component, rapid changes in mood in response to external events, somatization of symptoms, phobic symptoms, and diurnal mood swings (Tyrer 1982). The response of these anxious patients is difficult to reconcile with the stimulant effects of monoamine oxidase inhibitors on monoaminergic activity. Adaptive changes in receptor sensitivity following chronic drug use appears an equally doubtful explanation since the same changes occur with monoamine oxidase inhibitors (e.g., pargyline) which are not clinically effective antidepressants.

The evidence on the whole suggests that antidepressant effects of monoamine oxidase inhibitors are in some way connected with, but not necessarily directly related to, monoamine oxidase inhibition. There is no evidence of abnormal central monoamine oxidase activity in depression. Investigations of platelet monoamine oxidase activity in various studies have shown no change, increased activity, or decreased activity (Green and Costain 1979; Berger and Barchas 1977). As with tricyclic antidepressants, the crucial change produced by monoamine oxidase inhibitors may be an alteration of gain or an increase in stability in interacting central monoaminergic synapses. Tyrer (1982) notes from clinical observations that response to monoamine oxidase inhibitors, when it occurs, does not typically consist of a gradual improvement of symptoms, but of a sudden dramatic change which occurs over 24 h. 'It seems that a "switch mechanism" in the brain must be operating to produce such a qualitative change in such a short time' (Tyrer 1982, pp. 259–60).

Effects on sleep and EEG

The effects of monoamine oxidase inhibitors on sleep are reviewed by Kay *et al.* (1976). Many studies have shown that they cause marked reduction in REMS, and even complete suppression (Kupfer and Bowers 1972). Dunleavy and Oswald (1973) remarked upon the dramatic onset of REMS suppression caused by these drugs. The change from about 20 per cent to 100 per cent suppression could occur within 24 hours and coincided with a sudden improvement of mood in the patients. In most studies drug effects on SWS have been much less marked, but patients frequently complain of insomnia. Little tolerance to the effect on REMS appears to occur; phenelzine has been observed to depress REMS for up to 40 nights. However, a rebound in REMS occurs on discontinuation of the drug.

Phenelzine (60–90 mg daily) has also been reported to decrease REMS in patients with narcolepsy (Chapter 3), and to reduce the frequency of cataleptic attacks and the severity of hypersomnia. Orthodox sleep was also decreased in these patients and the drug maintained its clinical effectiveness over a whole year in which the effects were followed (Wyatt *et al.* 1971a).

These effects of monoamine oxidase inhibitors on sleep are similar to those of amphetamine, although there is a lesser general stimulant effect. The effects on the waking EEG are also similar but less marked (Itil and Soldatos 1980). There is an increase in alpha- and slow beta-activity with a decrease in both slower and faster potentials. Gogolek (1980) reports a generally increased arousal pattern in animals, while Lader and Bhanji (1980) found little effect on spontaneous EEG activity in man.

Effects on mood

Iproniazid, an early monoamine oxidase inhibitor, is a derivative of isoniazid and was used in the treatment of tuberculosis. The drug was noted occasionally to produce euphoric effects and to induce a feeling of subjective well-being not warranted by the X-ray findings. Apart from these tuberculous patients, and the patients with narcolepsy (who became more alert, but not usually euphoric), there is little information on the effects of monoamine oxidase inhibitors in psychiatrically normal subjects. However, some monoamine oxidase inhibitors, especially the non-hydrazines with amphetamine-like structure, can produce euphoric reactions in depressed patients. Occasional cases have been reported in which patients exceeded the prescribed dose in order to obtain the stimulant effects (Tyrer 1982). Like tricyclic antidepressants, monoamine oxidase inhibitors can precipitate mania in patients with bipolar disorders. However, general effect of these drugs in patients who respond is a fairly sudden normalization of mood with amelioration of depressive ideation, and a feeling of increased confidence and energy. This effect is reminiscent of the similar sensations produced by amphetamine in normal subjects (Chapter 4).

Therapeutic effects in depressive disorders

There has been some doubt whether monoamine oxidase inhibitors are effective drugs for depression. Early results in patients with retarded schizophrenia and depression were not promising (Kline and Cooper 1980). Several trials in severely depressed inpatients suggested that these responded less well to monoamine oxidase inhibitors than to other treatments, including electroconvulsive therapy, tricyclic antidepressants, and even placebo. However, some of these early negative results may have been due to inadequate dosage (Tyrer 1982). Later studies suggested that there was a definite response to monoamine oxidase inhibitors in patients with atypical facial pain (Chapter 6), and in selected patients with prominent anxiety (neurotic depression and anxiety/depression). Sheehan et al. (1980) found phenelzine to be superior to placebo for patients with anxiety states characterized by phobic, hypochondriacal, and hysterical symptoms, and some trials have shown that iproniazid and phenelzine were superior to placebo in the treatment of agoraphobia and social phobias (Tyrer 1982). These findings were confirmed in further studies which indicate that monoamine oxidase inhibitors have marked antiphobic and anxiolytic activity. Patients gain increased confidence, energy, and self-esteem. This reaction recalls the early description of monoamine oxidase inhibitors as 'psychic energizers' and Tyrer (1982) has described them as 'delayed psychostimulants'. Occasionally, monoamine oxidase inhibitors have been reported to bring about dramatic improvement in patients with obsessional neuroses which have failed to respond to other treatments.

Adverse effects

Anticholinergic effects

Anticholinergic effects are common, especially at the start of treatment, but a degree of tolerance develops with continued dosage.

Cardiovascular effects

Hypotension may occur and has been attributed to an alpha-adrenergic stimulant effect in the vasomotor centre (Rogers et al. 1981) or to the formation of false transmitters such as octopamine. Both these effects are consequences of the monoamine oxidase inhibition. Some subjects develop hypertensive crises (Tyrer 1982) and these can be precipitated by interactions with other drugs and certain foods, as described below. Headaches and oedema of the limbs and sometimes of the face may occur.

Central nervous system effects

Insomnia is common and some patients develop agitation, tremor, and hyperreflexia, occasionally with clonus. Monoamine oxidase inhibitors have been reported to convert retarded into agitated depression, to precipitate mania, confusion, or a schizophreniform psychosis. Some patients paradoxically develop drowsiness; this effect occurred in 6 per cent of 168 patients treated with monoamine oxidase inhibitors by Tyrer (1982).

Miscellaneous effects

Hepatotoxicity, skin rashes, and blood dyscrasias are rare adverse effects.

Acute overdose

After a latent period of 6–12 h, the effects of an acute overdose include agitation, hallucinations, hyperpyrexia, dilated pupils, hyperreflexia, convulsions proceeding to coma, and hypo- or hypertension.

Drug interactions

Indirectly acting sympathomimetic amines, including those contained in certain foods (Stewart 1976), can give rise to a serious interaction with monoamine oxidase inhibitors, due to increased release of catecholamines. The reaction consists of severe hypertension and hyperthermia and may terminate in fatal subarachnoid haemorrhage. Although monoamine oxidase inhibitors are said not to interact with directly acting sympathomimetic amines (Tyrer 1982), hypertensive reactions have been reported with intravenous adrenaline and noradrenaline (Kline and Cooper 1980; Matthew and Lawson 1979), presumably because of additive effects at catecholaminergic receptors. The combination of monoamine oxidase inhibitors with tricyclic, bicyclic, and tetracyclic antidepressants can interact to produce cerebral excitement which may be followed by coma and severe hyperthermia, and sometimes a hypertensive reaction (Rogers *et al.* 1981). Reserpine, methyldopa and L-dopa can also precipitate hypertension.

The inactivation of some drugs which are normally metabolized by oxidizing enzymes is inhibited by monoamine oxidase inhibitors, with the result that the effects of these drugs are potentiated and prolonged. Such drugs include narcotic analgesics, barbiturates, and to a lesser extent other hypnotics and sedatives. The effects of general anaethetics, suxamethonium, anticholinergic drugs, and caffeine may also be potentiated.

Drug dependence

Drug dependence can occur with monoamine oxidase inhibitors, especially those with amphetamine-like structure. Tolerance develops and some patients take large doses in order to maintain the stimulant and occasionally euphoric effects. A severe withdrawal reaction similar to that of amphetamine and cocaine withdrawal (Chapter 7) can occur on sudden cessation of these drugs. This phenomenon appears to be rare, but some patients have difficulty in stopping medication because of withdrawal symptoms, and the incidence of such symptoms is greater than that on withdrawal of tricyclic antidepressants (Tyrer 1984; Liskin *et al.* 1985). A rebound of REMS has also been noted.

Other drugs used in affective disorders

Monoamine precursors

Monoamine precursors have been tried in depression on the basis that they might have therapeutic effects by increasing the (hypothetically) low monoamine activity in the brain (Chapter 11). On the whole, the results have been far from dramatic. L-dopa , the precursor of dopamine, is of doubtful value for depression and may precipitate mania (van Praag 1980b). *Tyrosine* , which increases noradrenaline and dopamine synthesis, has so far not been clearly shown to be effective (van Praag 1982). However, Goldberg (1980a,b) was impressed by the response to L-tyrosine of two depressed patients with low urinary MHPG concentrations who had failed to respond to antidepressant drugs and electroconvulsive therapy. Prior to L-tryosine treatment, the patients had required up to 20 mg dexamphetamine daily to remain depression-free. *Tryptophan* and *5-hydroxytryptophan*, precursors of serotonin, may be of value in the subgroup of depressed patients with low cerebrospinal fluid concentrations of 5-HIAA (van Praag 1980a, 1982). 5-hydroxytryptophan (used with a peripheral decarboxylase inhibitor) and tryptophan (with a selective MAO-B inhibitor) may potentiate the anti-depressanteffects of serotonin reuptake blockers such as clomipramine.

Flupenthixol

Flupenthixol is a thioxanthine derivative with acknowledged antipsychotic properties, and is widely used in the treatment of schizophrenia (Chapter 14). A number of reports have suggested that, when given in much smaller doses, it may be effective in some forms of depression. Several open studies reviewed by Mindham (1979) reported a 70 per cent response rate to this drug in depressed patients, a result very similar to that obtained with amitriptyline, and double blind comparisons with placebo appeared to confirm these findings (Young *et al.* , (1976). Whether improvement with flupenthixol was due solely to its anxiolytic effect has been debated (Kellet 1976; Robertson and Trimble 1981), but it was as affective as amitriptyline on the Hamilton, Beck, and other depression rating scales. Other antipsychotic drugs including thioridazine and sulpiride have also been reported to be useful in depression, and as discussed below they are also effective in the treatment of mania.

Benzodiazepines

Benzodiazepines are discussed in Chapter 4. They have potent anxiolytic actions and are often used in mild depression and anxiety or, in combination with tricyclic and other antidepressant drugs, in more severe anxiety/ depression. Their use in affective disorders is reviewed by Feighner (1982), Fawcett and Kravitz (1982), and Costa and Silva (1980). In many controlled trials on depressed patients benzodiazepines have been shown to be inferior to standard antidepressants. However, an antidepressant action, separate from the anxiolytic action, has been claimed for two benzodiazepines: bromazepam and the triazolobenzodiazepine alprazolam (Costa and Silva 1980; Feighner 1982; Fawcett and Kravitz 1982). The place of benzodiazepines as antidepressant agents remains to be established, and as discussed in Chapter 4, the development of dependence suggests that they are not suitable for long-term use.

Carbamazepine

Carbamazepine is an interesting drug which may have a therapeutic potential in manic-depressive disorders. It has a wide spectrum of activity with uses in paroxysmal pain syndromes, some types of epilepsy, and diabetes insipidus. It is structurally related to the tricyclic antidepressants and has a similar spatial molecular configuration to the anticonvulsant phenytoin.

Pharmacokinetics

Carbamazepine is slowly but well absorbed although plasma concentrations fluctuate during absorption. It has a plasma elimination half-life of 25–60 h after single dosage, falling to 10 h on chronic administration, possibly due to enzyme induction. It is metabolized to an epoxide derivative which has anti-epileptic activity but a half-life of only 2 h.

Biochemical effects

The biochemical actions of carbamazepine are not well understood; they have recently been reviewed by Post and Uhde (1983). It has a weak noradrenaline uptake blocking action, about a quarter of that of imipramine. It also blocks the stimulation-induced release of noradrenaline in peripheral animal tissues. Its anticonvulsant effects are blocked by noradrenaline depletion and by the action of alpha$_2$-receptor stimulants. There is no evidence of significant activity on dopaminergic or serotonergic mechanisms, but it appears to decrease GABA turnover. It is possible that carmbamazepine interacts with benzodiazepine-GABA receptors (Chapter 4); it has been reported to increase the binding of tritiated diazepam to its receptors.

Carbamazepine has several effects on endocrine activity. It decreases circulating concentrations of tri- and tetraiodothyronine, but does not alter concentrations of thyroid stimulating hormone. It may act as a direct vasopressin agonist and has antidiuretic effects which have been used in the treatment of diabetes insipidus. In addition, it induces escape from dexamethasone suppression of cortisol (Chapter 11). This effect may be partly due to enzyme induction which enhances the metabolism of dexamethasone, but it also alters the circadian rhythm of urinary corticosteroid excretion and increases the 24-h excretion of cortisol in normal subjects and depressed patients. A possible effect on endogenous opioid systems is suggested by the observation that carbamazepine facilitates opiate and enkephalin-induced motor activity in the mouse, and it has also been observed to decrease cerebrospinal somatostatin concentration in patients with affective disorders.

Behavioural and neurophysiological effects in animals

Carbamazepine has a distinctive profile of effects on animal behaviour: it is active in some antidepressant tests but does not reverse the effects of reserpine. It is also active on some anxiolytic tests, showing a positive action in conflict procedures (Chapter 3). It has little or no dopamine or acetylcholine antagonist activity, but is active in inhibiting aggressive behaviour. Electrophysiological studies show that carbamazepine has marked effects on the limbic system. It inhibits after-discharges elicited by electrical stimulation from a variety of limbic areas. It is the most effective anticonvulsant in stabilizing limbic electrical activity, followed by valproic acid, phenobarbitone, and the benzodiazepines and succinimides.

Clinical effects

Anticonvulsant activity Carbamazepine is one of the treatments of choice for temporal lobe epilepsy (Chapter 9) and is also effective in grand mal epilepsy, although it has no effect in petit mal attacks. The effect is thought to be due to its actions on the limbic system where it possibly enhances GABA activity. It may be relevant that it is often beneficial for the mood and behavioural disturbances associated with complex partial seizures, even if the seizures are not fully controlled.

Paroxysomal pain disorders Carbamazepine is of value in trigeminal and other neuralgias (Swerdlow 1984). This effect may be partly due to its anticonvulsant activity or to a facilitating effect on endogenous opioid systems. The effect in these chronic pain syndromes is interesting in the light of their relationship to depressive disorders (Chapter 6).

Diabetes insipidus Carbamazepine has an antidiuretic effect possibly due to vasopressin agonist activity and has been used in diabetes insipidus.

Affective disorders The use of carbamazepine in affective disorders is discussed by Post and Uhde (1983), Ballenger and Post (1980), and Post *et al.* (1985). In a double-blind placebo controlled study of patients with bipolar disorder, carbamazepine was found to produce a marked or partial response in 8 of 12 manic patients. Several of these relapsed when placebo was substituted for the drug and improved again when carbamazepine was reinstated. In 12 of 25 unipolar and bipolar depressed patients there was an apparent response to carbamazepine and again some of these relapsed when placebo was substituted. Similar results have been obtained in open trials. The response appears to be dose-related in individuals but clinical improvement does not correlate with plasma or cerebrospinal fluid concentrations of carbamazepine, although there was a positive correlation with concentration of the epoxide metabolite. Some manic patients who have not responded to lithium appear to respond to carbamazepine.

The effects of carbamazepine in affective disorders may be related to its actions on noradrenergic activity. The drug was found to reduce noradrenaline concentration in the cerebrospinal fluid of manic patients in whom this value was raised before treatment, and to increase it in depressed patients who initially had low concentrations. These effects may be consistent with the dual effects of carbamazepine in both preventing noradrenaline release and also blocking its reuptake. It was also suggested that carbamazepine might have some prophylactic efficacy in preventing relapses in patients with bipolar disorders, especially those who have not responded to lithium. A prophylactic effect might be due to the dual action on noradrenaline and in addition the stabilising action on limbic system activity. Thus, carbamazepine may have a certain clinical utility, especially in bipolar disorders which have failed to respond to the more established treatments, but its role in affective disorders requires further investigation.

Adverse effects Adverse effects are common with carbamazepine and depend on dosage. Dizziness and ataxia were present in 20–30 per cent of patients with affective disorders treated by Ballenger and Post (1980) who used a dose of 800–1600 mg daily. Clumsiness, drowsiness, slurred speech and diplopia occurred in about 15 per cent of these patients. Less commonly skin rashes, acheing or weakness in the limbs, paraesthesiae, water retention and cardiac arrhythmias occur.

Lithium

Lithium is usually administered as lithium carbonate, and has been shown to have therapeutic actions in mania, and depression and in the prophylaxis of affective disorders. It is reviewed by Tyrer and Shaw (1982), Schildkraut (1973a,b), Gerbino *et al.* (1978), and Baldessarini (1980).

Pharmacokinetics

Lithium carbonate is readily and almost completely absorbed after oral administration. The lithium ion is initially distributed in the extracellular fluid and then more gradually enters most tissues. The serum elimination half-life varies between 18-20 h in young adults and 36-42 h in the elderly. At steady state, the concentration of lithium in the cerebrospinal fluid is about 40 per cent of that in blood. Elimination of lithium is almost entirely renal. It readily passes into the glomerular filtrate and 70-80 per cent is reabsorbed in the proximal tubules. This reabsorption is competitive with that of sodium, and sodium deficiency or sodium diuresis can increase lithium retention: for this reason diuretics may enhance the toxicity of lithium.

Because of the low therapeutic index of lithium, (therapeutic: toxic serum concentration = 1:2.5) it is necessary to monitor serum concentrations to ensure that they are kept within the therapeutic range of approximately 0.6-1.2 mmol/l. There is considerable variation between individuals in both the dosage required and the serum concentration which produces either therapeutic or toxic effects. Methods of estimating dosage requirements and for monitoring concentrations are discussed by Tyrer and Shaw (1982).

Pharmacological actions

The mechanisms of action of lithium is not known. It is a monovalent alkaline metal and its ion competes with sodium, potassium, magnesium, and calcium ions in biological tissues. It can also interact with ammonium groups, including those of the biogenic amines (Bunney *et al.* 1979). There have been many investigations of its actions on monoamine and other neurotransmitter systems, but the results are confusing.

Effects on catecholamines

Acute (up to 10 days) administration of lithium increases the turnover of noradrenaline in the brain in animals.

Chronic administration, however, does not affect the concentration or turnover of catecholamines in the rat brain. Limited data from humans have shown an increase of urinary MHPG excretion in the first few days of lithium administration in mania and an increase in VMA excretion in normal subjects treated acutely with lithium. In patients receiving chronic lithium treatment, the effects on MHPG excretion disappeared.

In isolated tissues, lithium decreases the release of exogenously administered 3H-noradrenaline in response to electrical stimulation. This effect has been shown in rat brain slices and in the isolated perfused cat's spleen. The decreased release of noradrenaline can be prevented by raising the concentration of calcium in the perfusing fluid, suggesting that lithium may interfere with the action of calcium in the stimulation-mediated release of noradrenaline. Chronic administration of lithium increases the uptake of noradrenaline across synaptosomal membranes.

The mechanisms for these effects of lithium are not known. Schildkraut (1973) suggests that lithium may compete with calcium and magnesium in various catecholamine transport and release systems. The net effect of lithium administration appears to be a decrease in the amount of noradrenaline available to receptors. Such an effect might possibly be a basis for its actions, at least in mania.

Effects on dopamine

The effects of lithium on dopaminergic systems are not clear, but inhibition of dopamine synthesis has been demonstrated in rats treated with lithium for 2 weeks. The electrically stimulated, calcium dependent, release of dopamine from nerve terminals is inhibited by lithium (Baldessarini 1980). The development of Parkinsonian symptoms in patients maintained on lithium also suggests dopaminergic underactivity (Tyrer 1982). Lithium also appears to prevent the development of dopamine receptor supersensitivity in patients treated with haloperidol (Tyrer 1982; Chapter 14). Bunney *et al.* (1979) discuss the possibility that dopamine receptor supersensitivity occurs in mania and that this abnormality is reversed or prevented by lithium. Gerbino *et al.* (1978) cited evidence that lithium may block the euphoriant effects of amphetamine, both in depressed patients and non-depressed amphetamine abusers.

Effects on serotonin

Short-term (1-5 days) administration of lithium to rats increases the high affinity uptake of tryptophan into forebrain synaptosomes. There is an associated increase in serotonin synthesis and turnover, and in tryptophan hydroxylase activity. The concentration of 5-HIAA in the forebrain in response to electrical stimulation of the raphe nuclei is also increased. With chronic lithium administration, the activity of tryptophan hydroxylase reverts to pre-treatment levels. The effects of chronic treatment on concentrations and turnover of serotonin varies between different parts of the brain: decreased serotonin concentrations have been reported in hypothalamus and brainstem, but increased concentrations and turnover with decreased release on electrical stimulation, in the forebrain. In humans, the administration of lithium has been found in some (e.g., Bowers and Heninger 1977), but not all, studies to increase cerebrospinal fluid concentrations of 5-HIAA in patients with low pre-treatment concentrations.

Effects on other systems

The effects of lithium on other neurotransmitters are not clear. It may decrease the synthesis and release of acetylcholine in the cortex (Friedman 1973), and it appears to have some effect on GABA metabolism, although the evidence is sparse (Tyrer and Shaw 1982). Lithium has little effect on catecholamine-sensitive adenylate cyclase activity or on the binding of ligands to catecholamine receptors (Baldessarini 1980). However, it inhibits hormone-sensitive adenylate cyclase and this may account for some of its endocrine effects.

Many studies have been devoted to elucidating the effects of lithium on membrane transport systems involving sodium, potassium, magnesium, and calcium, and on the extracellular and intracellular distribution of these ions (Friedman 1973; Bunney *et al.* 1979). So far it has not been possible to relate any of these effects to the mood-stabilising action of lithium. However, electrophysiological studies in animal preparations (reviewed by Small and Small 1973) show that lithium can partially substitute for sodium in the ionic exchange associated with the propagation of action potentials in nerves. The presence of lithium decreases the conduction velocity and amplitude of action potentials and blocks transmission through some synapses. It is conceivable that such an action may tend to stabilize certain neuronal circuits and prevent large swings of activity in either direction. Glen and Reading (1973) propose that lithium stabilizes central nervous system activity by regulating cell membrane ATPases concerned with the transfer of calcium ions across the cell wall.

Effects on EEG

The effects of lithium on the EEG are reviewed by Small and Small (1973) and Tyrer and Shopsin (1980). In animals, several days administration of lithium at doses producing serum concentration in the human therapeutic range causes a diffuse slowing of EEG activity which persists for several days after cessation of treatment. The main effects are observed in the orbital frontal cortex. The animals became less spontaneously active and responded less to stimulation. Decrease in aggressive behaviour has been noted in several animal species.

In man, acute administration of lithium produces a tendency towards synchronisation of the EEG. There is slowing of the dominant alpha-frequency with a general increase in amplitude. There is an increase in theta and delta, and also in beta activity. The pattern is similar to that produced by neuroleptics. The effects are dose-related and marked changes only occur when toxic concentrations are reached. On chronic administration of lithium to patients with affective disorders, these changes persist. In addition there is an accentuation of any pre-existing paroxysmal abnormalities. Patients with abnormal EEG records prior to treatment are liable to develop neurological and neurotoxic problems during lithium administration (Tyrer and Shopsin

1980). The amplitude of somatosensory and auditory evoked responses and the magnitude of the contingent negative variation have been reported to increase after lithium treatment. These effects may be related to clinical improvement since lithium in general tends to have depressant effects on EEG activity.

Effects on sleep

The effects of lithium on sleep are reviewed by Tyrer and Shopsin (1980), and Kay et al. (1976). No effects have been observed in normal subjects after 8 days treatment with lithium. In patients with mania or depression, lithium reverses the abnormal sleep pattern. It produces a decrease in REMS, an increase in REM latency, an increase in SWS, and an increase in total sleep. These effects are observed with 24 h of lithium administration and appear to reverse promptly, even after chronic treatment, with no evidence of rebound.

Clinical effects

Lithium in clinically used doses produces no discernible psychotropic effects in normal subjects. However, it has potent effects in a variety of affective disorders reviewed by Tyrer and Shaw (1982), Shaw (1979), and Gerbino et al. (1978).

Effects in mania

Early studies (Cade 1949) suggested that lithium might have a 'specific' pharmacological effect in mania. Many open and controlled trials have been conducted since then, but these have been beset with many problems including the relative rarity of mania, the difficulty of including patients with severe mania, the delay in response to lithium, the necessity for monitoring blood concentrations, and the frequency of adverse effects. Nevertheless, lithium has been compared with placebo in mild to moderate mania using various trial designs including the blind substitution of placebo for lithium at different times during treatment (Stokes et al. 1971). The general conclusion has been that lithium is superior to placebo; that there is a delay in the onset of its therapeutic effect; and that 75–80 per cent of patients with mild to moderate mania will respond to lithium in about 2 weeks. The problems of conducting controlled trials involving patients with severe mania are even greater.

However, several controlled trials have compared lithium with neuroleptics, usually chlorpromazine (Prien et al. 1972; Johnson et al. 1971). The general conclusion has been that neuroleptics are superior: the symptoms are controlled more rapidly, within days as opposed to 2 weeks, and the adverse effects are less dangerous. However, both neuroleptics and lithium terminate manic episodes within 3 weeks in patients who continue treatment.

Although the neuroleptics are clearly more practical drugs to use in the management of mania because of their more rapid onset of action, there are some interesting qualitative differences in the response to neuroleptics and lithium (Gerbino et al. 1978). The neuroleptics produce an early decrease in motor activity but this effect is accompanied by considerable central nervous system depression. There is no clear early break in the mania, and euphoria and excitement may still be apparent despite the drug effects which, initially at least, appear to allow the patient to be 'quietly manic'. In contrast, the mood change with lithium appears to be much sharper and more specific. Hyperactivity and affect return to normal without sedation, and once normality is achieved it is virtually complete with no accompanying central nervous system depression. These qualitative differences, which are difficult to rate objectively, have suggested that lithium affects some underlying neuronal dysfunction fundamental to mania, while neuroleptics merely override some of the symptoms, chiefly the overactivity. Byk (1976) notes that lithium can also block the euphoric 'highs' produced by amphetamine and cocaine, reduce the enjoyment of alcohol, and inhibit the behavioural activation induced by morphine in mice.

Effects in depression

Lithium has been investigated as a treatment for depression in several trials in which it has been compared with tricyclic antidepressants or placebo. Little or no antidepressant activity has been detected in most studies, but many of them have only covered short periods of less than three weeks. However Worall et al. (1979) and Mendels et al. (1972) found lithium to be superior or equal to imipramine in mixed groups of depressed patients, with a therapeutic effect appearing in the second or third week of treatment. Noyes et al. (1974) also reported a response to lithium in depressed patients with relapse on substitution of placebo. Further investigation of possible antidepressnt effects of lithium is required, but there is a suggestion that it may be of some value, especially in patients with bipolar disorders.

Prevention of recurrence

Several prolonged placebo controlled trials continued over several months to years have shown that long-term lithium treatment has a significant prophylactic effect in preventing, in attenuating the length or severity, or in reducing the frequency of relapses of affective illness. This effect appears to apply almost equally to recurrences of mania or depression, and to unipolar and bipolar depression (Baestrup et al. 1970; Hullin et al. 1972). Some investigations have suggested a lesser effect in unipolar depression but a large study by the Medical Research Council Drug Trials Subcommittee (1981) found lithium and amitriptyline equally effective, and superior to placebo as prophylactic agents in unipolar depression. Nevertheless, the relapse rate of affective disorders, even with maintenance drug treatment, is of the order of 30 per cent. There is no clear way of predicting response to the prophylactic effect of lithium and the high incidence of adverse effects limits the use of lithium in some patients.

Other disorders of affect

Lithium has been used in a number of other disorders associated with changes of affect, discussed by Tyrer and Shaw (1982), and Gerbino *et al.* (1978). In milder cases of schizoaffective disorder lithium has a possible therapeutic effect, but it is less effective than neuroleptics in more severe cases. Anti-aggressive actions of lithium have been demonstrated in impulsively aggress-ive male prisoners, and possibly in aggressive epileptics and mentally subnormal individuals. It has also been used in character disorders with emotional instability, hyperactive children, affective disorders associated with alcoholism, amphetamine abuse, prementrual tension (Chapter 11), Kleine-Levin syndrome (Chapter 3), and cluster headaches (Chapter 6).

Adverse effects

Lithium is a toxic drug and serious adverse effects can occur if serum con-centrations are excessive, and may also occasionally result from long-term therapy. Unwanted effects occurring during the first few days of treatment include fine tremor of the hands, gastrointestinal symtpoms, thirst, and polyuria. These symptoms can be minimized by starting with small doses which are then gradually increased until therapeutic serum concentrations are attained. Muscle weakness, fatigue, ataxia, and sometimes emotional blunting may also be seen in the first few weeks of treatment. Development of coarse tremor, confusion, spasticity, convulsions, and dehydration are indications of overdose and necessitate withdrawal of drug or adjustment of dosage. After 6 weeks or more, further symptoms may apear, including oedema, weight gain due to increased eating or drinking, alteration in taste (Himmelhoch and Hanin 1974), and less commonly, signs of hypothyroidism or impaired renal function. Many patients also complain of poor memory, although this symptom is equally common in patients maintained on tricyclic antidepressants (Coppen and Abou-Salek 1983). The incidence of unwanted effects in patients on long-term treatment is high: in a survey of 237 such patients (Vestergaard *et al.* 1980) only one-tenth had no symptoms attributed to the drug.

Renal effects

Polyuria and polydipsia are common at therapeutic serum concentrations of lithium, and probably result from inhibition of antidiuretic hormone-sensitive adenylate cyclase, resulting in decreased renal water reabsorption: nephrogenic diabetes insipidus. Such changes are readily reversible on cess-ation of treatment. Toxic doses are nephrotoxic, and can cause irreversible glomerular and tubular damage. Serious renal damage is rare in patients maintained on lithium as long as toxic concentrations are avoided (Tyrer and Shaw 1982).

Endocrine effects

About 10 per cent of patients on chronic lithium therapy develop hypothyroidism (Rogers *et al.* 1981). The mechanism may be inhibition of hormone-sensitive adenylate cyclase, resulting in decreased synthesis of thyroid hormone. The consequent increase in release of thyroid-stimulating hormone may induce a goitre. Occasionally thyrotoxicocis occurs. Parathyroid hormone effects mediated by adenylate cyclase may be similarly blocked by lithium treatment, and may result in loss of bone calcium and density after long-term treatment. The gain in weight is possibly due to insulin release by lithium while oedema and salt retention may result from increased aldosterone secretion (Baldessarini 1980).

Cardiovascular effects

Cardiovascular effects of lithium may be due to replacement of intracellular potassium by lithium, which is more slowly extruded through the cell membrane. Electrocardiographic changes, arrhythmias, heart block, and heart failure may occur, especially with toxic doses.

Central nervous system effects

At therapeutic concentrations central nervous system effects of lithium are usually mild, but problems may exist in treating patients with neurological disease. Lithium exacerbates paroxysmal EEG abnormalities, and fits may occasionally be precipitated in epileptics. In patients with Parkinsonism or cerebellar disease, lithium may exacerbate the symptoms.

Acute lithium toxicity

Acute toxicity develops if plasma concentrations exceed the therapeutic range, but susceptibility varies considerably between individuals. Toxic signs usually appear at a concentration about 1.3 mmol/l, but in susceptible individuals they may occur at 0.5–1 mmol/l. Concentrations of 3–5 mmol/l may be lethal. The development of toxicity is usually delayed because of the slow penetration of lithium into the brain, and may persist after plasma concentrations have declined. Initial symptoms include nausea, vomiting, and diarrhoea, followed by impairment of consciousness, coarse tremor, nystagmus, ataxia, and dysarthria. Muscle fasiculation, myoclonus, hyperreflexia, and convulsions develop, followed by renal failure, cardiac arrhythmia, coma, and death. The overall mortality from acute lithium overdose is about 12 per cent (Proudfoot 1982) and depressed patients are at particular risk from suicide attempts.

Effects in pregnancy and lactation

Lithium treatment in pregnancy and the postnatal period is reviewed by Weinstein (1980). Lithium probably has teratogenic effects, and foetal hypothyroidism and goitre may result from its use in later pregnancy. Maternal treatment with lithium in the last 2 weeks of pregnancy has resulted in foetal death, and in hypotonia, cyanosis, bradycardia, and arrhythmia in the neonate. These effects can occur when maternal serum lithium concentrations are within the therapeutic range. However, most cases are associated with the use of diuretics or salt restriction in the mother, measures which increase serum lithium concentrations. Lithium concentration in breast milk is 30–100 per cent of maternal serum concentration and breast-fed infants have serum lithium concentrations of 10–50 per cent of their mother's; breast feeding during lithium administration is thus inadvisable.

Drug interactions

Since the reabsorption of lithium in the proximal renal tubules is competitive with that of sodium, thiazide diuretics, which decrease proximal tubular reabsorption of sodium, may precipitate of lithium toxicity. Nephrotoxic drugs such as the aminoglycoside antibiotics may also increase the risk of lithium toxicity. Non-steroidal antiinflammatory drugs potentiate the effects of antidiuretic hormone and can lead to a rise in serum lithium concentration. Lithium decreases intracellular potassium concentration and may for this reason enhance digoxin toxicity.

Lithium may potentiate the extrapyramidal effects of neuroleptics and may itself in toxic concentrations produce extrapyramidal effects. Lithium can prolong the actions of suxamethonium, pancuronium, and d-tubocurarine.

Electroconvulsive therapy

A full discussion of electroconvulsive therapy is beyond the scope of this book: the subject is reviewed by Crow and Johnstone (1979), Gulevich (1977), and Fink (1979, 1981). However, electroconvulsive therapy is mentioned here because it remains an important treatment for patients in whom a rapid response is required because of the severity of the depression or the risk of suicide, and for those who have not responded adequately to drugs. Electroconvulsive therapy is effective in depressive disorders, as shown by numerous studies in which it has been compared with sham electroconvulsive therapy and antidepressant drugs (for example, Brandon et al. 1984; West 1981; Freeman et al. 1978; and other investigations cited in the above reviews). It is probably more effective than drugs in terminating attacks of depression and has a much quicker onset of action, although repeated treatments may be necessary. It appears to be most effective in endogenous depression. Most studies have found it of value in neurotic depression, but it is of doubtful value in schizoaffective disorders and not helpful in mania. Despite its effectiveness in current depressive episodes, electroconvulsive therapy is less effective than drugs in preventing recurrences of affective illness. However, the treatment can be combined with drugs, and there is some evidence that tricyclic antidepressants may potentiate the therapeutic effects of electroconvulsive therapy. Like drugs, the treatment carries a small mortality risk and some morbidity, although the latter may possibly be reduced with little loss of efficacy by the use of unilateral electroconvulsive therapy (Green 1978).

The mode of action of electroconvulsive therapy is not clear, but it appears to increase postsynaptic responsiveness to the effects of noradrenaline, serotonin, and dopamine (Grahame-Smith et al. 1978; Whalley et al. 1982; Costain et al. 1982; Green 1978), possibly by increasing receptor sensitivity. Green (1978) observed in animals that repeated convulsions decreased the concentration and synthesis of GABA in certain brain regions and suggested that the increased responsiveness to monoamines might result from a 'switching off' of GABA function. Electroconvulsive therapy is sometimes followed by a rapid and dramatic switch from a grossly abnormal to an apparently normal clinical state.

Part V
Schizophrenia

13
Schizophrenia: clinical features and brain mechanisms

Schizophrenia is to many the most fascinating and elusive of medical disorders. The strangeness of its psychiatric manifestations, particularly the thought distortion and the flatness or inappropriateness of affect, seems to set them apart from common experience. Yet, like the affective syndromes (Chapter 11), schizophrenia merges with the normal condition and with other psychiatric states. As in depression and mania, the seat of dysfunction is probably the limbic system and the aetiology is probably multiple, but in spite of a plethora of theories, the cellular mechanism remains obscure.

Symptoms

'Schizophrenia can only be defined in terms of its symptomatology' (Fairburn 1981, p. 1115). The diagnosis is made on clinical grounds, and depends largely on the presence of some of a variable collection of symptoms and the exclusion of others. Various sets of diagnostic criteria are discussed by Gelder *et al.* (1981) and Fairburn (1981); one of the most useful is probably that developed by Spitzer *et al.* (1975) (Table 13.1), which also takes into account the course of the illness. However, the exclusion of frank organic disease hinders rather than helps a search for common mechanisms underlying the symptomatology.

The symptoms of schizophrenia are vividly described in psychiatric text-books (for example Mayer-Gross *et al.* 1954; Gelder *et al.* 1981). They are conveniently divided into positive symptoms, which are characteristic of the acute schizophrenic syndrome, and negative symptoms, seen mainly in chronic schizophrenic states.

Positive symptoms

Hallucinations Auditory hallucinations are among the most common symptoms, occuring in nearly 75 per cent of patients with acute schizophrenia (World Health Organization 1979). Of particular importance for diagnosis are hallucinations of voices giving commands, speaking the patient's thoughts out loud, giving a running commentary on his actions, or discussing him in

Table 13.1.   Broad diagnostic criteria for schizophrenia (A, B, and C are required for the diagnosis to be considered)

A. At least one of the following symptoms:
    1. Thought broadcasting, insertion or withdrawal.
    2. Bizarre delusions such as delusions of control, multiple delusions.
    3. Delusions other than persecutory or jealousy, lasting at least one week.
    4. Delusions of any type if accompanied by hallucinations for at least one week.
    5. Auditory hallucinations including voices giving a running commentary on the subject's thoughts or behaviour, or voices conversing with each other.
    6. Non-affective verbal hallucinations spoken to the subject.
    7. Hallucinations lasting throughout the day for several days or intermittently for at least a month.
    8. Formal thought disorder, associated with blunted, flat or inappropriate affect.
    9. Catatonic motor behaviour.
B. A period of illness lasting at least two weeks.
C. Symptoms do not meet criteria for affective syndrome or organic mental disorder to such a degree as to form a prominent part of the illness.

References: Fairburn 1981; Gelder *et al.* 1983; Spitzer *et al.* 1975.

the third person. Similar auditory hallucinations without insight may occur in temporal lobe epilepsy (Trimble 1981) and this observation suggests temporal lobe involvement in schizophrenia. Visual, tactile, olfactory, gustatory, and somatic hallucinations are less common and also occur in temporal lobe epilepsy. Complex visual hallucinations are a feature of delirious states and can be provoked by psychotomimetic drugs (Chapter 14).

Delusions Delusions are chararacteristic of schizophrenia, particularly delusions concerning the possession of thoughts and delusions of outside control. Delusions of persecution and of grandeur occur in schizophrenia and are also seen in affective disorders and in organic brain disease.

Thought disorder Impairment or loss of the normal logical structure of thought is characteristic of schizophrenia, but also may be seen to some degree in affective disorders and dementia. The disorder of logical thought, difficulty in abstract conception, and distortion of language seen in schizophrenia suggests a cortical dysfunction particularly affecting the dominant hemisphere, a possibility which is discussed further below.

Disorders of affect Several abnormalities of mood are seen in schizophrenia. Flattening and incongruity of affect are characteristic, and lead to social withdrawal. However, considerable intensity of emotion which appears to be out of context may sometimes be displayed. Sustained abnormalities of mood, including anxiety, irritability, depression, or elation, also occur. As mentioned in Chapter 11, schizophrenia may merge with depressive and manic syndromes. Disorders of mood in schizophrenia, as in anxiety and the affective disorders, point to dysfunction of limbic arousal and reward/punishment systems controlling affect.

Negative symptoms

Chronic schizophrenia is sometimes referred to as the schizophrenic defect state. Patients display no drive or initiative, little emotion, poverty of thought and speech, and are slow in all their actions. There is evidence of cognitive impairment, and some 25 per cent have temporal disorientation and are unable to state their age, the current date, or the duration of their hospital stay. They are unable to acquire new information and for some time has apparently stood still since the onset of their illness (Crow and Johnstone 1980). Insight is lost and the patient does not recognize that his symptoms are due to illness. These symptoms suggest cortical and limbic degenerative changes.

Motor disturbances

Various disorders of motor activity, described as catatonia, occur rarely in schizophrenia. These include a form of stupor in which the patient is immobile, mute, and unresponsive although fully conscious, but may suddenly undergo a change to uncontrollable motor activity and excitement. Disorders of muscle tone may occur, such as muscle rigidity or flexibilatas cerea, in which the patient can passively be placed into awkward postures which he then maintains for long periods without any of the signs of discomfort which would be shown by normal subjects. Stereotyped movements, complex behavioural mannerisms, automatic obedience, and various other complex disorders of movement are occasionally seen. The catatonic syndrome may also occur in a number of other conditions reviewed by Gelenberg (1976): affective disorders and neuroses; neurological disorders involving the basal ganglia, limbic system, temporal lobes, diencephalon, and frontal lobes; metabolic conditions; and certain drugs (psychotomimetic drugs, amphetamine, phencyclidine, antipsychotic drugs, and others). A common factor in catatonic disorders appears to be dysfunction in striato-limbic pathways.

Clinical variations

The clinical picture in schizophrenia is variable and many patients present with or develop a mixture of both positive and megative symptoms. Borderline disorders between schizophrenia and depressive disorders (schizo-affective disorders) and between schizophrenia, neuroses and personality disorders (schizoptypal personality, borderline personality or borderline schizophrenia) may possibly exist. It is also possible that a number of states, both psychotic and non-psychotic, may constitute a genetic spectrum of schizophrenia (Reich 1975).

Incidence and clinical course

Schizophrenia is less common than the affective disorders. Surveys from 12 countries show a prevalence of 0.2–0.4 per cent (compared to 3–9 per cent for unipolar depressive disorders). The peak age of onset is 20–39 years; the age of onset is younger and the frequency slightly greater in males than females. Certain discrete populations have a higher or lower prevalence of schizophrenia than the general average.

The clinical course is variable. Schizophrenia usually presents as an acute syndrome with the sudden emergence of predominantly positive symptoms. Most patients respond to therapy but are liable to relapses of acute illness, even with antipsychotic drug treatment. In one study reported by Crow (1978a), over 70 per cent of schizophrenics treated with placebo relapsed within 12 months and 80 per cent by 2 years. The corresponding figures for antipsychotic drug-treated patients were approximately 33 per cent and 48 per cent.

Some patients with acute schizophrenia progress to a chronic state and develop negative symptoms or disabling degrees of anxiety or depression. Occasionally, negative symptoms appear insidiously without a preceding acute phase. Various follow-up studies reviewed by Gelder *et al.*, (1981) and Tsuang (1982) have shown that about 20 per cent of patients have complete remissions and 30 per cent make a good social readjustment, but the outcome for the remainder is poor. About 25 per cent remain severely disturbed, while up to 10 per cent of schizophrenic patients die by suicide.

Aetiological factors

Genetic factors

There is little doubt that there is a strong genetic basis in schizophrenia although the mode of inheritance is unknown (Murray *et al.* 1985). The risk of developing schizophrenia is greatly increased in the relatives of schizophrenics. While the lifetime risk for the general population is about 1 per cent, the risk for second degree relatives of schizophrenics is 3 per cent, for first degree relatives 10 per cent, and for children with both parents affected 40 per cent. Twin studies (Murray and Reveley 1983; Crow 1983; Kendler 1983) have shown concordance rates of 9–26 per cent for dizygous twins and 35–58 per cent for monozygous twins, regardless of whether they are reared together or apart. The incidence of schizophrenia is not increased in adoptive parents of children who become schizophrenic, and there is no increase in the incidence of schizophrenia among children with normal biologic parents but schizophrenic adoptive parents.

Personality

There has been much discussion as to whether genetically determined personality chacteristics predispose to schizophrenia. The spectrum concept of schizophrenia (Reich 1975) proposes that there is a genetic diathesis manifested in a range of personality disorders (variously labelled schizoid personality, schizotypal personality, borderline personality, borderline schizophrenia) which confers a vulnerability to develop schizophrenia under environmental stress. It has also been argued that there is a continuum between normal personality, schizoid personality, and schizophrenia, and that schizoid personality is a partial expression of the same psychological abnormalities that are seen in schizophrenia (Kretschmer 1936). These views were developed by Schulsinger (1985) who believed that schizophrenia does not suddenly arise in a previously normal individual, but that both schizophrenics and borderline schizophrenics have a premorbid personality disorder, and that the genetically transmitted abnormality is not schizophrenia itself, but borderline schizophrenia, a condition that carries vulnerability to stress.

There has been considerable difficulty in defining borderline states. Spitzer et al. (1979), in an analysis of questionnaire data, concluded that borderline states as clinically diagnosed include two district populations, only one of which, schizotypal personality (schizoid personality), might be genetically related to schizophrenia. Schizoid personality is described by Gelder et al. (1981). Individuals with this type of personality are lacking in emotional warmth, detached, and in extreme cases, cold, callous, seclusive, and friendless. Another personality dimension, psychoticism, is related to psychosis, crime, drug addiction, other behavioural abnormalities, and to certain physiological variables also seen in schizophrenia (Eysenck and Eysenck 1976; Claridge and Chappa 1973; Claridge and Birchall 1978; see below).

Although vulnerability to schizophrenia does appear to be inherited, the fact that the concordance rate for schizophrenia in monozygous twins is 50 per cent indicates that environmental factors must also be important in aetiology, and Gelder et al. (1981) emphasized that only a minority of individuals with schizoid personalities become schizophrenic.

Psychosocial stresses

Several psychosocial theories of schizophrenia have been advanced, suggesting that the disease arises as a reaction to abnormal relationships within the family, particularly the relationship with the mother. However, it is not clear whether such factors, when they exist, are the cause or result of schizophrenic behaviour. Life stresses have also been suggested to precipitate schizophrenia and it has been found that the rate of stressful life events was increased in the three months before a schizphrenic breakdown (Brown and Birley 1968); however, this is also true for depressive and anxiety disorders.

Social and environmental factors appear to influence the outcome of schizophrenia. Too little or too much social stimulation can aggravate symp-

toms in schizophrenics and relapse rates are higher in schizophrenics return-
ing to families with high emotional involvement in the patient's illness than
to less emotionally involved families. Stressful life events can also precipitate
relapses. The evidence in general indicates that psychosocial factors, although
important in schizophrenia, are not specific. The subject is reviewed by Leff
(1981), Vaughan and Leff (1976), Hirsch (1983), and Davis (1978).

Neurological diseases

Converging lines of evidence from many sources indicate the presence of
structural brain damage in many cases of schizophrenia. Typical schizophrenic features are seen in association with several neurological diseases,
particularly of the temporal lobe and diencephalon, such as temporal lobe
epilepsy, Huntingdon's chorea, Wilson's disease, brain tumours, head injury,
and encephalitis. In addition, as many as two-thirds of schizophrenics without obvious neurological disease show neurological abnormalities ('soft
signs'), such as defects in stereognosis, balance and proprioception, which
suggest defects in the integration of proprioceptive and other sensory information (Cox and Ludwig 1979). Similar soft signs are found in subjects with
schizoid personality characteristics (Quitkin et al. 1976).

Cerebral atrophy

The most direct evidence of structural brain damage in schizophrenia comes
from studies of cerebral ventricular size. Early reports from air encephalographic examination showing that some schizophrenic patients had
enlarged lateral ventricles (Haug 1962) have since been confirmed by investigations using computer tomography. Johnstone et al. (1976) Weinberger et
al. (1979a,b), Reveley et al. (1983), Marsden (1976), Crow et al. (1980), and
Johnstone (1985) all reported that, compared with normal controls and
patients with affective disorders, a proportion of schizophrenics have significantly enlarged lateral ventricles or widening of cerebral sulci, suggestive
of cerebral and cortical atrophy. Some also have evidence of cerebellar cortical atrophy (Weinberger et al. 1979c). These changes, which are usually
modest, but can be marked, are not due to age, treatment, or the presence of
dementia. Post-mortem studies also show lower brain weight and larger
ventricles in schizophrenia compared with affective disorders. There is a high
concordance rate of ventricular size amongst monozygous twins, but where
one twin has schizophrenia, this twin has the larger ventricles (Johnstone
1984).

The proportion of schizphrenics with cerebral atrophy is not known, but
it is probably considerable. Weinberger et al. (1979b) found some abnormality on computerised tomography brain scans in two-thirds of 75 chronic
schizophrenic patients. Cerebral atrophy appears to be more common in
chronic schizophrenia and is often related to the presence of negative symp-

toms, intellectual deterioration, and poor response to neuroleptics (Wein-berger and Wyatt 1980; Crow and Johnstone 1980). Crow (1980, 1982) suggested that there may be two types of schizophrenia: Type I with positive symptoms, little cognitive impairment, normal cerebral ventricular size, and good response to neuroleptics; and Type II with negative symptoms and structural brain damage (Table 13.2). Woods and Wolf (1983) suggested that there is a direct relationship between ventricular size and duration of schizophrenic illness. However, Schulz et al., (1983) reported that enlarged lateral ventricles are found in teenage patients during the first episode of acute schizophrenia. Revely et al. (1983) suggest that ventricular enlargement is confined to schizophrenics without a genetic predisposition. In their survey of 21 monozygous schizophrenic twins, only those without a family history of major psychiatric disorder had enlarged ventricles.

The finding of structural brain damage in schizophrenia is clearly of great importance (Hill 1976; Lancet 1982b), and has led to the exploration of possible environmental causes, other than the known neurological diseases mentioned above.

Table 13.2. Characteristics of Type I and Type II schizophrenia

	Type I	Type II
Characteristic symptoms	Positive symptoms (hallucinations, delusions, thought disorder)	Negative symptoms (flattening of affect poverty of speech, lack of drive)
Type of schizophrenia usually associated	Acute schizophrenia	Chronic schizophrenia
Intellectual impairment	Little impairment	Sometimes marked impairment
Postulated pathology	Increased dopaminergic activity in mesolimbic systems	Cell loss and structural brain changes, eventually with decreased dopaminergic activity
Response to neuroleptic drugs	Good	Poor
Outcome	Usually reversible; may progress to Type II	Irreversible

Reference: Crow 1982.

Birth injury

One factor which might cause cerebral atrophy and eventually precipitate schizophrenia in predisposed individuals is injury to the brain during birth. Mednick and Schulsinger (1983; see also Schulsinger 1985) undertook a prospective study of 207 apparently normal children of schizophrenic mothers (High Risk Group) and 104 control children. The age range of the children was 9–20 years. Among a number of factors analysed was the midwives' report on the delivery of all the children. Pregnancy or birth complications recorded included anoxia, prematurity, prolonged labour, placental difficulty, umbilical cord complications, mother's illness during pregnancy, multiple births, and breech presentations. Eight years after the start of the study, 20 of the High Risk Group had suffered major psychiatric breakdowns (mostly schizophrenia). These were matched with 20 control children and 20 from the High Risk Group who had remained normal. It was found that 70 per cent of the psychiatrically ill children had suffered birth complications, compared with 15 per cent of the High Risk Group without psychiatric breakdown and 33 per cent of the control group. Mednick and Schulsinger (1973) suggested from these results that perinatal complications may trigger some genetically predisposed characteristics that can lead to schizophrenia. They proposed that damage results from the extreme sensitivity of neural tissue to anoxia, and cited evidence that the most vulnerable brain area is the hippocampus.

Reveley et al. (1983), in a study of monozygous twins, found a correlation between larger cerebral ventricular size and perinatal complications which included birth weight of less than 1.5 kg, breech or difficult forceps delivery, and neonatal asphyxia. In 18 normal twins this relationship was highly significant ($P < 0.001$), but in 21 schizophrenic twins the relationship was less clear. Schizophrenic twins with a positive family history of schizophrenia had large ventricles, but no history of birth complications, while schizophrenic twins with a negative family history had large cerebral ventricles and a history of birth complications. These findings suggest that individuals with high genetic predisposition may develop schizophrenia without the additional precipitating factor of neonatal hypoxia. Where genetic predisposition is lower or absent, neonatal asphyxia may be an environmental precipitating factor. However, the effect is non-specific since many of the psychiatrically normal controls had larger than normal cerebral ventricles, and perinatal asphyxia is unlikely to be the whole explanation of cerebral atrophy in schizophrenia since many of the schizophrenics had large ventricles without a history of birth complications.

Viral infection

Another environmental agent which has excited considerable interest as a possible cause or precipitating agent of schizophrenia is a slow or latent virus infection. Viral infections of the nervous system are known to be capable of producing mental disorders, as in the case of Creutzfeld–Jacob disease (Chapter 9) and various forms of encephalitis. A viral infection might perhaps explain the curious seasonal distribution of schizophrenia: the illness presents most commonly in the early summer and patients who develop schizophrenia are more likely to have been born in the winter months than at other times of the year (Crow 1983). A similar phenomenon occurs in Japanese viral hepatitis, and is attributed to seasonal epidemics with variations in immunity and tolerance in the population. Episodes of mania and depression also show seasonal variation, being most common in the early summer.

Viruses are notoriously difficult to isolate, especially from the brain and cerebrospinal fluid, and none have yet been definitely associated with schizophrenia. Tyrrell et al. (1979) and Crow et al. (1979b) found a virus-like agent in the cerebrospinal fluid of 18 out of 47 patients with acute or chronic schizophrenia but Mered et al. (1983) failed to replicate these findings in 23 patients with chronic schizophrenia. However, Albrecht et al. (1980) found that the concentration of cerebrospinal fluid antibody against cytomegalovirus was significantly increased, compared with controls, in 68 per cent of 60 schizophrenics. The authors pointed out several characteristics of this virus that might link it with schizophrenia. For example, the virus can remain latent for years and shows an affinity for the limbic system. Histological changes in the brain, consisting of diffuse glial proliferation, are found in patients with generalized cytomegalovirus infection and have been reported in the brain of some schizophrenics. Kaufman et al. (1983) also found cytomegalovirus antibodies in the cerebrospinal fluid of some schizophrenics and the presence of antibody appeared to be related to cerebral atrophy as shown by computerized tomography studies.

A viral aetiology for schizophrenia, by cytomegalovirus or any other, is clearly far from proved. However, Crow (1985) has raised some interesting speculations which link a possible virus infection, genetic factors, and the considerable evidence (discussed below) that schizophrenia is a disease of the dominant cerebral hemisphere. He suggests that schizophrenia may result from the expression and perhaps replication of a retrovirus which has become incorporated in the genome, possibly a gene that determines cerebral dominance. The virus becomes preferentially located in the dominant hemisphere and results in asymmetric disturbance of cerebral function, especially in the left temporal lobe.

Another possibility suggested by Knight (1982) is that schizophrenia is an autoimmune disease in which the positive symptoms are due to the presence of dopamine receptor stimulating autoantibodies and the negative symptoms represent an autoimmune encephalitis-like syndrome in which a viral infection triggers a destructive autoimmune response against certain dopaminergic pathways in the limbic system. Knight pointed out that the pattern of inheritance of schizophrenia is similar to that of other autoimmune disorders. The importance of dopaminergic systems in schizophrenia is discussed below.

Hemispheric dysfunction

As described in Chapter 8, the normal human brain is functionally asymmetric. The dominant hemisphere, usually the left, is specialized for verbal-linguistic and analytic processing and the non-dominant (right) hemisphere for visual-spatial functions including pattern recognition. The right hemisphere may also be more involved than the left in emotional perception and expression and emotional concepts in general (Ross 1984). There seems little doubt that this asymmetry is both structurally and functionally disturbed in schizophrenia, and that the dominant hemisphere is primarily affected. The evidence gained from several types of investigation points to limbic structures as the main loci of dysfunction.

Post-mortem studies Post-mortem studies of schizophrenic brains have shown that ventricular enlargement when present is usually most marked in the inferior horn of the lateral ventricle, within the temporal lobe. Crow (1985) reported a decrease in cortical thickness, especially affecting the para-hippocampal gyrus, in the brains of schizophrenics compared with those of patients with affective disorders. The most marked differences were on the left side. Computer tomography studies have shown a tendency to decreased density of brain tissue in the left hemisphere especially in the frontal lobes (Mackay 1984; Roberts 1984). Diffuse gliosis and other cellular changes involving limbic structures have been reported in several studies of schizophrenic brains reviewed by Torrey and Petersen (1974). Thickening of the corpus callosum, which runs through the limbic system, has also been found in schizophrenic brains (Rosenthal and Bigelow 1972). The association of schizophrenic symtpoms with known neurological lesions, such temporal lobe epilepsy and tumours involving the dominant temporal lobe has already been mentioned (Trimble 1981; Flor-Henry 1976).

Reynolds (1983), in an examination of two separate series of brains, found that the concentration of dopamine (but not of noradrenaline) in the left amygdala was greatly increased in schizophrenic as compared with normal brains. In the schizophrenic brains, dopamine concentration in the right amygdala was normal, and dopamine and noradrenaline concentrations in the caudate nucleus were normal and symmetrical. This finding is of particular interest in view of the dopamine theory of schizophrenia, discussed below, and the fact that a major action of antipsychotic drugs used in schizophrenia is dopamine receptor blockade (Chapter 14). Whether the abnormality of dopamine distribution is a cause or effect of schizophrenia, and whether it reflects neuronal over- or underactivity is not revealed by this study.

Blood flow and cerebral metabolism Investigations of cerebral blood flow in schizophrenia are discussed by Ingvar (1982) and Sheppard *et al.* (1983; 1984). Total cerebral blood flow and brain metabolism appear to be normal in schizophrenia but there is evidence of regional abnormalities. Using [133]-xenon inhalation techniques, Ingvar (1982) reported decreased blood flow in frontal regions in chronic schizophrenics; this 'hypofrontality' correlated with clinical features of inactivity and autistic and catatonic behaviour. By contrast, an increased blood flow was noted in temporal and occipital regions, especially in patients with severe cognitive disturbance. Sheppard *et al.* (1983), using [15]-oxygen position emission techniques, found significant though complex differences in the lateral distribution of blood flow and brain metabolism in acute schizophrenics compared with controls. In the normal subjects, blood flow was generally greater in the right hemisphere than the left, while in the schizophrenics as a group there was little difference between the two sides. Combining blood flow and metabolic data from individual subjects showed that 7 of the 12 schizophrenics, but only one of the 12 controls had greater left-sided activity. There was no apparent relation between thought disorder and laterality in the schizophrenics (Sheppard *et al.* 1984), but cognitive state was not controlled during blood flow measurements (Kellett 1984).

Gur *et al.* (1983) attempted to correlate regional cerebral blood flow with types of cognitive activity. In 15 right-handed schizophrenics and a control group, blood flow in the right and left cerebral hemispheres was measured at rest, during a verbal task, and during a spatial task. The normal subjects showed the expected increase in left-sided flow during the verbal task and in right-sided flow during the spatial task. By contrast, the schizophrenics showed the same blood flow in both hemispheres during the verbal task and had a greater left-sided flow during the spatial task. The performance of the schizophrenics in the tests was poorer than that of the controls. The results were taken to support the hypothesis, developed from analysis of cognitive performance, that in schizophrenia there is both overactivation and dysfunction of the dominant left hemisphere (Gur 1978).

Further information on brain biochemical activity underlying cerebral blood flow distribution may shortly be forthcoming from functional brain tomographic scanning with labelled L-dopa and spiroperidol, which is now possible (Sheppard *et al.* 1984).

Cognitive performance Gur (1978, 1979a,b) discussed evidence derived from many psychometric studies that cognitive performance in schizophrenia reflects left hemispheric dysfunction. For example, in normal subjects linguistic stimuli, such as written syllables, are recognized better when presented (by tachistoscope) to the right visual field (left cerebral hemisphere) and visuospatial stimuli, such as patterns, are recognized better when presented to the left visual field (right cerebral hemisphere). In schizophrenia, the recognition of linguistic stimuli is poorer when presented on the right visual field; spatial stimuli, as in normal subjects, is recognised better from the left visual field, but recognition of both types of stimuli is poorer than in normal subjects. This finding, and results from various other tests including dichotic listening tasks (Wexler and Heninger 1979), suggest that in schizophrenia the left hemisphere is deficient in the initial processing of verbal information.

It can also be inferred that the left hemisphere is overactivated in schizophrenic patients. For example, in normal subjects, activation of each hemisphere is often accompanied by contralateral eye deviations. Thus, activation of the left hemisphere, produced by giving the subject a linguistic problem, produces an eye movement to the right and activation of the right hemisphere, during solution of a spatial problem, is accompanied by eye deviation to the left. Schizophrenic subjects make significantly more eye movements to the right, indicating left hemispheric activation, regardless of whether the cognitive task is linguistic or visuospatial. From these and other tests, Gur (1978, 1979a,b) suggested that schizophrenics tend to overuse the left hemisphere, even though its function is impaired. This combination may explain why schizophrenics appear to use faulty logic and have difficulty in problem solving. According to Gur (1979a), they 'are triply disabled by having a dysfunctional left hemisphere, by failing to shift processing to the right, and by overactivation of the dysfunctional hemisphere' (Gur 1979a; p. 273). These cognitive behaviours are also shown by patients with extensive damage in the right hemisphere, who are presumably forced to rely on the left hemisphere, and by normal subjects under conditions of stress, intoxication, and fatigue.

There is also some evidence of defective interhemispheric transfer of information in schizophrenics. Green (1978) and Butler (1979) described the results of various tests designed to assess this function. In one such test, the subject learns a tactile discrimination task with one hand and is then required to perform the task with the other hand, necessitating transfer of the information to the opposite hemisphere. Schizophrenics perform poorly on such tasks and manifest impaired ability to transfer information both from right to left and left to right hemispheres. Their performance is similar to that of 'split-brain' (divided hemisphere) monkeys. Green (1978) suggests that some schizophrenic symptoms may be related to defective interhemispheric communication. Possibly the incongruity of affect so characteristic of some types of schizophrenia results from failure of transfer of emotional concepts from right to left hemispheres, while the 'overuse' of the left hemisphere described by Gur (1979a,b) may result from similar lack of transfer of right cognitive functions to the dominant hemisphere.

Electroencephalographic studies Electroencephalographic (EEG) changes observed in schizophrenia are reviewed by Shagass *et al.* (1978), Gruzelier (1979), Saletu (1980), Venables (1981), and Spohn and Patterson (1979). On the whole, investigations show generalized abnormalities with some evidence of disturbed lateralization. In the resting EEG, increased paroxysmal activity, dysrhythmic activity, and spike and wave formation have frequently been reported, and some catatonic patients have abnormal EEGs reminiscent of epilepsy. Most of these findings date from earlier studies, and it is not entirely clear whether the inclusion of patients with epileptic psychoses influenced the results. However, several investigations using deep electrodes, discussed by Torrey and Petersen (1974), have shown abnormal electrical activity, including spike activity and high voltage paroxysmal activity, in the septal region, anterior hippocampus, amygdala, temporal lobes, and front-orbital area in schizophrenic patients. These abnormalities become more pronounced under thiopental anaesthesia. The advent of quantitative methods has allowed more specific evaluation of EEG findings. Frequency analysis has shown that the EEG in schizophrenia is in general characterised by a decrease in alpha activity and an increase in both fast beta activity, and slow delta and theta activity. The average frequency is increased and the average amplitude decreased. There is an increase in frequency variability and a decrease in amplitude variability (Table 13.3). It is of interest that similar changes are found in psychotic children, children at high genetic risk from schizophrenia, and also in normal adults under the influence of LSD. In schizophrenics the EEG tends to revert towards normality if the clinical

Table 13.3. Quantitative EEG findings in schizophrenia

EEG Variables			
Activity	Hz	Adult schizophrenics	High-risk children* for schizophrenia
delta	1–3.5	+	+
theta	3.6–5.5	+	
alpha	5.6–13	−	−
beta$_1$	1.4–26	+	+
beta$_2$	27–40	+	+
beta$_3$	>40	+	+
Average frequency		+	+
Frequency variability		+	+
Average amplitude		−	−
Amplitude variability		−	−

+: Increased compared with controls; −: decreased compared with controls.
* Non-psychotic children with schizophrenic parent or parents.
Reference: Saletu 1980.

condition responds to antipsychotic medication. Some schizophrenic patients show a 'hyponormal' EEG with a regular rhythmic, synchronized alpha pattern; patients with this type of EEG tend to be resistant to antipsychotic treatment.

With regard to lateralization, several studies have shown that the decrease in alpha-activity, the increase in theta- and beta-activity, and the frequency variability are most marked in the left temporal regions in schizophrenia, and it is this area which shows the greater difference from normal subjects. In addition, there appears to be less intra- and interhemispheric coherence of frequency in schizophrenics compared with normal subjects. The distinction between left and right hemispheric electroencephalographic activation according to type of cognitive task seems to be blurred in schizophrenia, with activation in both left and right hemispheres in both linguistic and visuospatial tasks (Alpert and Martz 1977). Serafetinides *et al.* (1981) found increased beta-activity in the left hemisphere of schizophrenic patients with predominant symptoms of thought disorder and increased beta activity in the right hemisphere in schizophrenics with predominant symptoms of anxiety or depression.

Sleep EEG studies in schizophrenia show reduced total sleeping time and reduced amounts of Stages 2, 3 and 4 sleep. REM sleep is approximately normal in amount, but its distribution may be somewhat altered. There is a disturbance of the normal rhythmicity of the 90–min. cycles of REMS, frequent changes of sleep stage, and different sleep patterns from night to night. In general sleep studies indicate instability and increased arousal in schizophrenics. The sleep pattern reverts towards normal in patients who respond to antipsychotics.

Investigations of averaged evoked potentials have shown many differences between schizophrenics and normal subjects, although the findings have often been conflicting. Some of the main differences are shown in Table 13.4. and are discussed by Shagass *et al.* (1978), Spohn and Patterson (1979), and Saletu, (1980). In general, the amplitude of the early components (before 100 ms) of the somatosensory, auditory, and visual evoked potentials is larger than normal in schizophrenics, while the amplitude of the later components (after 100 ms) is smaller, and there is an increase in variability. The latency of both early and late components is decreased, a finding also present in children at genetic risk of schizophrenia. Slow potentials, such as the contingent negative variation (CNV) are decreased in magnitude but there is prolonged negativity after the CNV and after motor reactions in general. Abraham *et al.* (1976) have reported that the reduced CNV in schizophrenics does not return to normal on clinical recovery and that CNV magnitude is also reduced in psychiatrically normal relatives of schizophrenics. Some investigations have revealed alterations in laterality of evoked potentials (Serafetinides *et al.* 1981).

Table 13.4.   Averaged evoked potential findings in schizophrenia

Somatosensory evoked potentials (SEP)	
Auditory evoked potential (AEP)	
Visual evoked potential (VEP)	
early components (before 100 msec)	increased amplitude
late components (after 100 msec)	decreased amplitude
	greater variability
latency	some early and late
	components faster
P300 (positive wave at about 300 msec, related to stimulus uncertainty)	reduced or absent
Contingent negative variation (CNV)	decreased magnitude
Post-imperative negative variation (PINV)	prolonged
Readiness potential	reduced or absent
Post-motor negativity	prolonged

Reference: Shagass *et al.* 1978; Saletu 1980.

The meaning of the abnormal evoked responses in schizophrenia is not clear, since the electrogenesis of these potentials is not understood. However, they may reflect alterations both in arousal activity and in central processing mechanisms (Venables 1981). Prolonged negativity after motor actions may be connected with the tendency to perseveration. Reduced amplitude of the somatosensory evoked potential induced by painful stimuli has been interpreted to suggest an abnormality of endogenous opioid systems in schizophrenia, as discussed below.

Autonomic responses Autonomic variables have been assiduously studied in schizophrenia and evidence has been sought of altered levels of tonic or phasic arousal and attention. Variables measured include electrodermal, pupillary, and cardiovascular activity, and smooth pursuit eye movements. The results have been variable, conflicting and difficult to interpret. They are reviewed in detail by Venables (1973, 1977, 1980, 1981), Spohn and Patterson (1979).

Electrodermal responses have perhaps given the most informative results. These responses are of interest because they appear to be under the major control of influences from the reticular formation and limbic system; abnormalities of response thus suggest involvement of these systems in schizophrenia. In normal subjects, the electrodermal response to a mental stimulus, such as a tone, is a momentary increase in skin electrical conductance due to a phasic increase in sweat gland activity. On successive repetitions of the tone, the response becomes smaller and may virtually disappear, a phenomenon attributed to habituation. This response is altered in schizophrenics: there is a bimodal distribution consisting of 50 per cent of patients who show no skin conductance responsivity and 50 per cent who show hyper-responsivity and a remarkable lack of habituation (Venables 1980). Mednick and Schulsinger (1973), in their study of children of schizophrenic mothers, found that one of the features which distinguished between children who later developed schizophrenia from children who remained well was hyper-responsivity and slow habituation of the skin conductance response. These children, as mentioned above, had a high incidence of birth complications, and it was suggested that these might have caused anoxic damage to limbic structures. Some of the abnormal electrodermal responses, both in these children and in adult schizophrenics, were asymmetric and suggested left hemisphere limbic dysfunction (Venables 1977).

Limbic lesions in monkeys cause changes in electrodermal responses similar to those seen in schizophrenic patients. Lesions of the amygdala can cause electrodermal non-responsivity, hypo-responsivity or hyper-responsivity, and bilateral removal of the hippocampus results in failure of habituation of electrodermal responses. Alterations of electrodermal response in schizophrenia have therefore been interpreted as reflecting involvement of limbic arousal control systems, perhaps predominantly affecting the left side of the brain.

The relation between autonomic and central nervous system responses have been explored in various experiments reviewed by Claridge (1978). It appears that although schizophrenics as a group may not differ markedly from normal subjects in any one measure of arousal, they do differ in the correlation or integration between various measures. For example, in normal subjects the skin potential, a measure of autonomic arousal, correlates with measures of central arousal, such as the two-flash threshold (the ability to perceive as separate two closely spaced brief light flashes); the higher the skin potential the sharper the perception. In most schizophrenics this relationship is reversed, so that when skin potential is high the ability to perceive separately two closely spaced light flashes is decreased. In a subgroup of paranoid schizophrenics the ability to separate light flashes is abnormally high for a given level of autonomic arousal. Thus, an important characteristic of schizophrenics may be that for a particular level of autonomic arousal their degree of perceptual responsivity (central arousal) is either abnormally high or low. Claridge (1978) suggested that these results are due to a failure of integration between various types of arousal.

An interesting observation in relation to these studies is that relationships similar to those found in schizophrenics also occur in normal subjects with high psychoticism scores on the Eysenck Personality Questionnaire (Eysenck and Eysenck 1976), and in normal subjects under the influence of the psychotomimetic drug LSD (Claridge 1978; Claridge and Chappa 1973). The results lead to three important conclusions. Firstly, there appears to be a disorder in the central integration of arousal functions in schizophrenia. Although not actually measured, the abnormality may include a lack of integration of emotional, goal-directed, arousal with general or autonomic arousal. Secondly, the studies suggest that 'psychoticism as a normal personality dimension (has), as its biological basis, a particular kind of nervous typological organisation seen, in its extreme form, in the psychotic disorders' (Claridge and Chappa 1973; p. 175). Such individuals may be those with a particular vulnerability to develop schizophrenia under stress, as postulated in the spectrum concept of schizophrenia mentioned above. Thirdly, the fact that similar changes can be induced in normal subjects by LSD suggests a biochemical basis for schizophrenia, a question discussed below.

Motor laterality If schizophrenia reflects altered function in the dominant hemisphere, it might be associated with alterations in motor laterality (handedness). This proposition (Flor-Henry 1979) appears to be true, although in a complex manner. Flor-Henry (1979) reviewed many studies related to sinistrality and dextrality in schizophrenia. Investigations involving large (over 1200) and small (54) numbers of schizophrenic patients show an excess of sinistrality compared with controls. Schizophrenics also have a high representation of intermediate states with left/right confusion. Estimates of the incidence of left handedness in schizophrenia vary, but overall about 60 per cent of schizophrenics are left-handed compared with 20 per cent of control subjects.

The relationship between handedness and the occurrence of schizophrenic illness in schizophrenic twins is interesting. Crow (1985) reanalysed the data from several twin studies and found that in monozygous twins concordant for handedness and dextral, the concordance for schizophrenia was 93 per cent. In twins discordant for handedness, the concordance for schizophrenia was only 23 per cent, but the left-handed twins had a higher incidence of schizophrenia (74 per cent) than the right-handed twins (47 per cent). In dizygotic twins, none of the associations found in monozygotic twins are present.

These studies of handedness in schizophrenia are consistent with the other evidence indicating a disturbance of cerebral laterality. However, they give no evidence of whether the excess in sinistrality is a cause or effect of schizophrenia. It is possible that early injury to the left side of the brain is one cause of both schizophrenia and sinistrality; equally, there may be a genetic link between handedness and vulnerability to schizophrenia. It is not clear whether cerebral dominance for other functions shifts with motor laterality in normal subjects. Many normal left-handers have left sided speech representation similar to dextral subjects, while some have a less clear lateralization of speech, with both hemispheres contributing to language processing (Beaumont 1983). The latter condition appears to be the case in some schizophrenics.

Brain mechanisms in schizophrenia

Brain systems in schizophrenia

It is clear from the clinical and physiological evidence described above that brain systems regulating arousal, affect, and cognition are all disturbed in schizophrenia. Perception of external stimuli, central processing of information, motivation, affective state, muscle tone, tonic and phasic central and autonomic arousal, and other diverse functions may all be distorted simultaneously and to varying degrees. Thus, it is not possible to classify the syndrome as a primary disorder of any one functional system. Probably no clinical condition demonstrates more clearly that the various systems modulating behaviour cannot be operationally isolated. Indeed, the salient feature of schizophrenia appears to be a fault in the interrelationships between different functional systems; it seems to reflect a breakdown of communications both within the brain, and between the brain and the outside world.

There is abundant evidence pointing to the approximate anatomical site of dysfunction in schizophrenia. All the symptoms can occur in organic disorders involving the temporal lobes, limbic structures, and frontal cortex. *Post-mortem* studies and measurements of blood flow, cerebral metabolism, and EEG again point to a disturbance of function in limbic structures, and frontal and temporal lobes. Biochemical and pharmacological investigations (discussed below) point in the same direction. Neurological 'soft' signs found in schizophrenics suggest a dysfunction of frontal and parietal lobes (Cox and Ludwig 1979).

There is in addition considerable evidence suggesting that the dysfunction is most marked in the left (dominant) hemisphere, although not limited to one side. In computer assisted tomography brain scans, air encephalography, EEG and cerebral blood flow studies, and *post-mortem* examinations, the maximal pathological changes are usually found in the left temporal and frontal regions. Cognitive testing suggests excessive use of a dysfunctioning left hemisphere (Gur 1978). The same multiple methods of examination also suggest a defect of interhemispheric transfer, and many manifestations of schizophrenia, such as incongruity of affect and abnormal covariance between perception and autonomic response (Claridge 1978), testify to poor integration between systems.

Thus, the site of dysfunction in schizophrenia can be roughly localized to the limbic system and its cortical connections, mainly in the left hemisphere. It is in this intercourse of phylogenetically ancient and modern neural pathways that the main functional systems determining behaviour—arousal, reward and punishment, learning, memory and cognition—are normally integrated to produce meaningful and goal-directed responses, and it is here too, it seems, that there is a failure of integration in schizophrenia. Arguments for regarding schizophrenia as an asymmetric, predominantly left-sided dysfunction of the anterior limbic system are marshalled by Flor-Henry (1979).

Within the limbic system, it is not at present possible to delineate precisely the pathways concerned, and in any case these may not be identical in all schizophrenics. The connections of the limbic system are not fully worked out; some recent studies on corticolimbic connections are described by Pandya and Seltzer (1982) and Iverson (1984). Pharmacological evidence, discussed below, suggests the prime importance of dysfunction in dopaminergic mesolimbic, mesocortical, and corticostriatal pathways. The importance of the ventral tegmental area, which contains the cell bodies of the dopaminergic mesolimbic neurones, is stressed by Stevens (1979) and Cooper (1984).

As to the nature and direction of the limbic perturbation in schizophrenia, the answers are even less clear. It seems likely that the condition reflects a whole spectrum of neural states ranging from markedly increased to markedly reduced activity in the affected pathways. Symptoms such as hallucinations and certain types of thought disorder suggest an excess of uncontrolled cerebral activity, while symptoms such as anhedonia, loss of drive, poverty of thought and speech suggest loss of function in some systems. Acute schizophrenia reflects perhaps an irritative lesion with stimulation of activity and loss of synaptic control, while chronic schizophrenia reflects a structural brain lesion with neural loss and irreversible reduction of function. These states would correspond with Type I and Type II schizophrenia (Crow 1982; Table 12.2). Yet the two types of schizophrenia merge, and positive and negative symptoms can co-exist.

The penumbra of schizophrenia also merges with a number of other states. As already mentioned, it merges with a normal state in which certain personality characteristics are prominent, and with a spectrum of personality disorders. It merges with mania and depression which, as discussed in Chapter 11, are also disorders of the limbic system (Chapter 11). In some cases it is difficult to sustain a distinction between schizophrenia and dementia: in both there is structural damage and cell loss in the brain and any clinical differences presumably depend on the degree and distribution of cell loss. Finally, schizophrenia merges with a variety of neuropathological states caused by lesions, infections, metabolic states, and drugs.

From these considerations it is possible to conclude that schizophrenia can be precipitated by any agent which leads to dysfunction in the (mainly left) anterior limbic system. There is no reason to suppose that there is only one such precipitating factor, and schizophrenia is almost certainly a condition of multiple aetiology expressed through a final common pathway in the limbic system (Richter 1978). It seems likely that certain individuals are genetically predisposed to schizophrenia, possibly by virtue of their inherent limbic system organization and balance of cerebral laterality. These individuals may have schizoid or psychotic personality traits which conceivably have an adaptive value for survival under certain conditions, but which render them relatively susceptible to the development of schizophrenia when exposed to non-specific factors such as environmental stress. Other individuals may develop schizophrenia when exposed to factors which specifically damage the limbic system. Such specific agents may include birth trauma, neurological lesions, drug effects, and neurotropic viruses.

Having identified functional brain systems, anatomical locations, some predisposing factors and precipitating agents that may be involved, is it possible to identify a mechanism for schizophrenia in terms of cellular events in neurones? The answer to this question has been sought by biochemical and pharmacological approaches aimed at defining neurotransmitter and neuromodulator systems in which disturbance of function is fundamental to the disease process. The results of these efforts, which also offer a hope of pharmacological treatment of schizophrenia, are discussed below.

Neurotransmitters in schizophrenia

As stated in previous chapters, neurotransmitter systems in the brain do not operate in isolation. They interact with other neurotransmitter pathways acting synergistically and antagonistically, and the release and receptor actions of many neurotransmitters is controlled by several other transmitter and modulators. Nevertheless, it is possible that in schizophrenia, as in Parkinson's disease and Alzheimer's disease, the neurones of one transmitter system may be primarily or mainly affected. The search for a specific primary abnormality has generated many biochemical theories of schizophrenia.

Dopamine

Of the various biochemical theories of schizophrenia, those involving dopamine are supported by the most abundant evidence. The 'classical' dopamine theory, which suggested that schizophrenia results from absolute or relative dopaminergic overactivity at critical brain sites, has a history similar to that of the various monoamine theories of depression (Chapter 11). It stemmed from the observation that antipsychotic drugs, which are effective in controlling some schizophrenic symptoms, have in common a dopamine receptor blocking action, and that dopamine receptor agonists and drugs which release dopamine can precipitate schizoid psychotic reactions, and greatly aggravate the symptoms of existing schizophrenia. Subsequent advances in the understanding of the distribution and physiology of dopamine receptors have, if anything, strengthened the idea that dopaminergic dysfunction may account for at least some of the clinical features of schizophrenia.

Antipsychotic drugs Antipsychotic drugs (Chapter 14) do not cure schizophrenia, but can greatly improve many of the symptoms and it is generally accepted they they affect fundamental features including thought disorder (Snyder 1982). These drugs are chemically heterogeneous and have actions on many neurotransmitter systems, but their antagonist actions at certain dopamine receptors (discussed below) correlate very closely with their clinical potency. Furthermore, in the case of flupenthixol and butaclamol, which exist in two isomeric forms, only one isomer (alpha-flupenthixol and (+) -butaclamol) has antipsychotic potency and only this isomer has dopamine blocking activity. Hence, it seems that the antipsychotic effects result from dopamine receptor blockade and this in turn suggests the possibility of dopaminergic overactivity in schizophrenia.

Dopaminergic drugs Amphetamine, which releases dopamine and noradrenaline from monoaminergic nerve terminals, and probably also has some receptor agonist activity, can in normal subjects precipitate a psychotic state which is indistinguishable from acute paranoid schizophrenia (Chapter 4). In schizophrenics, low doses of amphetamine can exacerbate schizophrenic symptoms, and the degree to which this effect occurs correlates with the degree of the patient's response to antipsychotic drugs (Snyder 1982). L-dopa, which increases dopamine synthesis, and bromocriptine, a dopamine receptor agonist, can similarly precipitate psychotic reactions and aggravate schizophrenic symptoms. The psychotic symptoms caused by all these drugs are dramatically reversed by small doses of neuroleptics. These observations indicate that schizophrenic symptoms can be caused by activation of dopamine receptors.

Dopamine release Could dopaminergic overactivity in schizophrenia result from increased transmitter release? The evidence related to this question is discussed by Crow (1978b). The concentration of the dopamine metabolite homovanillic acid (HVA) in the cerebrospinal fluid has been measured after loading with probenecid (which blocks removal of HVA). Increased concentrations of cerebrospinal fluid HVA are found in amphetamine psychosis, but several studies have shown that in schizophrenia HVA concentrations are lower than normal, especially in patients with severe illness. Thus, this test suggests decreased rather than increased dopamine release in schizophrenia. Post-mortem studies of schizophrenic brains have revealed little difference from normal in the concentration of dopamine metabolites (Crow *et al.* 1979a; Owen *et al.* 1978).

Secondly, psychosis with schizophreniform features has been described in patients with idiopathic and post-encephalitic Parkinson's disease, in which dopamine deficiency has been shown to occur in mesolimbic structures as well as in the corpus striatum. Thus, increased dopamine release does not appear to be necessary for the presence of schizophrenia-like symptoms. Thirdly, the release of prolactin by the anterior pituitary is under inhibitory dopaminergic control from the tuberoinfundibular system of the hypo-thalamus. Antipsychotic drugs cause an increase in prolactin secretion. If dopaminergic hyperactivity extended to this system in schizophrenia, decreased prolactin secretion would be expected. However, plasma prolactin concentration has been found to be normal in schizophrenia.

Three lines of investigation have thus failed to demonstrate increased dopamine release in schizophrenia. On the other hand, there remains the finding of increased concentrations of dopamine in the left amygdala in post-mortem schizophrenic brains (Reynolds 1983). Such a localized and asymmetric increase seems unlikely to be due to medication, and its sig-nificance remains to be assessed. Meanwhile, a more promising possibility appears to be an alteration of dopamine receptor sensitivity in schizophrenia.

Dopamine Receptors Dopamine receptors, however, like those for other monoamine neurotransmitters, are heterogeneous, and there has been much discussion over which of them might be involved in producing schizophrenic symptoms. The characterization of dopamine receptors is far from complete, and their properties and classification have been discussed and described by many authors (for example, Kebabian and Calne 1979; Iverson 1978; Iverson *et al.* 1980; Snyder 1981b; Offermeier and van Rooyen 1982; Laduron 1981; Kebabian and Cote 1981; Calne 1981; Cools 1982; Beart 1982; Creese 1982).

At present it seems likely that there are at least three types of dopamine receptors (Fig. 13.1, Table 13.5). Post-synaptic receptors include dopamine-1 (DA-1) receptors which are linked to adenylate cyclase and dopamine-2 (DA-2) receptors which are usually not linked to this enzyme (though some may inhibit it; Creese 1982). These receptor subtypes have different phar-macological profiles and binding characteristics, and may mediate different responses (excitatory or inhibitory) as shown on Table 13.5. In addition, presynaptic and somatodentritic autoreceptors (dopamine-3, DA-3) recep-tors may modulate the synaptic release of dopamine (Tepper *et al.* 1985), although their existence has been debated (Laduron 1984; Dourish and Cooper 1985). It is possible that the dopamine receptor consists of a single macromolecular complex in which the conformation (and therefore the effec-tive subtype) varies according to the presence or absence of co-operatively linked serotonergic or noradrenergic subunits (Cools 1982).

Dopaminergic pathways The functions of the various dopamine receptor subtypes are not clearly understood. Both DA-1 and DA-2 post-synaptic receptors and dopamine autoreceptors are found in many parts of the brain. Dopaminergic pathways have a widespread distribution and can be divided into four separate systems (Fig. 13.2). The *nigrostriatal system* arises from cell bodies in the substantia nigra (cell groups $A_{8,9}$) and projects to the corpus striatum. The fact that degeneration of these dopaminergic cell bodies occurs

Multiple dopamine receptors

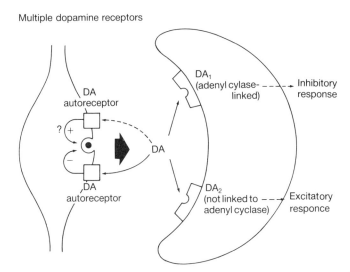

Fig. 13.1. Pre-synaptic and post-synaptic receptors for dopamine. DA, dopamine. Post-synaptic receptors mediate tissue responses and include dopamine-1 (DA_1) receptors linked to adenylate cyclase and dopamine-2 (DA_2) receptors not linked to this enzyme. Pre-synaptic autoreceptors may modulate dopamine release.

in Parkinson's disease (Hornykiewicz 1973) indicated that this system is concerned with the control of muscle tone and movement. In addition, some dopaminergic cells from cell group A_9 project to the cingulate cortex (Bunney 1984). Both DA-1 and DA-2 receptors have been demonstrated in the corpus striatum (Snyder 1981a,b). Exactly how the receptor subtypes are involved in motor control is not known. Parkinsonism occurs as an adverse effect of neuroleptic drugs which antagonize both DA-1 and DA-2 receptors (phenothiazines) and also with those which are relatively selective DA-2 receptor antagonists (butyrophenones). However, there is no correlation between the propensity of neuroleptic drugs to cause Parkinsonism and their antipsychotic action

The *tuberoinfundibular* pathway arises from cells in the median eminence which project within the hypothalamus. This system exerts an inhibitory control on the pituitary release of prolactin and other hormones (Chapter 11). The receptors involved are DA-2 receptors, but their activity in this area does not appear to be related to psychiatric symptoms.

The *chemoreceptor trigger* zone of the medullary vomiting centre is under dopaminergic control. The receptors involved are probably DA-2 receptors since selective DA-2 agonists (apomorphine and bromocriptine) cause vomiting while DA-2 antagonists including neuroleptics have antiemetic effects. The actions of neuroleptic drugs at this site have no relation to their antipsychotic efficacy.

Table 13.5. Characteristics of dopamine receptor subtypes

	Dopamine-1 receptors (DA-1, D-1, DA i*) cell bodies	Dopamine-2 receptors (DA-2, D-2, DA e*) axons, terminals, ?cell bodies	Dopamine-3 receptors (DA-3, D-3, autoreceptors) cell bodies, dendrites, terminals
Neuronal location			
Adenylate cyclase linkage	yes–stimulate adenylate cyclase formation	unassociated (sometimes inhibit adenylate cyclase formation)	unassociated
Radioligands (relatively selective)	^{3}H-thioxanthenes	^{3}H-butyrophenones	^{3}H-dopamine
Agonists	bromocriptine (micromolar concentrations) dopamine (micromolar concentrations)	bromocriptine (nanomolar concentrations) apomorphine (nanomolar concentrations) dopamine (nanomolar concentrations)	3-PPP** apomorphine (extremely low concentrations) dopamine (extremely low concentrations)

Antagonists	?piribedil bromocriptine (partial) phenothiazines	sulpiride	?phenothiazines ?butyrophenones ?other neuroleptics
Function	?motor control (corpus striatum)	phenothiazines butyrophenones molindone inhibition of prolactin release (hypothalamus) control of pituitary secretion of other hormones stimulation of emesis (medulla) motor control (corpus striatum) (may mediate some schizophrenic symptoms)	negative feedback control of dopamine release

* DA i and DA e receptors have been postulated to mediate inhibitory and excitatory dopaminergic effects, respectively (Kebabian and Calne 1979).

** 3-PPP = 3-(3-hydroxyphenyl)-N-*n*-propylpiperidone

References: Creese 1982; Kebabian and Calne 1979; Offermeier and van Rooyen 1982.

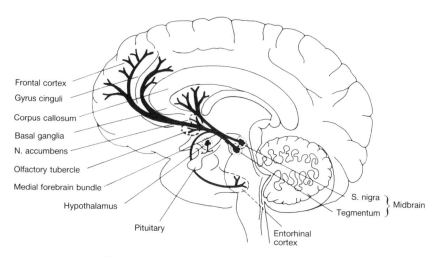

Fig. 13.2. Dopaminergic pathways in the brain.

The *mesolimbic pathway* arises from cell group A_{10} in the ventral tegmental area and projects via the median forebrain bundle to many limbic structures including the nucleus accumbens, amygdala, and in the *mesocortical pathways* (Glowinski *et al.* 1985) to the frontral entorhinal cortex. There are many reasons for suspecting that this system is the seat of dysfunction in schizophrenia. As already discussed, evidence from physiological studies of limbic function, clinical conditions producing schizophrenic symptoms, and from post-mortem, blood flow, EEG, and computer tomography investigations in schizophrenia all points towards dysfunction of the limbic system and its frontal lobe connections, although it gives no information on which transmitter systems might be involved. Limbic structures and prefrontal cortex contain DA-1, DA-2, and DA-3 receptors. The clinical potency in schizophrenia of different types of neuroleptics correlates very closely with their DA-2 receptor antagonistic activity and their affinity for DA-2 receptors as measured by ^{3}H-haloperidol or ^{3}H-Spiroperidol binding (Table 13.5; Chapter 14). These findings thus relate antipsychotic potency of drugs to DA-2 receptor antagonism and suggest that DA-2 receptor sensitivity might be increased in schizophrenia. Accordingly, there have been many recent studies of dopamine receptor density in post-mortem specimens of schizophrenic brains.

Dopamine receptor density in schizophrenia The binding of DA-1 and DA-2 receptor ligands has now been measured in several samples of schizophrenic brains and compared with that of controls (Owen *et al.* 1978; 1981; Lee and Seeman 1980 a,b; MacKay *et al.* 1980; Cross *et al.* 1981; Reynolds *et al.* 1980). No differences have been found in DA-1 receptor binding between the two groups, but most studies have shown a significant increase in DA-2 receptor binding in schizophrenic brains. This difference has been shown for the binding of the DA-2 receptor ligands ^{3}H-haloperidol, ^{3}H-spiroperidol, and ^{3}H-spiperone and is mainly due to increased density of DA-2 receptors although there is also some increase in affinity. The brain areas showing this change include the caudate nucleus, putamen, nucleus accumbens, and olfactory tubercle. Although there was considerable overlap in receptor density between schizophrenics and controls, Owen *et al* (1978) found a mean increase of 100 per cent in ^{3}H-spiroperidol binding in the caudate nucleus of a series of 19 schizophrenic brains, and similar increases were found by Lee and Seeman (1980a,b) in a series of 50 schizophrenic brains. Reynolds *et al* (1980) failed to replicate these findings in a study of ^{3}H-spiperone binding in the putamen in 12 schizophrenic specimens. This negative finding could have been due to differences in technique or in the type of schizophrenic patient studied. A later study (Reynolds *et al.* 1981) suggested that patients with paranoid psychosis tend to show an increase in DA-2 receptor density while patients with non-paranoid psychosis show a significant decrease. Thus, changes in DA-2 receptor density may be related to the type of schizophrenia.

There has been considerable discussion as to whether this finding reflects an abnormality related to the schizophrenic process itelf, or whether it is the result of antipsychotic medication. As discussed in Chapters 6 and 11, chronic exposure to receptor antagonists leads to increases in the density of the antagonized receptors, and the DA-2 antagonist activity of the neuroleptics might be followed by an increase in the numbers of DA-2 receptors. Increases in DA-2 receptor binding have been observed in animals treated chronically with neuroleptics but the increases have been of the order of 25 per cent rather than the 100 per cent increases found in some schizophrenic brains (Snyder 1982).

Several authors have examined the differences in DA-2 receptor density between the brains of neuroleptic treated schizophrenics and those of schizophrenics who either have not had neuroleptic treatment (a sample difficult to obtain) or have had no treatment for some time before death. Results from these studies are conflicting. MacKay *et al.* (1980) found that ^{3}H-spiperone binding in the brains from seven schizophrenic patients who had received no neuroleptic treatment for a month or more before death did not differ from controls, although 21 treated schizophrenics in the same study did show increased binding in the caudate nucleus and nucleus accumbens. This finding suggested that DA-2 receptor density was related to treatment, a view also expressed by Snyder (1981a,b). On the other hand, Owen *et al.* (1978) and Lee and Seeman (1980 a,b) found that DA-2 receptor density was still significantly increased in the brains from schizophrenic patients who had never received neuroleptic medication or who had had no such treatment for at least a year (a total of 16 patients in the two studies). In the study of Lee and Seeman (1980a,b) there was no significant difference in ^{3}H-spiperone and

^{3}H-haloperidol binding in the caudate nucleus or putamen between treated and untreated schizophrenics, and both groups showed a highly significant increase in DA-2 receptor density compared with controls ($P < 0.001$).

The numbers involved in these studies are small and differences in DA-2 receptor density could be due to clinical heterogeneity between treated and untreated groups. However, it is interesting that there is no evidence of an increase in DA-1 receptor density in either treated or untreated schizophrenics. If the rise in DA-2 receptor density is due to neuroleptic medication, a concomitant rise in DA-1 receptors would be expected in at least some patients since many neuroleptics (phenothiazines) also block DA-1 receptors. Cross *et al.* (1981), and Lee and Seeman (1980 a,b) specifically assessed DA-1 receptor binding in schizophrenic brains and found no difference from controls in either treated or untreated subjects. Analysis of DA-2 receptor binding studies in these patients showed that drug-treated subjects showed increases in both DA-2 receptor density and affinity, but drug-free subjects showed increases only in DA-2 receptor density. Thus, increased DA-2 receptor density in limbic structures in schizophrenia may not always be due to neuroleptic medication and there may be a selective increase in DA-2 receptors associated with the disease process in schizophrenia. Such an increase does not appear to be present in all subjects and may be limited to a subgroup of patients or to particular symptoms.

Drawbacks of dopamine theory Despite the findings which seem to suggest supersensitivity of DA-2 receptors in limbic structures in schizophrenia, and a relationship between antagonism of these receptors and the antipsychotic potency of neuroleptic drugs, the dopamine theory of schizophrenia suffers from serious drawbacks. One of these is that antipsychotic drugs do not alleviate all schizophrenic symptoms. Significant drug effects are apparent only for positive symptoms, such as hallucinations, delusions, and thought disorder; there is very little effect on negative symptoms including poverty of speech and flatness of affect (Johnstone *et al.* 1978). Even in patients who respond to drugs, the response is often only partial, and in many instances the drugs appear to control rather than to normalize the psychiatric state. These findings indicate that increased dopamine receptor activation, if present in schizophrenia, is responsible only for some symptoms seen most commonly in the acute forms of the condition. In chronic schizophrenia, dopaminergic overactivity may not be involved at all. Indeed, it has been suggested that negative symptoms may result from dopaminergic underactivity and that they may respond to dopaminergic agonists (Alpert and Friedhof 1980; Chouinard and Jones 1978). Yet positive and negative symptoms may co-exist in both acute and chronic schizophrenia. It is clear that the dopamine hypothesis cannot explain all the phenomena of schizophrenia.

A second drawback of the classical dopamine theory is that, like the antidepressants (Chapter 11), the antipsychotic drugs are associated with a therapeutic time-lag. The antipsychotic effects do not become manifest for some weeks, although the DA-2 receptor antagonism occurs quickly. As shown in Fig. 13.3, the rise in serum prolactin concentration (due to DA-2 receptor blockade in the tuberoinfundibular system) is maximal within 1 week of starting treatment, while the therapeutic effect takes at least 3 weeks to develop (Crow 1979). The discrepancy does not appear to be due to pharmacokinetic factors and suggests that immediate DA-2 receptor antagonism is not directly responsible for antipsychotic effects, which may result from some secondary process with a longer time course. Two such possibilities have been considered: the slow induction of depolarization block of dopamine neurones by neuroleptics, and homeostatic receptor changes involving dopamine autoreceptors.

Depolarization block Recent electrophysiological studies in animals reported by Bunney (1984) indicate that in the neurones of cell group A_{10} (the origin of the mesolimbic pathway) antipsychotic drugs produce a slowly developing depolarization block which has a much greater effect in reducing dopaminergic transmission than the initial dopamine receptor antagonism. The

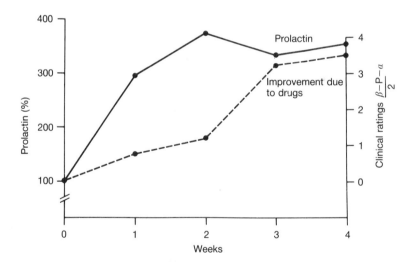

Fig. 13.3. Time course of clinical improvement in schizophrenia and of rise in serum prolactin concentration during antipsychotic treatment. Clinical improvement occurs considerably later than rise in serum prolactin, which is due to dopamine-2 receptor blockade in the tuberoinfundibular system. Improvement due to antipsychotic medication (clinical rating) calculated as scores in patients on active treatment (α-flupenthixol) versus inactive medication (β-flupenthixol, or placebo, P). (From Crow 1979.)

development of this state requires chronic drug administration and occurs over approximately the same time course as the therapeutic delay. Bunney (1984) suggests that the therapeutic effects coincide with this delayed and potent blocking action which affects both pre-synaptic and post-synaptic neuronal sites. It is of interest that with antipsychotic drugs which do not produce extrapyramidal effects (such as clozapine, sulpiride, molindone: Chapter 14), this depolarization block is limited to A_{10} cells, while the other neuroleptics produce depolarization block of A_9 cells in addition.

Dopamine autoreceptors The release of dopamine at synapses (and also its synthesis and metabolism) appears to be partly controlled by complex feedback loops involving cholinergic and GABA-ergic neurones (described later), and partly by dopaminergic autoreceptors (DA-3 receptors, Fig. 13.1, Table 13.5). The evidence for the existence of such autoreceptors and for their functional importance in man and animals is reviewed by Roth (1979) and Meltzer (1980), although their existence is disputed by Laduron (1984). Nevertheless, DA-3 receptors have been identified by behavioural, electrophysiological, pharmacological, and radioligand binding studies. They are located on neuronal cell bodies, dendrites, and nerve terminals, and are present in the nigrostriatal and mesolimbic systems and in the cerbral cortex.

Stimulation of DA-3 receptors by dopamine and dopaminergic agonists decreases dopamine release and hence reduces dopaminergic activity. Autoreceptors are more sensitive than post-psynaptic dopamine receptors to the actions of dopaminergic agonists. Hence, very low concentrations of such agonists can produce 'paradoxical' effects which are the opposite of those of post-psynaptic dopamine receptor stimulation. Very small doses of dopamine agonists (apomorphine and bromocriptine) have been reported (Meltzer 1980) to produce several such effects in man including: (a) sedative effects in normal subjects and in excited psychiatric and neurological states, (b) a specific antischizophrenic effect, (c) a specific antimanic effect, (d) the production of Parkinsonian symptoms in schizophrenics when combined with low doses of a dopamine antagonist, and (e) improvement of symptoms in tardive dyskinesia, Huntingdon's disease and spasmodic torticollis.

Meltzer (1980) cited several studies in which 1 mg of apomorphine given subcutaneously or intramuscularly to unmedicated schizophrenics has produced a rapid, but transient (20–50 min) improvement of many psychotic symptoms including delusions, cognitive disturbances, and bizarre, suspicious, and aggressive behaviour. However, several other studies using different dosages and routes of administration of apomorphine or bromocriptine reported no antipsychotic effects. The use of neuroleptics appears to prevent the antipsychotic effects of apomorphine. These preliminary and rather inconclusive studies suggest that there might be a subgroup of schizophrenics with subsensitive DA-3 receptors and in addition raise the possibility that specific dopamine autoreceptor agonists might have a therapeutic potential in schizophrenia. One such substance, 3-(3-hydroxyphenyl)-N-*n*-propyl-piperidone (3-PPP; Chapter 14) is at present under investigation for this purpose (Nilsson and Carlsson 1982).

It is possible that the delayed therapeutic effects of antipsychotic agents in schizophrenia are due to the development of DA-3 receptor hypersensitivity following continuous receptor antagonism produced by chronic administration. There is some evidence from biochemical studies in animals that neuroleptics have antagonistic actions at DA-3 receptors, although they are less potent than at post-synaptic sites. Loxapine, haloperidol, and spiroperidol appear to have the most potent DA-3 receptor antagonist effects, while chlorpromazine, fluphenazine, and thioridazine are less potent. However, the results have differed in different investigations and it is not clear whether DA-3-blocking potency correlates with antipsychotic potency. There is some biochemical evidence that dopamine autoreceptors can become supersensitive following chronic neuroleptic administration (Meltzer 1980). However in binding studies with ^{3}H-dopamine and ^{3}H-apomorphine, Snyder (1982) found no evidence of increased DA-3 receptor binding following chronic neuroleptic administration in animals, and no increase in DA-3 receptor bindings in post-mortem specimens of brains from schizophrenics who had been treated with antipsychotics.

The importance of DA-3 receptors in schizophrenia and in the antipsychotic actions of antipsychotic drugs is unresolved at present. It remains possible however, that subsensitivity of DA-3 receptors rather than supersensitivity of DA-2 receptors may account for some schizophrenic symptoms or some clinical subtypes of schizophrenia. Schizophrenia could, as has been proposed for affective disorders (Chapter 11), be a reflection of instability of synaptic control mechanisms. DA-3 receptors appear normally to be most active in inhibiting dopamine release when impulse traffic through dopaminergic synapses is high (Meltzer 1980). Presumably, their activity under these conditions prevents excessive stimulation of post-synaptic dopamine receptors. Subsensitivity of DA-3 receptors might render the subject more vulnerable to extremes of dopaminergic hyperactivity. However, the control of dopamine release at synapses is influenced not only by DA-3 receptors but also other neurotransmitter systems, any one of which could be involved in schizophrenia.

GABA and acetylcholine

The release of dopamine from nerve terminals in some parts of the brain appears to be modulated not only by DA-3 receptor activity but also by multitransmitter negative feedback loops (Fig. 13.4). Released dopamine stimulates post-synaptic dopamine receptors situated on cholinergic neurones. These synapse onto GABA-ergic neurones which in turn inhibit

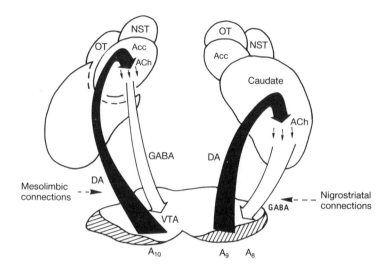

Fig. 13.4. Central cholinergic and GABAergic feedback loops controlling dopamine release. Acc, nucleus accumbens; OT, olfactory tubercle; NST, bed nucleus of the stria terminalia; VTA, ventral tegmental area; $A_{8,9,10}$, cell groups in VTA and substantia nigra; ACh, acetylcholine; DA, dopamine. (Adapted from Stevens 1979.)

the dopamine-releasing neurones. Such feedback loops are thought to constitute a major influence on the firing rate of dopaminergic neurones in the central tegmental area, which project to limbic nuclei, and in the substantia nigra, which project to the corpus striatum (Meltzer 1980; Stevens 1979). Other transmitters and modulators are probably also involved in these feedback loops, but it has been suggested that GABA deficiency in limbic pathways might be a characteristic of some forms of schizophrenia. In one post-mortem study, Perry *et al.* (1979) found reduced concentrations of GABA in the nucleus accumbens and thalamus in the brains of schizophrenic patients. GABA concentrations were similar to those found in Huntingdon's chorea, a known GABA-deficiency disease. However, later investigations have failed to replicate these results (Cross *et al.* 1979; Bennett *et al.* 1979). Treatment of schizophrenia with the GABA analogue baclofen, or with benzodiazepines, which enhance GABA activity, have not given consistently successful results (Davis *et al.* 1976; Frederiksen 1975; Nistri 1975; Trabucchi and Ba 1975) and the importance of GABA-ergic systems in schizophrenia is doubtful.

Similarly, cholinergic dysfunction does not appear to be primarily involved in schizophrenia. Although many neuroleptics have anticholinergic affects, there is no relation between these and antipsychotic potency.

Noradrenaline

The possibility that noradrenergic activity may be altered in schizophrenia has been considered by many authors. Farley *et al.* (1980) reported that concentrations of noradrenaline were significantly increased above control values in specific areas (stria terminalis, ventral septum, and nucleus accumbens) in the brains of four patients dying with chronic paranoid schizophrenia. Lake *et al.* (1980) found that cerebrospinal fluid concentrations of noradrenaline were significantly elevated compared with controls in a series of 35 schizophrenic patients. The elevation of noradrenaline was most marked in patients with paranoid features.

Whether such abnormalities represent overactivity or underactivity of noradrenergic systems is not clear. The fact that many antipsychotic drugs have alpha- and beta-adrenoceptor antagonistic activity suggests that part of their antipsychotic action may be due to adrenoceptor blocking effects. There is no overall correlation between antipsychotic potency and adrenoceptor antagonism, although some drugs such as clozapine are weak dopamine receptor antagonists and yet are effective in schizophrenia, possibly because of alpha-adrenergic effects (Snyder 1982). Clonidine, which stimulates alpha$_2$-adrenergic receptors and hence reduces noradrenaline release, was found to be as effective as neuroleptics in alleviating positive schizophrenic symptoms in a small preliminary placebo-controlled trial (Freedman *et al.* 1982). Therapeutic effectiveness has also been claimed for the beta adrenoceptor antagonist propranolol (Gruzelier and Yorkston 1978; Yorkstone *et al.* 1974, 1977a,b). Propranolol also appears to increase the therapeutic efficiency of neuroleptics, although this may be due to pharmacokinetic factors (Peet 1981); high doses of propranolol may in addition have central anti-serotonergic activity (Harrison-Read 1984). The results suggest that increased noradrenergic activity might be a feature of some forms of schizophrenia, especially since antidepressant drugs (Chapter 12) and amphetamine, which releases noradrenaline as well as dopamine, can aggravate schizophrenia.

However, Mason (1983), on the basis of an animal model, proposed the opposite hypothesis and suggested that schizophrenic symptoms may result from underactivity of noradrenergic pathways in the dorsal bundle, which contains fibres originating in the locus coeruleus, projects to many parts of the brain, and forms part of the reward system of the brain (Chapter 5). This hypothesis, which has been criticized by Reynolds (1984) and Harrison-Read (1984), awaits further evidence. Stein *et al.* (1977) also suggested that lack of noradrenergic activity in reward pathways from the locus coeruleus might account for the anhedonia and perhaps other features of chronic schizophrenia, while Hartmann (1976) proposed that deficient functioning in brain noradrenergic systems night account for a deficit in central feedback processing of sensory input in schizophrenia. An imbalance between activity of functionally interdependent dopaminergic, noradrenergic, and serotonergic pathways connected in series in limbic pathways has also been suggested to occur in schizophrenia (Cools 1975). However, there is no clear evidence of noradrenergic under- or over-activity in schizophrenia, or of a direct causal link between noradrenergic systems and this condition.

Transmethylation and endogenous psychotogens

Catecholamines are normally metabolized by orthomethylation and there has been considerable interest in the past in various theories suggesting that aberrant methylation in schizophrenia might result in the accumulation of psychotomimetic substances. These theories, which are reviewed by Gillin *et al.* (1978), Baldessarini *et al.* (1979), Bowers (1980), Barchas *et al.* (1977), and Smythies (1984), are based on the observation that some drugs which produce psychotomimetic effects have close structural similarities to endogenous substances. For example, mescaline is structurally related to catechol amines, amphetamine differs little from phenylethylamine, and LSD has structural similarities to serotonin. Potentially hallucinogenic substances including phenylethylamine (Sandler and Reynolds 1976), dimethyl-tryptamine (Murray and Oon 1976), and O-methylbufotenin (Smythies 1984), are formed endogenously in small amounts in humans. The psychotic symptoms produced by these compounds respond to neuroleptic drugs; however, there is no evidence that the production of such endogenous psychotogens is increased in schizophrenia.

A modification of the older hypotheses has been proposed by Smythies (1984) who suggests that schizophrenia, as well as psychotic depression and mania, may be associated with alterations in the kinetics of the transmethylation system. The overall rate of transmethylation was found to be slower than normal in some schizophrenics and faster than normal in some depressives. Some schizophrenics therefore appear to have under-active methylation systems, a defect which would presumably lead to decrease in the rate of metabolism by orthomethylation of catechol amines. In contrast, some patients with depression appear to have over-active methylation systems. It has always been a mystery why methionine, a methyl donor, produces an acute psychotic reaction in 40 per cent of schizophrenics (Reynolds *et al.* 1984). Smythies (1984) suggests that these represent the subgroup with under-active methylation systems.

Serotonin

The effects of LSD (Chapter 14), have been claimed to have important similarities to schizophrenic symptomatology. LSD can produce psychotic reactions in normal subjects and can aggravate symptoms in schizophrenia. Young (1974) made a phenomenological comparison of LSD effects and schizophrenic states and concluded that the similarities were more striking than the differences. Claridge (1978) found that LSD produced changes in the covariance between measures of central perception and autonomic arousal that were similar to these found in schizophrenic patients and normal subjects with high psychoticism scores. LSD appears to facilitate impulse flow in the afferent collaterals into the reticular formation (Chapter 2, Bradley 1957). It may therefore have the effect of flooding the reticular formation with unfiltered sensory information and cause alterations in perception and arousal which are similar to those which occur in schizophrenia.

Since LSD acts on serotonergic receptors (Chapter 14), it has been suggested that there might be a disorder of serotoninergic activity in schizophrenia. However, no abnormalities have been found in the concentrations of serotonin, serotonin metabolites, or the serotonin precursor tryptophan in schizophrenic brains (Crow 1978c). A report of alterations in serotonin receptor binding in schizophrenic brains (Bennett *et al.* 1979) was not confirmed in a later study (Whitaker *et al.* 1981). At present there is no definite evidence that serotonergic mechanisms are of central importance in schizophrenia.

Opioids and other endogenous polypeptides

There are many reasons for suspecting that endogenous opioids are somehow involved in schizophrenia. Enkephalins and other opioids coexist in monoaminergic neurones and are coreleased with dopamine and noradrenaline in limbic areas, including the ventral tegmental area and the locus coeruleus (Lundberg and Hokfelt 1983). Opioid receptors are present on dopaminergic nerve terminals in the corpus striatum and mesolimbic regions (Reisine *et al.* 1980). Endogenous opioids have been shown to stimulate dopaminergic activity in the mesolimbic system (Koob and Bloom 1983). Such opioid-dopamine interactions provide a possible interface by which opioid systems could affect activity in pathways which appear to be involved in schizophrenia (Koob and Bloom 1983).

Large doses of opiate narcotics administered systemically, and intra-cisternally injected enkephalin and beta-endorphin, produce in animals a naloxone reversible state of immobilization and generalized muscular rigidity. This state is accompanied by seizure discharges in the limbic system (Smith and Copolov 1979) and bears a certain resemblance to the catatonic syndrome seen in some forms of schizophrenia, an observation which led to the suggestion that schizophrenia might be associated with excessive endogenous opioid activity in the brain. However, the postural rigidity also has a similarity to a cataleptic state induced by high doses of neuroleptics; this interpretation led to the suggestion that schizophrenia might be associated with a deficiency of endogenous neuroleptic opioids. The evidence relating to these theories is discussed by MacKay (1981), Koob and Bloom (1983),

Smith and Copolov (1979), van Ree and de Wied (1981), and van Praag and Verhoeven (1981).

Opioid excess hypothesis Terenius (1980), Rimon *et al.* (1980), and Wahlstrom and Terenius (1981) found increased cerebrospinal fluid concentrations of Fraction I and II endorphin-like substance in acute schizophrenic patients compared with control subjects. Concentrations of these fractions decreased after neuroleptic treatment and clinical improvement. However, the precise nature of these fractions has not been determined and they do not correspond to known endogenous polypeptides. Domschke *et al.* (1979) reported a significant increase compared with controls in cerebrospinal fluid concentrations of beta-endorphin in five acute schizophrenics, and a significant decrease in seven chronic schizophrenics. Dupont *et al.* (1978) also reported a decrease in cerebrospinal fluid concentration of enkephalin-like material in chronic schizophrenics. These studies are limited by technological difficulties in identifying endogenous opioids but suggest that central opioid-like activity may be increased in acute but decreased in chronic schizophrenia.

Studies of post-mortem schizophrenic brains have not revealed changes in beta-endorphin-like immunoreactivity (Lightman *et al.* 1979). However, Reisine *et al.* (1980) studied opioid receptor binding with ³H-naloxone in the brains of schizophrenics and found a significant decrease in binding in the caudate nucleus in neuroleptic-free patients. It was suggested that this could be due to an adaptive response to abnormally high concentrations of endogenous opioids during life.

If schizophrenic symptoms result from an increase in endogenous opioid concentrations, they would be expected to respond to opioid antagonists. Naloxone in very high doses has been reported to cause a reduction in hallucinations in a few controlled studies, and improvement in catatonic stupour after high dose (up to 400 mg) infusions of naloxone has also been observed (Smith and Copolov 1979). Smaller doses of naloxone (0.4–20 mg) in several other studies have produced variable results but a transient antihallucinogenic effect has been observed in about 30 per cent of patients (van Ree and de Wied 1981). Naloxone is very short-acting (Chapter 7) but naltrexone, a long-acting opioid antagonist, (200–800 mg daily for 1 or 2 weeks) was compared with placebo in schizophrenic patients by Gitlin *et al.* (1981) and Watson *et al.* (1979). There was no alteration in schizophrenic symptoms and no effect suggestive of an opiate withdrawal syndrome. On the whole, drug studies have not produced impressive clinical results in schizophrenia, apart from a possible reduction of hallucinations in some patients.

In spite of the inconclusive clinical results, physiological studies suggest that there may be functional over-activity in some opioid-mediated systems in schizophrenia. Relative insensitivity to pain and reduced somatosensory evoked potentials to painful stimuli have been clearly demonstrated in schizophrenic patients (Davies and Buchsbaumm 1981; Davies *et al.* 1979). In these patients, naltrexone has analgesic effects and increases the magnitude of the somatosensory evoked potentials. However, visual and auditory evoked potentials may also be reduced in amplitude in schizophrenia, and increased activity in endogenous opioid pathways may be a non-specific phenomenon related to stress. Amir *et al.* (1981) proposed that certain genetically predisposed (schizoid) individuals have an inherently labile endogenous opioid system which responds to stress by hypersecretion. Repeated hypersecretion following recurrent psychological stress may lead to increased dopaminergic activity in the brain and precipitate psychotic symptoms.

Opioid deficiency hypothesis Studies of the cerebrospinal fluid concentration of endogenous opioids, mentioned above, have suggested a possible deficiency of these substances in some chronic schizophrenics. The decreases in naloxone binding in the brain in schizophrenics reported by Reisine *et al.* (1980) could be interpreted as a primary deficiency of opioid receptors rather than as an adaptive change. If a deficiency of endogenous opioids does occur in schizophrenia, a therapeutic response to opioid drugs would be expected. Narcotic analgesics such as morphine and methadone, however, do not appear to have antipsychotic effects. In several studies (cited in van Ree and de Wied 1981, and van Praag and Verhoeven 1981) intravenous beta-endorphin produced an initial worsening of symptoms in schizophrenics, followed by a delayed but slight improvement for several days. A longer-acting synthetic analogue of enkephalin (FK 33-824) has been tested in a few studies on schizophrenic patients and found to produce an initial aggravation of symptoms, accompanied by morphine-like adverse effects, followed by a delayed, but undramatic improvement. In some of these patients the drug caused a striking reduction of hallucinations (Jorgensen *et al.* 1979). On the whole, however, the results with opioid treatment in schizophrenia have been unpromising.

Gamma-type endorphins Although neither opioid excess nor opioid deficiency have been convincingly demonstrated in schizophrenia, some interesting data has emerged concerning the possible involvement of (Des-tyrosynyl-1) -gamma-endorphin (DT gamma endorphin). This polypeptide is a daughter fragment of beta-endorphin; it has been demonstrated in the rat brain and pituitary, and in human cerebrospinal fluid. Its actions in animals and man are described by van Ree *et al.* (1981 1982), van Ree and de Wied (1982), van Ree (1982a,b,c), Verhoeven *et al.* (1979), van Praag and Verhoeven (1981), and Lamberts *et al.* (1982).

DT gamma endorphin is almost devoid of morphine-like activity, but it produces naltrexone-reversible behavioural effects in animals which are very similar to the behavioural effects exerted by neuroleptic drugs. The compound (1 mg DT gamma endorphin phosphate injected intramuscularly for 8 days) appeared to produce definite and sometimes marked overall improvement in schizophrenic patients who had not responded to antipsychotic drugs (Verhoeven *et al.* 1978 1979). The effects were apparent in acute schizophrenia, but only small numbers of patients have been treated in open and double blind trials, and Manchanda and Hirsch (1981) were unable to confirm the results.

The actions of DT gamma endorphin may be mediated by an effect on dopaminergic neurones. The polypeptide appears to antagonize selectively opioid-induced dopamine release by increasing the sensitivity of dopamine autoreceptors (van van Ree and de Wied 1981). These authors suggest that in schizophrenia a metabolic error (either decreased formation or increased inactivation) leads to a deficiency of DT gamma endorphin. As a result, dopamine autoreceptors are subsensitive and the set point for feedback regulation of neurones in the mesolimbic system is abnormal, causing a sustained increase in dopaminergic activity. This theory, which has yet to be substantiated, links endogenous gamma endorphin polypeptides to dopamine theories of schizophrenia and suggests that acute schizophrenia, like the affective disorders (Chapter 11), might result from disturbance of synaptic homeostatic mechanisms.

Other biochemical theories

Many other hypotheses of schizophrenia have been advanced. The condition has been linked *inter alia* with zinc deficiency, folate deficiency, gluten sensitivity, hyperallergy, and pineal gland dysfunction. Some of these ideas have been synthesized by Horrobin (1977 1979) who proposed an underlying metabolic error leading to a deficiency of prostaglandins of the I series. At present no strong evidence for any of these theories has appeared and prostaglandin E concentrations have been found to be higher than normal in the cerebrospinal fluid of schizophrenics (Mathe *et al.* 1980). The numerous theories no doubt reflect the presence of many non-specific factors in schizophrenia and the probable heterogeneity of its causes.

At present the strongest biochemical and pharmacological evidence, which cannot be lightly dismissed, suggests an involvement of dopaminergic mesolimbic and mesocortical pathways, perhaps mediated through an endogenous opioid-related polypeptide mechanisms, in schizophrenia. Such pathways may be vulnerable to structural or functional disruption by anoxia and many other factors. An initial hyperactive phase, responding to antipsychotic medication, may be followed by a phase of permanent damage which is resistant to pharmacological manipulation. The actions of antipsychotic drugs and psychotomimetic agents, discussed in the next chapter, provide further evidence on this question.

14
Antipsychotic and psychotomimetic drugs

The antipsychotic drugs are a chemically heterogenous group with the property of controlling certain psychotic symptoms in man. The earlier drugs, reserpine and chlorpromazine, were described by Delay and Deniker (1952) as neuroleptics, a term which differentiated their effects from those of classical central nervous system depressants. The neuroleptic syndrome consisted of suppression of spontaneous movements, disinterest in the environment, lack of emotional response, but little change in the level of consciousness. At the same time, neurological effects resembling Parkinsonism were described in the early reports, and for a while it was thought that these effects were inevitably connected with the antipsychotic effects. Some of the newer drugs, however, are relatively free of extrapyramidal effects and the term antipsychotic applies better than the term neuroleptic to the whole range of drugs.

Classification

The pharmacological profiles of the antipsychotic agents have many similarities which, as discussed below, depend on their ability to antagonize dopamine receptors in the brain. There are, however, considerable differences in potency and in the liability to produce adverse effects. Structure-activity relationships are discussed by Schmutz and Picard (1980).

The drugs are classified by chemical group, as shown in Table 14.1, which also indicates frequency of incidence of various adverse effects. Classical or standard antipsychotic drugs include the phenothiazines, butyrophenones, and thioxanthines. Pimozide, a long acting agent, is more specific in its antipsychotic effects than the standard agents. Some more recently introduced agents, such as molindone and sulpiride, also seem to be more specific in their actions and are sometimes termed atypical antipsychotic agents. Thioridazine, a phenothiazine, which is less likely than others of this group to produce extrapyramidal effects, is sometimes classed as an atypical agent. Clozapine, another atypical agent, was the subject of many studies and is mentioned below although it has since been withdrawn. Finally there are several new experimental agents such as 3-PPP [3-(3-hydroxyphenyl)-N-*n*-propylpiperidine] under investigation.

407

Table 14.1. Some antipsychotic drugs

Drugs and chemical groups	Incidence of effects at antipsychotic dosage[1]			
	Extrapyramidal effects	Antiemetic effects	Sedative effects	Hypotensive effects
Phenothiazines				

Aliphatic side-chain
    chlorpromazine
    promazine
	++	++	+++	++

Piperidine side-chain
    thioridazine
    mesoridazine
	+	+	++	++

Piperazine side-chain
    trifluoperazine
    perchlorperazine
    perphenazine
    fluphenazine[2]
	+++	+++	++	+

Butyrophenones
  haloperidol
  benperidol
  droperidol
  trifluperidol
	+++	+++	++	+

Thioxanthines
  chlorprothixine
  thiothixine
  flupenthixol
  clopenthixol
	++	++	++	++

Diphenylbutylpiperazines
  pimozide
  fluspirilene[2]
	++	+	+	+

Dibenzodiazepines
  loxapine
  clozapine[3]
	+	+	+	+

Dihydroindole molindone	+	o	++	o
Substituted benzamide sulpiride	+	+	+	o

1. Incidence of effects: + =low; + + =moderate; + + + =high.
2. Depot preparations.
3. Withdrawn from clinical use.
References: Rogers *et al.*1981; Baldessarini 1980.

Pharmacokinetics

The pharmacokinetics of the antipsychotic drugs have not been fully worked out because of technical difficulties in measurement and the multiplicity of metabolites. However, sensitive radioreceptor assay methods are now available and further pharmacokinetic information is becoming available. Reviews are provided by Muller-Oerlinghansen (1980) and Breyer-Pfaff (1980). In general, the drugs tend to be erratically absorbed, have large apparent volumes of distribution, and are concentrated in the brain. In blood, they are highly protein bound and have long elimination half-lives. They are extensively metabolized in the liver to form several metabolites, some of which may be pharmacologically active. Steady state plasma concentration varies at least ten-fold between individuals on the same dose.

Steady-state plasma concentration and therapeutic effect

The problems of relating steady state plasma concentration of antipsychotic drugs to their therapeutic effects in schizophrenia have been discussed by Grahame-Smith and Orr (1978). One of the problems is the heterogeneity of the schizophrenic syndrome. Some patients will not respond to drugs whatever the plasma concentration; others may improve irrespective of medication. There may nevertheless be a group of patients in whom clinical response is related to plasma drug concentrations and pharmacodynamic drug effects. Yet within the group, some symptoms may respond to drugs but not others, and the improvement may be related to the formation of active metabolites rather than to the effects of the parent drug. In general it appears that the best response to antipsychotic drugs occurs in patients with acute schizophrenic episodes and positive symptoms. In these patients there is probably an optimal therapeutic range of antipsychotic drug concentration.

Depot preparations

Compliance with oral medication is particularly low in schizophrenia; the absorption of most oral preparations is erratic; and in many cases the requirement for medication is indefinite. For these reasons, depot preparations offer considerable advantages for maintenance therapy. These preparations consist of fatty acid esters of phenothiazines in an oily solution. When injected intramuscularly the duration of action is 2–4 weeks. Long acting depot neuroleptics have proved successful in preventing relapses of schizophrenia (Daniels 1976; Capstick 1980, Zander et al. 1981; Nishikawa et al. 1982). They can also be used in acutely disturbed paients, but are unsuitable for initiation of therapy.

Biochemical actions

Dopamine receptor antagonism

The antipsychotic drugs exert a wide range of biochemical effects which differ between drug groups, but an action common to them all is antagonism of dopamine receptors in the central nervous system. It is this action which appears to be related to their therapeutic effects in schizophrenia.

Acute effects The evidence for dopamine receptor antagonism by antipsychotic drugs is summarized by Iverson and Iverson (1981), Carlsson (1978), Bunney (1984), Baldessarini (1980), Bartholini and Lloyd (1980), and Ackenheil (1980). The drugs selectively increase the rate of release and turnover of dopamine in the animal brain, as shown by increased formation of dopamine metabolites and increased incorporation of radioactively labelled tyrosine into dopamine. Increased concentrations of dopamine metabolites have also been demonstrated in the cerebrospinal fluid in man after administration of antipsychotic drugs. This increase in dopamine turnover has been interpreted as the consequence of increased firing rates of dopaminergic neurones responding homeostatically to receptor blockade through cholinergic and GABAergic feedback loops (Chapter 13). Direct neurophysiological recordings of the activity of dopaminergic neurones in cell groups A_9 and A_{10} have shown an increase in firing rate after acute administration of drugs which have antipsychotic effects but not after administration of chemical analogues without antipsychotic potency (Bunney 1984).

Secondly, antipsychotic drugs antagonize the physiological and behavioural effects of drugs which directly or indirectly stimulate dopamine receptors. For example, the psychotic reaction induced in man by high doses of amphetamine is readily reversed by antipsychotic agents. Similarly, the emetic effect of apomorphine, which is due to direct stimulation of dopamine receptors in the chemoreceptor trigger zone of the medullary vomiting centre, can be prevented by antipsychotic agents. In animals, a variety of behavioural effects of dopamine receptor agonists are reversed by antipsychotic agents, and this effect is of predictive value in screening for new antischizophrenic drugs (Carlsson 1978). The increased release of prolactin and the extrapyramidal effects exerted by most antipsychotic drugs have likewise been shown to be due to dopamine receptor antagonism.

Biochemical studies also demonstrate antagonism of dopamine receptors in the central nervous system. Some antipsychotic agents inhibit the dopamine-stimulated formation of cyclic AMP in homogenates of dopamine-rich brain areas (Iverson and Iverson 1981). This effect is due to antagonism of dopamine-1 (DA-1) receptors which are coupled to adenylate cyclase (Chapter 13). For many phenothiazines and thioxanthenes the potency of this effect correlates with clinical potency in schizophrenia. Of particular importance was the finding that only the alpha isomer of flupenthixol and only the (+) isomer of butaclamol (a drug with a related tricyclic structure) have dopamine antagonist activity, and only these isomers have antipsychotic effects.

However, the butyrophenones and benzamides, which are clinically potent, have only weak DA-1 receptor antagonist activity. Later studies showed that these drugs, as well as all other antipsychotics, compete with radioligands such as ^{3}H-haloperidol and ^{3}H-Spiperone for dopamine-2 (DA-2) binding sites in the brain and the rank order of potency of antipsychotics in inhibiting ^{3}H-haloperidol binding correlates very closely with their clinical potency in schizophrenia (Fig. 14.1). As discussed in Chapter 13, this finding suggested that the antipsychotic effects of these drugs are due to antagonism of DA-2 receptors and raised the possibility that schizophrenia is associated with increased DA-2 receptor sensitivity.

The antipsychotic drugs also antagonize dopamine autoreceptors (Creese 1983; Chapter 13), which are found on dopaminergic terminals in the corpus striatum and on the cell bodies of the dopaminergic neurones in the A_9 and A_{10} cell groups. Their normal effect on stimulation is inhibition of dopamine synthesis and release, and part of the increase in dopamine turnover found on acute administration of antipsychotic drugs (mentioned above) is due to drug antagonism at dopamine autoreceptors. Acute administration of all antipsychotic drugs increases the firing rate of A_{10} cells, but it is interesting that those which give rise to extrapyramidal effects also increase the firing rate of A_9 cells, while atypical antipsychotics such as clozapine and thioridazine, which rarely cause extrapyramidal effects, appear to have selective actions on A_{10} cells only (Creese 1983).

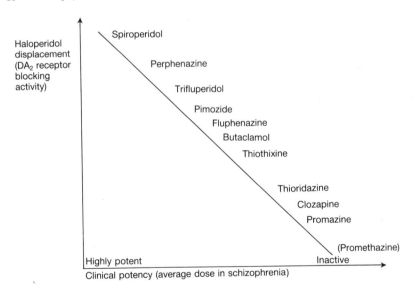

Fig. 14.1. Diagram of the relationship between dopamine-2 receptor binding activity and clinical potency of antipsychotic drugs. DA-2 receptor binding (measured as potency of haloperidol displacement from binding sites) plotted against clinical potency (measured as average therapeutic dose in schizophrenia).

The evidence seems clear that all the antipsychotic drugs in clinical use block dopamine receptors in the brain. Many of the drugs have antagonist activity over the full range of DA-1, DA-2, and dopamine autoreceptors. Antagonism at DA-1 receptors does not appear to be necessary for an antipsychotic effect, while there is a good correlation, which includes all the drugs, between DA-2 receptor binding affinity and antischizophrenic potency. The importance of antagonism at dopamine autoreceptors is not yet clear.

A feature of most of the drugs is that they are non-selective in their sites of action, antagonizing dopamine receptors in all the dopaminergic pathways (Chapter 13). This widespread effect gives the drugs their characteristic profile of pharmacological effects, both adverse and therapeutic. Dopamine receptor antagonism in the nigrostriatal pathway may be related to the development of Parkinsonism and other extrapyramidal effects. Antagonism in the tubero-infundibular pathway results in neuroendocrine effects including a rise in prolactin secretion. Dopamine receptor antagonism at the chemoreceptor trigger zone confers on many antipsychotic drugs their antiemetic property. Finally, antagonistic effects on dopamine receptors in the mesolimbic and mesocortical pathways appears to be associated with antipsychotic effects. Several of the atypical, antipsychotic drugs have relatively selective actions at this site.

A new approach to the development of antypsychotic agents is a search for drugs which selectively stimulate dopamine autoreceptors, thus reducing dopamine synthesis and release. The properties of such a dopamine auto-receptor agonist, 3-PPP (3-(3-hydroxyphenyl)-N-n-propyldiperidine) are described by Nilsson and Carlson (1982).

Chronic effects Dopamine receptor antagonism in the mesolimbic pathway does not, however, by itself explain the therapeutic effects of antipsychotic drugs in schizophrenia. As discussed in Chapter 13, there is a delay of some weeks before therapeutic effects are apparent, although dopamine receptor blockade occurs immediately, as demonstrated in behavioural, biochemical, and electrophysiological studies. The different time course of the increase in prolactin secretion (due to dopamine receptor blockade in the hypothalamus) and clinical improvement in schizophrenic patients treated with alpha-flupenthixol is shown in Fig. 13.4. The Parkinsonian effects of antipsychotic drugs are also slow to develop and tend to coincide with the onset of antipsychotic activity, while tardive dyskinesia (described below) takes even longer to appear. Yet neither Parkinsonism nor tardive dyskinesia are essential for therapeutic response in schizophrenia; some patients never develop these adverse reactions while some effective antipsychotic agents rarely produce them.

Could the therapeutic time lag, and the delayed development of Parkinsonism and tardive dyskinesia be a result of adaptive changes in dopamine receptors induced by chronic administration of antipsychotic drugs? The subject of receptor modulation following long-term drug treatment has been discussed in general in Chapter 6 and in relation to antidepressant drugs in Chapter 11. There is no doubt that antipsychotic drugs cause changes in receptor density and sensitivity when repeatedly administered. The possible relationship of such changes to their effects in schizophrenia are discussed by Creese and Snyder (1980).

(i) Post-synaptic receptors. Many investigations have shown that dopamine receptors in the corpus striatum become supersensitive when chronically deprived of agonist supply. Thus denervation by injection of 6-hydroxy-dopamine into the substantia nigra, inhibition of dopamine synthesis by alpha-methyl-paratyrosine, or dopamine depletion with reserpine, all produce behavioural supersensitivity to the motor effects of dopamine agonists in animals, and an increase by 100–120 per cent in the binding of DA-2 receptor ligands (such as ^{3}H-haloperidol) in the corpus striatum. Similarly, chronic treatment with many antipsychotic drugs is followed by apomorphine supersensitivity and a 20–30 per cent increase in striatal ^{3}H-haloperidol binding which is due mainly to increased receptor density (Creese and Snyder 1980). Drugs such as promethazine which have little dopamine antagonistic activity and little antipsychotic potency do not produce these changes.

As discussed in Chapter 13, chronic neuroleptic treatment in man also appears to increase DA-2 receptor binding in both striatal and limbic structures, (Snyder 1981a,b). It is possible that increased receptor density is also associated with the schizophrenic process itself since some studies have shown increased DA-2 receptor density in a small number of unmedicated schizophrenic patients (Lee and Seeman 1980a,b). However, receptor binding appears to be higher in patients who have received antipsychotic drugs than in those who have not (Reynolds et al. 1981). No changes have been observed in DA-1 receptor density in schizophrenic brains.

Animal and human studies thus agree that chronic treatment with antipsychotic drugs can lead to adaptive increases in DA-2 receptor sensitivity. It is possible that this change accounts for the late appearance of tardive dyskinesia (see below), but it is highly unlikely that such a change could account for the therapeutic effects of the drugs in schizophrenia or for the development of Parkinsonism. Considerable evidence, discussed in Chapter 13, suggests that some schizophrenic symptoms are associated with increased DA-2 receptor activation in the limbic system, while it is well established that Parkinson's disease results from a dopaminergic deficit in the nigrostriatal system. The development of DA-2 receptor supersensitivity in response to drug treatment would therefore be expected to aggravate rather than ameliorate schizophrenic symptoms and to reverse rather than precipitate Parkinsonian symptoms.

(ii) Autoreceptors. An alternative possibility is a long-term effect on dopamine autoreceptors, which are also antagonized by antipsychotic drugs (Creese 1983). The development of dopamine autoreceptor hypersensitivity would result in a decrease of dopamine synthesis and release, and a consequent reduction of activity in dopaminergic pathways. There is some evidence that such an effect does occur. In both humans and animals the increase in dopamine synthesis and turnover initially produced by antipsychotic drugs becomes attenuated with continued treatment, possibly as a result of increased dopamine autoreceptor sensitivity (Bartholini and Lloyd 1980; Ackenheil 1980; Belleroche and Bradford 1981). List and Seeman (1980) found that chronic treatment with antipsychotic agents produced a 28 per cent increase in ^{3}H-dopamine binding in the rat brain. This ligand binds preferentially to dopamine autoreceptors and the finding thus suggests an increase in their density. Gallagher et al. (1978) produced electrophysiological evidence of pre-synaptic supersensitivity in dopaminergic neurones of the rat substantia nigra following chronic haloperidol treatment. Total inhibition of firing of these cells was induced by intravenous dosage with 80 g/kg of apomorphine before haloperidol treatment; after chronic haloperidol dosing, total inhibition of firing occured after only 10 g/kg of apomorphine. The development of supersensitivity was blocked by the chronic administration of lithium. Meltzer (1980) discusses other biochemical evidence for dopamine autoreceptor hyperresponsivity in rats following chronic antipsychotic drug medication. On the other hand, Snyder (1982) found no increase in autoreceptor binding in rats and no increase in post-mortem brains of schizophrenic patients who had received long-term medication with antipsychotic drugs.

The question remains unresolved at present. However, it is probable that both pre- and post-synaptic receptor hypersensitivity is a normal adaptive response to chronic treatment with antipsychotic drugs and to dopamine receptor antagonists in general. The situation may be similar to the effects of antidepressant drugs at noradrenergic synapses (Chapter 11). The opposing receptor adaptations would tend to cancel out in terms of overall dopaminergic transmission, but it is possible that together they would confer a greater stability at dopaminergic synapses. This effect may be of therapeutic value for some schizophrenic symptoms (Chapter 13), but it does not convincingly account for all the delayed actions of the antipsychotic drugs.

(iii) Depolarization blockade. Another explanation for the time dependent effects of these drugs is provided by recent electrophysiological recordings of dopaminergic neurone activity in the substantia nigra (A_9 cells) and ventral tegmentum (A_{10} cells; Bunney 1984; White and Wang 1983; Creese 1983). The acute effect of antipsychotic drugs is an increase in firing rate of dopaminergic neurones, as a consequence of pre- and post-synaptic receptor antagonism. Chronic treatment, however, is followed by an almost complete silencing of these neurones. This electrical silence was shown to be due to depolarization blockade since activity could be reinstated by hyperpolarizing agents such as GABA, but not by depolarizing agents such as glutamate. Direct intracellular recording confirmed the presence of tonic depolarization, and the cells could be induced to fire by the injection of a hyperpolarizing current. Lesioning studies show that the depolarization block is not due to a local effect on neurone cell bodies but depends on the presence of innervated pathways. It is presumed that the block develops as a result of post-synaptic and possibly presynaptic dopamine receptor antagonism.

Examination of the brain sites involved in depolarization block showed that all the antipsychotic drugs studied produced depolarization in cells of the A_{10} area, the origin of the mesolimbic and mesocortical pathways (Table 14.2). Classical antipsychotic drugs (chlorpromazine, haloperidol) also silenced cells of the A_9 area, but the firing of these cells was not affected by atypical antipsychotic agents (thioridazine, sulpiride) which have a low liability to produce Parkinsonism. Drugs without antipsychotic activity (metoclopramide, promethazine) did not affect the firing of A_{10} cells, although metoclopramide, which can produce extrapyramidal effects, did decrease the firing of A_9 cells. Thus there was a relationship between the pharmacological profiles of the drugs and their blocking affects on A_{10} and A_9 cells. The tonic depolarization began to develop after a week of treatment and was observed to be still maintained at 8 weeks. There was a subpopulation of cells in both A_9 and A_{10} areas which continued to fire despite chronic treatment. These cells were shown to project to the prefrontal or cingulate cortex and to lack autoreceptors. It is possible that the absence of autoreceptors may be connected with resistance to antipsychotic-induced depolarization block.

These results can tentatively be extrapolated to account for the clinical effects of antipsychotic drugs in schizophrenia (Bunney 1984; Creese 1983). The acute action of the drugs in blocking post-synaptic dopaminergic receptors leads to a compensatory increase in dopaminergic activity, as observed in the initial increase in neuronal firing rate. This increased activity, combined with the drug's blocking effect on autoreceptors, results in an increased synaptic release of dopamine. The extra molecules of released dopamine compete with the drug for receptor sites and so reduce the effectiveness of the drug-induced receptor antagonism. Under these circumstances the drug is not very effective in producing either therapeutic or extrapyramidal effects. However, as depolarization block develops with chronic administration, the homeostatic mechanisms fail; the neurones become inactivated, and synaptic dopamine release is reduced. At this stage, the blockade of the dopamine receptor by the drug becomes increasingly effective, allowing clinical improvement and neurological adverse effects to emerge. Clinical improvement is related to the development of depolarization block in A_{10} cells and their terminals, and extrapyramidal effects to depolarization block in A_9

Table 14.2. Effects of antipsychotic drugs and therapeutically inactive analogues on spontaneous firing rates of midbrain dopaminergic neurones after acute and chronic administration

Change in number of cells firing spontaneously

	A_{10} cells; ventral tegmental area (projections to mesolimbic and mesocortical pathways)		A_9 cells; substantial nigra (projections to nigrostriatal and nigrocortical pathways)	
	Acute	Chronic	Acute	Chronic
Antipsychotic drugs				
chlorpromazine	increase	decrease	increase	decrease
haloperidol	increase	decrease	increase	decrease
clozapine	increase	decrease	?increase?no change*	?increase?no change*
molindone	increase	decrease	no change	no change
thioridazine	increase	decrease	no change	no change
L-sulpiride	increase	decrease	?increase?no change*	?increase?no change*
Inactive analogues				
promethazine	no change	no change	no change	no change
D-sulpiride	no change	no change	no change	no change
metoclopramide	no change	no change	increase	decrease

* Conflicting results from different studies.
Reference: Bunney 1984.

cells. The fact that atypical antipsychotic drugs which lack neurological adverse effects fail to inactivate A_9 cells, but (like classical antipsychotics) produce depolarization block in A_{10} cells is consistent with this interpretation. The time-course of the depolarization block also coincides roughly with the time-course of clinical effects.

This explanation remains speculative and the mechanism whereby depolarization block is produced by the drugs is not known. However, the electrophysiological findings strengthen the evidence from other sources that the therapeutic effects of the antipsychotic drugs are, eventually, due to dopamine receptor blockade in mesolimbic pathways, Nevertheless, these drugs also have effects in many other neurotransmitter systems which, as discussed in Chapter 13, may be involved in schizophrenia.

Effects on cholinergic activity

As mentioned in Chapter 13 (see also Fig. 13.5), there are reciprocal feedback connections between dopaminergic, cholinergic, and GABAergic neurones in many parts of the brain. Activity in these circuits is influenced in a complex manner by the actions of antipsychotic drugs. In the corpus striatum, some cholinergic interneurones appear to be under a tonic inhibitory influence from dopaminergic neurones. Dopamine receptor blockade by antipsychotic agents releases these neurones from inhibitory control and results in an increase in striatal turnover of acetylcholine (Bartholini and Lloyd 1980). This effect is not due to anticholinergic properties of the neuroleptics since it occurs with haloperidol which has little anticholinergic activity, and does not occur with potent anticholinergic drugs such as atropine. By contrast, dopamine receptor agonists and electrical stimulation of dopaminergic neurones in the substantia nigra decrease acetylcholine liberation while dopamine receptor blockers, including drugs without antipsychotic effects (metoclopramide), increase striatal acetylcholine turnover. The production of Parkinsonian symptoms such as rigidity and tremor by antipsychotic drugs is probably the consequence of striatal cholinergic hyperactivity secondary to the dopamine receptor blockade (Bartholini and Lloyd 1980). These drug-induced symptoms are markedly alleviated by anticholinergic drugs.

In addition to these indirect effects on cholinergic transmission, many antipsychotic drugs, especially phenothiazines, have direct cholinergic (muscarinic) receptor antagonistic activity. In general the likelihood of production of extrapyramidal effects is inversely related to potency of anticholinergic action (Richelson 1981). The lack of Parkinsonian effects of atypical antipsychotic agents such as clozapine and thioridazine may be partially due to their anticholinergic effects (Carlsson 1978), as well as to their relative lack of striatal activity as discussed above.

In the limbic system, dopamine receptor blockade by antipsychotic drugs does not alter acetylcholine turnover, as shown by direct measurements of acetylcholine liberation in the nucleus acccumbens, septum, and dorsal and ventral hippocampal formation (Bartholini and Lloyd 1980). It appears that, unlike striatal cholinergic neurones, those in the limbic system do not receive a dopaminergic input. In contrast, cholinergic neurones appear to influence dopaminergic activity, since anticholinergic compounds block the increase in limbic dopamine turnover produced acutely by antipsychotic drugs.

In the cortex, acetylcholine turnover parallels changes in dopaminergic transmission. Thus, dopaminergic agonists enhance cortical acetylcholine liberation, an effect which is blocked by antipsychotic agents. The differential effects of antipsychotic drugs on cholinergic activity in different brain areas presumably depends on the neuronal network peculiar to each region. Cholinergic mechanisms do not appear to be involved in the therapeutic effects of the antipsychotic drugs in schizophrenia, but as mentioned above, they may be of importance in the development of Parkinsonism and possibly play a role in tardive dyskinesia. In addition many antipsychotic drugs (particularly phenothiazines) have peripheral anticholinergic activity, due to muscarinic receptor blockade, which may give rise to adverse effects.

Effects on GABAergic activity

Both limbic and striatal dopaminergic neurones receive an inhibitory GABA-ergic input. This influence may be affected by antipsychotic drugs, although it is not clear whether the drugs act directly on GABA receptors or indirectly via their actions on dopaminergic activity. It is noteworthy that some antipsychotic drugs (the butyrophenones) contain the GABA moiety in their molecular structure. Antipsychotic drugs of diverse structures cause increases in central GABA turnover and alterations in GABA receptor binding (Bartholini and Lloyd 1980). However, GABA systems do not appear to be directly involved in schizophrenic symptoms (Chapter 13) or in the therapeutic effects of antipsychotic drugs. Nevertheless, GABAergic pathways from the forebrain synapsing in the ventral tegmental area may be important in regulating certain limbic-related behaviours including locomotor activity, aggression, and food intake (Arnt and Scheel-Kruger 1979).

Effects on noradrenaline, serotonin and histamine receptors

Some antipsychotic drugs have significant central and peripheral alpha- and beta-adrenoceptor antagonistic activity (Snyder 1982). They stimulate the synthesis and turnover of noradrenaline in the brain, presumably by a receptor-mediated feedback mechanism (Carlsson 1978), and can block or reverse the pressor effects of noradrenaline. However, this action does not appear to be necessary for an antischizophrenic effect: it is not shared by all antipsychotic agents and adrenergic blockade does not correlate with therapeutic potency over the range of drugs. Adrenergic blocking actions, however, produce postural hypotension and may contribute to the sedative and possibly to the antipsychotic effects (Robinson *et al.* 1979a,b) of some of these drugs.

Many of the antipsychotic agents have blocking effects at serotonergic receptors, although they have little effect on central serotonin turnover and are not very effective in reversing the effects of increased central serotonin concentration in animals (Carlsson 1978). It is possible that a serotonergic receptor antagonism contributes to the effect of antipsychotic drugs in reversing the actions of some psychotomimetic agents. The importance of serotonergic mechanisms in schizophrenia is not clear (Chapter 13).

Some of the agents have fairly potent antagonistic actions at histamine-1 and histamine-2 receptors (Richelson 1981). At present, it does not seem likely that this is important for the antischizophrenic actions but it may contribute to sedative effects.

Effects on endogenous opioids

Hong *et al.* (1980) showed that chronic administration of haloperidol, pimozide, and chlorpromazine selectively increased the concentration of methionine enkephalin in the corpus striatum and nucleus accumbens of rats. This effect was thought to be an indirect result of dopamine receptor blockade, since there are close interconnections between dopaminergic and opioid activity in the striatal and limbic systems. The importance of this effect of antipsychotic drugs in schizophrenia is not clear, although as discussed in Chapter 13, it is possible that endogenous opioid or related polypeptides may be disturbed in this condition.

Effects on mood and behaviour

Normal subjects

In psychiatrically normal subjects, antipsychotic drugs typically produce an ataractic state, characterized by diminution in emotional responsiveness, indifference to environmental stimuli, and reduction in initiative and spontaneous activity. Although tiredness and sedation may be present, the subject remains rousable and intellectual performance is little impaired. Even very large doses of most antipsychotic drugs do not produce coma and the lethal dose is extraordinarily high (Baldessarini 1980). Normal individuals treated with high doses of antipsychotic agents become more tractable, compliant, and suggestible: these effects have led to the misuse of the drugs on political dissidents in the USSR.

Acute psychotic states

In excited or agitated psychotic states, such as acute episodes of schizophrenia, mania, and organic or drug-induced delirium, the drugs have an immediate calming effect, and reduce aggressive and impulsive behaviour.

This effect is exerted without pronounced sedation, so that the patient remains accessible and becomes more amenable and easier to handle. More gradually, psychotic symptoms of hallucinations, delusions, and thought disorder diminish and finally disappear. These effects are not confined to subjects with schizophrenia as defined by strict diagnostic criteria, but occur in any disorder, organic or functional, in which positive schizophreniform symptoms, excitement, agitation, or delirium are prominent. The use of antipsychotic drugs in manic episodes of bipolar affective disorders is described in Chapter 12. The psychosis induced by amphetamine or LSD responds rapidly to antipsychotic drugs, usually within hours, an observation which casts some doubt on the relation of these psychoses to schizophrenia, in which the therapeutic effect is delayed for some weeks.

Anxiety and depression

Patients with acute severe anxiety states and panic reactions who have failed to respond to sedative/anxiolytic drugs may respond to antipsychotic agents, especially those with sedative effects such as chlorpromazine and haloperidol (Chapter 4). Some depressed patients respond to flupenthixol, thioridazine, or sulpiride in low doses (Chapter 12). Apart from controlling agitation; the drugs may have an affect on psychotic delusions in affective disorders (Baldessarini 1980). However, depression has also been reported as an adverse effect of antipsychotic agents.

Therapeutic efficacy in schizophrenia

Antipsychotic drugs do not cure schizophrenia. Some patients do not respond at all; few among those who do respond revert to complete or permanent normality, and even the best drug responders tend to relapse when treatment is stopped. Nevertheless, it is generally agreed that the antipsychotic drugs have unique and relatively specific effects on certain schizophrenic symptoms, effects which are not due to general sedation. Phenothiazines have been found in carefully controlled trials involving thousands of schizophrenic patients to be superior to barbiturates, which are no more effective than placebo (Klein and Davis 1969). More recently developed antipsychotic drugs have similar effects to phenothiazines, although many of them are more potent.

Spontaneous improvement (social recovery) occurs in about 20 per cent of schizophrenics: with antipsychotic drug treatment this figure is increases to 50–60 per cent in those who have been ill for less than 3 years (Rogers *et al.* 1981). Improvement is seen mainly in certain symptoms including thought insertion, thought broadcasting, thought block, delusions, feelings of passivity, and auditory hallucinations. Klein and Davis (1969) reported improvement in blunted affect, withdrawal, and autistic behaviour. However, most authors report little effect on negative symptoms (Rogers *et al.* 1981; Johnstone *et al.* 1978; Angrist *et al.* 1980). On the whole, drug treatment does not increase the number of symptom-free patients, but shifts patients with overt psychotic symptoms into the group with residual symptoms (Rogers *et al.* 1981). Maintenance of this degree of recovery requires long-term treatment, perhaps for life, since if drug therapy is stopped 25 per cent of patients relapse within a week and 75-95 per cent within a year. Even on continued drug treatment the relapse rate is over 25 per cent within 1 year. Patients maintained on long-term antipsychotic therapy may complain of lack of emotional responsivity: although better able of cope socially they feel cut off from emotional experiences, either pleasurable or painful.

As discussed above, the beneficial effects of the antipsychotic drugs on the positive symptoms of schizophrenia are thought to be a result of competitive antagonism at dopaminergic receptors. It is interesting in this connection that patients with acute schizophrenia require much larger doses than normal subjects to produce the ataractic state (Okuma *et al.* 1976).

Effects on animal behaviour

The effects of antipsychotic drugs on animals are, as far as can be judged, very similar to those on psychiatrically normal humans. Exploratory behaviour and locomotor activity are reduced. Emotional responses to a variety of pharmacological and environmental stimuli are fewer, smaller, and slower, and the animal appears indifferent to the external environment. However, the ability to discriminate stimuli is not lost; the animal will still withdraw from painful or noxious stimuli and can perform learned behaviours if sufficient stimulation and motivation is provided. Aggressive reactions are diminished. Intracranial self-stimulation behaviour is reduced as tested with electrodes in the median forebrain bundle and other rewarding brain areas. Other rewarding behaviours, including food and water intake, sexual activity, and self-injection of reinforcing drugs such as cocaine and amphetamine, are diminished.

Conditioned as opposed to unconditioned responses are selectively impaired. For example, it was shown by Corvoisier *et al.* (1953) that rats treated with chlorpromazine would no longer climb a pole in order to avoid an electric shock, the impending delivery of which was signalled by a learned cue (conditioned active avoidance task). The animals would ignore the warning stimulus although they would still exhibit escape behaviour once the shock (unconditioned stimulus) occurred. This behaviour contrasted with that produced by general central nervous system depressants which reduced equally both the conditioned avoidance and unconditioned escape responses. Conditional passive avoidance is similarly suppressed by chlorpromazine, and also conditioned behaviour involving positive reinforcement (Iverson and Iverson 1981). These conditioned behaviours are impaired in a dose-dependent manner by a variety of antipsychotic drugs and have proved useful as a screening test in developing new drugs with antipsychotic actions in humans. However, their relevance to human psychosis is doubtful since the responses are blocked by anticholinergic drugs and tolerance also develops. Furthermore, atypical agents, such as clozapine and sulpiride, which are effective in schizophrenia, do not affect conditioned responses in animals (Baldessarini 1980). It is thought that the effect is mediated by drug actions in the nigrostriatal rather than the mesolimbic system.

Large doses of standard antipsychotic drugs produce a state of catalepsy in animals. This state, which resembles the catatonia and flexibilitas cerea seen in schizophrenia and some neurological disorders (Chapter 13), consists of immobility and an alteration of muscle tone which allows the animal to be placed in abnormal postures that persist. Catatonia is not produced by atypical drugs such as sulpiride.

Effects on arousal

The effects of antipsychotic drugs on arousal are of interest in view of the evidence that some schizophrenic patients appear to be hyperaroused. For example, in schizophrenia sleep is disturbed; EEG frequency is increased; the sedation threshold is raised, higher doses of central nervous system depressants being required to produce a given degree of sedation in schizophrenics than in normal subject (Okuma et al. 1976); and skin conductance responses may be exaggerated with poor habituation. It has been suggested that the social withdrawal of schizophrenia may be a defence against a feeling of being bombarded with sensory stimuli, a state similar to that produced by psychotomimetic drugs such as LSD (Shore 1979). Clinical observations have shown that over-zealous attempts at rehabilitation or a high degree of emotional involvement by relatives provokes relapse in schizophrenia, suggesting a heightened sensitivity to the quality of the environment (Fairburn 1981). Acute psychotic episodes in schizophrenia may resemble the hyperexcited states of mania. As discussed in Chapter 13, the disorder of arousal in schizophrenia may be due not simply to overarousal but to a lack of co-ordination between various arousal systems in the brain (cortical, limbic, autonomic, etc.).

Bradley and Key (1958) found in animals that chlorpromazine and other phenothiazines inhibit arousal responses in the electrocorticogram, decrease spontaneous electrical activity of neurones in the brainstem reticular formation, and decrease the response of these neurones to stimulation via peripheral sensory pathways. Phenothiazines were also shown to block the increase in reticular formation activity provoked by amphetamine and LSD. These experiments provided electrophysiological evidence that antipsychotic drugs dampen the central arousing effects of afferent and pharmacological stimulation. In addition, Killam and Killam (1956) showed that the arousal threshold of neurones in the limbic system to electrical stimulation of the reticular formation was raised by phenothiazines, while cortical arousal in response to reticular formation stimulation was less affected. This finding is consistent with the behavioural evidence that emotional responses to external stimuli are reduced with little alteration in consciousness or decrement of cognitive performance. This action is probably of prime importance in determining the therapeutic benefit of antipsychotic drugs in schizophrenia. These early studies fit in well with the later work (described above) showing that antipsychotic drugs decrease the firing rates of A_{10} cells in the ventral tegmental area due to dopamine receptor anatagonistic activity. It is possible that some also have antagonistic activity in the synapses from afferent collaterals into the reticular formation.

At the opposite extreme, chronic schizophrenics show evidence of underarousal, such as non-responsiveness of electrodermal activity (Chapter 13). As would be expected from the electrophysiological evidence, antipsychotic drugs are of little benefit in these cases.

Effects on sleep Antipsychotic drugs tend to normalize the disturbed sleep pattern (Chapter 13) in psychotic patients. Chlorpromazine increases SWS and REMS initially, in both normal and schizophrenic subjects. The increased SWS persists with chronic use, but tolerance apparently develops to the effect on REMS (Kay *et al.* 1976).

Effects on EEG Antipsychotic drugs produce characteristic effects on the EEG which are of predictive value in screening for new drugs with antipsychotic potency (Fig. 2.9). These effects are reviewed by Fink (1975) and Roubicek (1980). Typically the drugs produce EEG slowing and increased synchronization; there is an increase in delta and theta activity and a decrease in fast beta activity (22–33 Hz). The amplitude of EEG waves is increased and variability of rhythm reduced. Arousal reactions, such as alpha-blocking on external stimulation, are decreased. There is an increase in spike activity and bursts of spikes may be induced. This finding is in keeping with the observation that antipsychotic drugs lower the seizure threshold.

The effects of antipsychotic drugs on evoked potentials are reviewed by Shagass and Straumanis (1978). Coinciding with clinical improvement in schizophrenia, they have a normalizing effect especially on the variability of somatosensory and visual evoked potentials. In general, they tend to reduce the amplitude and increase the latency of these potentials. In normal subjects, somatosensory evoked potentials may occasionally be increased in amplitude, but the effect of chlorpromazine on the contingent negative variation is usually a decrease in magnitude (Tecce *et al.* 1975).

Effects on perception and cognitive performance
The effects of single small doses of antipsychotic drugs on perception, cog-

nitive function, and psychomotor performance in normal subjects are reviewed by Janke (1980). There is no evidence of a specific effect on perception. Performance in IQ tests may be improved in schizophrenics, but is not altered in normal subjects. Learning and memory are not affected in doses below 100 mg chlorpromazine, and in particular it has not been possible to show in man a specific action on conditioned responses, in spite of the predictive power of this effect in animals (see above). There is little published information on the effects of large doses or chronic medication in normal subjects. As mentioned above, schizophrenic patients have a much higher tolerance to the sedative and other effects of antipsychotic drugs and cognitive function may be improved by therapeutic doses in these patients.

Adverse effects
The acute toxicity of antipsychotic drugs is very low and they have a high therapeutic index. Nevertheless, the incidence of adverse effects is high and gives rise to considerable morbidity. The relative frequency at which various adverse effects are produced by different drugs is shown in Table 14.1

Extrapyramidal effects
Several types of involuntary movements and disorders of muscle tone can be caused by antipsychotic drugs. These all result directly or indirectly from perturbations in dopaminergic function in the corpus striatum. Extrapyramidal effects are produced drugs with prominent dopamine receptor antagonist activity at A_9 cells, and are less likely to occur with the atypical drugs, which have a more selective action on A_{10} cells (Table 14.2). Some extrapyramidal effects occur at the start of drug treatment, others may be delayed for weeks or months, while some may not appear for months or years, or may even emerge when treatment is stopped. At present there is no explanation for the fact that only some patients develop these syndromes while others can with impunity take similar doses of antipsychotic drugs for similar periods of time.

Acute dystonic reactions Acute dystonic reactions can affect any muscle group but commonly take the form of spasms of the tongue, neck or back muscles, or oculogyric crises. The greatest period of risk is the first 5 days of treatment. Dystonic reactions are more common at higher drug dosage but there is a large interindividual variation in susceptibility and they may sometimes be precipitated by small or even single doses. The exact mechanism by which the drugs cause localized spasm in particular muscle groups is unknown, but the symptoms respond dramatically to parenteral administration of anticholinergic drugs and are presumably largely due to striatal cholinergic overactivity secondary to dopamine receptor blockade. Possibly central histamine receptors are also involved since acute dystonic reactions also respond to intramuscular diphenhydramine, although this drug also has anticholinergic properties.

Akathisia Akathisia, an uncontrollable motor restlessness, may occur between 5 and 60 days from the start of treatment. The response to anticholinergic or antihistamine agents is only partial and a reduction in dosage is usually necessary. Akathisia may respond to propranolol (Wilbur and Kulik 1983). It may be relevant that injection of GABA agonists into the ventral tegmental area of rats induces compulsive hypermotility, while injection of dopamine agonists or anticholinergic agents into this area produces sedation and catalepsy (Arnt and Scheel-Kruger 1979).

Parkinsonism A Parkinsonian syndrome, which may be indistinguishable from idiopathic Parkinsonism, develops in some patients. Its onset is usually delayed for two weeks or more and its appearance often coincides with signs of clinical improvement in schizophrenia. Bunney, (1984) and Creese, (1983) suggest that Parkinsonism results from drug-induced depolarisation blockade in A_9 dopaminergic neurones in the substantia nigra.

However, other neurotransmitter systems may also be involved. There is an inverse relationship between the liability of an antipsychotic drug to produce Parkinsonism and its potency in blocking muscarinic cholinergic receptors. Many of the manifestations of Parkinsonism may be due to cholinergic hyperactivity secondary to dopaminergic blockade, and the syndrome responds to anticholinergic drugs. Richelson (1981) suggests that increased cholinergic activity in the corpus striatum in turn increases the release of GABA (since excitatory cholinergic and inhibitory GABAergic neurones appear to be linked in series in this region). Increased release of GABA from neurones projecting to the thalamus is suggested to cause the akinesia and bradykinesia associated with the Parkinsonian syndrome.

A certain degree of tolerance seems to develop to the Parkinsonian effects of antipsychotic drugs. The symptoms may disappear or improve after some weeks or months of continued treatment, or they may merge with or be replaced by the quite different syndrome of tardive dyskinesia. Tolerance to the antischizophrenic actions of the drugs does not appear to develop to the same extent as that to the extrapyramidal actions although psychiatric symptoms which are possibly rebound effects may occur on drug withdrawal (see below).

Tardive dyskinesia Tardive dyskinesia is a delayed adverse effect which appears months or sometimes several years after the start of antipsychotic drug treatment. The clinical features (described by Paulson 1975; McClelland 1985; Berger and Dunn 1985) consist of bizarre movements involving oral, lingual, buccal, facial, trunk, or limb muscles. The incidence of tardive dyskinesia has been variously estimated but it probably develops in 10–20 per cent of patients receiving antipsychotic drugs for over a year (*British Medical Journal* 1981a). The syndrome is not confined to patients with schizophrenia but may also occur in psychiatrically normal subjects taking antipsychotic drugs. The relative risk of producing tardive dyskinesia with different antipsychotic drugs is not known. It has been associated with all the classical drugs but so far the risk connected with the atypical antipsychotics appears to be very low (Baldessarini 1980). The syndrome may be caused by non-antipsychotic agents with DA-2 receptor antagonistic actions (meto-clopramide). There is only a weak correlation between the incidence of tardive dyskinesia and length of drug exposure or drug dose, and the presence of or treatment for Parkinsonism does not appear to be related (*British Medical Journal* 1981a). In most cases cessation of medication is followed by sub-stantial improvement in the condition, but this may take several months or up to 2 years and there is often an initial exacerbation. In a significant number of patients the disorder appears to be irreversible (Paulson 1975; Creese 1983).

The underlying mechanism of tardive dyskinesia is not clear. One factor may be the development of DA-2 receptor supersensitivity in the corpus striatum, which has been demonstrated in rats after long-term treatment with antipsychotic agents that cause tardive dyskinesia in man (Clow *et al.* 1979a,b; Rupniak *et al.* 1984a,b). However, Waddington (1985) found no differences in DA-2 receptor density (^{3}H-spiperone binding) in post-mortem brains between schizophrenic patients with or without tardive dyskinesia during life. Nevertheless, the condition is temporarily ameliorated by increas-ing receptor blockade and aggravated by decreasing dopamine receptor blockade and by L-dopa and amphetamine (Baldessarini 1980). The slowly developing depolarization blockade observed by Bunney (1984) would encourage the development of dopamine receptor supersensitivity and, as Creese (1983) observes, this might be sufficient to cause tardive dyskinesia if a few molecules of released dopamine manage to reach supersensitive postsynaptic dopamine receptors. However White and Wang (1983) observed, after chronic antipsychotic agent treatment in rats, an increased number of dopaminergic cells in the A_9 and A_{10} cell areas with an unusual firing pattern. It is possible that an abnormal release of dopamine from these cells onto supersensitive dopamine receptors might produce the bizarre movements of tardive dyskinesia.

Richelson (1981) stressed the importance of other neurotransmitters in tardive dyskinesia, pointing out that increased dopaminergic activity as a result of dopamine receptor supersensitivity might lead to decreased chol-inergic and GABAergic activity. Fibiger and Lloyd (1984) produce evidence of neuroleptic-induced degeneration of GABAergic systems in the corpus striatum in rats after long-term administration, and Tamminga *et al.* (1979)

point out that GABA receptor agonists can temporarily relieve tardive dyskinesia in man. Jeste *et al.* (1982) suggested that abnormal drug metabolism might be involved in some patients.

Treatment of tardive dyskinesia is unsatisfactory. Increasing the dose of antipsychotic drugs provides only temporary relief; results with cholinergic drugs (choline, lecithin, deanol) are not impressive; GABA-enhancing drugs (benzodiazepines, sodium valproate, muscimol) provide only partial relief; benzodiazepines may precipitate tardive dyskinesia (Rosenbaum and de la Fuente 1979); and muscimol may produce psychiatric symptoms (Tamminga *et al.* 1979) Stopping the antipsychotic drug is probably the best solution once the condition has developed, but for patients in whom the psychosis is thereby aggravated it may be necessary to continue treatment despite the presence of tardive dyskinesia. Substitution of more selective atypical antipsychotic drugs which spare the nigrostriatal system may be a practical alternative (Casey *et al.* 1979), and the use of these drugs may perhaps prevent the occurrence of tardive dyskinesia in patients requiring long-term treatment.

Neuroleptic malignant syndrome The neuroleptic malignant syndrome (*Lancet* 1984a) is a rare idiosyncratic response which has been observed after treatment with phenothiazines and butyrophenones. It is characterized by akinesia, muscle rigidity, hyperthermia, autonomic instability, and altered consciousness. The cause of the syndrome is unknown, but it is thought to be related to dopamine receptor blockade in the basal ganglia.

Neuroendocrine effects

Many antipsychotic drugs exert a wide range of neuroendocrine effects, reviewed by Sachar *et al.* (1976), Sulsman and Givant (1980) and Nathan and van Kammen (1985). The effects stem from dopamine receptor antagonist actions in the tuberoinfundibular system (Chapter 13) resulting in alterations in the secretion of hypothalamic releasing factors which are normally under inhibitory or excitatory dopaminergic control. Consequently, the release of several anterior pituitary hormones is either increased or decreased. Some of the effects may also result from drug actions or dopamine receptors localized to cells in the anterior pituitary.

The most studied effects are those on prolactin (Meltzer and Fang 1976). Serum concentrations of prolactin are increased after administration of most of the commonly used antipsychotic agents. The effect is almost immediate and provides a measure of the drug's DA-2 receptor blocking potency, since there are no DA-1 receptors in this region (Creese 1982). Although, as mentioned above (Fig. 13.4), the effects on prolactin secretion and the anti-schizophrenic effects do not appear at the same time, there is a good correlation between the rise in prolactin secretion and clinical potency in schizophrenia for many of the antipsychotic drugs. The effect on prolactin, however, is not necessary for an antischizophrenic action, since some agents (pimozide, clozapine; Kane *et al.* 1981) do not affect prolactin secretion. Raised prolactin secretion is responsible for adverse effects including breast engorgement and galactarrhoea which may occur in male and female patients.

Other effects on pituitary hormones include a decrease in gonodotropin release, which may cause amenorrhoea and testicular atropy; a decrease in growth hormone release; and a decrease in corticotropin secretion, which may reduce the adrenal corticosteroid response to stress. Hypothalamic dysfunction may explain the increase in appetite and weight gain which is sometimes caused by phenothiazines.

Cardiovascular effects

The commonest cardiovascular effect of phenothiazines is postural hypotension due to peripheral and central alpha-adrenoceptor blockade. This is combined with a reflex tachycardia and peripheral vasodilatation which can lead to hypothermia. Tolerance develops to the hypotensive effect with continued administration. Phenothiazines also exert quinidine-like antiarrhythmic and cardiodepressant effects, and sudden cardiac arrhythmia or cardiac arrest occurs rarely. Butyrophenones and thioxanthines also have alpha-adrenoceptor blocking effects, but these are virtually absent with the atypical antipsychotic agents. Phenothiazines also consistently raise plasma cholesterol concentrations.

Anticholinergic effects

The anticholinergic affects of antipsychotic drugs, due to cholinergic muscarinic blocking activity, may give rise to dry mouth, nasal stuffiness, constipation, blurred vision, and other manifestations of cholinergic blockade. Pimozide and the newer agents have very few autonomic effects.

Sedation and depression

Sedation with drowsiness and confusion may occur with phenothiazines and butyrophenones. Thioxanthines, diphenylpiperazines, and the newer drugs are less sedative. Prolonged use of antipsychotic drugs can cause depression.

Hypersensitivity reactions

Jaundice due to intrahepatic cholestasis occurs in 2–4 per cent of patients treated with chlorpromazine; this is thought to be a hypersensitivity reaction and is associated with eosinophilia. Allergic skin rashes occur in about 5 per cent of patients on chlorpromazine and contact dermatitis, and photosensitivity may develop. Rarely, phenothiazines cause blood dyscrasias including agranulocytosis.

Oculodermal melanosis

Long-term administration of high doses of phenothiazines, especially chlor-promazine, may give rise to pigmentary changes in the skin and eyes, termed oculodermal melanosis. Areas of skin exposed to sunlight become excessively pigmented with grey-blue discoloration and biopsy shows deposits of melanin along with dehydroxylated metabolites of chlorpromazine. Similar deposits may cause corneal and lens opacities. Pigmentary retinopathy which may cause irreversible visual impairment only occurs after high doses (1000 mg daily) of thioridazine. The mechanism is unknown, but may involve stimulation of melatonin secretion from the pineal gland or melanocyte stimulating hormone from the pituitary.

Drug interactions

Antipsychotic drugs with sedative effects potentiate the effects of other central nervous system depressants including alcohol, hypnotics, narcotic analgesics, and general anaesthetics. The analgesic actions of opiates may be potentiated by an additive effect in dampening the emotional reaction to pain. However, Hanks et al. (1983) dispute that haloperidol has an opioid-sparing effect and produce evidence from 424 patients with cancer showing that the administration of low doses (5 mg daily) or larger doses (20–30 mg daily) of haloperidol had no effect on the patient's morphine requirements for pain relief. Nevertheless, it is claimed that antipsychotic drugs increase the respiratory depressant, meiotic, and sedative effects of narcotic analgesics (Baldessarini 1980; Rogers et al. 1981). The antiemetic effect of antipsychotic drugs is useful for countering narcotic-induced nausea and vomiting. As would be expected, antipsychotic drugs inhibit the action of dopamine agonists.

Chlorpromazine inhibits the metabolism of alcohol, by an effect on alcohol dehydrogenase, and also inhibits the metabolism of tricyclic antidepressants, increasing their plasma concentrations. It is a moderately potent enzyme inducer.

Tolerance and dependence

Tolerance develops to the sedative, hypotensive, and even the Parkinsonian actions of antipsychotic drugs, although tolerance to the antipsychotic effects seems to be much less. A degree of physical dependence is produced and dosage reduction or sudden cessation of these drugs may cause withdrawal dyskinesias, usually of the tardive dyskinesia type with choreo-athetosis. It is not clear whether the rapid psychotic relapse seen in some patients within a week of stopping antipsychotic medication is always due to re-emergence of the underlying illness or whether it may sometimes represent a withdrawal reaction characterized by anxiety, sleeplessness, and agitation (Davis and

Rosenberg 1979; Berger and Dunn 1985). The question of whether non-psychotic patients taking antipsychotic agents experience withdrawal effects does not appear to have been seriously investigated. The drugs are not 'rewarding' and are not abused, but it is possible that those with sedative effects might induce withdrawal anxiety in susceptible individuals.

Other drugs used in schizophrenia

The incomplete effect of antipsychotic agents in schizophrenia has prompted trials with other drugs. Some of these may benefit individual patients, but none so far represent a pharmacological breakthrough. At present it seems doubtful if cure, as opposed to symptomatic control, of schizophrenia will ever be attainable by pharmacological means. Nevertheless, the pursuit of drugs which can improve control of symptoms while exerting lesser adverse effects than present antipsychotic agents is a worthwhile objective.

Benzodiazepines

Benzodiazepines in usual anxiolytic doses are not effective in schizophrenia, but it has been suggested that high doses may be beneficial in certain patients. Beckmann and Haas (1980) studied the effects of diazepam (400 mg daily) in an open trial in 15 schizophrenic patients. In the group as a whole, the drug produced a marked decrease in anxiety, a gradual mood-elevating effect, and in 12 patients enhanced feelings of well-being and euphoria. There was a notable absence of sedation (except after the first 50 mg dose). In nine patients with paranoid delusions and hallucinations there was a significant therapeutic effect. However, the five patients with marked affective symptoms on admission (depression, euphoria, psychotic anxiety) either failed to respond or became worse because of hyperactivity, excitation, and sleep difficulties. It was proposed that benzodiazepines might alleviate symptoms in paranoid schizophrenia either through GABA-enhancement (which would also inhibit dopaminergic systems in the brain) or by enhancement of central opioid activity. No signs of tolerance were shown during continued treatment for several months and there were no withdrawal signs during stepwise reduction of dosage. However, the possibility of dependence may be a risk with long-term benzodiazepine treatment (Chapter 4), and controlled comparisons between high dose benzodiazepines and antipsychotic drugs are needed before this treatment can be evaluated.

Beta adrenoceptor antagonists

Early uncontrolled studies suggested that propranolol might have a therapeutic effect in schizophrenia (Yorkston *et al.* 1974; 1977a,b), although these results were criticized (Tyrer 1977; Schiff 1977). In a later controlled investigation it was found that large doses of propranolol (over 600 mg daily) was as effective as chlorpromazine (300 mg daily) in newly admitted patients with florid schizophrenic symptoms (Yorkston *et al.* 1981). Patients were randomly assigned to each drug and followed for 6–12 weeks. The amount and rate of improvement were similar in both groups but neither drug proved very effective, only 18 out of the total of 46 patients remitting or showing marked improvement. Propranolol may increase the therapeutic efficacy of antipsychotic drugs when used in combination, but this is probably through a pharmacokinetic interaction (Peet 1981). Beta-adrenoceptor antagonists can also cause hallucinations in normal subjects and may precipitate a frank psychotic disorder (Steinert and Pugh 1979). Their place in the treatment of schizophrenia remains doubtful.

Clonidine, an alpha$_2$-noradrenergic receptor stimulant, which decreases noradrenaline release, was reported to be as effective as antipsychotic drugs and more effective than placebo in a small trial in eight schizophrenic patients (Freedman *et al.* 1982). Patients were selected because they had tardive dyskinesia; this condition improved during substitution of clonidine or placebo for antipsychotic drugs.

Opioid and related polypeptides

The possible involvement of opioid systems in schizophrenia is discussed in Chapter 13. Naloxone and the longer-acting naltrexone have been investigated for antipsychotic activity but the results have been variable (van Ree and de Weid 1981; Gitlin *et al.* 1981; Freeman and Fairburn 1981). A World Health Organization collaborative study (Pickar 1983), found a naloxone-related improvement in schizophrenic patients concurrently treated with antipsychotic drugs, but not in medication-free patients, suggesting the possibility of a synergistic effect of dopamine and endogenous opioid receptor blockade. Results with beta-endorphin and synthetic enkephalin analogues in schizophrenia have been undramatic (van Ree and de Wied 1981; Jorgensen *et al.* 1979). Initial promising results with des-tyrosynyl-gamma endorphin (Verhoeven *et al.* 1978 1979) (Chapter 13) have not been confirmed in some later studies (Manchanda and Hirsch 1981). The role of opioid-related polypeptides in the management of schizophrenia probably merits further investigation.

Miscellaneous agents

Other suggestions for improving the pharmacological treatment of schizophrenia include piracetam or vasopressin for cognitive disorders (Kabes *et al.* 1979; Dimond *et al.* 1979; Korsgaard *et al.* 1981), dopamine agoninsts for negative symptoms (Gerlach and Luhdorf 1979), vitamins and benzopyrones (Casley-Smith 1983), and dietary measures.

Psychotomimetic drugs

Classification

The psychotomimetic drugs (sometimes described as hallucinogenic or psychodelic agents) are a miscellaneous group of substances, often of plant origin, which can produce effects sometimes resembling psychiatric states in man. Many of these substances exist in nature and some are widely used for recreational and religious purposes in various parts of the world. They have few therapeutic uses, but have generated considerable interest as possible models for schizophrenia. Examples of the main groups of psychotomimetic agents are shown in Table 14.3. Some of these drugs have already been described (amphetamine: Chapter 4; phencyclidine and organic solvents: Chapter 7; anticholinergic drugs: Chapter 10). There is no sharp distinction between drugs classed as psychotomimetic and other centrally acting drugs: for example amphetamine, bromides, ACTH, opioids, alcohol, and many drugs classified under diverse headings can, in suitable doses, produce psychotomimetic effects. In this chapter, the properties of d-lysergic acid diethylamide (LSD) and of cannabis are considered.

Table 14.3. Some psychotomimetic drugs

Agents	Plant source
Substances related to serotonin	
mescaline	peyote cactus (Lopophora williamsii)
psilocybin, psilocin	'magic mushrooms' (Psilocybe mexicanum, stropharia cubensis)
d-lysergic acid diethylamide (LSD)	ergot (Claviceps purpura)
dimethyltryptamine	alkaloid in New World snuff
harmaline	bata-carboline (Banisteriopsis)
Cannabis preparations	marihuana, hashish (Cannabis sativa)
Anticholinergic drugs	
atropine	(Atropa belladonna)
hyoscine	(Hyosycyamus niger)
strammonium	(Datura strammonium)
Amphetamine derivatives	
Miscellaneous	
methylphenidate	
phenmetrazine	
phencyclidine	
organic solvents	
amyl nitrite	

d-*Lysergic acid diethylamide* (*LSD*)

LSD is one of the most potent of known drugs; an oral dose of 25 μg can produce central nervous system effects in man. The drug enjoyed a temporary vogue as a recreational agent, and in 1977 approximately 20 per cent of people aged 18–25 in the United States had sampled it (Jaffe 1980). Its popularity has now precipitously declined although it is still available illicitly. Mescaline, psylocin, and other drugs in this group produce similar effects, but are less potent.

Pharmacokinetics

LSD is rapidly absorbed after oral or parenteral administration, and rapidly distributed in the body. Only very small amounts reach the brain, and brain concentrations remain 1000 times lower than plasma concentrations even after intrathecal administration in man (Freedman and Boggan 1982). However, peak brain concentrations are reached within minutes after injection and the drug has been shown to be selectively concentrated in the visual and limbic areas, and also in the pineal gland, in the rat and monkey. Clearance from the brain follows the same time course as that from the plasma. The plasma elimination half-life is about 3–4 h in man but is dose-dependent, high doses having longer half-lives. The onset, severity, and duration of clinical effects correlate with brain and plasma concentrations, although symptoms may considerably outlast the half-life of the drug. LSD is metabolized in the body and subsequently eliminated by the kidney. No active metabolites are formed.

Clinical effects

LSD produces three characteristic types of symptoms in man: somatic, perceptual, and psychological (Hollister 1982; Jaffe 1980). The somatic symptoms, which appear within a few minutes, include dizziness, weakness, tremor, nausea, drowsiness, paraesthesiae, and blurred vision. They are accompanied by few somatic alterations, although pupillary dilatation, increased reflexes, incoordination, and ataxia may occur and there may be signs of sympathetic and parasympathetic stimulation.

Perceptual and mood effects appear within an hour and last for several hours. Perceptual symptoms include complex, changeable alterations in shapes and colours, difficulty in focussing, heightened perception of hearing and of visual detail, distortion of space with macropsia and micropsia, and sometimes a running together of sensory modalities (synaesthesia). There is a distortion of body image and of time, perceived time being much faster than clock time. These sensory distortions undergo wave-like recurrences, and the environment is perceived in a novel way. Changes in mood depend on personality and setting. Euphoria, elation, anxiety, fear, irritability or depression may predominate. Often several of these feelings coexist or rapidly change from one to another, accompanied by alternate laughing or crying. The subject may appear hypervigilant or withdrawn and may display irritability on interruption. Not uncommonly there is a fear of fragmentation and of loss of control of perceptions, thoughts, and memories.

After about 4 h, major disturbances in cognition are apparent. Initially, thought patterns are altered and thoughts become difficult to express, accompanied by deterioration in performance tests involving reasoning and memory. Later, feelings of depersonalization, unreality, and dreamlike sensations are prominent. Subjects may feel that their thoughts are of great clarity and meaningfulness. Metaphysical preoccupations dominate, and there may be a feeling of disembodiment and oneness with the world or the cosmos. Hallucinations (visual or auditory) may occur, but these may represent sensory illusions or distortions. A feeling of omnipotence may supervene with irrational beliefs, such as a belief in the ability to fly. During this time, the subject may be in a trance-like state which gradually clears over the next few hours. The entire syndrome may last 12–24 h. This variegated syndrome was well described by Hofmann (quoted in Brecher 1972, pp. 346–7), who supplied the first personal report of the effects of 0.25 mg of LSD taken by mouth.

Biochemical actions

The structural similarity of LSD to serotonin suggests an interaction with serotonergic mechanisms in the brain. Much evidence indicates that such an interaction occurs, although its precise nature is not clear. Serotonin has complex effects throughout the body: it increases anxiety and inhibits reward by actions in limbic pathways (Chapters 3 and 5); suppresses pain sensation through descending pathways from the periaqueductal grey matter, but in the periphery stimulates nociceptors (Chapter 5); promotes sleep through pathways from the raphe nuclei (Chapter 2). Through the raphe nuclei, it may also play a part in general perception by inhibiting ascending traffic in the reticular formation and in secondary sensory areas, thus protecting the brain from being overwhelmed by sensory information.

Biochemical investigations (reviewed by Freedman and Boggan 1982) show that LSD decreases the release, turnover, synthesis, and utilization of serotonin. This effect occurs immediately after administration and is sustained for several hours or days. The biochemical effects are to some degree independent of changes in neuronal activity, since they still occur after destruction of serotonin containing raphe neurones, and they may involve intracellular as well as membrane changes. Neurophysiological studies (reviewed by Aghajanian 1982) show that LSD has a direct inhibitory effect on the activity of serotonergic neurones in the raphe nuclei. Their firing rate is decreased by LSD administered intravenously or by local iontophoretic application, and electrical activity in these neurones in freely moving cats is decreased in a dose-dependent manner which coincides with the onset of behavioural manifestations. However, the behavioural effects tend to outlast the depression of raphe neuronal activity.

Possible interactions of LSD with serotonin receptors are discussed by Aghajanian (1982). Serotonin receptors include both presynaptic auto-receptors and two types of post-synaptic receptors (Chapter 11). The auto-receptors operate a negative feedback control system for serotonin synthesis and release; the post-synaptic receptors are inhibitory and excitatory, respect-ively. It is suggested that LSD binds preferentially to and has a relatively selective stimulant action on serotonin autoreceptors, situated on raphe neurones. Post-synaptic serotonin receptors in limbic and visual areas which receive an input from these neurones are thought to be of the inhibitory type. The effect of the decreased serotonin release from raphe neurones, induced by the autoreceptor action of LSD, is thus a disinhibition of activity in the limbic system and secondary visual brain areas (Fig. 14.2). Such an effect may constitute the general mechanism for the perceptual distortion and hallucinations produced by LSD. LSD may also sensitize excitatory post-synaptic serotonin receptors leading to an increase in perceptual reactivity.

LSD also has both an agonist and antagonist activity at dopaminergic and noradrenergic receptors, and activates noradrenergic neurones in the locus coeruleus (Aghajanian 1982; Watson 1977). Binding studies show that it

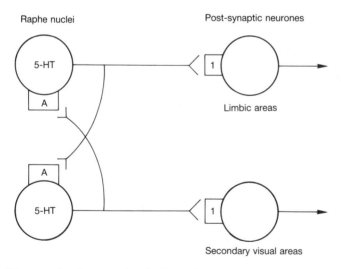

Fig.14.2. Diagram showing postulated effects of LSD at serotonin receptor subtypes in the brain. A, autoreceptors: stimulation inhibits serotonin release. I, inhibitory post-synaptic serotonin receptors: stimulation inhibits firing of post-synaptic neurone. LSD is postulated to stimulate A preferentially, thus disinhibiting post-synaptic neurones in limbic and sensory areas. (Adapted from Aghajanian 1982.)

binds to dopamine receptors, alpha- and beta-adrenergic receptors, and histamine-2 receptors in the brain (Freedman and Boggon 1982). Neuroleptics such as haloperidol displace LSD from its binding sites in the brain. The importance of these effects on non-serotonergic transmitter systems in mediating its pharmacological actions is not known. However, they may be important since mescaline, a related drug with similar effects, does not act on serotonin autoreceptors, while lisuride, an analogue of LSD, has similar effects on serotonin activity yet is not a psychotomimetic agent.

Adverse effects

The acute toxicity of LSD is low and deaths attributable to direct effects of the drug have not been reported in man (Jaffe 1980). However, acute dysphoric reactions ('bad trips') occur in about 20 per cent of drug exposures. These usually consist of panic attacks and feelings of loss of control or of going insane. They are influenced by the prevailing mood and personality of the subject and by the environmental setting, but sometimes occur in users who have previously experienced 'good trips'. Acute delusional or paranoid states and hallucinations are sometimes seen and suicide, self-injury, or fatal accidents may occur in these subjects. 'Flashbacks', consisting of recurrence of drug effects without repeated drug dosage, occur occasionally. These unpredictable episodes, weeks or months after drug exposure, are unexplained. In a few individuals who are presumably constitutionally susceptible, LSD and related drugs may precipitate prolonged psychotic states persisting for weeks or months. The clinical picture may resemble dementia, depression, or schizophrenia. Whether or not such states would have occurred without the drug is debatable. In schizophrenic subjects the drugs aggravate the symptoms. Homicide has been reported on several occasions during psychotic states precipitated by LSD (Hollister 1982).

Tolerance and dependence

Tolerance to the behavioural and biochemical effects of LSD occurs extremely rapidly in man and animals and can be seen after three or four daily doses. Cross-tolerance to psilocin and other related drugs occurs but not to central stimulants such as amphetamine (Appel *et al.* 1982). LSD does not support intracranial self-stimulation and is not self-administered by animals, nor does it appear to produce a withdrawal syndrome on abrupt cessation after chronic administration. Its dependence-producing potential in man appears to be very low. The pattern of drug use in man is usually one of a small number of exposures (often only a single exposure) over a brief time-span, followed by complete or nearly complete abstinence (Poling and Appel 1982). The occasional chronic user typically takes the drug once or twice a week and eventually discontinues it on his own volition (Jaffe 1980).

Relationship to schizophrenia

There is no particular reason to link LSD and its analogues specifically with schizophrenia. It is interesting, as discussed in Chapter 13, that it can, in individuals with schizoid personality types, produce a similar dissociation between autonomic and cortical (perceptual) arousal to that seen in schizophrenia (Claridge 1978). However, this may represent a non-specific disturbance of limbic activity. The ability of LSD to produce a psychotic state is shared by many other drugs with different modes of action, although it suggests that a disturbance of serotonergic mechanisms may be one of the factors contributing to perceptual, attentional, emotional, and autonomic disruption in schizophreniform states.

Cannabis

The use of cannabis preparations has been increasing in the western world since the 1960s. By 1977, 60 per cent of young adults in the United States reported some experience with marihuana; in Great Britain the practice is somewhat less common, but still considerable in a similar age-group. In this country and North America, cannabis preparations are usually smoked in cigarettes which deliver, in relatively small, but variable quantities, several psychoactive cannabinoids, as well as substances which both enhance and inhibit their actions (Fairburn and Pickens 1979 1980). The most potent psychotropic agent is delta-9-tetrahydrocannabinol (delta-9-THC). This substance can be obtained pure and has been used in much experimental work. In North Africa, Greece, the Middle East, and the Far East, much larger quantitites of cannabinoids are smoked or ingested, and drug effects observed in these countries does not necessarily apply to populations in the United States and Great Britain.

Much research has been devoted to the chemistry and pharmacology of cannabinoids in recent years. Earlier work is reviewed by Mesulam (1973), Paton and Crown (1972), Nahas and Paton (1979), Jaffe (1980) and Meyer (1978), and more recent work by Mesulam (1982) and Coper (1982).

Pharmacokinetics

Cannabinoids are highly fat soluble and are quickly and completely absorbed through cell membranes. They are rapidly metabolized in the liver and lungs so that their bioavailability is lower after oral administration or inhalation than after intravenous injection (Agurell et al. 1979). On reaching the blood, delta-9-THC is rapidly distributed, following a similar pattern to thiopentone and other strongly lipophilic substances and reaching high initial concentrations in areas with the highest blood flow. It is gradually taken up by fat depots and the brain, and from these sites it is only slowly released back into the blood. The heart rate changes produced by delta-9-THC tend to parallel the blood concentration changes, but the psychological effects develop as the drug passes out of the blood stream into the brain (Fig. 14.3).

Metabolism of cannabinoids is largely by hydroxylation and some of the metabolites, including the 7-hydroxy and 11-hydroxy derivatives, are pharmacologically active. The elimination half-life of delta-9-THC is 56 h. Traces of this compound and its metabolites persist in the plasma for several days and can be detected in the fat and brain of animals for days after a single administration. Metabolites have been found in the human urine weeks after administration. Because of this extremely slow elimination, repeated use of cannabis can lead to cumulation of cannabinoids in the body. Repeated administration of cannabis may inhibit microsomal function, further reducing the rate of metabolism (Rogers *et al.* 1981), but it is also claimed that chronic marihuana smokers metabolize delta-9-THC more rapidly than non-smokers (Jaffe 1980).

The distribution of delta-9-THC and the 7-hydroxy metabolite within the brain has been studied in the monkey by McIsaac *et al.* (1971) (Table 14.4). Over the time course corresponding with the behavioural effects, the drug was concentrated in the frontal cortex and limbic areas, including hippocampus and amygdala, and in areas concerned with auditory and visual perception, the geniculate bodies, and superior and inferior colliculi. Accumulation of the drug in these areas might account for some of the

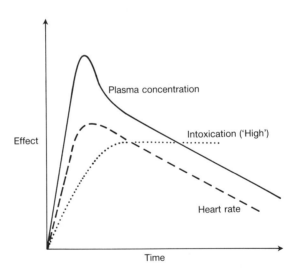

Fig. 14.3. Diagram of the relationship between plasma concentration of delta-9-tetrahydrocannabinol (after inhalation or intravenous injection) and heart rate changes and subjective 'high'. Heart rate changes parallel changes in blood concentration, but the psychological effects develop as the drug passes out of the bloodstream and into the brain. (Reference: Agurell *et al.* 1979.)

Table 14.4.   Distribution of ^{3}H-delta-9-tetrahydrocannabinol in the monkey brain after intravenous administration*

Neocortical areas, especially frontal cortex
Limbic areas, especially hippocampus and amygdala
Sensory areas, including geniculate nuclei, superior and inferior colliculi, visual and parietal cortex
Motor areas, caudate nucleus, putamen, cerebellum
Pons
Highest concentrations occur at 15 min and coincide with maximal behavioural effects

* ^{3}H-delta-9-tetrahydrocannabinol   and   its   7-hydroxy   metabolite   detected   by autoradiography and liquid scintillation.
Reference: McIsaac *et al.* 1971.

psychotropic effects discussed below. The drug was also found in the pons where it may exert cardiovascular effects, and in the cerebellum and caudate nucleus, which may account for the ataxia and inco-ordination.

Clinical effects

Pharmacologically-active cannabinoids have a marked sedative effect which contrasts with the arousing effect of LSD. Apart from this difference, the clinical effects of cannabis are similar to, though usually less intense than, those produced by LSD. They follow a similar temporal sequence: the initial symptoms are mainly somatic, appearing within minutes of the start of smoking. Then follows a 'high' characterized by changes in perception and mood, which reaches a peak in about 30 min and may continue for some hours. Finally, with higher doses a variety of psychotic states may be produced. All these effects are influenced by dosage, personality characteristics, starting state, surroundings, and expectation. Some of the complex interactions between these variables are described by Ashton *et al.* (1981).

The most consistent somatic effects are on the cardiovascular system. There is a dose-related increase in heart rate, sometimes accompanied by hypo- or hypertension and often followed by reddening of the conjuctiva due to vasodilatation. Dry mouth, decreased sweating, and symptoms of gastrointestinal and bronchial irritation may occur, especially in unaccustomed smokers.

Perceptual changes affect all sensory modalities. There may be heightened perception of colour and subjects may see patches or patterns of colours, dimming, brightening, and flowing. Sounds seem more vivid and musical appreciation is increased. General bodily sensations include feelings of float-ing, weightlessness, heaviness or swelling, hot and cold sensations, numbness, and tingling. Spatial perception is distorted: objects can seem abnormally small or large, distances immense or minute, and the surroundings may apear to advance and recede. The perception of time is disturbed, so that felt or reported time is greater than clock time. Feelings of timelessness, of time standing still, and blurring of past, present, and future may come and go. As with LSD, all these symptoms characteristically wax and wane in fluctuating surges.

Mood alterations accompany the perceptual changes. A dose-related euphoria is common; this may vary from contentment and a sense of well-being to exhilaration and ecstasy. When, as commonly practised, small doses are taken at social gatherings, a pleasant euphoria and loquaciousness may be the only symptoms experienced: these effects are very similar to those produced by social doses of alcohol. Fatuous giggling commonly occurs with social doses and paroxysmal attacks similar to some types of 'laughing epilepsy' have been described. The euphoric effect depends to a large degree on the surroundings: it is less common in naive subjects and is most likely to occur when the drug is taken in company. Dysphoria is also common and includes feelings of anxiety and panic, unpleasant somatic sensations and paranoid feelings. Euphoria and dysphoria, laughing and crying, may alter-nate with each other.

Thought processes are initially characterized by a feeling of increased speed of thought, rapid and racing thoughts, flight of ideas, crowding of perceptions, and flooding with thoughts. Thoughts may get out of control, become fragmented, and lead to mental confusion. There are corresponding difficulties in concentrating and impairment of performance in complex tasks occurs even after very small doses. Performance is affected by a combination of increased distractibility, impairment of selective attention and difficulty in shifting from one focus of attention to another. Memory, especially short-term memory, is impaired.

Accompanying the changes in perception, mood, and cognition is an initial state of excitement and increased motor activity. This is followed by a dose-related central nervous system depression, leading to drowsiness and sleep. Initially, the EEG shows a combination of increased fast activity and hyper-synchronization. The effect on the sleeping EEG is similar to that of other hypnotics, including a suppression of REMS. Motor changes induced by cannabis include a state of physical inertia with inco-ordination, ataxia, and dysarthria, which accompanies the sedative effects. In animals a state of catalepsy may occur, but this is rare in man except after high doses.

With higher doses, cannabis can produce frank psychotic changes. Visual and auditory hallucinations may occur. Feelings of unreality and deper-sonalization are common. The subject may feel disembodied, or feel that he is divided into two individuals, one watching the other. Feelings of great insight and significance may occur, and may alternate with sensations of utter meaninglessness. Anxiety, mounting to panic, severe depression, paranoid delusions, and schizophreniform and psychotic states have been described.

Mechanism of action

The mechanism of action of cannabis is completely unknown. It does not appear to react specifically with any neurotransmitter system and, in spite of the similarity of the clinical effects to those of LSD, there is no evidence that delta-9-THC or any other cannabinoid has a special effect on serotonergic systems. Cannabis has been shown in various studies to alter the uptake of dopamine, noradrenaline, serotonin, and GABA into synaptosomes in various parts of the brain in animals. A stereospecific interaction between delta-9-THC with some dopamine receptors in the brain and an action on DA-sensitive adenylate cyclase has been described (Hershkowitz 1978). Interactions occur between delta-9-THC and tricyclic antidepressants, amphetamines, beta adrenoceptor antagonists, and neuroleptics, and it may block acetylcholine release or affect its uptake (Miller 1979). Similarities have also been described between some cannabis actions and those of opiates (Kaymakcalan 1979), suggesting an interaction with endogenous opioids or their receptors. Paton (1979) suggests that low doses of delta-9-THC may act on some specific receptor to produce many of its psychotropic effects because of its high potency and because small changes in structure and the use of optical isomers results in marked loss of activity. However, the chemical structure of delta-9-THC does not immediately suggest an interaction with one of the known neurotransmitters. Higher doses of delta-9-THC probably exert non-specific central nervous system depressant actions as a result of generalized uptake into lipoid cell membranes, similar to general anaesthetics and alcohol. It bears a general structural resemblance to some steroid compounds with central nervous system depressant activity (Gill *et al.* 1972).

Although the mechanism of action is not clear, the site of action for many of the psychological effects is probably in the limbic system and secondary sensory areas (Table 14.4). Ultrastructural abnormalities, including widening of synaptic gaps and clumping of synaptic vesicules have been demonstrated in the septal region, hippocampus and amygdala after delta-9-THC treatment in rats (McGeer and Jakubovic 1979). Cannabis has also been observed to produce electrophysiological changes in these regions. Heath (1972) showed high voltage slow wave activity in the septal area of a human subject after cannabis, the effect coinciding with mood elevation and 'rushes' of euphoria, and dying down as the 'rushes' subsided. Bursts of high amplitude spindles were also noted in the septum, temporal cortex and hippocampus. In animals, cannabinoids disrupt hippocampal theta-rhythm (Miller 1979) and have both stimulant and depressant effects on hippocampal seizures (Feeney 1979).

Biochemical studies (Izquierdo *et al.* 1973) have shown that cannabis blocks potassium efflux from the afferently stimulated hippocampus and impairs the normal increase in RNA concentration following afferent stimulation. Finally, lesions of the hippocampus can reproduce many of the functional impairments seen with cannabis (Miller 1979; Stiglick *et al.* 1984).

Adverse effects

The acute toxicity of cannabis preparations is low and deaths from overdose almost never occur (Paton *et al.* 1973). 'Bad trips' with acute panic reactions occur in some subjects and 'flashbacks' of psychological symptoms despite periods of abstinence have been reported. Acute psychotic reactions can occur with high doses. Paton *et al.* (1973) concluded that any subject could be made to pass through a reversible schizophrenia-like state with an appropriate dose of cannabis. Cannabis aggravates the symptoms of schizophrenia. Many cases have been reported in which the use of cannabis caused a recurrence of acute psychotic symptoms in patients well controlled with antipsychotic drugs. Several cases have also been described in which the taking of cannabis appeared to initiate schizophrenia in apparently normal subjects. Rottanburg *et al.* (1982) reported that heavy cannabis use is associated with a rapidly resolving psychotic illness which resembles schizophrenia and includes marked hypomanic features. Whether cannabis *per se* causes this psychosis or merely acts as a precipitant in predisposed individuals is not clear.

Long-term chronic cannabis use has been said to cause an amotivational syndrome which includes apathy, dullness, impairment of concentration and memory, and general unwillingness to undertake complex tasks or to make long-term plans. Others have claimed permanent intellectual impairment and personality change. It is still debatable whether such alterations are due to the effects of cannabis (Meyer 1978; Murray 1986). However, the very slow elimination of cannabinoids and extended half-life of psychoactive principles, as well as possible cumulative effects of repeated cannabis use are likely to lead to considerable impairment of performance in regular users. Other health risks are reviewed by Maykut (1985).

Tolerance and dependence

There is little doubt that a marked degree of tolerance of cannabis occurs both in animals and man (Coper 1982). This applies to the autonomic, sedative, and psychological effects. Cross-tolerance with alcohol and some other central nervous system depressants occurs, but there is no cross-tolerance to LSD or other psychotomimetic agents. The so-called 'reverse tolerance' in which experienced users obtain psychological effects from smaller doses than previously necessary may be due to learning, placebo effects, saturation of lipid binding sites, increased formation of active metabolites, or practice at inhaling the drug (Rogers *et al.* 1981).

Delta-9-THC is rewarding in animals who can be trained to self-administer it (Chapter 4). In man, a degree of dependence can occur although its dependence-producing potential appears to be relatively low. Abrupt withdrawal of cannabis after chronic high dose usage leads to a syndrome of irritability, restlessness, anxiety, anorexia, weight loss, insomnia, tremor, and hyperpyrexia. There is a rebound in REMS which is suppressed by cannabis (Jaffe 1980). Occasional social doses, however, do not seem to lead to severe drug-dependence in the vast majority of individuals.

Relationship to schizophrenia

The relationship of cannabis actions to schizophrenia has been discussed by Paton *et al.* (1973) and by Ashton (1982). As with LSD, there are certain similarities between the clinical symptoms of the psychosis and the pscyhotic symptoms produced by large doses of cannabis. It is well documented that cannabis, like LSD and amphetamines, can aggravate the symptoms of established schizophrenia and may possibly precipitate the condition in predisposed subjects. However, the mechanisms of action of cannabis are unknown and the vast amount of research devoted to this drug in the past 15 years has contributed little to the understanding of schizophrenia. At present it appears that any agent, pharmacological or non-pharmacological, which disrupts limbic integrative functions may produce similar symptoms. Psychotomimetic drugs may act primarily on serotinergic (LSD), dopaminergic or noradrenergic (amphetamine, cocaine), opioid (phencyclidine, alcohol, narcotics), or other pathways. The clinical picture produced may depend on the anatomical site and the functional state of the pathways affected. To understand why some individuals develop depression or mania, some anxiety states, some schizophrenia, and some intermediate states when exposed to similar circumstances requires a greater knowledge of the way limbic functions are organized than is at present available.

References

Abraham, P., McCallum, W. C., and Gourley, J. (1976). The CNV and its relation to specific psychiatric syndromes. In *The Responsive Brain* (eds J. R. Knott, and W. C. McCallum), pp. 144-9. John Wright, Bristol.

Ackner, B. (1956). The relationship between anxiety and the level of peripheral vasomotor activity. *J. Psychosom. Res.* **1**, 21-48.

Ackenheil, M. (1980). Biochemical effects (in man). In *Psychotropic Agents Part I: Antipsychotics and Antidepressants* (eds F. Hoffmeister, and G. Stille), pp. 213-23. Springer-Verlag, Berlin.

Adam, K., Adamson, L., Brezinova, V., Hunter, W. M., and Oswald, I. (1976). Nitrazepam: lastingly effective but trouble on withdrawal. *Br. Med. J.* **1**, 1558-62.

Adam, K., Allen, S., Carruthers-Jones, I., Oswald, I., and Spence, M. (1976). Mesoridazine and human sleep. *Br. J. clin. Pharmac.* **3**, 157-63.

Adam, K., and Oswald, I. (1977). Sleep is for tissue restoration. *J. Roy. Coll. Physns.* **11**, 376-88.

Agarwal, D. P., Harada, S., Goedde, H. W., and Schrappe, O. (1983). Cytosolic aldehyde dehydrogenase and alcoholism. *Lancet*, **1**, 68.

Agarwal, R. A., Lapierre, Y. D., Rastogi, R. B., and Singhal, R. C. (1977). Alterations in brain 5-hydroxy-tryptamine metabolism during the 'withdrawal' phase after chronic treatment with diazepam and bromazepam. *Br. J. Pharmac.* **60**, 3-9.

Aghajanian, G. K. (1982). Neurophysiological properties of psychotomimetics. In *Psychotropic Agents Part III* (eds F. Hoffmeister, and S. Stille), pp. 89-109. Springer-Verlag, Heidelberg.

Aghajanian, G. K., and Rogawski, M. A. (1983). The physiological role of alpha-adrenoceptors in the CNS: new concepts from single cell studies. *Trends in Pharmic. Sci.* **4**, 315-17.

Agnew, H., Webb, W. B., and Williams, R. L. (1967). Comparison of stage 4 and 1-REM sleep deprivation. *Perceptual Motor Skills*, **24**, 851-8.

Agranoff, B. W., Burrell, H. R., Dokas, L. A., and Springer, A. D. (1978). Progress in Biochemical approaches to learning and memory. In *Psychopharmacology: A Generation of Progress* (eds M. A. Lipton, A. DiMascio, and K. F. Killam), pp. 623-35. Raven Press, New York.

Agurell, S., Lindgren, J. E., and Ohlsson, A. (1979). Introduction to quantification of cannabinoids and their metabolites in biological fluids. In *Marihuana: Biological Effects* (eds G. G. Nahas, and W. D. M. Paton), pp. 3-15. Pergamon Press, Oxford.

Ahlquist, R. P. (1948). A study of the adrenotropic receptors. *Am. J. Physiol.* **153**, 586-600.

Akil, H., Richardson, D. E., Barchas, J. D., and Li, C. H. (1978a). Appearance of beta-endorphin-like immunoreactivity in human ventricular cerebrospinal fluid upon analgesic electrical stimulation. *Proc. Natl. Acad. Sci.* **75**, 5170-2.

Akil, H., Richardson, D. E., Hughes, J., and Barchas, D. (1978b). Enkephalin-like material in ventricular cerebrospinal fluid of pain patients after analgesic focal stimulation. *Science*, **201**, 463–5.

Albrecht, P., Torrey, E. F., Boone, E. Hicks, J. T., and Daniel, N. (1980). Raised cytomegalovirus—antibody level in cerebrospinal fluid of schizophrenic patients. *Lancet*, **ii**, 767–72.

Alexander, B. K., and Hadaway, P. F. (1982). Opiate addiction: the case for an adaptive orientation. *Psychol. Bull.* **92**, 367–81.

Almay, B. G. L., Johansson, F., von Knorring, L., Sedvall, G., and Terenius, L. (1980). Relationships between CSF levels of endorphins and monoamine metabolites in chronic pain patients. *Psychopharmacology*, **62**, 139–42.

Alpern, H. P., and Jackson, S. J. (1978). Stimulants and depressants: drug effects on memory. In *Psychopharmacology: A Generation of Progress* (eds M. A. Lipton, A. DiMascio, and K. F. Killam), pp. 663–75. Raven Press, New York.

Alpert, M., and Friedhoff, A. J. (1980). An un-dopamine hypothesis of schizophrenia. *Schizophrenia Bull.* **6**, 387–90.

Alpert, M., and Martz, J. (1977). Cognitive views of schizophrenia in light of recent studies of brain asymmetry. In *Psychopathology and Brain Dysfunction* (eds C. Shagass, S. Gershon, and A. J. Friedhoff), pp. 1–13. Raven Press, New York.

Altman, H. J., Nordy, D. A., and Ogren, S. O. (1984). Role of serotonin in memory: facilitation by alaprocate and zimeldine. *Psyhopharmacology*, **84**, 496–502.

Amir, S., Amit, Z., and Brown, Z. W. (1981). Stress, endorphins and psychosis. *Mod. Prob. Pharmacopsychiat.* **17**, 192–201.

Amsterdam, J., Brunswick, D., and Mendels, J. (1980). The clinical application of tricyclic antidepressant pharmacokinetics and plasma levels. *Am. J. Psychiat.* **137**, 653–62.

Amsterdam, J. D., Winokur, A., Bryant, S., Larkin, J., and Rickels, K. (1983). The dexamethasone suppression test as a predictor of antidepressant response. *Psychopharmacology*, **80**, 43–5.

Anderson, J. M., and Hubbard, B. M. (1981). Age-related changes in Alzheimer's disease. *Lancet*, **ii**, 1261.

Anderson, P. (1982). Cerebellar synaptic plasticity—putting theories to the test. *Trends Neurosci.* **5**, 324–5.

Anderson, P., Cremona, A., and Wallace, P. (1984). What are safe levels of alcohol consumption? *Br. Med. J.* **289**, 1657–8.

Andersson, K. (1975). Effects of cigarette smoking on learning and retention. *Psychopharmacologia, (Berl.)* **41**, 1–5.

Andersson, K., and Hockey, G. R. J. (1977). Effects of cigarette smoking on incidental memory. *Psychopharmacology*, **52**, 223–6.

Ando, K., and Yanagita, T. (1981). Cigarette smoking in rhesus monkey. *Psychopharmacology*, **72**, 117–27.

Angrist, B., Rotrosen, J., and Gershon, S. (1980). Differential effects of amphetamine and neuroleptics on negative vs. positive symptoms in schizophrenia. *Psychopharmacology*, **72**, 17–9.

Anisman, H., Kokkinidis, L., and Sklar, L. S. (1981). Contribution of neurochemical change to stress-induced behavioural deficits. In *Theory in Psychopharmacology*, Vol.I. (ed S. J. Cooper), pp. 65–102. Academic Press, London.

Annear, W. C., and Vogel-Sprott, M. (1985). Mental rehearsal and classical conditioning contribute to ethanol tolerance in humans. *Psychopharmacology*, **87**, 90–3.

Antelman, S. M., and Chiodo, L. A. (1981). Repeated antidepressant treatments induce a long-lasting dopamine autoreceptor subsensitivity: is daily treatment necessary for clinical efficiency? *Psychopharmacology Bull.* **17,** 92–4.

Appel, J. B., Poling, A. D., and Kuhn, D. M. (1982). Psychotomimetics: behavioural pharmacology. In *Psychotropic Agents Part III* (eds F. Hoffmeister and S. Stille) pp. 45–55. Springer-Verlag, Heidelberg.

Appleyard, M. E., Smith, A. D., Wilcock, G. K., and Esiri, M. M. (1983). Decreased CSF acetylcholinesterase activity in Alzheimer's disease. *Lancet,* **ii,** 452.

Aranko, K., Mattila, M. J., and Seppala, T. (1983). Development of tolerance and cross-tolerance to the psychomotor actions of lorazepam and diazepam in man. *Br. J. clin. Pharmac.* **15,** 545–52.

Arbuthnott, G. W. (1980). The dopamine synapse and the return of 'pleasure centres' in the brain. *Trends Neurosci.* **3,** 199–200.

Arendt, T., Bigl, V., Waltther, F., and Sonntag, M. (1984). Decreased ratio of CSF acetylcholinesterase to butyrylcholinesterase activity in Alzheimer;s disease. *Lancet,* **i,** 173.

Armitage, A. K., Hall, G. H., and Morrison, C. (1968). Pharmacological basis for the tobacco smoking habit. *Nature,* **217,** 331–4.

Armitage, A. K., Hall, G. H., and Sellers, C. M. (1969). Effects of nicotine on electrical activity and acetylcholine release from the cat cerebral cortex. *Br. J. Pharmac.* **35,** 152–60.

Arnt, J., and Scheel-Kruger, J. (1979). GABA in the ventral tegmental area: differential regional effects on locomotion, aggression and food intake after microinjection of GABA agonists and antagonists. *Life Sciences,* **25,** 1351–60.

Ary, T. E., and Komiskey, H. L. (1982). Phencyclidine-induced release of [³³H] dopamine from chopped striatal tissue. *Neuropharmacol.* **21,** 639–45.

Asberg, M., Cronholm, B., Sjoqvist, F., and Tuck, D. (1971). Relationship between plasma level and therapeutic effect of nortriptyline. *Br. Med J.* **3,** 331–4.

Asberg, M., and Sjoqvist, F. (1981) Therapeutic monitoring of tricyclic antidepressants—clinical aspects. In *Therapeutic Drug Monitoring.* (eds A. Richens, and V. Marks), pp. 224–38. Churchill Livingstone, Edinburgh.

Asberg, M., Thoren, P., Trasken, L., Bertilsson, L., and Ringberger, V. (1976). 'Serotonin depression' —a biochemical subgroup within the affective disorders? *Science,* **191,** 478–80.

Aserinsky, E., and Kleitman, N. (1953). Regularly occurring periods of eye motility and concomitant phenomena during sleep. *Science,* **118,** 273–4.

Ashton, H. (1982). Actions of cannabis: do they shed light on schizophrenia?. In *Biological Aspects of Schizophrenia and Addiction* (ed G. Hemmings), pp. 225–41. John Wiley and Sons, London.

Ashton, H. (1983a). Drugs and driving. *Adverse Drug Reaction Bull.* **98,** 360–3.

Ashton, H. (1983b). Teratogenic drugs. *Adverse Drug Reaction Bull.* **101,** 372–5

Ashton, H. (1984). Benzodiazepine withdrawal: an unfinished story. *Br. Med J.* **288,** 1135–40.

Ashton, H. (1985a). Disorders of the foetus and infant. In *Textbook of Adverse Drug Reactions.* (ed D. M. Davies), pp. 77–127. Oxford University Press, Oxford.

Ashton, H. (1985b). Benzodiazepine overdose: are specific antagonists useful? *Br. Med J.* **290,** 805–6.

Ashton, H. (1986). Adverse effects of prolonged benzodiazepine use. *Adverse Drug Reaction Bull.* **118,** 440–3.

Ashton, H., Golding, J. F., Marsh, V. R., Millman, J. E., and Thompson, J. W. (1981). The seed and the soil: effects of dosage, personality and starting state on the response to delta⁹tetrahydrocannabinol in man. *Br. J. Pharmac.* **12,** 705–20.

Ashton, H., Golding, J. F., Marsh, V. R., and Thomspon, J. W. (1985). Somatosensory evoked potentials and personality. *Person. individ. Diff.* **6,** 141–3.

Ashton, H., Marsh, V. R., Millman, J. E., Rawlins, M. D., Telford, R., and Thompson, J. W. (1980). Biphasic dose-related responses of the CNV (contingent negative variation) to IV nicotine in man. *Br. J. clin. Pharmac.* **10,** 579–89.

Ashton, H., Millman, J. E., Telford, R., and Thompson, J. W. (1974). The effect of caffeine, nitrazepam and cigarette smoking on the contingent negative variation in man. *Electroenceph. clin. Neurophysiol.* **37,** 59–71.

Ashton, H., Millman, J. E., Telford, R., and Thompson, J. W. (1976). A comparison of some physiological and psychological effects of propranolol and diazepam in normal subjects. *Br. J. clin. Pharmac.* **3,** 551–9.

Ashton, H., Millman, J. E., Telford, R., and Thompson, J. W. (1978). A comparison of some physiological and psychological effects of Motival (fluphenazine and nortriptyline) and diazepam in normal subjects. *Br. J. clin. Pharmac.* **5,** 141–7.

Ashton, H., Savage, R. D., Telford, R., Thompson, J. W., and Watson D. W. (1972). The effects of cigarette smoking on the response to stress in a driving simulator. *Br. J. Pharmac.* **45,** 546–56.

Ashton, H., and Stepney, R. (1982). *Smoking: Psychology and Pharmacology.* Tavistock Publications, London.

Ashton, H., and Watson, D. W. (1970). Puffing frequency and nicotine intake in cigarette smokers. *Br. Med. J.* **3,** 679–81.

Atweh, S. F., and Kuhar, M. J. (1983). Distribution and function of opioid receptors. *Br. Med. Bull.* **39,** 47–52.

Averback, P. (1983). Two new lesions in Alzheimer's disease. *Lancet,* **ii,** 1203.

Ayd, F. J. (1986). Five to fifteen years' maintenance doxepin therapy. *Int. Clin. Psychopharmacol.* **1,** 53–65.

Azmitia, E. (1978). Reorganisation of the 5-HT projections to the hippocampus. *Trends Neurosci.* **1,** 45–8.

Baastrup, P. C., Poulsen, J. C., Schou, M., Thomsen, K., and Amdisen, A. (1970). Prophylactic lithium: double blind discontinuation in manic-depressive and recurrent depressive disorders. *Lancet,* **ii,** 326–30.

Badawy, A. A-B., and Evans, M. (1981). The mechanism of the antagonism by naloxone of acute alcohol intoxication. *Br. J. Pharmac.* **74,** 514–6.

Baldessarini, R. J. (1980). Drugs and the treatment of psychiatric disorders. In *The Pharmacological Basis of Therapeutics.* (eds A. G. Gilman,. L. S. Goodman, and A. Gilman), pp. 391–447. Macmillan Co., New York.

Baldessarini, R. J., Stramentolini, G. and Lipinski, J. F. (1979). Methylation hypothesis. *Arch. Gen. Psychiat.* **36,** 303–7.

Ball, M. J., Fisman, M. Hachinski, V., Blume, W., Fox, A., Kral, V. A., Kirshen, A. J., Fox, H., and Merskey, H. (1985). A new definition of Alzheimer's disease: a hippocampal dementia. *Lancet,* **i,** 14–6.

Ballenger, J. C., and Post, R. M. (1980). Carbamazepine in manic-depressive illness: a new treatment. *Am. J. Psychiat.* **137,** 782–90.

Ban, T. A. (1978). Vasodilators, stimulants, and anabolic agents in the treatment of geropsychiatric patients. In *Psychopharmacology: A Generation of Progress.* (eds M. A. Lipton, A. DiMascio, and K. F. Killam), pp. 1525–33. Raven Press, New York.

Bandler, R. (1984). Indentification of hypothalamic and midbrain periaquaductal grey neurones mediating aggressive and defensive behaviour by intracerebral microinjections of excitatory amino acids. In *Modulation of Sensorimotor Activity During Alterations in Behavioural States*. (ed R. Bandler), pp. 369-91. Alan R. Liss Inc. New York.

Banki, C. M. (1977). Correlation of anxiety and related symptoms with cerebrospinal fluid 5-hydroxyindolacetic acid in depressed women. *J. Neurol. Transm.* **41**, 135-43.

Banks, W. A., and Kastin, A. J. (1983) Aluminium increases permeability of the blood-brain barrier to labelled D.S.I.P. and beta-endorphin: possible implications for senile and dialysis dementia. *Lancet*, **ii**, 1227-1229.

Barbaccia, M. L., Chuang, D-M., Gandolfi, O., and Costa, E. (1983). Trans-synaptic mechanisms in the actions of imipramine. In *Frontiers in Neuropsychiatric Research*. (eds E. Usdin, M. Goldstein, A. J. Friedhoff, and A. Georgatas), pp. 19-31. Macmillan Co., London.

Barbaccia, M. L., Reggiani, A., Spano, P. F., and Trabucchi, M. (1981). Ethanol-induced changes of dopaminergic function in three strains of mice characterised by a different population of opiate receptors. *Psychopharmacology*, **74**, 260-2.

Barchas, J. D., Elliott, G. R., and Berger, P. A. (1977). Biogenic amine hypotheses of schizophrenia. In *Psychopharmacology: From Theory to Practice* (eds J. D. Barchas, P. A. Berger, R. D. Ciaranello, and Elliott, G. R.), PP. 100-20. Oxford University Press, New York.

Barker, J. L., and Mathers, D. A. (1981). GABA receptors and the depressant action of pentobarbitol. *Trends Pharmac. Sci.* **4**, 10-3.

Barnard, E. A., and Demoliou-Mason, C. (1983). Molecular properties of opioid receptors. *Br. Med. Bull.* **39**, 37-46.

Barnes, P. J. (1981). Radioligand binding studies of adrenergic receptors and their clinical relevance. *Br. Med. J.* **282**, 1207-10.

Barnes, T. R. E., and Bridges, P. K. (1982). New generation of antidepressants. In *Drugs in Psychiatric Practice*. (ed P. J. Tyrer), pp. 219-48. Butterworth & Co. London.

Bartholini, G., and Lloyd, K. G. (1980). Biochemical effects of neuroleptic drugs. In *Psychotropic Agents Part I: Antipsychotics and Antidepressants*. (eds F. Hoffmeister, and G. Stille), pp. 193-212. Springer-Verlag, Berlin.

Baskin, D. S., and Hosobuchi, Y. (1981) Naloxone reversal of ischaemic neurological deficits in man. *Lancet*, **ii**, 272-5.

Batini, C., Moruzzi, G., Palestrini, M., Rossi, G. R., and Zanchetti, A. (1959). Effects of complete pontine transection on the sleep-wakefulness rhythm: The mid-pontine pretrigeminal section. *Arch. Ital. Biol.* **97**, 1-12.

Bear, D., Levin, K., Blumer, D., Chatham, D., Ryder, J. (1982). Interictal behaviour in hospitalised temporal lobe epileptics: relationship to idiopathic psychiatric syndromes. *J. Neurol. Neurosurg. Psychiat.* **45**, 481-8.

Beart, P. M. (1982). Multiple dopamine receptors-new vistas. In *More about Receptors*. (ed J. W. Lamble), pp. 87-92. Elsevier Biomedical Press, Amsterdam.

Beary, M. D., Lacey, J. H., and Bhat, A. V. (1983). The neuroendocrine impact of 3-hydroxy-diazepam (temazepam) in women. *Psychopharmacology*. **79**, 295-7.

Beaumont, J. G. (1983). *Introduction to Neuropsychology*. Blackwell Scientific Pubs. Oxford.

Beck, A. T. (1967). *Depression: Clinical Experimental and Theoretical Aspects*. Harper and Row, New York.

Beckmann, H., and Goodwin, F. K. (1975). Antidepressant responses to tricyclics and urinary MHPG in unipolar patients. *Arch. Gen. Psychiat.* **32**, 17–21.

Beckmann, H., and Haas, S. (1980). High dose diazepam in schizophrenia. *Psychopharmacology*, **71**, 79–82.

Beecher, H. K. (1959). *Measurement of Subjective Responses.* Oxford University Press, Oxford.

Beeley, L. (1978). Drugs in early pregnancy. *J. Pharmacother.* **1**, 189.

Behar, M., Magora, F., Olshwang, D., and Davidson, J. T. (1979). Epidural morphine in treatment of pain. *Lancet*, **i**, 527–8.

Bejerot, N. (1980). Addiction to pleasure: a biological and social-psychological theory of addiction. In *Theories on Drug and Abuse.* (eds D. J. Lettieri, M. Sayers, and H. W. Pearson), pp. 246–55. Dept. of Health and Human Services, National Institute of Drug Abuse, Rockville, Md., U.S.A.

Belleroche, J. S., de and Bradford, H. F. (1981). Evidence for an inhibitory presynaptic component of neuroleptic drug action. *Br. J. Pharmac.* **72**, 427–33.

Benedetti, M.S., and Dostert, P. (1985). Stereochemical aspects of MAO interactions: reversible and selective inhibitors of monoamine oxidase. *Trends Neurosci.* **6**, 246–7.

Benedittis, G., de., and Gonda, F., de., (1986). Hemispheric specialisation and the perception of pain: a task-related EEG power spectrum analysis in chronic pain patients. *Pain*, **22**, 375–84.103.

Bennett, J. P., Enna, S. J., Bylund, D. B., Gillin, J. C., Wyatt, R. J., and Snyder, S. (1979). Neurotransmitter receptors in frontal cortex of schizophrenics. *Arch. Gen. Psychiat.* **36**, 927–34.

Benton, D., and Rick, J. T. (1976). The effect of increased brain GABA produced by amino-oxyacetic acid on arousal in rats. *Psychopharmacology*, **49**, 85–9.

Berger, P. A. (1977). Antidepressant medications and the treatment of depression. In *Psychopharmacology: from Theory to Practice.* (eds J. D. Barchas, P. A. Berger, R. D. Ciaranello, and G. R. Elliott), pp. 174–207. Oxford University Press, New York.

Berger, P. A., and Barchas, J. D. (1977). Biochemical hypotheses of affective disorders. In *Psychopharmacology: from Theory to Practice.* (eds J. D. Barchas, P. A. Berger, R. D. Ciaranello, and G.R. Elliott), pp. 151–73. Oxford University Press, New York.

Berger, P. A., and Dunn, M. J. (1985). Tardive dyskinesia: the major problem with antipsychotic maintenance therapy. In *Drugs in Psychiatry.* (eds G. D. Burrows, T. R. Norman, and B. Davies), Vol.3, pp. 185–212. Elsevier Science Publishers BV, Amsterdam.

Berger, T., French, E. D., Siggins, G. R., Shier, W. T., and Bloom, F. F. (1982). Ethanol and some tetrahydroisoquinolines alter the discharge of cortical and hippocampal neurones: relationship to endogenous opioids. *Pharmacol. Biochem. Behav.* **17**, 813–21.

Bergman, U., and Griffiths, R. R. (1986). Relative abuse of diazepam and oxazepam: prescription forgeries and theft/loss reports in Sweden. *Drug and Alcohol Dependence* **16**, 293–301.

Berntson, G. G., Beattie, M. S., and Walker, J. M. (1976). Effects of nicotine and muscarinic compounds in biting attack in the cat. *Pharmacol. Biochem. and Behav.* **5**, 235–9.

Berridge, M. J. (1981). Receptors and calcium signalling. In *Towards Understanding Receptors.* (ed J. W. Lamble), pp. 122–31. Elsevier/North Holland Biomed. Press.

Besson, J. (1983). Dementia: biological solution still a long way off. *Br. Med. J.* **287,** 926–7.

Betts, T. A., and Birtle, J. (1982). Effects of two hypnotic drugs on actual driving performance next morning. *Br. Med J.* **285,** 852.

Bevan, P., Bradshaw, C. M., and Szabadi, E. (1975). The effect of tricyclic antidepressants on cholinergic responses of single cortical neurones. *Br. J. Pharmac.* **53,** 29–36.

Bevan, P., Bradshaw, C. M., and Szabadi, E. (1977). The pharmacology of adrenergic neuronal responses in the cerebral cortex: evidence for excitatory alpha and inhibitory beta receptors. *Br. J. Pharmac.* **59,** 635–41.

Bialos, D., Giller, E., Jatlow, P., Docherty, J., and Harkness, M. S. W. (1982). Recurrence of depression after long-term amitriptyline treatment. *Am J. Psychiat.***139,** 325–7.

Bickel, M. H. (1980). Metabolism of antidepressants. In *Psychotropic Agents Part I: Antipsychotics and Antidepressants.* (eds F. Hoffmeister, and G. Stille), pp. 551–72. Springer-Verlag, Berlin.

Bickford, R. G., Mulder, D. W., Dodge, H. W., Svien, H. J., and Rome, P. R. (1958). Changes in memory function produced by electrical stimulation of the temporal lobe in man. *Res. Publ. Ass. Res. nerv. ment. Dis.* **36,** 227.

Biegon, A., and Samuel, D. (1980). Interaction of tricyclic antidepressants and opiate receptors. *Biochem. Pharmacol.* **29,** 460–2.

Bierness, D., and Vogel-Sprott, M. (1984). Alcohol tolerance in social drinkers: operant and classical conditioning effects. *Psychopharmacology,* **84,** 393–7.

Bird, E. D. (1978). Huntingdon's disease (chorea). *Trends Neurosci.* **1,** 57–9.

Bird, K. D., Chesher, G. B., Perl, J., and Starmer, G. A. (1982). Naloxone has no effect on ethanol-induced impairment of psychomotor performance in man. *Psychopharmacology,* **76,** 193–7.

Birkmayer, W., and Riederer, P. (1975) Biochemical postmortem findings in depressed patients. *Adv. Biochem. Psychopharmacol.* **11,** 397–97.

Bjorkelund, A., and Stenevi, U. (1979) Regeneration of monoaminergic and cholinergic neurones in the mammalian central nervous system. *Physiol. Rev.* **59,** 62–100.

Black, D. (1982). Misuse of solvents. *Health Trends.* **14,** 27–8.

Blake, D. R., Dodd, M. J., and Grimley-Evans, J. (1978). Vasopressin in amnesia. *Lancet,* **i** , 608.

Blaustein, M. P., and Ector, A. C. (1975). Barbiturate inhibition of calcium uptake by depolarised nerve terminals *in vitro. Molecular Pharmacol.* **11,** 369–78.

Blier, P., Montigny, C., de and Tardif, D. (1984). Effects of the two antidepressant drugs mianserin and indalpine on the serotonergic system: single cell studies in the rat. *Psychopharmacology,* **84,** 242–9.

Bliss, T. V. P. (1979). Synaptic plasticity in the hippocampus. *Trends Neurosci.* **2,** 42–5.

Bliss, T. V. P., and Dolphin, A. C. (1982). What is the mechanism of long-term potentiation in the hippocampus? *Trends Neurosci.* **5,** 289–90.

Bliss, T. V. P., and Gardner-Medwin, A. R. (1973). Long-lasting potentiation of synaptic transmission in the denstate area of the unanaesthetised rabbit following stimulation of the perforant path. *J. Physiol. Lond.* **232,** 357–74.

Bloch, V., and Bonvallet, M. (1960). Le controle inhibiteur bulbaire des responses electrodermales. *C. R. Soc. Biol.* **154,** 42–5.

Bloom, F. E. (1985). Neurotransmitter diversity and its functional significance. *J. Roy. Soc. Med.* **78**, 189–92.

Bloom, G., Euler, U. S. von., and Frankenhaeuser, M. (1963). Catecholamine excretion and personality traits in paratroop trainees. *Acta. Physiol. Scand.* **58**, 77–89.

Blum, K., Hamilton, M. G., Hirst, M., and Wallace, J. E. (1978). Putative role of isoquinoline alkaloids in alcoholism: a link to opiates. *Alcoholism: clinical and Exp. Res.* **2**, 113–20.

Boeuf, L. le., Lodge, A., J, and Eames, P. G. (1978). Vasopressin and memory in Korsakoff's syndrome. *Lancet*, **ii**, 570.

Bohus, B., Gispen, W. H., and Wied, D. de., (1973). Effect of lysine vasopressin and ACTH4-10 on conditional avoidance behaviour of hypophysectomised rats. *Neuroendocrinology*, **11**, 137–43.

Bohus, B., Kovacs, G. L., and Wied, D. de., (1978). Oxytocin, vasopressin and memory: opposite effects on consolidation and retrieval processes. *Brain Research*, **157**, 414–7.

Bolles, R. C., and Fanselow, M. S. (1982). Endorphins and behaviour. *Ann. Rev. Psychol.* **33**, 87-101.

Bond, A. J., James, C. C., and Lader, M. H. (1974). Physiological and psychological measures in anxious patients. *Psychol. Med.* **4**, 364–73.

Bond, A., and Lader, M. (1981). After-effects of sleeping drugs. In *Psychopharmacology of Sleep.* (ed D. Wheatly), pp. 177–97. Raven Press, New York.

Bond, M. R. (1979). *Pain: its Nature, Analysis and Treatment.* Churchill Livingstone, Edinburgh.

Bond, M. R. (1980). Personality and Pain. In *Persistent Pain: Modern Methods of Treatment.* (ed S. Lipton), Vol.2, pp. 1–26. Academic Press, London and Grune and Stratton, New York.

Bondareff, W. (1983). Age and Alzheimer disease. *Lancet*, **i**, 1447.

Bondareff, W., Mountjoy, C. Q., and Roth, M. (1981) Selective loss of neurones of origin of adrenergic projection to cerebral cortex (nucleus locus coeruleus) in senile dementia. *Lancet*, **i**, 783–4.

Bonn, J. A., Readhead, C. P. A., and Timmons, B. H. (1984). Enhanced adaptive behavioural response in agoraphobic patients pretreated with breathing retraining. *Lancet*, **ii**, 665–9.

Bonn, J. A., Turner, P., and Hicks, D. (1972). Beta-adrenergic-receptor blockade with practolol in treatment of anxiety. *Lancet*, **i**, 814–5.

Borland, R. G., and Nicholson, A. N. (1975). Comparison of the residual effects of two benzodiazepines (nitrazepam and flurazepam hydrocholoride) and pentobarbitone on human performance. *Br. J. clin. Pharmac.* **2**, 9–17.

Bottjer, S. W., and Arnold, A. P. (1984). Hormones and structural plasticity in the adult brain. *Trends Neurosci.* **7**, 168–71.

Bourne, H. R., Bunney, W. E., Colburn, R. W., Davis, J. M., Davis, J. N., Shaw, D. M., and Coppen, A. J. (1968). Noradrenaline, 5-hydroxytryptamine, and 5-hydroxyindolacetic acid in hind brains of suicidal patients. *Lancet*, **ii**, 805–8.

Bousfield, D. (1982). Old age, dementia and the brain. *New Scientist.* **94**, 648.

Bousigue, Y. X., Girand, L. Fournie, D., and Tremoulet, M. (1982). Naloxone reversal of neurological deficit. *Lancet*, **ii**, 618–9.

Bowen, D. M., and Davison, A. N. (1984). Dementia in the elderly: biochemical aspects. *J. Roy. Coll. Physicians*, **18**, 25–7.

Bowers, M. B. (1980). Biochemical processes in schizophrenia: an update. *Schizophrenia Bull.* **6**, 393–403.

Bowers, M. B., and Heminger, G. R. (1977). Lithium: clinical effects and cerebrospinal fluid monoamine metabolites. *Commun. Psychopharmacol.* **1**, 135-45.

Bowery, N. G. (1976). Reversal of the action of gamma-aminobutyric acid (GABA) antagonists by barbiturates. *Br. J. Pharmac.* **58**, 456P.

Bowker, R. M. (1984). Chemically identified pathways in the brainstem and their possible roles in sleep-arousal mechanisms. In *Modulation of Sensorimotor Activity During Alterations in Behavioural States.* (ed R. Bandler), pp. 76-95. Alan R. Liss Inc., New York.

Bowman, W. C., Rand, M. J., and West. G. B. (1968). *Textbook of Pharmacology.* Blackwell Scientific Publications. Oxford.

Bowsher, D. (1978a). Pain pathways and mechanisms. *Anaesthesia*, **33**, 935-44.

Bowsher, D. (1978b). *Mechanisms of Nervous Disorder: an Introduction.* Blackwell Scientific Publications, Oxford.

Bradley, P. B. (1958). The central action of drugs in relation to the reticular formation of the brain. In *Reticular Formation of the Brain.* (eds H. H. Jasper, L. D. Proctor, R. S. Knighton, W. C. Noshay, and R. T. Costello) pp. 123-50. Churchill, London.

Bradley, P. B. (1961). The pathophysiology of consciousness. In *Bewusstseinsstorung.* (eds H. Staub, and H. Tholen), pp. 14-22. Georg Thieme Verlag, Stuttgart. Symposium von 10 January. St. Moritz, Schweiz.

Bradley, P. B., and Key, B. J. (1958). The effect of drugs on arousal responses produced by electrical stimulation of the reticular formation of the brain. *Electroenceph. clin. Neurophysiol.* **10**, 97-110.

Bradshaw, C. N., Roberts, M. H. T., and Szabadi, E. (1974). Effects of imipramine and desipramine on responses of single cortical neurones to noradrenaline and 5-hydroxytryptamine. *Br. J. Pharmac.* **52**, 349-58.

Braestrup, C., and Nielsen, M. (1980). Benzodiazepine Receptors. *Arzneimittelforschung*, **30**, 852-7.

Braestrup, C., Nielsen, M., Jensen, L. H., Honore, T., and Petersen, E. N. (1983). Benzodiazepine receptor ligands with positive and negative efficacy. *Neuropharmacol.* **22**, 1451-8.

Braestrup, C., Nielsen, M., and Olsen, C. E. (1980). Urinary and brain beta-carboline-3-carboxylates as potent inhibitors of brain benzodiazepine receptors. *Proc. Natl. Acad. Sci., U.S.A.* **77**, 2288-92.

Braestrup, C., Nielsen, M., and Squires, R. F. (1979). No changes in rat benzodiazepines receptor after withdrawal from continuous treatment with lorazepam and diazepam. *Life Sci.* **24**, 347-50.

Braithwaite, R., Montgomery, S., and Dawling, S. (1978). Nortriptyline in depressed patients with high plasma levels II. *Clin. Pharm. Therap.* .**23**, 303-8.

Branchey, M.H., Branchey, L. B., and Richardson, M. A. (1981). Effects of neuroleptic adjustment on clinical condition and tardive dyskinesia in schizophrenic patients. *Am. J. Psychiat.* **13**, 608-12.

Branconnier, R. J., and Cole, J. O. (1977). Effects of chronic papaverine administration on mild senile Organic Brain Syndrome. *J. Am. Geriatr. Soc.* **25**, 458-62.

Brandon, S., Cowley, P., McDonald, C., Neville, P. Palmer, I. C., and Wellstood-Eason, S. (1984). Electroconvulsive therapy: results in depressive illness from the Leicestershire trial. *Br. Med J.* **288**, 22-5.

Brazier, M. A. B. (1977). *Electrical Activity of the Nervous System.* Pitman Medical Publishing Co. Ltd. Tunbridge Wells, Kent.

Brecher, E. M. (1972). *Licit and Illicit Drugs.* Consumers Union, Mount Vernon, New York.

Breckon, B., (1983). Mainline to hell. *B.M.A. News Review*, **9**, 29–32.

Breimer, D. D., and Jochemsen, R. (1981). Pharmacokinetics of hypnotic drugs. In *Psychopharmacology of Sleep* (ed D. Wheatley), pp. 135–52. Raven Press, New York.

Bremer, F. (1935). Cerveau isolé et physiologie du sommeil. *C. R. Soc. Biol. (Paris)*, **118**, 1235–42.

Bremer, F. (1970). Preoptic hypnogenic focus and mesencephalic reticular formation. *Brain Res.* **21**, 132–4.

Breuker, E., Dingledine, R., and Iverson, L. L. (1976). Evidence for naloxone and opiates as GABA antagonists. *Br. J. Pharmac.* **58**, 458P.

Breyer-Pfaff, V. (1980) Metabolism and Kinetics. In *Psychotropic Agents Part I: Antipsychotics and Antidepressants.* (eds F. Hoffmeister, and G. Stille), pp. 228–304, Springer-Verlag, Berlin.

Bridges, P. K., Barlett, J. R., and Sepping, P. (1976). Precursors and metabolites of 5-hydroxytryptamine and dopamine in the ventricular cerebrospinal fluid of psychiatric patients. *Psychol. Med.* **6**, 399–405.

Brierley, J.B. (1977) Neuropathology of amnesic states. In *Amnesia.* (eds C. W. M. Whitty, and O. L. Zangwill), pp. 199–23. Butterworth, London, Bost.

British Medical Bulletin (1983). *Opioid Peptides.* (ed J. Hughes),**39**, PP. 1–100.

British Medical Journal (1968). Sleep disorder. *Br. Med. J.* **2**, 450.

British Medical Journal (1971). Terrors of sleep. *Br. Med. J.* **2**, 507–8.

British Medical Journal (1972). Neonatal behaviour and maternal barbiturates. *Br. Med. J.* **4**, 63–4.

British Medical Journal (1973). Thyrotrophin-releasing hormone in use. *Br. Med. J.* **2**, 465.

British Medical Journal (1975). Depression and curtailment of sleep. *Br. Med. J.* **4**, 543.

British Medical Journal (1977). Depression in men and women. *Br. Med. J.* **2**, 849–50.

British Medical Journal (1980a). Alcoholism: an inherited disease? *Br. Med. J.* **281**, 1301–2.

British Medical Journal (1980b). Phencyclidine: the new American street drug. *Br. Med. J.* **281**, 1511–2.

British Medical Journal (1981a). Tardive dyskinesia. *Br. Med. J.* **282**, 1257–8.

British Medical Journal (1981b). Minor brain damage and alcoholism. *Br. Med. J.* **2**, 455–6.

British Thoracic Society Research Committee (1983). Comparison of four methods of smoking withdrawal in patients with smoking related diseases. *Br. Med. J.* **286**, 595–87.

Brixen-Rasmussen, L., Halgrener, J., and Jorgensen, A. (1982). Amitriptyline and nortriptyline excretion in human breast milk. *Psychopharmacology*, **76**, 94–5.

Brockaway, A. L., Glaser, G., Winokur, G., and Ulett, G. A. (1984). The use of control population in neuropsychiatric research (psychiatric, psychological and EEG evaluation of a heterogeneous sample). *Am. J. Psychiat.* **111**, 248–62.

Brodie, N. H. (1977). A double blind trial of naftidrofuryl in treating confused elderly patients in general practice. *Practitioner* **218**, 274–8.

Broughton, R., and Gastaut, H. (1973). Memory and sleep . In *Sleep: Physiology,*

Biochemistry, Psychology, Pharmacology, Clinical Implications (eds W.P. Koella, and P. Levin) pp. 53-8. S. Karger, Basel.

Brown, G. M. and Birley, J. L. T. (1968). Crises and life changes at the onset of schizophrenia. *J. Health and Soc. Behav.* **9,** 203-24.

Bruce, M., Scott, N., Lader, M., and Marks, V. (1986). The psychopharmacological and electrophysiological effects of single doses of caffeine in healthy human subjects. *Br. J. Clin. Pharmac* **22,** 81-7

Buchsbaum, M. (1976). Self-regulation of stimulus intensity: augmenting/reducing and the averaged evoked response. In *Consciousness and Self-regulation.* (eds G. E. Scwartz, and D. Shapiro), Vol.1, p.101-35. John Wiley and Sons, London.

Buchsbaum, M. S., Davis, G. C., Naber, D., and Pickar, D. (1983). Pain enhances naloxone-induced hyperalgesia in humans as assessed by somatosensory evoked potentials. *Psychopharmacology,* **79,** 99-103.

Buchsbaum, M., Goodwin, F., Murphy, D., and Borge, G. (1971). Average evoked responses in affective disorders. *Am. J. Psychiat.* **128,** 17-25.

Bunney, B. S. (1984). Antipsychotic drug effects on the electrical activity of dopaminergic neurones. *Trends Neurosci.* **7,** 212-5.

Bunney, W. E. (1978). Psychopharmacology of the switch process in affective illness. In *Psychopharmacology: A Generation of Progress.* (eds M. A. Lipton, A. DiMascio and K. F. Killam), pp.1249-59. Raven Press, New York.

Bunney, W. E., and Davis, J. M. (1965). Noreprinephrine in depressive reactions. *Arch. Gen. Psychiat.* **13,** 483.

Bunney, W. E., Pert, A., Rosenblatt, J., Pert, C. B., and Gallaper, D. (1979). Mode of action of lithium. *Arch. Gen. Psychiat.* **36,** 898-901.

Bureseva, O., and Bures, J. (1976). Piracetam-induced facilitation of interhemispheric transfer of visual information in rats. *Psychopharmacologia,* **46,** 93-102.

Burian, E. (1974). An ergot alkaloid preparation (Hydergine) in the treatment of presenile brain atrophy (Alzheimer's disease): a case report. *J. Am. Geriat. Soc.* **22,** 126-8.

Burkard, W. P., Keller, H. H., Da Prada, M., and Haefely, W. (1983). Neurochemical effects of the atypical antidepressant disclofensine in the rat. In *Frontiers in Neuropsychiatric Research.* (eds E. Usdin, M. Goldstein, A. J. Friedhoff, and A. Georgatas), pp. 109-20. MacMillan Press Ltd., London.

Burn, J. H. (1961). The action of nicotine and the pleasure of smoking. *Advanc. Sci.* **17,** 494-8.

Burrows, G. D., and Davies, B. (1984). Recognition and management of anxiety.. In *Antianxiety Agents.* (eds G. D. Burrows, T. R. Norman, and B. Davies), pp. 1-11. Elsevier Science Publishers BV, Amsterdam.

Bush, H. D., Bush, M. F., Miller, M. A. (1976). Addictive agents and intracranial self-stimulation: daily morphine and lateral hypothalamic self-stimulation. *Physiol. Psychol.* **14,** 79-85.

Butler, S. (1979) Interhemispheric relations in schizophrenia. In *Hemisphere Asymmetries of Function in Psychopathology.* (eds J. Gruzelier, and P. Flor-Henry), pp. 47-59. Elsevier/North Holland Biomedical Press, Amsterdam.

Butler, S. H., Colpitts, Y. H., Gagliardi, G. J., Chen, A. C. N., and Chapman, C. R. (1983). Opiate analgesia and its antagonism in dental event-related potentials: evidence for placebo antagonism. *Psychopharmacology,* **79,** 325-8.

Byck, R. (1976). Peptide transmitters: a unifying hypothesis for euphoria, respiration, sleep, and the action of lithium. *Lancet,* **ii,** 72-3.

Cade, J. F. J. (1949). Lithium salts in the treatment of psychotic excitement. *Med. J. Aust.* **2**, 349–52.

Caine, E. D., Weingartner, H., Ludlow, C. L., Cudahy, E. A., and Wehry, S. (1981). Qualitative analysis of scopolamine-induced amnesia. *Psychopharmacology*, **74**, 74–80.

Calloway, S. P. (1982). Endocrine changes in depression. *Hospital Update*, **8**, 1345–50.

Calloway, S. P., Dolan, R. J., Fonagy, P., Souza, V. F. A. de., and Wakeling, A. (1984a). Endocrine changes and clinical profiles in depression: I. The dexamethasone suppression test. *Psychol. Med.* **14**, 749–58.

Calloway, S. P., Dolan, R. J., Fonagy, P., Souza, V. F. A. de., and Wakeling, A. (1984b). Endocrine changes and clinical profiles in depression: II. The thyrotropin-releasing hormone test. *Psychol. Med.* **14**, 759–65.

Calne, D. B. (1981). Clinical relevance of dopamine receptor classification. In *Towards Understanding Receptors*. (ed J.W. Lamble), pp. 118–21. Elsevier/North-Holland Biochemical Press, Amsterdam.

Campbell, I. C., and Durcan, M. J. (1982) Genetic variation in response of central adrenoceptors to stress.? *Br. J. clin. Pharmac.* Vol. 75, 32P.

Candy J. M., Edwardson, J. A., Klinowski, J., Oakley, A. E., Perry, E. K., and Perry, R. H. (1985). Co-localisation of aluminium and silicon in senile plaques: implications for the neurochemical pathology of Alzheimer's disease. In *Ageing of the Brain*. (eds W. H. Crispen, and J.Traber), Springer Verlag, Berlin.

Candy, J. M., and Key, B. J. (1977). A presynaptic site of action within the mesencephalic reticular formation for (+)-amphetamine-induced electrocortical desynchronisation. *Br. J. Pharmac.* **61**, 331–8.

Candy, J. M., Klinowski, J., Perry, R. H., Perry, E. K., Fairbairn, A., Oakley, A. E., Carpenter, T. A., Atack, J. R., Blessed, G., and Edwardson, J. A. (1986). Aluminosilicates and senile plaque formation in Alzheimer's disease. *Lancet*, **i**, 354–7.

Candy, J. M., Oakley, A. E., Atak, J., Perry, R. H., Perry, E. K., and Edwardson, J. A. (1984). New observations on the nature of senile plaque cores. In *Regulation of Transmitter Function. Proc. 5th Meeting Eur. Soc. Neurochem. Budapest*. (eds E.S. Vizi, and K. Magyar), Academic Press, New York.

Canon, W. B. (1936). *Bodily Changes in Pain, Hunger, Fear and Rage*. (2nd edition). Appleton-Century-Crofts, New York.

Canon, W. B., and Rosenbleuth, A. (1949). *The Supersensitivity of Denervated Structures*. Macmillan Co., New York.

Capell, P. J. (1978). Trends in cigarette smoking in the U.K. *Health Trends*, **10**, 49–54.

Capstick, N. (1980). Long-term fluphenazine deconoate maintenance dosage requirements of chronic schizophrenic patients. *Acta Psychiat. Scan.* **61**, 256–62.

Carlsson, A. (1978). Mechanism of action of neuroleptic drugs. In *Psychopharmacology: A Generation of Progress*. (eds M. A. Lipton, A. DiMascio, and K. F. Killam), pp. 1057–70. Raven Press, New York.

Carlton, P. L., and Wolgin, D. C. (1971). Contingent tolerance to the anorexigenic effect of amphetamine. *Physiol. Behav.* **7**, 331–3.

Carmichael, F. J., and Israel, Y. (1975). Effects of ethanol on neurotransmitter release by rat brain cortical slices. *J. Pharmac. Exp. Therap.* **193**, 824–34.

Carr, G. D., and White, N. M. (1986). Anatomical dissociation of amphetamine's rewarding and aversive sites: an intracranial microinjection study. *Psychopharmacology*, **89**, 340-6.

Carroll, B. J. (1978). Neuroendocrine function in psychiatric disorders. In *Psychopharmacology: A Generation of Progress*. (eds M. A. Lipton, D. DiMascio, and K. M. Killam), pp.487-97. Raven Press, New York.

Carroll, B. J., Feinberg, M., Greden, J. F. (1981). A specific laboratory test for the diagnosis of melancholia. *Arch. Gen. Psychiat.* **38**, 15-24.

Carroll, B. J., Mowbray, R. M., and Davies, B. (1970). Sequential comparison ofL-tryptophan with ECT in severe depression. *Lancet*, **i**, 967-9.

Casey, D. E., Gerlach, J., and Simmelsgaard, H. (1979). Sulpiride in tardive dyskinesia. *Psychopharmacology*. **66**, 73-7.

Casley-Smith, J. R. (1980). Benzopyrones in the treatment of schizophrenia. *Lancet*, **i**, 421.

Castleden, C. M. (1984). Therapeutic possibilities in patients with senile dementia. *J. Roy. Coll. Physicians*. **18**, 28-31.

Catalan, J., and Gath, D. H. (1985). Benzodiazepines in general practice: time for decision. *Br. Med J.* **198**, 1374-6.

Catley, D. M., Lehane, J. R., Jones, J. G. (1981). Failure of naloxone to reverse alcohol intoxication. *Lancet*, **i**, 1263.

Caulfield, M. P., Straughan, D. W., Cross, A. S., Crow, T., and Birdsall, N. J. M. (1982). Cortical muscarinic receptor subtypes and Alzheimer's disease. *Lancet*, **ii**, 1277.

Changeaux, J-P., and Danchin, A. (1976). Selective stabilisation of developing synapses as a mechanism for the specification of neuronal networks. *Nature*, **264**, 705-12.

Charney, D. S., Heninger, G. R., Sternberg, D. E., and Landis, H. (1982). Abrupt discontinuation of tricyclic antidepressant drugs: evidence for noradenergic hyperactivity. *Br. J. Psychiat.* **141**, 377-86.

Charney, D. S., Heninger, G. R., Sternberg, D. E., Redmond, D. E., Leckman, J. F., Maas, J. W., and Roth, R. H. (1981a). Presynaptic adrenergic receptors sensitivity in depression. *Arch. Gen. Psychiat.* 38, 1334-40.

Charney, D. S., Menkes, D. B., and Heninger, G. R. (1981b). Receptor sensitivity and the mechanism of action of antidepressant treatment. *Arch. Gen. Psychiat.* **38**, 1160-80.

Chase, M. H., and Morales, F. R. (1984). Supraspinal control of spinal cord motoneuron membrane potential during active sleep. In *Modulation of Sensorimotor Activity During Alterations in Behavioural States*. (ed R. Bandler), pp. 167-78. Alan R. Liss Inc., New York.

Chen, C. N. Kalucy, R. S., Hartmann, M. K., Lacey, J. H., Crisp, A. H., Bailey, J. E., Eccleston, E. G., and Coppen, A. (1974). Plasma tryptophan and sleep. *Br. Med J.* **4**, 564-6.

Cherry, N., and Kiernan, K. (1976) Personality scores and smoking behaviour. *Br. J. Prevent. Soc. Med.* **30**, 123-31.

Chiu, T. H., and Rosenberg, H. C. (1978). Reduced diazepam binding following chronic benzodiazepine treatment. *Life Sci.* **23**, 1153-8.

Chouinard, G., and Jones, B. D. (1978) Schizophrenia as a dopamine deficiency disease. *Lancet*, **ii**, 99-100.

Christie, M. J., Little, B. C., and Gordon, A. M. (1980). Peripheral indices of depressive states. In *Handbook of Biological Psychiatry Part II. Brain Mechanisms and*

Abnormal Behaviour—Psychopharmacology. (ed V. M. van Praag), pp. 145–82. Marcel Dekker Inc., New York and Basel.

Chu, N. S., and Bloom, F. E. (1973). Norepinephrine-containing neurone changes in spontaneous discharge patterns during sleep and waking. *Science*, **179**, 908–10.

Cicero, T. J. (1978). Tolerance to and physical dependence on alcohol: behavioural and neurobiological mechanisms. In *Brain and Pituitary Peptides*, Ferring Symposium, Munich, 1979, pp 1603–17. Karger, Basel.

Claridge, G. (1978). Animal models of schizophrenia: the case for lsd-25. *Schizophrenia Bull.* **4**, 186–209.

Claridge, G., and Birchall, P. (1978). Bishop, Eysenck, Block, and Psychoticism. *J. Abnorm. Psychol.* **87**, 664–8.

Claridge, G., and Chappa, H. J. (1973). Psychoticism: a study of its biological basis in normal subjects. *Br. J. clin. Psychol.* **12**, 175–87.

Claridge, G. S. (1967). *Personality and Arousal.* Pergamon Press, Oxford

Clark, C. R., Geffen, L. B., and Geffen, G. M. (1984). Monoamines in the control of state-dependent cortical functions: evidence from studies of selective attention in animals and humans. In *Modulation of Sensorimotor Activity During Alterations in Behavioural States.* (ed R. Bandler), pp. 487–502. Alan R. Liss Inc., New York.

Clark, M. S. G. (1969). Self-administered nicotine solution preferred to placebo by the rat. *Br. J. Pharmac.* **35**, 367.

Clarke, C. H., and Nicholson, A. N. (1978). Immediate and residual effects in man of the metabolites of diazepam. *Br. J. clin. Pharmac.* **6**, 325–33.

Clement-Jones, V., and Besser, G. M. (1983). Clinical perspectives in opioid peptides. *Br. Med. Bull.* **39**, 95–100.

Clement-Jones, V., McLoughlin, L., Lowry, P. J., Besser, G. M., Rees, L. H., and Wen, L. H. (1979). Acupuncture in heroin addicts; changes in met-enkephalin and beta endorphin in blood and cerebrospinal fluid. *Lancet*, **ii**, 380–2.

Clement-Jones, V., McLoughlin, L., Tomlins, S. Besser, G. M., Rees, L. H., and Wen, H. L. (1980). Increased beta-endorphin but not met-enkephalin levels in human cerebrospinal fluid after acupuncture for recurrent pain. *Lancet*, **ii**, 946–8.

Clow, A., Jenner, P., and Marsden, C. D. (1979a). Changes in dopamine-mediated behaviour during one year's neuroleptic administration. *Eur. J. Pharmacol.* **57**, 363–75.

Clow, A., Jenner, P., Theodorou, A., and Marsden, C. D. (1979b). Striatal dopamine receptors become supersensitive while rats are given trifluoperazine for six months. *Nature*, **278**, 59–61.

Coble, P., Foster, F., and Kupfer, D. J. (1976). Electroencephalographic sleep diagnosis of primary depression. *Arch. Gen. Psychiat.* **33**, 1124–7.

Cohen, R. M., Campbell, I. C., Dauphin, M., Tallman, J. F., and Murphy, D. L. (1982). Changes in alpha and beta receptor densities in rat brain as a result of treatment with monoamine oxidase inhibiting antidepressants. *Neuropharmacology*, **21**, 293–8.

Cohen, M. R., Cohen, R. M., Pickar, D., Weingartner, H., Murphy, D. L., and Bunney, W. E. (1981). Behavioural effects after high dose naloxone administration to normal volunteers. *Lancet*, **ii**, 1110.

Cohen, S. I., Silverman, A. J., Wadell, W., and Zuidema, G. D. (1961). Urinary catechol amine levels, gastric secretion and specific psychological factors in ulcer and non-ulcer patients. *J. Psychosomatic. Res.* **5**, 90–115.

Cohn, J. B. (1981). Multicenter double-blind efficacy and safety study comparing alprazolam, diazepam and placebo in clinically anxious patients. *J. clin. Psychiat.* **42,** 347–51.

Collins, M. A. (1982). A possible neurochemical mechanism for brain and nerve damage associated with chronic alcoholism. *Trends Pharmac. Sci.* **3,** 373–5.

Collins, M. A., Nijm, W. F., Borge, G. F., Teas, G., and Goldfarb, C. (1979). Dopamine-related tetrahydroisoquinolines: significant urinary excretion by alcoholics after alcohol consumption. *Science,* **206,** 1184–6.

Cook, P. (1979). How drug activity is altered in the elderly. *Geriatric Medicine,* **9,** 45–6.

Cookson, J. C. (1982). Post-partum mania, dopamine and oestrogens. *Lancet,* **ii,** 672.

Cools, A. R. (1975). An integrated theory of the aetiology of schizophrenia. In *On the Origin of Schizophrenic Psychoses.* (ed H.M. van Praag), pp. 58–80. De Ervan Bohn, B.V. Amsterdam.

Cools, A. R. (1982). The puzzling 'cascade' of multiple receptors for dopamine: an appraisal of the current situation. In *More About Receptors.* (ed J. W. Lamble), pp. 76–86. Elsevier Biomedical Press, Amsterdam.

Cooper, J. R., Bloom, F. E., and Roth, R. H. (1978). *The Biochemical Basis of Pharmacology.* Oxford University Press, Inc. New York.

Cooper, R., Newton, P., and Reed, M. (1985). Neurophysiological signs of brain damage due to glue sniffing. *Electroenceph. clin. Neurophysiol.* **60,** 23–6.

Cooper, R., Osselton, J. W., and Shaw J. C. (1980). *EEG Technology.* (3rd edn). Butterworth, London.

Cooper, S. J. (1983). Benzodiazepine-opiate antagonist interactions in relation to anxiety and appetite. *Trends Pharmac. Sci.* **4,** 456–8.

Cooper, S. J. (1984). Neural substrates for opiate-produced reward: solving the dependency puzzle. *Trends Pharmac. Sci.* **5,** 49–50.

Coper, H. (1982). Pharmacology and Toxicologic of cannabis. In *Psychotropic Agents Part III.* (eds F. Hoffmeister, and S. Stille), pp. 135–58. Springer-Verlag, Heidelberg.

Coppen, A. (1972). Indoleamines and the affective disorders. *J. Psychiat. Res.* **9,** 163–71.

Coppen, A., and Abou-Saleh, M. T. (1983). Lithium in the prophylaxis of unipolar depression: a review. *J. Roy. Soc. Med.* **76,** 297–301.

Coppen, A., and Peet, M. (1979). The long-term management of patients with affective disorders. In *Psychopharmacology of Affective Disorders.* (eds E. S. Paykel, and A. Coppen), pp. 248–56. Oxford University Press, Oxford.

Coppen, A., and Wood, K. (1978). Tryptophan and depressive illness. *Psychol. Med.* **8,** 49–57.

Coppen, A., Whybrow, P. C., Noguera, R., Maggs, R., and Prange, A. J. (1972). The comparative antidepressant value of L-tryptophan and imipramine with and without attempted potentiation by liothyronine. *Arch. Gen. Psychiat.* **26,** 234–7.

Corcoran, D. W. J. (1965). Personality and the Inverted-U Relation. *Br. J. Psychol.* **56,** 267–73.

Corkin, S. (1981). Acetylcholine, ageing and Alzheimer's disease: implications for treatment. *Trends Neurosci.* **4,** 287–90.

Corvoisier, S. J., Fournel, J., Ducrot, R., Kolsky, M., and Koetschet, P. (1953) Proprietes pharmacodynamiques du chlorhydrate de chloro-3 (dimethylamino-3-propyl)-10 phenothiazines (4.560R.P.) *Arch. Intern. Pharmacodynam.* **92,** 303–61.

Costa, E. (1981a). The role of gamma-aminobutyric acid in the action of 1,4 benzo-diazepines. In *Towards Understanding Receptors*. (ed J.W. Lamble), pp. 176-83. Elsevier/North Holland, Amsterdam.

Costa, E. (1981b). Receptor plasicity: biochemical correlates of pharmacological significance. In *Long-term Effects of Neuroleptics*. Adv. Biochem. Psycho-pharmacol. Vol.24 (ed F. Cattabeni), pp. 363-77. Raven Press, New York.

Costa, E., Corda, M. G., and Guidotti, A. (1983). On a brain polypeptide functioning as a putative effector for the recognition sites of benzodiazepine and beta-carboline derivatives. *Neuropharmacol.* **22,** 1481-92.

Costa, E., and Silva, J. A. (1980). Benzodiazepines and depression. In *Benzo-diazepines: Today and Tomorow.* (eds R. G. Priest, U. V. Filho, R. Amrein and M. Skreta), pp. 131-42. MTP Press Ltd., Lancaster, England.

Costain, C. W., Cowen, P. J., Gelder, M. G., and Grahame-Smith, D. G. (1982). Electroconvulsive therapy and the brain: evidence for increased dopamine-mediated responses. *Lancet*, **ii,** 400-4.

Cousins, M. J., Mather, L. E., Glynn, C. J., Wilson, P. R., and Graham, J. R. (1979). Selective spinal analgesia. *Lancet*, **i,** 1141.

Cowe, L., Lloyd, D. J., and Dawling, S. (1982). Neonatal convulsions caused by withdrawal from maternal clomipramine. *Br. Med J.* **284,** 1837-8.

Cowen, P. J., and Nutt, D. J. (1982). Abstinence symptoms after withdrawal from tranquillising drugs: is there a common neurochemical mechanisms? *Lancet*, **ii,** 360-2.

Cox, S. M., and Ludwig, A. M. (1979). Neurological soft signs and psychopathology. I. Findings in Schizophrenia. *J. Nerv. Ment. Dis.* **167,** 161-5.

Coyle, J. T., Price, D. L., and DeLong, M. R. (1983a). Anatomy of cholinergic projections to cerebral cortex: implications for the pathophysiology of senile dementia of the Alzheimer's type. *Trends Pharmac. Sci.* Suppl. 90-3.

Coyle, J. T., Price, D. L., and DeLong, M. R. (1983b). Alzheimer's disease: a disorder of cortical cholinergic innervation. *Science.* **219,** 1184-90.

Crabbe, J. C., and Rigter, H. (1980). Learning and the development of alcohol tolerance and dependence. The role of vasopressin-like peptides. *Trends Neurosci.* **3,** 20-3.

Cramer, H., Rudolph, J., Consbruch, U., and Kendel, K. (1974). On the effects of melatonin on sleep and behaviour in man. In *Serotonin—New Vistas*, Adv. Biochem. Psychopharmacol. Vol.II, (eds E. Costa, G. L. Gessa and M. Sandler), pp. 181-6. Raven Press, New York.

Crawley, J. N., Maas, J. W., Roth, R. H. (1979). Increase in plasma 3-methoxy-4-hydroxyphenethylene glycol following stimulation of the nucleus locus coeruleus. *Psychopharm. Bull.* **15,** 27-9.

Crawley, J. N., Marangos, P. J., Stivers, J., Goodwin, F. K. (1982). Chronic clon-azepam administration induces benzodiazepine receptor subsensitivity. *Neur-opharmacology*, **21,** 85-9.

Creese, I. (1982). Dopamine receptors explained. *Trends Neurosci.* **5,** 40-3.

Creese, I. (1983). Classical and atypical antipsychotic drugs: new insights. *Trends Neurosci.* **6,** 479-81.

Creese, I., and Sibley, D. R. (1981). Receptor adaptations to centrally acting drugs. *Ann. Rev. Pharmacol. Toxicol.* **21,** 357-91.

Creese, I., and Snyder, S. H. (1980). Chronic neuroleptic treatment and dopamine receptor regulation. In *Long-Term Effects of Neuroleptics*, Adv. Biochem. Psy-chopharmacol. Vol.24. (ed F. Cattabeni), pp. 89-94. Raven Press, New York.

Crews, F. T., and Smith, C. B. (1978). Presynaptic alpha-receptor subsensitivity after long-term antidepressant treatment. *Science*, **202**, 322-4.

Crick, F. (1982). Do dendritic spines twitch? *Trends Neurosci.* **5**, 44-6.

Crick, F., and Mitchison, G. (1983). The function of dream sleep. *Nature*, **304**, 111-4.

Criswell, H. E., and Levitt, R. A. (1975). Cholinergic drugs. In *Psychopharmacology: A Biological Approach*. (ed R.A. Levitt), pp. 91-117. Hemisphere Publishing Corporation, Washington D.C.

Cross, A. J., Crow, T. J., and Owen, F. (1979). Gamma-aminobutyric acid in the brain in schizophrenia. *Lancet*, **i**, 560-1.

Cross, A. J., Crow, T. J., and Owen, F. (1981). ^{3}H-flupenthixol binding in post-mortem brains of schizophrenics: evidence for a selective increase in dopamine D 2 receptors. *Psychopharmacology*, **74**, 122-4.

Crow, T. J. (1972). Catecholamine-containing neurones and electrical self-stimulation: 1. A review of some data. *Psychol. Med.* **2**, 414-21.

Crow, T.J. (1978a). Rational drug treatment in schizophrenia. In *Biological Basis of Schizophrenia*. (eds G. Hemmings, and W. A. Hemmings), pp. 113-6. MTP Press Ltd., Lancaster.

Crow, T. J. (1978b). An evaluation of the dopamine hypothesis of schizophrenia. In *The Biological Basis of Schizophrenia*. (eds G. Hemmings, and W. A. Hemmings), pp. 63-78. MTP Press Ltd., Lancaster.

Crow, T. J. (1978c). The biochemistry of schizophrenia. *Br. J. Hosp. Med.* **26**, pp. 532-44.

Crow, T.J. (1979). What is wrong with dopaminergic transmission in schizophrenia? *Trends Neurosci.* **2**, 52-4.

Crow, T. J. (1980). Molecular pathology of schizophrenia: more than one diease process? *Br. Med J.* **1**, 66-8.

Crow, T. J. (1982). Two syndromes in schizophrenia? *Trends Neurosci.* **5**, 351-4.

Crow, T. J. (1983). Is schizophrenia an infectious disease? *Lancet*, **i**, 173-5.

Crow, T.J. (1985). Integrated viral genes as the cause of schizophrenia: a hypothesis. In *Psychopharmacology; Recent Advances and Future Prospects*. (ed S. D. Iverson), pp. 228-42. Oxford University Press, Oxford.

Crow, T. J., Baker, H. F., Cross, A. J., Joseph, M. H., Lofthouse, R., Longden, A., Owen, F., Riley, G. J., Glover, R., and Killpack, W. S. (1979a). Monoamine mechanisms in chronic schizophrenia: post-mortem neurochemical findings. *Br.J. Psychiat.* **134**, 249-56.

Crow, T. J., Ferrier, I. N., Johnstone, E. C., Macmillan, J. F., Owens, D. G. C., Parry, R. P., and Tyrell, D. A. J. (1979b). Characteristics of patients with schizophrenia or nuerological disorder and virus-like agent in cerebrospinal fluid. *Lancet*, **i**, 842-4.

Crow, T. J., Frith, C. D., Johnstone, E. C., and Owen, D. G. C. (1980). Schizophrenia and cerebral atrophy. *Lancet*, **i**, 1129-30.

Crow, T. J., and Johnstone, E. C. (1979). Electroconvulsive therapy—efficacy, mechanism of action and adverse effects. In *Psychopharmacology of Affective Disorders*. (eds E. S. Paykel, and A. Coppen), pp. 108-22. Oxford University Press, Oxford.

Crow, T. J., and Johnstone, E. C. (1980). Dementia praecox and schizophrenia: was Bleuler wrong? *J. Roy. Coll. Physicians*. **14**, 238-40.

Cuello, A. C. (1983). Central distribution of opioid peptides. *Br. Med. Bull.* **39**, 11-6.

Cuello, A. C., and Sofroniew, M. V. (1984). The anatomy of the CNS cholinergic neurones. *Trends Neurosci.* **7**, 74-8.

Culebras, A. (1976). Effect of papaverine on cerebral electrogenesis. *Neurol.* **26,** 673–79.

Cumin, R. Bandle, E. F., Gamzu, E., and Haefely, W. E. (1982). Effects of the novel compound aniracetam (RO 13-5057) upon impaired learning and memory in rodents. *Psychopharmacology,* **28,** 104–11. Effects of the novel compound aniracetam (RO 13-5057) upon impaired learning and memory in rodents. *Psychopharmacology,* **28,** 104–11.

Dahl, L. E., Dencker, S. J., and Lundin, P. (1981). A double-blind study of dothiepin hydrochloride (prothiaden) and amitriptyline in outpatients with masked depression. *J. Int. Med. Res.* **9,** 103–7.

Dalton, K. (1964). *The Premenstrual Syndrome.* Heinemann, London.

Damasio, A. R. (1983). Language and the basal ganglia. *Trends Neurosci.* **6,** 442–4.

Damasio, A. R. (1985). Prosopagnosia. *Trends Neurosci.* **8,** 132–5.

Daniel, G. R. (1976). Assessment of depot neuroleptics. *Br. J. clin. Pharmac.* Suppl. 2, **3,** 417–21.

Daniels, A. M., and Latcham, R. W. (1984). Petrol sniffing and schizophrenia in a Pacific Island paradise. *Lancet,* **i,** 389.

Dannenberg, P., and Weber, K. H. (1983). Chemical structure and biological activity of the diazepines. *Br. J. clin. Pharmac.* Suppl. 2, **16,** 231–43S.

Darragh, A., Lambe, R., Kenny, M., Brick, I., Taaffe, W., and O'Boyle, C. (1982). RO 15-1788 antagonises the central effects of diazepam in men without altering diazepam bioavailability. *Br. J. clin. Pharmac.* **14,** 677–82.

Darragh, A., Lambe, R., O'Boyle, C., Kenny, M., and Brick, I. (1983). Absence of central effects in man of the benzodiazepine antagonist RO 15-1788. *Psychopharmacology,* **80,** 192–5.

Davidson, J., McLeod, M. N., and Blum, M. R. (1978). Acetylation phenotype, platelet monoamine oxidase inhibition and the effectiveness of phenelzine in depression. *Am. J. Psychiat.* **135,** 467–9.

Davies, G. C., and Buchsbaum, M. S., van Kammon, D. P., and Bunney, W. E. (1979). Analgesia to pain stimuli in schizophrenics and its reversal by naltrexone. *Psychiatry Res.* **1,** 61–9.

Davies, G. C., and Buchsbaum, M. S. (1981). Pain sensitivity in the functional psychoses. *Mod. Probl. Pharmacopsychiat.* **17,** 97–108.

Davies, P. (1983). Neurochemical aspects in Alzheimer's disease. *Trends Pharmac. Sci.* Suppl.98–9.

Davis, D.R. (1978). Family processes in schizophrenia. *Br. J. Hosp. Med.* **20,** 524–31.

Davis, K. L., and Rosenberg, G. (1979). Is there a limbic system equivalent of tardive dyskinesia? *Biol. Psychiat.* **14,** 699–703.

Davis, M., and Menkes, D. B. (1982). Tricyclic antidepressants vary in decreasing alpha$_2$-adrenoceptor sensitivity with chronic treatment: assessment of clonidine inhibition of acoustic startle. *Br. J. Pharmac.* **77,** 217–22.

Davison, A. N. (1982). Ageing research matures. *Trends Neurosci.* **5,** 217–8.

Deakin, J. F. W. (1983). Alzheimer's disease: recent advances and future prospects. *Br. Med. J.* **287,** 1323–4.353.

DeFelice, E., and Sunshine, A. (1981). Basic principles and management of pain. *Triangle (Sandoz),* **20,** 43–8.

Dehen, H., Willer, J. C., Boureau, F., and Cambier, J. (1977). Congenital insensitivity to pain, and endogenous morphine-like substances. *Lancet,* **ii,** 293–4.

Delay, J., and Deniker, P. (1952). Trente-hiut cas de psychoses traitees par la cure prolongee et continue de 4560RP. *Le Congres des Al. et Neurol. de Langue Fr. Compte rendu de Congres.* Masson et Cie, Paris.

Delgado, J.M. R., Roberts, W. W., and Miller, N. (1954). Learning motivated by electrical stimulation of the brain. *Am. J. Physiol.* **179**, 587–9.

Delini-Stula, A., Vassont, A., Hauser, K., Bittiger, H., Buech, U., and Olpe, H-R. (1983). Oxaprotaline and its enantiomers: do they open new avenues in the research on the mode of action of antidepressants? In *Frontiers in Neurophyschiatric Res.* (eds E. Usdin, M. Goldstein, A. J. Friedhoff, and A. Georgatas), pp. 121–34. Macmillan Co., London.

Demellweek, C., and Goudie, A.J. (1983) Behavioural tolerance to amphetamine and other psychostimulants: the case for considering behavioural mechanisms. *Psychopharmacology*, **80**, 287–307.

Dement, W. (1960). The effect of dream deprivation. *Science*, **131**, 1705–7.

Deneau, G., and Inoki, C. (1967). Nicotine Self-administration in monkeys. *Ann. N.Y. Acad. Sci.* **142**, 277–9.

Deneau, G., Yanagita, T., and Seevers, M. H. (1969). Self-administration of psychoactive substances by the monkey. *Psychopharmacologia*, (*Berl.*) **16**, 30–48.

Department of Health and Social Security (1985). Limited list of medical products in certain categories available in the NHS after 1 April 1985. *D.H.S.S. Store.* Health Publications Unit. Lancs.

Desai, N., Taylor-Davies, A., and Barnett, D. B. (1983). The effects of diazepam and oxprenolol on short term memory in individuals of high and low state anxiety. *Br. J. clin. Pharmac.* **15**, 197–202.

Desarmenien, M. Feltz, P., Occhipinti, G., Santangelo, F., and Schlichter, R. (1984). Coexistence of GABA A and GABA B receptors on A delta and C primary afferents. *Br. J. Pharmac.* **81**, 327–33.

Deutsch, J. A. (1971). The cholinergic synapse and the site of memory. *Science*, **174**, 788–94.

Dimond, S. J., and Bronwers, E. Y. M. (1976). Increase in the power of memory in normal man through the use of drugs. *Psychopharmacology*, **49**, 307–9.

Dimond, S. J., Scammell, R. E., Pryce, I. G., Huws, D., and Gray, C. (1979). Some effects of piracetam (UCB 6215 Nootropyl) on chronic schizophrenia. *Psychopharmacology*, **64**, 341–8.

Ditch, M., Kelly, F. J., and Resnick, O. (1971). An ergot preparation (Hydergine) in the treatment of cerebrovascular disorders in the geriatric patient: a double blind study. *J. Am. Geriat. Soc.* **19**, 208–217.

Docherty, J. P., and Parloff, N. B. (1984). Psychotherapy, *Lancet*, **i**, 1074.

Domino, E. F. (1979). Behavioural, electrophysiological, endocrine and skeletal muscle actions of nicotine and tobacco smoking. In *Electrophysiological Effects of Nicotine.* (eds A. Remond, and C. Izard), pp. 136–46. Elsevier/North Holland Biochemical Press. Amsterdam.

Domschke, W., Dickschas, A., and Mitzney, P. (1979). C.S.F. beta-endorphin in schizophrenia. *Lancet*, **i**, 1979.

Dongier, M. (1973). Event-related slow potential change in psychiatry. In *Biological Diagnosis of Brain Distorders.* (ed S. Bogoch), pp. 47–59. Spectrum, New York.

Dongier, M., Dubrovsky, B., and Engelsmann, L. (1977). Event-related slow potentials in psychiatry. In *Psychopathology and Brain Dysfunction.* (eds C. Shagass, S. Gershon, and A.J. Friedhoff), pp. 291–352. Raven Press, New York.374.

Dorman, T. (1985) Toxicity of tricyclic antidepressants: are there important differences? *J. Int. Med. Res.* **13**, 77–83

Douglas, R. J. (1967). The hippocampus and behaviour. *Psychol Bull.* **67**, 416–42.

Douglas, R. J. (1975). The development of hippocampal function; implications for theory and for therapy. In *The Hippocampus.* (eds R. L. Isaacson, and K. H. Pribram), pp. 327–57. Plenum Press, New York.

Douglas, R. J., and Pribram, K. H. (1966). Learning and limbic lesions. *Neuropsychologia,* **4**, 197–220.

Dourdain, G., Peuch, A. J., and Simon, P. (1980). Triazolam compared with nitrazepam and with oxazepam in insomnia: two double-blind, crossover studies analysed sequentially. *Br. J. clin. Pharmac.* **11,** Suppl. 1, 43, 9S

Dourish, C. T., and Cooper, S.J. (1985) Behavioural evidence for the existence of dopamine autoreceptors. *Trends Pharmac. Sci.* **6**, 17–8.

Dowson, J. H. (1982). Neuronal lipofuscin accumulation in ageing and Alzheimer dementia: a pathogenic mechanism? *Br. J. Psychiat.* **140**, 142–8.

Drachman, D. A. (1978). Central cholinergic system and memory. In *Psychopharmacology: A Generation of Progress.* (eds M. A. Lipton, A. DiMascio, and K. F. Killam), pp. 651–62. Raven Press, New York.

Drucker-Colin, R. (1981). Endogenous sleep peptides. In *Psychopharmcology of Sleep* (ed D. Wheatly), pp. 53–71. Raven Press, New York.

Drug Newsletter (1981). Adverse reactions to solvent abuse. *Drug Newsletter.* **11**, 42–3.

Drug Newsletter (1983). Benzodiazepine dependence and withdrawal. *Drug Newsletter* Suppl. April 1983, 77–80.

Drug Newsletter (1985). Benzodiazepine dependence and withdrawal—an update. *Drug Newsletter,* **31**, 125–8.

Drug Newsletter (1986). From the region's yellow cards ... drugs and nightmares. *Drug Newsletter,* **38**, 155.

Drug and Therapeutics Bulletin (1979). Triazolam (Halcion) psychological disturbances. *Drug Therap. Bull.* **17**, 76.

Drug and Therapeutics Bulletin (1980). The CRM on benzodiazepines. *Drug Therap. Bull.* **18**, 97–8.

Drug and Therapeutics Bulletin (1983). Drugs which can be given to nursing mothers. *Drug Therap. Bull.* **21**, 5–8.

Duggan, A. W. (1982). Brain stem control of the responses of spinal neurones to painful skin stimuli. *Trends Pharmac. Sci.* **5**, 127–30.

Duggan, A. W. (1983). Electrophysiology of opioid peptides and sensory systems. *Br. Med. Bull.* **39**, 65–70.

Duggan, A. W., Hall, J. G., and Headley, P. M. (1977a). Suppression of transmission of nociceptive impulses by morphine: selective effects of morphine administered in the region of the substantia gelatinosa. *Br. J. Pharmac.* **61**, 65–76.

Duggan, A. W., Hall, J. G., and Headley, P. M. (1977b). Enkephalins and dorsal horn neurones of the cat: effects on responses to noxious and innocuous skin stimuli. *Br. J. Pharmac.* **61**, 399–408.

Dunleavy, D. L. F., and Oswald, J. (1973). Phenelzine, mood response and sleep. *Arch. Gen. Psychiat.* **28**, 353–56.

Dunn, A. (1980). Neurochemistry of learning and memory: an evaluation of recent data. *Ann. Rev. Psychol.* **31**, 343–90.

Dunn, W. L. (1978). Smoking as a possible inhibitor of arousal. In *Behavioural Effects of Nicotine.* (ed K. Battig), pp. S. Karger, Basel.

Durie, D. J. (1981). Sleep in animals. In *Psychopharmacology of Sleep*. (eds D. Wheatly), pp. 1–18. Raven Press, New York.

Eccles. J. C. (1977). An instruction-selection theory of learning in the cerebellar cortex. *Brain Res.* **127,** 327–52.

Edelman, G. M. (1978). Group selection and phasic reentrant signalling: a theory of higher brain function. In *The Mindful Brain*. (eds G. M. Edelman, and V. B. Mountcastle), pp. 51–100. MIT Press, Cambridge, Mass.

Edwards, F., Schabinsky, V. V., Jackson, D. M., Starmer, G. A., and Jenkins, O. (1983). Involvement of catechol amines in acute tolerance to ethanol in mice. *Psychopharmacology*, **79,** 246–50.

Ekstrand, B. R., Barrett, T. R., West, J. N., and Maier, W. (1977). The effect of sleep on human long term memory. In *Neurobiology of Sleep and Memory*. (eds R. Drucker-Colin, and J. L. McGough), pp. 419–39. Academic Press, New York.

Elde, R., Hokfelt, T., Johansson, O., and Terenius, L. (1976). Immunohistological studies using antibodies to leucine enkephalin: initial observations on the nervous system of the rat. *Neuroscience*, **1,** 349–52.

Ellingboe, J. (1978). Effects of alcohol on neurochemical processes. In *Psychopharmacology: A Generation of Progress*. (eds M. A. Lipton, A. DiMascio, and K. F. Killam), pp. 1653–64. Raven Press, New York.

Elmadjinan, F., Hope, J. M., and Lamson, E. T. (1957). Excretion of epirephrine and norepinephrine in various emotional states. *J. clin. Endocrinol.* **17,** 608–20.

Emery, F. E., Hilgendorf, E. L., and Irving, B. L. (1968). The psychological dynamics of smoking. *Tobacco Research Council*. Research Paper **10,** London.

Enna, S. J. (1981). GABA receptors. In *Towards Understanding Receptors* (ed J.W. Lamble), pp. 171–5. Elsevier/North Holland, Amsterdam.

Enna, S. J., and Andree, T. (1982). GABA receptor heterogeneity: relationship to benzodiazepines. In *Pharmacology of Benzodiazepines*. (eds E. Usdin, P. Skolnick, J. F. Tallman, D. Greenblatt, and S. M. Paul), pp. 121–32. Macmillan Co., London.

Erickson, C. K., and Graham, D. T. (1973). Alteration of cortical and reticular acetylcholine release by ethanol *in vivo. J. Pharmacol. Exp. Therap.* **185,** 583–93.

Eriksson, E., Eden, S., and Modigh, K. (1982). Up- and down-regulation of central postsynaptic alpha$_2$receptors reflected in the growth hormone response to clonidine in reserpine-pretreated rats. *Psychopharmacology*, **77,** 327–31.

Evans, D. A. P., Davidson, K., and Pratt, R. T. C. (1965). The influence of acetylator phenotype on the effects of treating depression with phenelzine. *Clin. Pharm. Therap.* **6,** 430–5.

Evans, J. I., Lewis, S. A., Gibb, I. A. M., Cheetham, M. (1968). Sleep and barbiturates: some experiments and observations. *Br. Med J.* **4,** 291–3.

Evans, J. I., and Ogunremi, O. (1970). Sleep and hypnotics—further experiments. *Br. Med. J.* **3,** 310–3.

Everitt, B. J., and Keverne, E. B. (1980). Models of depression based on behavioural observations of experimental animals. In *Psychopharmacology of Affective Disorders*. (eds E. S. Paykel, and A. Coppen), pp. 41–59. Oxford University Press, Oxford.

Ewusi-Mensah, F., Saunders, J. B., Wodak, A. D., Murray, R. M. and Williams, R. (1983). Psychiatric morbidity in patients with alcoholic liver disease. *Br. Med. J.* **287,** 1417–9.

Exton-Smith, A. N., and McLean, A. E. M. (1979). Uses and abuses of chlormethiazole. *Lancet*, **i,** 1093.

Eysenck, H. J. (1957). *The Dynamics of Anxiety and Hysteria*. Routledge and Kegan Paul, London.

Eysenck, H. J. (1967). *The Biological Basis of Personality*. C. C. Thomas, Springfield, Illinois.

Eysenck, H. J. (ed) (1981). *A Model for Personality*. Springer-Verlag, Berlin.

Eysenck, H. J. (ed) (1983). *A Model for Intelligence*. Springer-Verlag, Berlin

Eysenck, H. J., and Eaves. L. J. (1980). *The Causes and Effects of Smoking*. Maurice Temple Smith, London.

Eysenck, H. J., and Eysenck, S. B. G. (1963). *Eysenck Personality Inventory*. University of London Press.

Eysenck, H. J., and Eysenck, S. B. G. (1975). *Eysenck Personality Questionnaire*. Hodder and Stoughton, Essex.

Eysenck, H. J., and Eysenck, S. B. G. (1976). *Psychoticism as a dimension of personality*. Hodder and Stoughton, London.

Faber, J. and Havrdova, Z. (1981). Differential effect of REM stimulating and REM inhibiting drugs (reserpine and amitriptyline) on memory. *Activ. nerv. sup. (Praha.)*, **23**, 169–71.

Fairbairn, J. W., and Pickens, J. T. (1979). The oral activity of delta¹-tetrahydrocannabinol and its dependence on prostaglandin E_2. *Br. J. Pharmacol.* **67**, 379–85.

Fairbairn, J. W., and Pickens, J. T. (1980). The effect of conditions influencing endogenous prostaglandins on the activity of delta¹-tetrahydrocannabinol in mice. *Br. J. Pharmacol.* **69**, 491–5.

Fairburn, C. G. (1981). Schizophrenia. *Hospital Update*, **7**, 1115–27.

Farhoumand, N., Harrison, J., Pare, C. M. B., Turner, P. and Wynn, S. (1979). The effect of high dose oxprenolol on stress-induced physical and psychological variables. *Psychopharmacology*, **64**, 365–9.

Farley, I. J., Shannak, K. S. and Hornykiewicz, O. (1980). Brain monoamine changes in chronic paranoid schizophrenia and their possible relation to increase a dopamine receptor sensitivity. In *Receptors for Neurotransmitters and Peptide Hormones*. (eds G. Pepeu, M. J. Kuhar, and S. J. Enna), pp. 427–33. Raven Press, New York.

Fawcett, J. A. and Kravitz, H. M. (1982). Alprazolam: pharmacokinetics, clinical efficacy and mechanism of action. *Pharmacotherapy*, **2**, 243–54.

Feighner, J. P. (1982). Benzodiazepines as antidepressants. In *Modern Problems of Pharmacopsychiatry*. (ed T. A. Ban), pp. 196–212. S. Karger, Basel.

Feeney, D. M. (1979). Marihuana and epilepsy: paradoxical anticonvulsant and convulsant effects. In *Psychotropic Agents Part III*. (eds F. Hoffmeister, and S. Stille), pp. 643–59. Springer-Verlag, Heidelberg.

Feinmann, C., Harris, M. and Cawley, R. (1984). Psychogenic facial pain: presentation and treatment. *Br. Med. J.* **288**, 436–8.

Fenton, G. W. (1984). The electroencephalogram in psychiatry: clinical and research applications. *Psychiatric Developments*, **2**, 53–75.

Ferrero, P., Guidotti, B., Conti-Tronconi, B. and Costa, E. (1984). A brain octadecaneuropeptide generated by tryptic digestion of DBI (diazepam binding inhibitor) functions as a proconflict ligand of benzodiazepine recognition sites. *Neuropharmacol.* **23**, 1359–62.

Ferrier, B. M., Kennett, D. J. and Devlin, M. C. (1980). Influence of oxytocin on human memory processes. *Life Sci.* **27**, 2311–7.

Feudis, F. V. de. (1982). Gamma-aminobutyric acid and analgesia. *Trends Pharmac. Sci.* **3**, 444–6.

Feyerabend, C., and Russell, M. A. H. (1978). Effect of urinary pH and nicotine excretion on plasma nicotine during cigarette smoking and chewing nicotine gum. *Br. J. clin. Pharmac.* **5**, 293–7.

Fibiger, H. C., and Lloyd, K. G. (1984). Neurobiological substrates of tardive dyskinesia: the GABA hypothesis. *Trends Neurosci.* **7**, 462–4.

Fields, H. L., and Levine J. D. (1984). Placebo analgesia—a role for endorphins? *Trends Neurosci.* **7**, 271–3.

Fifkova, E., and Delay, R. J. (1982). Cytoplasmic action in neuronal processes as a possible mediator of synaptic plasticity. *J. Cell. Biol.* **95**, 345–50.

File, S., Lister, R. G., and Nutt, D. J. (1982). The anxiogenic action of benzodiazepine antagonists. *Neuropharmacol.* **21**, 1033–7

File, S. E., and Pellow, S. (1983). RO 5-4864, a ligand for benzodiazepine micromolar and peripheral binding sites: antagonism and enhancement of behavioural effects. *Psychopharmacology*, **80**, 166–70.

File, S., and Pellow, S. (1986). Intrinsic actions of the benzodiazepine receptor agonist RO 15-1788. *Psychopharmacology*, **88**, 1–11.

File, S. E., and Silverstone, T. (1981). Naloxone changes self-ratings but not performance in normal subjects. *Psychopharmacology*, **74**, 353–4.

Fink, M. (1969). EEG and human psychopharmacology. *Ann. Rev. Pharmacol. 9*, 241–51.

Fink, M. (1975). Cerebral electrometry in Phase-1 assessment of psychoactive drugs. In *Current Developments in Psychopharmacology*. (eds W. B. Essman, and W.B. Valzelli), Vol.1, pp. 301–15. Spectrum Publications, New York.

Fink, M. (1978). Psychoactive drugs and the waking EEG. In *Psychopharmacology: A Generation of Progress*. (eds M. A. Lipton, A. DiMascio, and K. F. Killam), pp. 691–8. Raven Press, New York.

Fink, M. (1979). *Convulsive Therapy: Theory and Practice*. Raven Press, New York.

Fink, M. (1981). Convulsive and drug therapies of depression. *Ann. Rev. Med.* **32**, 405–12.

Flood, J. F., Bennett, E. L., Orme, A. E., Rosenzweig, M. P., and Jarvik, M. E. (1978). Memory: modification of anisomycin-induced amnesia by stimulants and depressants. *Science*, **199**, 324–6.

Flor-Henry, P. (1976). Lateralised temporo-limbic dysfunction and psychopathology. *Ann. N.Y. Acad. Sci.* **280**, 777–97.

Flor-Henry, P. (1979). Laterality, shifts of cerebral dominance, sinistrality and psychosis. In *Hemisphere Asymmetries of Function in Psychopathology*. (eds J. Gruzelier, and P. Flor-Henry), pp. 3–19. Elsevier/North Holland Biomedical Press, Amsterdam.

Fludder, J. M., and Leonard, B.E. (1979). Chronic effects of mianserin on noradrenaline metabolism in the rat brain: evidence for presynaptic alpha-adrenolytic action in vivo. *Psychopharmacology*, **64**, 329–32.

Fowler, M. J., Sullivan, M. J., and Ekstrand, B.R. (1973). Sleep and memory. *Science*, **179**, 302–4.

Frankenhaeuser, M., and Jarpe, G. (1962). Psychophysiological reactions to infusions of a mixture of adrenaline and noradrenaline. *Scand. J. Psychol.* **3**, 21–9.

Franks, N. P., and Lieb, W. R. (1982). Molecular mechanisms of general anaesthesia. *Nature*, **300**, 487–93.

Frederiksen, P. K. (1975). Baclofen in the treament of schizophrenia. *Lancet*, **i**, 702–3.

Freedman, D. X., and Boggan, W.O. (1982). Biochemical pharmacology of psychotomimetics. In *Psychotropic Agents Part III*. (eds F. Hoffmeister, and S. Stille), pp. 57–88. Springer-Verlag, Heidelberg.

Freedman, R., Kirch, D., Bell, J., Adler, L. E., Pecerich, M., Pachtman, E. and Denver, P. (1982). Clonidine treatment for schizophrenia—a double blind comparison of placebo and neuroleptic drugs. *Acta Psychiat. Scand.* **65**, 35–45.

Freeman, C. P. (1984). Prophylaxis against unipolar depression. *Br. Med. J.* **289**, 512–14.

Freeman, C. P. L., Basson, J. V., and Crighton, A. (1978). Double-blind controlled trial of electroconvulsive therapy (E.C.T.) and simulated E.C.T. in depressive illness. *Lancet*, **i**, 738–40.

Freeman, C. P. L., and Fairburn, C. G. (1981). Lack of effect of naloxone in schizophrenic auditory hallucinations. *Psychol. Med.* **11**, 405–7.

Freemon, F. R. (1972). *Sleep research: A critical series*. Charles C. Thomas. Springfield Ill.

Frid, M., and Singer, G. (1979). Hypnotic analgesia in conditions of stress is partially reversed by naloxone. *Psychopharmacology*, **63**, 211–5.

Friedman, E. (1973). Pharmacology—lithium's effects on cyclic AMP, membrane transport and cholinergic mechanisms. In *Lithium: Its Role in Psychiatric Research and Medical Treatment*. (eds S. Gershon, and B. Shopsin), pp. 75–82. Plenum Press, New York.

Fuxe, K., Ogren, S-O., and Agnati, L. F. (1981). Long term zimelidine leads to a reduction in 5-hydroxytryptamine neurotransmission within the central nervous system of the mouse and rat. *Neurosci. Lett.* **21**, 57–62.

Fuxe, K., Ogren, S-O., Agnati, L. F., Benfenati, F., Cavicchioli, L., Fredholm, B., Andersson, K. Farabegoli, C. and Eneroth, P. (1983). Regional variations in 5-HT receptor populations and ^{3}H-imipramine binding sites in their responses to chronic antidepressant treatment. In *Frontiers in Neurophysichatric Research*. (eds E. Usdin, M. Goldstein, A. J. Friedhoff, and A. Georgatas), pp. 33–54. Macmillan Co., London.

Gadea-Ciria, M., Stadler, H., Lloyd, K. G., and Bartholini, G. (1973). Acetylcholine release within the cat striatum during sleep-wakefulness cycles. *Nature*, **243**, 518–9.

Gaffan, D. (1972). Loss of recognition memory in rats with lesions of the fornix. *Neuropsychologia*. **10**, 327–41.

Gaillard, J. M. (1979). Brain catecholaminergic activity in relation to sleep. In *Sleep Research*, (eds R. G. Priest, A. Pletscher, and J. Ward), pp. 35–41. MTP Press, Ltd., Lancaster.

Gaillard, J. M. (1983). Biochemical pharmacology of paradoxical sleep. *Br. J. clin. Pharmac.* **16**,B Suppl.2, 205– 30S.

Gaillard, J. M., and Blois, R. (1983). Effect of the benzodiazepine antagonist RO 15-1788 on flunitrazepam-induced sleep changes. *Br. J. clin. Pharmac.* **15**, 529–36.

Gallagher, D. W., Pert, A., and Bunney, W. E. (1978). Haloperidol-induced presynaptic dopamine supersensitivity is blocked by chronic lithium. *Nature*, **273**, 309–12.

Gallagher, D. W., and Tallman, J. F. (1983). Consequences of benzodiazepine receptor occupancy. *Neuropharmacol.* **22**, 1493–8.

Garcia-Sevilla, J. A., Zis, A. P., Hollingsworth, P. J., Greden, J. F., and Smith, C. B. (1981). Platelet alpha$_2$-adrenergic receptors in major depressive disorder. *Arch. Gen. Psychiat.* **38**, 1327–33.

Garriott, J. and Petty, C. S. (1980). Death from inhalant abuse: toxicological and pathological evaluation of 34 cases. *Clin. Toxicol.* **16**, 305–15.

Garruto, R. M., Fukatsu, R., Yanagihava, R., Gajdusek, D. C., Hook, G., and Fiori, C. E. (1984). Imaging of calcium and aluminium in neurofibrillary tangle bearing neurones in Parkinsonian-dementia of Guam. *Proc. Natl. Acad. Sci.* **81**, 1875–9.

Gash, D. M., and Thomas, G. J. (1983). What is the importance of vasopressin in memory processes? *Trends Neurosci.* **6**, 197–8.

Gash, D. M., and Thomas, G. J. (1984). The importance of vasopressin in memory. *Trends Neurosci.* **7**, 64–6.

Geaney, D. P., Elliott, J. M., Rutterford, M. G., Schachter, M., and Grahame-Smith, D. G. (1984). Headache and depression. *Lancet*, **i**, 1076.

Gebhart, G. F. (1982). Opiate and opioid peptide effects on brainstem neurons: relevance to nociception and antinociceptive mechanisms. *Pain*, **12**, 93–140.

Gee, K. W., and Yamamura, H. I. (1982). Benzodiazepine receptor heterogeneity: a consequence of multiple conformation states of a single receptor or multiple population of structurally distinct macomolecules?. In *Pharmacology of Benzodiazepines* (eds E. Usdin, P. Skolnick, J. F. Tallman., D. Greenblatt, and S. M. Paul), pp. 93–107. Macmillan Co., London.

Gelder, M., Gath, D. and Mayou, R. (1983). *Oxford Textbook of Psychiatry*. Oxford University Press, Oxford.

Gelenberg, A.J. (1976) The catatonic syndrome. *Lancet*, **i**, 1339–41.

Gellman, R. S., and Miles, F. A. (1985). A new role for the cerebellum in conditioning? *Trends Neurosci.* **8**, 181–2.

George, K. A., and Dundee, J. W. (1977). Relative amnestic actions of diazepam, flunitrazepam and lorazepam in man. *Br. J. clin. Pharmac.* **4**, 45–50.

George, R., Haslett, W.L., and Jenden, D.J. (1964). A cholinergic mechanism in the brainstem reticular formation: induction of paradoxical sleep. *Int. J. Neuropharmacol.* **3**, 541–52.

Gerbino, L., Oleshansky, M., and Gersham, S. (1978). Clinical use and mode of action of lithium. In *Psychopharmacology: A Generation of Progress.* (eds M. A. Lipton, A. DiMascio, and K. F. Killam), pp. 1261–75. Raven Press, New York.

Gerlach, J., and Luhdorf, K. (1979). The effect of L-dopa on young patients with simple schizophrenia, treated with neuroleptic drugs. *Psychopharmacologia*, **44**, 105–10.

German, D.C., and Bowden, D.M. (1974). Catecholamine systems as the neural substrate for intracranial self-stimulation: a hypothesis. *Brain Res.* **73**, 381–419.

Geschwind, N. (1975). Focal disturbances of higher nervous function. In *Textbook of Medicine.* (eds P. B. Beeson, and W. McDermott), p. 557. W.B. Saunders Company, Philadelphia.

Geschwind, N. (1983). Biological foundations of cerebral dominance. *Trends Neurosci.* **6**, 354–6.

Geschwind, N., and Levitsky, W. (1968). Human brain: left-right asymmetries in temporal speech region. *Science (Wash. D.C.).* **161**, 186–7.

Ghoneim, M. M., Mewaldt, S. P., Berie, J. L., and Hinruchs, J.V. (1981). Memory and performance effects of single and 3-week administration of diazepam. *Psychopharmacology*, **73**, 147–51.

Ghose, K. (1980). Biochemical assessment of antidepressive drugs. *Br. J. clin. Pharmac.* **10**, 539–50.

Gilbert, C. D. (1985). Horizontal integration in the neocortex. *Trends Neurosci.* **8**, 160–5.

Gilbert, P. (1984). *Depression: from Psychology to Brain State.* Lawrence Erlbaum Associates, Hillsdale, New Jersey.

Gill, E. W., Jones, G., and Lawrence, D. K. (1972). Chemical mechanisms of action of THC. In *Cannabis and its Derivatives.* (eds W. D. M. Paton, and J. Crown), pp. 76–87. Oxford University Press, Oxford.

Gilliland, K., and Andress, D. (1981). *Ad lib* caffeine consumption, symptoms of caffeinism, and academic performance. *Am. J. Psychiat.* **138**, 512–14.

Gillin, J. C., and Stoff, D. M., and Wyatt, R. J. (1978). Transmethylation hypothesis; a review of progress. In *Psychopharmacology: A Generation of Progress.* (eds M. A. Lipton, A. DiMascio, and K. F. Killam), pp. 1097–112. Raven Press, New York.

Gitlin, M. J., Gerner, R.H., and Rosenblatt, M. (1981). Assessment of naltrexone in the treatment of schizophrenia. *Psychopharmacology*, **74**, 51–3.

Giurgea, C. (1976). Piracetam: nootropic pharmacology of neurointegrative activity. In *Current Developments in Psychopharmaoclogy.* (eds W. B. Essman, and L. Valzelli), Vol. 3, pp. 223–73. Spectrum Publications, New York.

Glatt, M. A. (ed) (1977). *Drug Dependence: Current Problems and Issues.* MTP Press Ltd., Lancaster.

Glen, A. M., and Reading, H. W. (1973). Regulatory action of lithium in manic-depressive illness. *Lancet*, **ii**, 1239–41.

Glowinski, J., Tassin, J.P., and Thierry, A.M. (1985). The mesocortical—prefrontal dopaminergic neurones. In *Neurotransmitters in Action.* (ed D. Bousefield), pp. 233–41. Elsevier Biomedical Press, Amsterdam.

Godschalk, M., Dzoljic, M. R., and Bonta, I. L. (1977). The role of dopaminergic systems in gamma-hydroxybutyrate-induced electrocorticogram hypersynchronisation in the rat. *J. Pharm. Pharmac.* **29**, 605–8.

Gogolak, G. (1980). Neurophysiological properties (in animals) In *Psychotropic Agents Part I: Antipsychotics and Antidepressants.* (eds F. Hoffmeister, and G. Stille), pp. 415–35. Springer-Verlag, Berlin.

Gold, M. S., Redmond, D. E., and Donabedian, R. K. (1978a). Prolactin secretion, a measurable central effect of opiate-receptor antagonists. *Lancet*, **i**, 323–4.

Gold, M. S., Redmond, D. E., and Kleber, H. D. (1978b). Clonidine blocks acute opiate-withdrawal symptoms. *Lancet*, **ii**, 599–601.

Gold, M. S., Redmond, D. E., and Kleber, H. D. (1979a) Noradrenergic hyperactivity in opiate withdrawal supported by clonidine reversal of opiate withdrawal. *Am. J. Pshchiat.* **136**, 100–2.

Gold, P. E., and McGaugh, J. L. (1975). A single-trace, two-process view of memory storage processes. In *Short-Term Memory.* (eds D. Deutsch, J. A. Deutsch), pp. 355–78. Academic Press, New York.

Gold, P. W., Weingartner, H., Ballenger, J. C., Goodwin, F. K., and Post, R. M. (1979b). Effects of 1-desamo-8-D-arginine vasopressin on behaviour and cognition in primary affective disorder. *Lancet*, **ii**, 992–4.

Goldberg, I. (1980). Dexamethasone suppression test as indicator of safe withdrawal of antidepressant therapy. *Lancet*, **i**, 376.

Goldberg, I. K. (1980).L-tyrosine in depression. *Lancet*, **ii**, 364.

Golding, J. F., Harpur, T. and Brent-Smith, H. (1983). Personality and drug taking correlates of cigarette smoking. *Person. individ. Diff.* **4**, 703-6.

Golding, J. F. and Richards, M. (1985). EEG spectral analysis, visual evoked potentials and photic-driving correlates of personality and memory. *Person. individ. Diff.* **6**, 67-76.

Goldstein, A., Fischli, W., Lowney, L. I., Hunkapiller, M. and Hood, L. (1981). Porcine pituitary dynorphin, complete amino and sequence of the biologically active heptadecapeptide. *Proc. Natl. Acad. Sci. U.S.A.* **78**, 7219-23.

Goldstein, I. B. (1972). Electromyography. In *Handbook of Psychophysiology.* (eds N. S. Greenfield, and R. S. Sternbach), pp.329-65. Holt, Rinehart and Winston, Inc. New York.

Goldstein, M., Engel, J., Regev, I., and Mino, S. (1983). The possible role of central epinephrine alpha$_2$-adrenoceptors and presynaptic dopamine receptors in affective disorders. In *Frontiers in Neuropsychiatric Research.* (eds E. Usdin, M. Goldstein, A. J. Friedhoff, and A. Georgatas), pp. 55-64. Macmillan Co., London.

Goodwin, F. K., Brodie, H. K., Murphy, D. L. and Bunney, W. E. (1970). Administration of a peripheral decarboxylase inhibitor withL-dopa to depressed patients. *Lancet*, **i**, 908-11.

Goodwin, F. K., Cowdry, R. W., and Webster, M. H. (1978). Predictors of drug response in the affective disorders: towards an integrated approach. In *Psychopharmacology: A Generation of Progress.* (eds M. A. Lipton, A. DiMascio, and K. F. Killam), pp. 1277-88. Raven Press, New York.

Goodwin, F. K., and Post, R. M. (1983). 5-Hydroxytryptamine and depression: a model for the interaction of normal variances and pathology. *Br. J. clin. Pharmac.* **15**, 393-405.

Gottfries, C. G. (1980). Biochemistry of dementia and normal ageing. *Trends Neurosci.* **23**, 55-7.

Gozzani, J. L., and Izquierdo, I. (1976). Possible peripheral adrenergic and central dopaminergic influences in memory consolidation. *Psychopharmacology*, **49**, 109-11.

Grahame-Smith, D. G. (1985). Pharmacological adaptive-responses occurring during drug therapy and in disease. *Trends Pharmac. Sci.* **6**, 38-41.

Grahame-Smith, D. G., Green, A. R., and Costain, D. W. (1978). Mechanism of the antidepressant action of electroconvulsive therapy. *Lancet*, **i**, 254-6.

Grahame-Smith, D. G., and Orr, M. W. (1978). Cinical psychopharmacology. In *Recent Advances in Clinical Pharmacology.* (eds P. Turner, and D. G. Shand), pp.163-87. Churchill Livingstone, Edinburgh.

Grandison, L. (1983). Actions of benzodiazepines on the neuroendocrine system. *Neuropharmacol.* **22**, 1505-10.

Gray, J. A. (1970). The psychophysiological basis of Introversion/Extraversion. *Behav. Res. and Therapy.* **8**, 249-66.

Gray, J. A. (1977). Drug effects on fear and frustration: possible limbic site of action of major tranquillisers. In *Handbook of Psychopharmacology.* (ed. L. L. Iverson, S. D. Iverson, and S. H. Snyder), Vol.8, pp. 433-529. Plenum Press, New York.

Gray, J. A. (1981a). Anxiety as a paradigm case of emotion. *Br. Med. Bull.* **37**, 193-7.

Gray, J. A. (1981b). A critique of Eysenck's theory of personality. In *A Model for Personality.* (ed H. J. Eysenck), pp. 246-76. Springer-Verlag, Berlin.

Gray, J. A. (1982). *The Neuropsychology of Anxiety.* Clarendon Press, Oxford and Oxford University Press, New York.

Gray, J. A. (1985). A whole and its parts: behaviour, the brain, cognition and emotion. *Bull. Br. Psychol. Soc.* **38**, 99–110.

Greden, J. F. (1974). Anxiety or caffeinism: a diagnostic dilemma. *Am. J. Psychiat.* **131**, 1089–92.

Green, A. R. (1978). ECT—how does it work? *Trend Neurosci.* **1**, 53–4.

Green, A. R., and Costain, D.W. (1979). The biochemistry of depression. In *Psychopharmacology of Affective Disorders.* (eds E. S. Paykel, and A. Coppen), pp. 14–40. Oxford University Press, Oxford.

Green, A. R., Heal, D. J., Johnson, P., Laurence, B. E., and Nimgaonker, V.L. (1983). Antidepressant treatments: effects in rodents on dose-response curves of 5-hydroxytrptamine- and dopamine-mediated behaviours and 5-HT2 receptor number in frontal cortex. *Br. J. Pharmac.* **80**, 377–85.

Green, A. R., Heal, D. J., Lister, S., and Molyneux, S. (1982). The effect of acute and repeated desmethylimipramine administration on clonidine-induced hypoactivity in rats. *Br. J. Pharmac.* **75**, p. 33P.

Green, P. (1978). Defective interhemispheric transfer in schizophrenia. *J. Abnormal Psychol.* **87**, 472–80.

Greenberg, B. D., and Segal, D. S. (1986). Evidence for multiple opiate receptor involvement in different phencyclidine-induced unconditioned behaviours in rats. *Psychopharmacology*, **88**, 44–53.

Greenblatt, D. J., Divoll, M., Abernethy, D. R., Ochs, H. R., and Shader, R. (1983). Clinical pharmacokinetics of the newer benzodiazepines. *Clin. Pharmacokinet.* **8**, 233–52.

Greenblatt, D. J., Shader, R. I., Divoll, M., and Harmatz, J. S. (1981). Benzodiazepines; a summary of pharmacokinetic properties. *Br. J. clin. Pharmac.* **11**, 11–6S.

Greene, L. A. (1984). The importance of both early and delayed response to the biological actions of nerve growth factor. *Trends Neurosci.* **7**, 91–4.

Greenough, W. T. (1984). Structural correlates of information storage in the mammalian brain: a review and hypothesis. *Trends Neurosci.* **7**, 229–35.

Griffiths, R. R., Bigelow, G. E., Stitzer, M. L., and McLeod, D. R. (1983). Behavioural effects of drugs of abuse. In *Application of Behavioural Pharmacology in Toxicology.* (eds G. Zbinden, V. Cuomo, G. Racagini, and B. Weiss), pp. 367–82. Raven Press, New York.

Griffiths, R. R., McLeod, D. R., Bigelow, G. E., Liebson, I. A. and Roache, J. D. (1984). Relative abuse liability of diazepam and oxazepam: behavioural and subjective dose effects. *Psychopharmacology*, **84**, 141–54.

Grossman, A., and Rees, L. H. (1983). Neuroendocrinology of opioid peptides. *Br. Med. Bull.* **39**, 83–8.

Grosz, H. J. (1973). Effect of propranolol on active users of heroin. *Lancet*, **ii**, 612.

Gruzelier, J. (1979). Synthesis and critical reviews of the evidence for hemisphere asymmetries of function in psychopathology. In *Hemisphere Asymmetries of Function in Psychopathology.* (eds G. Gruzelier, and P. Flor-Henry), pp. 647–72. Elsevier/North Holland Biomedical Press. Amsterdam.

Gruzelier, J. H., and Yorkston, N. J. (1978). Propranolol and schizophrenia: objective evidence of efficacy. In *Biological Basis of Schizophrenia.* pp. 127–46.

Guidotti, A., Corda, M. G., Wise, B. C., Vaccarino, F., and Costa, E. (1983). GABA-ergic synapses. Supramolecular organisation and biochemical regulation. *Neuropharmacol.* **22**, 1471–80.

Guidotti, A., Toffano, G., and Costa, E., (1978). An endogenous protein modulates the affinity of GABA and benzodiazepine receptors in the rat brain. *Nature*, **275**, 553–5.

Guillard, J. M. (1979). Brain catecholaminergic activity in relation to sleep. In *Sleep Research*. (eds R. G. Priest, A. Platscher, and J. Ward), pp. 35–41. MTP Press Ltd., Lancaster.

Guilleminault, C., Eldridge, F., and Dement, W. (1973). Insomnia with sleep apnoea: a new syndrome. *Science*, **181**, 856–85

Guilleminault, C., and Tilkian, A. (1976). The sleep apnoea syndrome. *Ann. Rev. Med.* **27**, 465–83.

Guilleminault, C. Winkle, R., Connolly, S., Melvin, K., & Tilkian, A. (1984). Cyclical variation of the heart rate in sleep apnoea syndrome. *Lancet*, **i**, 126–31.

Gur, R. E. (1978). Left hemisphere dysfunction and left hemisphere overactivation in schizophrenia. *J. Abn. Psychol.* **87**, 226–38.

Gur, R. E. (1979a). Cognitive concomitants of hemispheric dysfunction in schizophrenia. *Arch. Gen. Psychiat.* **36**, 269–74.

Gur, R. (1979b). Hemispheric overactivation in schizophrenia. In *Hemisphere Asymmetries of Function in Psychopathology*. (eds G. Gruzelier, and P. Flor-Henry), pp. 113–23. Elsevier/North Holland Biomedical Press. Amsterdam.

Gur, R. E., Skolnick, B. E., and Gur, R. C. (1983). Brain function in psychiatric disorders. *Arch. Gen. Psychiat.* **40**, 1250–4.

Guyenet, P. G., and Aghajanian, G. K. (1979). ACh, Substance P and metenkephalin in the locus coeruleus; pharmacological evidence for independent sites of action. *Eur. J. Pharmacol.* **53**, 319–28.

Haefely, W. (1978). Behavioural and neuropharmacolgical aspects of drugs used in anxiety and related states. In *Psychopharmacology: A Generation of Progress*. (eds M. A. Lipton, A. DiMascio, and K. F. Killam) pp. 1359–74. Raven Press, New York.

Haefley, W., Pieri, L., Pole, P., and Schaffer, R. (1981). General pharmacology and neuropharmacology of benzodiazepine derivatives. In *Handbook of Experimental Pharmacology*. Vol.55, II (eds H. Hoffmeister, and G. Stille), pp. 13–262. Springer-Verlag, Berlin.

Haider, I. and Oswald, I. (1970). Late brain recovery after drug overdose. *Br. Med. J.* **2**, 318–22.

Hall, G. H. (1970). Effects of nicotine and tobacco smoke on the electrical activity of the cerebral cortex and olfactory bulb. *Br. J. Pharmac.* **38**, 271–86.

Hall, G. H., and Morrison, C. F. (1973). New evidence for a relationship between tobacco smoking, nicotine dependence and stress. *Nature*, **243**, 199–201.

Hall, G. H., and Turner, D. M. (1972). Effects of nicotine on the release of ^{3}T H-noradrenaline from the hypothalamus. *Biochem. Pharmacol.* **21**, 1829–38.

Hallstrom, C., and Lader, M. (1981). Benzodiazepine withdrawal phenomena. *Int. Pharmacopsychiat.* **16**, 235–44.

Hamburger, R., Sela, A., and Belamker, R. H. (1985). Differences in learning and extinction in response to vasopressin in six inbred mouse strains. *Psychopharmacology*, **87**, 124–5.

Hamilton, M. (1979). Mania and depression; classification, description and course. In *Psychopharmacology of Affective Disorders*. (eds E. S. Paykel, and A. Coppen), pp. 1–13. Oxford University Press, Oxford.

Hamilton, M. J., Smith, P. R., and Peek, A. W. (1983). Effects of bupropion, nomifensine and dexamphetamine on performance, subjective feelings, autonomic variables and electroencephalogram in healthy volunteers. *Br. J. clin. Pharmac.* **15,** 367–74.

Hamon, M., Nelson, D. L., Herbet, A. and Glowinski, J. (1980). Multiple receptors for serotonin in the rat brain. In *Receptors for Neurotransmitters and Peptide Hormones.* (eds G. Pepeu, M. J. Kuhar, and S. J. Enna), pp. 223–33. Raven Press, New York.

Han, J. S., and Terenius, L. (1982). Neurochemical basis of acupuncture analgesia. *Ann. Rev. Pharmacol. Toxicol.* **22,** 193–220.

Handler, C. E., and Perkin, G. D. (1983). Wernicke's encephalopathy. *J. Roy. Soc. Med.* **76,** 339-41.

Handley, S. L., Dunn, T. L., and Baker, J. M. (1977). Mood changes in puerperium and plasma trypophan and cortisol concentrations. *Br. Med. J.* **2,** 18–22.

Hanks, G. W., Thomas, P. J., Trueman, T., and Weeks, E. (1983). The myth of haloperidol potentiation. *Lancet,* **ii,** 523–42.

Harper, C. G., Kril, J. J., and Holloway, R. L. (1985). Brain shrinkage in chronic alcoholics: a pathological study. *Br. Med. J.* **290,** 501–4.

Harris, R. A., and Hood, W. F. (1980). Inhibition of synaptosomal calcium uptake by ethanol. *J. Pharmac. Exper. Therap.* **213,** 562–8.

Harrison, N. L., and Simmonds, M. A. (1983). Two distinct interactions of barbiturates and chlormethiazole with the GABA A receptor complex in rat cuneate nucleus in vitro. *Br. J. Pharmac.* **80,** 387–94.

Harrison, P. J. (1986) Pathogenesis of Alzheimer's disease—beyond the cholinergic hypothesis: discussion paper. J. Roy. Soc. Med., **79,** 347–52

Harrison-Read, P. E. (1981). Synaptic and behavioural actions of antidepressant drugs. *Trends Neurosci.* **4,** 28–34.

Harrison-Read, P. E. (1984). Noradrenergic and other strategies for devising new drug treatments of schizophrenia. *Trends Pharmac. Sci.* **5,** 139–41.

Hartmann, E. (1971). L-tryptophan as a physiological hypnotic. *Lancet,* **i,** 807.

Hartmann, E. (1976a). Schizophrenia: a theory. *Psychopharmacology,* **49,** 1–15.

Hartmann, E. (1976b). Long term administration of psychotropic drugs: effects on human sleep. In *Pharmacology of Sleep.* (eds R. L. Williams, and I. Karacan), pp. 211–24. John Wiley & Sons Inc., New York.

Hartmann, E. L. (1979). L-tryptophan and sleep. In *Pharmacology of the States of Alertness.* (eds P. Passouant, and I. Oswald), pp. 75–84. Pergamon Press Ltd., Oxford.

Hartmann, E. L. (1980). Sleep and the sleep disorders. In *Handbook of Biological Psychiatry, Part II. Brain Mechanisms and Abnormal Behaviour—Psychopharmacology.* (ed H. M. van Praag), pp. 331–57. Marcel Dekker, New York.

Hartmann, E. L. (1982). Insomnia. In *Pharmacology of Benzodiazepines.* (eds E. Usdin, P. Solnick, J. F. Tallman, D. Greenblatt, and S. M. Paul), pp. 187-98. Macmillan Co., London.

Harvey, S. C. (1980). Hypnotics and Sedatives. In *The Pharmacological Basis of Therapeutics.* (eds A. G. Gilman, L. S. Goodman, and A. Gilman), pp. 339–75. Macmillan Co., New York.

Hatsukami, D. K., Hughes, J. R., Pickens, R. W., and Srikis, D. (1984). Tobacco withdrawal symptoms: an experimental analysis. *Psychopharmacology,* **84,** 231–6.

Haug, J. O. (1962). Pneumoencephalographic studies in mental disease. *Acta Psychiatrica Scand.* Suppl. **165,** 1–114.

Hayflick, L. (1979). Cell ageing. In *Physiology and Cell Biology of Age.* Ageing, Vol.

8. (eds A. Cherkin, C. E. Finch, N. Kharasch, T. Makindon, and F. L. Scott), pp. 3–9. Raven Press, New York.

Hayward, M. (1977). Headache and pain in the head and neck. In *Persistent Pain: Modern Methods of Treatment*. (ed. S. Lipton) Vol.1, pp.35–60. Academic Press, London and Grune and Stratton, New York.

Hazra, J. (1970). Effect of hemicholinium-3 on slow wave and paradoxical sleep of the cat. *Eur. J. Pharmacol.* **11**, 395–7.

Health Education Council (1983). *That's the limit*. London.

Heath, R. G. (1964). Pleasure responses of human subjects to direct stimulation of the brain: physiological and psychodynamic considerations. In *The Role of Pleasure in Behaviour*. (ed R. G. Heath), Harper and Row, New York.

Heath, R. G. (1972). Marihuana effects on deep and surface electroencephalograms of man. *Arch. Gen. Psychiat.* **26**, 577–84.

Hebb, D. O. (1949). *The Organisation of Behaviour*. Wiley, New York.

Heimstra, N. W. (1973). The effects of smoking on mood change. In *Smoking Behaviour: Motives and Incentives*. (ed W. L. Dunn), pp. 197–207. Winston, Washington.

Henderson, G. (1982). Phencyclidine: a widely abused but little understood psychomimetic agent. *Trends Pharmac. Sci.* **3**, 248–50.

Henderson, G. (1983). Electrophysiological analysis of opioid action. *Br. Med. Bull.* **39**, 59–64.

Hendrickson, A. E. (1983a). The biological basis of intelligence. Part I: theory In *A Model for Intelligence*. (ed H. J. Eysenck), pp. 151–196. Springer-Verlag, Berlin.

Hendrickson, D. E. (1983b). The biological basis of intelligence. Part II: measurement. In *A Model for Intelligence*. (ed H. J. Eysenck), pp. 197–230. Springer-Verlag, Berlin.

Henriksen, S., Dement, W., and Barchas, J. (1974). The role of serotonin in the regulation of a phasic event of rapid eye movement sleep: the pontogeniculo-occipital wave. In *Serotonin—New Vistas*. Adv. in Biochem. Psychopharmacol. Vol.II. (eds E. Costa, G. L. Gessa, and M. Sandler), pp. 169–79. Raven Press, New York.

Henry, J. L. (1980). Substance P and pain: an updating. *Trends Neurosci.* **3**, 95–7.

Herberg, L. J., Stephens, D. N., and Franklin, K. B. J. (1976). Catecholamines and self stimulation: evidence suggesting a reinforcing role for noradrenaline and a motivating role for dopamine. *Pharmacol. Biochem. Behav.* **4**, 575–82.

Herbert, J. (1984). Behaviour and the limbic system with particular reference to sexual and aggressive interactions. In *Psychopharmacology of the Limbic System*. (eds M. R. Trimble, and E. Zorifian), pp. 51–67. Oxford University Press, Oxford.

Herning, R. I., Jones, R. T., Hooker, W. D., Mendelson, J., and Blackwell, L. (1985). Cocaine increases EEG beta: a replication and extension of Hans Berger's historic experiments. *Electroenceph. clin. Neurophysiol.* **60**, 470–7.

Hershkowitz, M. (1979). The effect of in vivo treatment with (-)delta-1-tetrahydrocannabinol and other drugs in the *in vitro* uptake of biogenic amines. In *Marihuana: Biological Effects*. (eds G. G. Nahas, and W. D. M. Paton), pp. 351–9. Pergamon Press, Oxford.

Herz, A. (1981). Role of endorphins in addiction. *Mod. Probl. Pharmaco-psychiat.* **17**, 175–80.

Herz, A., and Hollt, V. (1982). On the role of endorphins in addiction. In *Advances in Pharmacology and Therapeutics II. Vol.1. CNS Pharmacology - Neuropeptides*. (eds H. Yoshida, Y.Hagihara, and S. Ebashi), pp. 67–76. Pergamon Press, Oxford.

Herz, A., Hollt, V., and Przewlocki, R. (1980a). Endogenous opioids and addiction.

In *Brain and Pituitary Peptides*. Ferring Symposium, Munich, 1979, pp. 183–9. Karger, Basel.

Herz, A., Schulz, R., and Wuster, M. (1980b). Some aspects of opiate receptors. In *Receptors for Neurotransmitters and Peptide Hormones*. (eds G. Pepeu, M. J. Kuhar, and S. J. Enna), pp. 329–37. Raven Press, New York.

Herzberg, J. L., and Wolkind, S.N. (1983). Solvent sniffing in perspective. *Br. J. Hosp. Med.* **29,** 72–6.

Heston, L. L., and Mastri, A.R. (1977). The genetics of Alzheimer's disease. *Arch. Gen. Psychiat.* **34,** 976–81.

Hibbert, G. A. (1984). Hyperventilation as a cause of panic attacks. *Br. Med. J.* **288,** 263–4.

Higgitt, A., Lader, M., and Fonagy, P. (1986) The effects of the benzodiazepine antagonist R_0 15–1788 on psychophysiological performance and subjective measures in normal subjects. *Psychopharmacology* **89,** 395–403.

Hill, D. (1976). Cerebral atrophy and cognitive impairment in chronic schizophrenia. *Lancet,* ii, 1132.

Himmelhoch, J. M., and Hanin, I. (1974). Side effects of lithium carbonate. *Br. Med. J.* **2,** 233.

Hinde, R. A. (1977). Mother-infant separation and the nature of inter-individual relationships; experiments with rhesus monkeys. *Proc. Roy. Soc. Lond. (ser. B),* **196,** 29–50.

Hirsch, S. R. (1983). Psychosocial factors in the cause and prevention of schizophrenia. *Br. Med. J.* **286,** 1600–1.

Ho, I. K. (1980). Effects of acute and chronic administration of pentobarbitol on GABA system. *Brain Res. Bull.* **5,** (Suppl. 2) 913–7.

Ho., I. K., Brase, D. A., Loh, H. H., and Way, E.L. (1975). Influence of L-tryptophan on morphine analgesia, tolerance and physical dependence. *J. Pharmac. Exp. Therap.* **193,** 35–43.

Hockings, N., and Ballinger, B.R. (1983). Hypnotics and anxiolytics. *Br. Med. J.* **286,** 1949–51.

Hoehn-Saric, R. (1983). Effects of THIP on chronic anxiety. *Psychopharmacology,* **80,** 338–41.

Hoffman, B. B., and Lefkowitz, R. J. (1980). Radioligand binding studies of adrenergic receptors: new insights into molecular and physiological regulations. *Ann. Rev. Pharmacol. Toxicol.* **20,** 581–608.

Holaday, J. W., and Faden, A. I. (1982). Endorphins and thyrotropin releasing hormone in shock and trauma. In *CNS Pharmacology Neuropeptides*. (eds H. Yoshida, Y. Hagihara, and S. Ebashi), pp. 45–56. Pergamon Press, Oxford

Hollister, L. E. (1982). Pharmacology and toxicology of psychotomimetics. In *Psychotropic Agents Part III. Alcohol and Psychotomimetics, Psychotropic Effects of Central Acting Drugs*. (eds F. Hoffmeister, and G. Stille), pp. 321–44. Springer-Verlag, Berlin.

Holmes, S. W., and Sugden, D. (1982). Effects of melanotonin on sleep and neurochemistry in the rat. *Br. J. Pharmac.* **76,** 95–101.

Hong, J. S., Yang, H-Y. T., Gillin, J. C., and Costa, E. (1980). Effects of long-term administration of antipsychotic drugs on enkephalinergic neurons. In *Long-Term Effects of Neuroleptics*. Adv. Biochem. Psychopharmacol. Vol.24 (ed. F. Cattabeni), pp. 223–32. Raven Press, New York.

Hore, B. D., and Ritson, E. B. (1982). *Alcohol and Health*. Medical Council on Alcoholism, London.

Horel, J. A. (1978). The neuroanatomy of amnesia: a critique of the hippocampal memory hypothesis. *Brain*, **101**, 403–45.

Horne, J. A. (1976a). Recovery sleep following different visual conditions during total sleep deprivation in man. *Biolog. Psychol.* **4**, 107–18.

Horne, J. A. (1976b). Hail slow wave sleep: goodbye REM. *Bull. Br. psychiat. Soc.* **29**, 74–9.

Horne, J. A. (1979). Restitution and human sleep: a critical review. *Physiol. Psychol.* **7**, 115–25.

Horne, J. A. (1983). Human sleep in tissue restitution: some qualifications and doubts. *Clin. Sci.* **65**, 569–78.

Horne, J. A., and Wilkinson, S. (1985). Chronic sleep reduction: daytime vigilance, performance and EEG measures of sleepiness, with particular reference to 'practice' effects. *Psychophysiology*, **22**, 69–78.

Hornykiewicz, O. (1973). Dopamine in the basal ganglia. *Br. Med. Bull.* **29**, 172–8.

Horrobin, D. F. (1977). Schizophrenia as a prostaglandin deficiency disease. *Lancet*, **i**, 936–7.

Horrobin, D. F. (1979). Schizophrenia: reconciliation of the dopamine, prostaglandin, and opioid concepts and the role of the pineal. *Lancet*, **i**, 529–31.

Horvath, T., and Meares, R. (1979). The sensory filter in schizophrenia; a study of habituation, arousal and the dopamine hypothesis. *Br. J. Psychiat.* **134**, 39–45.

Houde, R. W. (1979). Systemic analgesics and related drugs: narcotic analgesics. In *Advances in Pain Research and Therapy*. (eds J. J. Bonica, and V. Ventafridda), Vol. 2, pp. 263–73. Raven Press, New York.

Howe, J. F. (1983). Phantom limb pain—a re-afferentation syndrome. *Pain*, **15**, 101–7.

Hu, H-Y. Y., Davis, J. M., and Pandey, G. N. (1981). Characterisation of alpha-adrenergic receptors in guinea pig cerebral cortex: effect of chronic antidepressant treatments. *Psychopharmacology*, **74**, 201–3.

Hubbard, B. M., and Anderson, J. M. (1983). Sex differences in age-related brain atrophy. *Lancet*, **i**, 1447–8.

Hubel, D. H., and Wiesel, T. N. (1977). Ferrier Lecture: Functional architecture of macaque monkey visual cortex. *Proc. Roy. Soc. Ser. B.* **198**, 1–59.

Hudgson, P. (1984). Alcoholic myopathy. *Br. Med. J.* **288**, 1984–5.

Hughes, J. (1983). Biogenesis, release and inactivation of enkephalins and dynorphins. *Br. Med. Bull.* **39**, 17–24.

Hughes, J., and Kosterlitz, H. W. (1983). Introduction. *Br. Med. Bull.* **39**, 1–3.

Hughes, J., Smith, T. W., Kosterlitz., H. W., Fothergill, L. A., Morgan, A. and Morris, H. R. (1975). Identification of two related pentapeptides from the brain with potent opiate agonist activity. *Nature*, **258**, 577–9.

Hullin, R. P., McDonald, R., and Allsopp, M. N. E. (1972). Prophylactic lithium in recurrent affective disorders. *Lancet*, **i**, 1044–6.

Hunkeler, W., Mohler, H., Pieri, L., Pole, P., Bonetti, E. P., Cumin, R., Schaffner, R., and Haefely, W. (1981). Selective antagonists of benzodiazepines. *Nature*, **290**, 514–6

Hussain, S. M. A., Gedye, J. L., Naylor, R., and Brown, A. L. (1976). The objective measurement of mental performance in cerebrovascular disease. *Practitioner*, **216**, 222–8.

Hutchison, R. R., and Emley, G. S. (1973). Effects of nicotine on avoidance, conditioned suppression and aggression response measures in animals and man. In

Smoking Behaviour: Motives and Incentives. (ed. W. L. Dunn), pp.171–96. Winston, Washington.

Ingvar, D. H. (1979). Cerebral circulation and metabolism in sleep. In *Sleep Research.* (eds R. G. Priest, A. Pletscher, and J. Ward), pp. 13–8. MTP Press Ltd., Lancaster.

Ingvar, D. H. (1982). Mental illness and regional brain metabolism. *Trends Neurosci.* **5,** 199–203.

Inque, S., Uchizono, K., and Nagasaki, H. (1982). Endogenous sleep-promoting factors. *Trends Neurosci.* **5,** 218–20.

Isaacson, R. L. (1974). *The Limbic System.* Plenum Press, New York.

Isaacson, R. L. (1982). *The Limbic System.* (2nd edn.) Plenum Press, New York.

Itil, T. M. (1975). Computer EEG profiles of antidepressants. In *Antidepressants.* (ed. S. Fielding, and H. Lal), pp. 319–51. Futura Publishing Co., New York.

Itil, T. M., and Soldatos, C. (1980). Clinical neurophysiological properties of antidepressants. In *Psychotropic Agents Part I: Antipsychotics and Antidepressants.* (eds F.Hoffmeister, and G. Stille), pp. 437–69. Springer-Verlag, Berlin.

Iversen, L. L. (1978). Biochemical pharmacology of GABA. In *Psychopharmacology: A Generation of Progress.* (eds D. Lipton, A. DiMascio, K. Killam) pp. 25–38. Raven Press, New York.

Iversen, L. L., and McKay, A. V. P. (1979). Pharmacodynamics of antidepressants and antimanic drugs. In *Psychopharmacology of Affective Disorders.* (eds E. S. Paykel, and A. Coppen), pp. 60–90. Oxford University Press, New York.

Iversen, L. L., Quick, M., Emson, P. C., Dowling, J.E., and Watling, R. (1980). Further evidence for the existence of multiple receptors for dopamine in the central nervous system. In *Receptors for Neurotransmitters and peptide Hormones.* (eds G. Pepeu, M. J. Kuhar, and S. J. Enna), pp. 193–202. Raven Press, New York.

Iversen, S. D. (1977). Temporal lobe amnesia. In *Amnesia.* (eds C. W. M. Whitty, and O. L. Zangwill), pp. 136–82. Butterworth, London, Boston.

Iversen, S. D. (1980). Models of anxiety and benzodiazepine actions. *Arzneimittelforschung, Drug Research,* **30,** (I) 862–8.

Iversen, S. D. (1984). Recent advances in the anatomy and chemistry of the limbic system. In *Psychopharmacology of the Limbic System.* (eds M. R. Trimble, and E. Zarifian), pp. 1–16.

Iversen, S. D., and Iversen, L. L. (1981). *Behavioural Pharmacology.* Oxford University Press, New York.

Izquierdo, I. (1982a). Beta-Endorphin and forgetting. *Trends Pharmacol. Sci.* **3,** 455–547.

Izquierdo, I. (1982b). Memory modulation, the sympathoadrenal system and the effect of drugs. *Trends Pharmac. Sci.* **3,** 352–3.

Izquierdo, I. (1983). Naloxone facilitation of memory. *Trends Pharmac. Sci.* **4,** 410.

Izquierdo, I. (1984). Memory enhancing drugs: a drug boom of the near future? *Trends Pharmac. Sci.* **5,** 493–4.

Izquierdo, I., Onsinger, O. A., and Berardi, A. C. (1973). Effect of cannabidiol and of other cannabis sativa compounds on hippocampal seizure discharges. *Psychopharmacologia,* **28,** 95–102.

Jack, M. L. (1981). Pharmacokinetics and metabolism of anxiolytics. In *Handbook of Experimental Pharmacology, Psychotroptic Agents.* Vol.55, II (eds F. Hoffmeister, and G. Stille), pp. 321–58. Springer-Verlag, Berlin.

Jacobs, B. L. (1984). Single unit activity of brain monoaminergic neurones in freely moving animals: a brief review. In *Modulation of Sensorimotor Activity During*

Alterations in Behavioural States. (ed R. Bandler), pp.99–120. Alan R. Liss Inc., New York.

Jaffe, J. H. (1980). Drug Addiction and drug abuse. In *The Pharmacological Basis of Therapeutics.* (eds A. G. Gilman, L. S. Goodman, and A. Gilman), pp. 535–607. Macmillan Co., New York.

Jaffe, J. H., and Martin, W.R. (1980). Opioid analgesics and antagonists. In *The Pharmacological Basis of Therapeutics.* (eds A. G. Gilman, L. S. Goodman, and A. Gilman), pp. 494–534. Macmillan Co., New York.

James, I. M., Griffith, D. N. W., Pearson, R.M., and Newberry, P. (1977). Effect of oxprenolol on stage-fright in musicians. *Lancet*, **ii**, 952–4.

Jancsar, S., and Leonard, B. E. (1983). Olfactory bulbectomised rat as a model of depression. In *Frontiers in Neuropsychiatric Res.* (eds E. Usdin, M. Goldstein, A. J. Friedhoff, and A. Georgatas), pp. 357–72. Macmillan Co., London.

Janke, W. (1980). Psychometric and psychophysiological actions of antipsychotics in man. In *Psychotropic Agents. Part I: Antipsychotics and Antidepressants* (eds F.Hoffmeister, and G. Stille), pp. 305–36. Springer-Verlag, Berlin.

Janowsky, D. S., El-Yousef, M. K., Davis, J. M., and Sekerke, H. J. (1972). A cholinergic adrenergic hypothesis of mania and depression. *Lancet*, **ii**, 632–5.

Janssen, D. and Bever, W. F. M. van. (1980) Butyrophenones and diphenylbutylpiperidines. In *Psychotropic Agents Part I: Antipsychotics and Antidepressants.* (eds F.Hoffmeister, and G. Stille), pp. 27–41. Springer-Verlag, Berlin.

Jarvik, M. E. (1967). Tobacco smoking in monkeys. *Ann. N. Y. Acad. Sci.* **142**, 280–94.

Jarvik, M. (1983). Further observations on nicotine as the reinforcing agent in smoking. In *Smoking Behaviour: Motives and Incentives.* (ed. W. L. Dunn), pp. 39–49. Winston, Washington.

Jarvis, M. J., Raw, M. , Russell, M. A. H., and Feyerabend, C. (1982). Randomised controlled trial of nicotine chewing gum. *Br. Med. J.* **285**, 537–40.

Jasinski, D. R., Johnson, R. E., and Henningfield, J.E. (1984). Abuse liability assessment in human subjects. *Trends Pharmac. Sci.* **5**, 196–200.

Jasper, H. H., Khan, R. T., and Elliott, K. A. C. (1965). Amino acids released from cerebral cortex in relation to its state of activation. *Science*, **147**, 1448–51.

Jasper, H. H., and Tessier, J. (1971). Acetylcholine liberation from cerebral cortex during paradoxical (REM) sleep. *Science*, **172**, 601–2.

Jeffcoate, W. J., Herbert, M., Cullen, M. H., Hastings, A. G., and Walder, C.P. (1979). Prevention of effects of alcohol intoxication by naloxone. *Lancet*, **i**, 1157–9.

Jeffreys, D. B., Flanagan, R. J., Volans, G. N. (1980). Reversal of ethanol-induced coma with naloxone. *Lancet*, **i**, 308–9.

Jenkins, J. S., Mather, H. M., Coughlan, A. K., and Jenkins, D. G. (1979). Desmopressin in post-traumatic amnesia. *Lancet*, **ii**, 1245–6.

Jenkins, W. J., Cakebread, K., and Palmer, K. R. (1982). Hepatic aldehyde dehydrogenase and alcoholism. *Lancet*, **ii**, 1275.

Jenkins, W. J., Cakebread, K., and Palmer, K.R. (1984). Effect of alcohol consumption on hepatic aldehyde dehydrogenase activity in alcohol patients. *Lancet*, **i**, 1048–9.

Jensen, K., Fruensgaard, K., Ahlfors, V-G., Pihkanan, T. A., Tuomikosni, S., Ose, E., Dencker, S. J., Linberg, D., and Nagy, A. (1975). Tryptophan/imipramine in depression. *Lancet*, **ii**, 920.

Jessell, T. M. (1982). Pain. *Lancet,* **ii,** 1084-7.

Jeste, D. V., Linnoila, M., Wagner, R. L., and Wyatt, R. J. (1982). Serum neuroleptic concentrations and tardive dyskinesia. *Psychopharmacology,* **76,** 377-80.

Jhamandas, K., and Sutak, M. (1976). Morphine-naloxone interaction in the central cholinergic system: the influence of subcortical lesioning and electrical stimulation. *Br. J. Pharmac.* **58,** 101-7.

Johansson, O., Hokfelt, T., Pernow, B., Jeffcoate, S. L., White, N., Steinbusch, H. W. M., Verhofsted, A. A. S., Emson, A. A. J., and Spindel, E. (1981). Immuno-histological support for three putative transmitters in one neurone: coexistence of 5-hydroxytryptamine, substance P and thyrotropin releasing hormone-like reactivity in medullary neurones projecting to the spinal cord. *Neurosci.* **6,** 1857-81.

Johansson, F., and von Knorring, L. (1979). A double blind controlled study of a serotonin uptake inhibitor (zimelidine) versus placebo in chronic pain. *Pain,* **7,** 69-78.

Johns, M. W. (1977). Self-poisoning with barbiturates in England and Wales during 1959-74. *Br. Med. J.* **i,** 1128-30.

Johnson, G., Gershson, A., Burdock, E. T., Floyd, A., and Hekimian, L. (1971). Comparative effects of lithium and chlorpromazine in the treatment of acute manic states. *Br. J. Psychiat.* **119,** 267-76.

Johnson, L. C., and Chernik, D. A. (1982). Sedative-hypnotics and human performance. *Psychopharmacology,* **76,** 101-13.

Johnson, L. C., Naitoh, P., Moses, J. M., and Lubin, A. (1974). Interaction of REM deprivation and stage 4 deprivation with total sleep loss. *Psychophysiology,* **11,** 147-59.

Johnstone, E. C. (1985). Schizophrenia: structural changes in the brain. In *Psychopharmacology: Recent Advances and Future Prospects.* (ed S. D. Iverson), pp. 196-203. Oxford University Press, Oxford.

Johnstone, E. C., Crow, T. J., Frith, C. D., Carney, M. W. P., and Price, J. S. (1978). Mechanism of the antipsychotic effect in the treatment of acute schizophrenia. *Lancet,* **i,** 848-51.

Johnstone, E. C., Crow, T. J., Frith, C. D., Husband, J., and Kreel, L. (1976). Cerebral ventricular size and cognitive impairment in chronic schizophrenia. *Lancet,* **ii,** 924-6.

Johnstone, E. C., and Marsh, W. (1973). Acetylator status and response to phenelzine in depressed patients. *Lancet,* **i,** 567-70.

Johnstone, G. A. R., and Willow, M. (1982). GABA and barbiturate receptors. *Trends Pharmac. Sci.* **3,** 328-30.

Jonas, J. M., and Gold, M. S. (1986). Cocaine abuse and eating disorders. *Lancet,* **i,** 390-1.

Jones, D. M., Jones, M. E. L., Lewis, M. J., and Spriggs, T. L. B. (1979). Drugs and human memory: effects of low doses of nitrazepam and hyoscine on retention. *Br. J. clin. Pharmac.* **7,** 479-83.

Jones, D. M., Lewis, M. J., and Spriggs, T. L. B. (1978). The effects of low doses of diazepam on human performance in group administered tasks. *Br. J. clin. Pharmac.* **6,** 333-7.

Jones, H. S., and Oswald, I. (1968). Two cases of healthy insomnia. *Electroenceph. clin. Neurophysiol.* **24,** 378-80.

Jones, K.L., Smith, D.W., and Myrianthopoulos, N.C. (1974). Outcome of offspring of chronic alcoholic women. *Lancet,* **i,** 1076-8.

Jorgensen, A., Fog, R. and Veilis, B. (1979). Synthetic enkephalin analogue in treatment of schizophrenia. *Lancet*, **i**, 935.

Joseph, M. H., Risby, D., Crow, T. J., Deakin, J. R. W., Johnstone, E. C., and Lawler, P. (1985). MHPG excretion in endogenous depression: relationship to clinical state and the effects of ECT. *Psychopharmacology*, **87**, 4428.

Jouvet, M. (1967). Neurophysiology of states of sleep. *Physiol. Rev.* **47**, 117-77.

Jouvet, M. (1969). Biogenic amines and the states of sleep. *Science*, **163**, 32-41.

Jouvet, M. (1972). The role of monoamines and acetylcholine containing neurons on the regulation of the sleep-waking cycle. *Ergebnisse der Physiologie.* **64**, 166-307.

Jouvet, M. (1973). Telencephalic and rhombencephalic sleep in the cat. In *Sleep: An Active Process; Research and commentary.* (ed W. B. Webb), pp. 12-32. Scott Foresman, Glenview Ill.

Jouvet, M. (1977). Neuropharmacology of the sleep-waking cycle. In *Handbook of Psychopharmacology Vol.8 Drugs, Neurotransmitters and Behaviour.* (eds L. L. Iverson, S. D. Iverson, S. H. Snyder), pp. 233-93. Plenum Press, New York.

Jouvet, M., and Pujol, J. F. (1974). Effects of central alterations of serotonergic neurons upon the sleep-waking cycle. In *Serotonin—New Vistas.* Adv. Biochem. Psychopharmacol. Vol. II. (eds E. Costa, G. L. Gessa, and M. Sandler), pp. 199-209. Raven Press, New York.

Kabes, J., Erban, L., Hanzlicek, L. and Skondia, V. (1979). Biological correlates of piracetam: clinical effects in psychotic patients. *J. Int. Med. Res.* **7**, 277-84.

Kales, A., Scharf, M. B. and Kales, J. D. (1978). Rebound insomnia: a new clinical syndrome. *Science*, **201**, 1039-41.

Kales, A., Tan, T., Kollar, E. J., Naitoh, P., Preston, T., and Malstrom, E. J. (1970). Sleep patterns following 205 hours of sleep deprivation. *Psychosom. Med.* **32**, 189-200.

Kalsner, S., and Quillan, M. (1984). A hypothesis to explain the presynaptic effects of adrenoceptor antagonists. *Br. J. Pharmac.* **82**, 515-22.

Kametani, H., Nomura, S., and Shimizu, J. (1983). The reversal effect of antidepressants on the escape deficit induced by inescapable shock in rats. *Psychopharmacology*, **80**, 206-8.

Kandel, E. R. (1978). Environmental determinants of brain architecture and of behaviour: early experience and learning. In *Principles of Neural Sciences.* (eds E. R. Kandel, and J. H. Schwartz), pp. 620-32. Edward Arnold Publishers Ltd., London.

Kandel, E. R. (1979). Small Systems of Neurones. *Scientific Am.* **241**, 61-70.

Kandel, E. R. (1983). From metapsychology to molecular biology: exploration into the nature of anxiety. *Am. J. Psychiat.* **140**, 1277-93.

Kandel, E. R., and Schwartz, H. (1982). Molecular biology of an elementary form of learning: modulation of transmitter release. *Science*, **218**, 433-43.

Kane, J. M., Cooper, T. B., Sachar, E. J., Holpern, F. S., and Bailine, S. (1981). Clozapine: plasma levels and prolactin response. *Psychopharmacology*, **73**, 184-7.

Kanno, O., and Clarenbach, P. (1985). Effect of clonidine and yohimbine on sleep in man: polygraphic study and EEG analysis by normalised slope descriptors. *Electroenceph. clin. Neurophysiol.* **60**, 478-84.

Kapp, B. S., and Gallagher, M. (1979). Opiates and memory. *Trends Neurosci.* **2**, 172-80.

Karli, P. (1984). Complex dynamic interrelations between sensorimotor activities and so-called behavioural states. In *Modulation of Sensorimotor Activity During*

Alterations in Behavioural States. (ed. R. Bandler), pp. 1–21. Alan R. Liss Inc., New York.

Karras, A., and Kane, J. M. (1980). Naloxone reduces cigarette consumption. Life *Science*, **27**, 1541–5.

Katz, R. J. (1980). Behavioural effects of dynorphin—a novel opioid neuropeptide. *Neuropharmacol.* **19**, 801–3.

Kaufmann, C. A., Weinberger, D. R., Yolken, R. N., Torrey, E. F., and Potkin, S. G. (1983). Viruses and schizophrenia, *Lancet*, **ii**, 1136–7.

Kay, D. C., Blackburn, A. B., Buckingham, J. A., and Karacan, J. (1976). Human pharmacology of sleep. In *Pharmacology of Sleep.* (eds R. L. Williams, and I. Karacan), pp. 83–210. John Wiley & Sons Inc., New York.

Kaymakcalan, S. (1972). Physiological and psychological dependence on THC in Rhesus monkeys. In *Cannabis and its Derivatives.* (eds W. D. M. Paton, and J. Crown), pp. 142–9. Oxford University Press, Oxford.

Kaymakcalan, S. (1979). Pharmacological similarities and interactions between cannabis and opioids. In *Marihuana: Biological Effects.* (eds G. G. Nahas, and W. D. M. Paton), pp. 591–605. Pergamon Press, Oxford.

Kebabian, J. W., and Calne, D. F. (1979). Multiple receptors for dopamine. *Nature*, **277**, 93–6.

Kebabian, J. W., and Cote, T. E. (1981). Dopamine receptors and cyclic AMP: a decade of progress. In *More About Receptors.* (ed J. W. Lamble), pp. 112–7. Elsevier Biomedical Press, Amsterdam.

Kellett, J. M. (1976). Flupenthixol for depression. *Br. Med. J.* **2**, 1405.

Kellett, J. M. (1984). Right-hemisphere dysfunction and schizophrenia. *Lancet*, **i**, 344.

Kemperman, C. J. F. (1982). Salsolinol in the brain. *Lancet*, **i**, 927.

Kemperman, C. J. F. (1983). Beta-carbolines, alcohol and depression. *Lancet*, **i**, 124–5.

Kendler, K. S. (1983). Overview: a current perspective of twin studies of schizophrenia. *Am. J. Psychiat.* **140**, 1413–25.

Keshavan, M. S., and Crammer, J. L. (1985). Clonidine in benzodiazepine withdrawal. *Lancet*, **i**, 1325–6.

Kesner, R. P., and Hardy, J. D. (1983). Long-term memory for contextual attributes: dissociation of amygdala and hippocampus. *Behav. Brain Res.* **8**, 139–42.

Kessler, K. A. (1978). Tricyclic antidepressants: Mode of action and clinical use. In *Psychopharmacology: A Generation of Progress.* (eds M. A. Lipton, A. DiMascio, and K. F. Killam), pp. 1289–302. Raven Press, New York.

Kety, S. S. (1970). The biogenic amines in the central nervous system: their possible roles in arousal, emotion, learning . In *The Neurosciences: Second Study Program.* (ed. F. O. Schmitt), pp. 324–6. Rockefeller University Press, New York.

Key, B. J., and Krzywosinski, L. (1977). Electrocortical changes induced by the perfusion of noradrenaline, acetylcholine and their antagonists directly into the dorsal raphe nucleus of the cat. *Br. J. Pharmac.* **61**, 297–305.

Keyser, J. de., Michotte, A., and Ebinger, G. (1984). Television induced seizures in alcoholics. *Br. Med J.* **289**, 1191–2.

Khachaturian, H., Lewis, M. E., Schafer, M. K-H., and Watson, S. J. (1985). Anatomy of the CNS opioid systems. *Trends Neurosci.* .**8**, 111–9.

Khan, A. V. (1981). A comparison of the therapeutic and cardiovascular effects of a single nightly dose of prothiaden (dothiepin, dosulepin) and lentizol (substained-release amitriptyline) in depressed elderly patients. *J. Int. Med. Res.* **9**, 108–12.

Kiianmaa, K., Hoffman, P. L., and Tabakoff, B. (1983). Antagonism of the behavioural effects of ethanol by naltrexone in BALB/C, C57BL/6 AND DBA/2 mice. *Psychopharmacology*, **79**, 291-4.

Killam, E. K., and Killam, K. F. (1956). A comparison of the effects of reserpine and chlorpromazine to those of barbiturates on central afferent systems in the cat. *J. Pharmacol. Exp. Therap.* **116**, 35-41.

King, C. D. (1974). 5-hydroxytryptamine and sleep in the cat: a brief overview. In *Serotonin—New Vistas*. Adv. Biochem. Psychopharmacol. Vol. II. (eds E. Costa, G. L. Gessa, and M. Sandler), pp. 211-6. Raven Press, New York.

King, M. D., Day, R. E., Oliver, J. S., Lush, M., and Watson, J. M. (1981). Solvent encephalopathy. *Br. Med. J.* **283**, 663-5.

Kirkegaard, C. (1981). The thyrotropin response to TRH in endogenous depression. *Psychopharmacology*, **6**, 189-212.

Klatsky, A. L., Friedman, G. D., Siegelaub, A. B., and Gerard, M. J. (1977). Alcohol consumption and blood pressure. Kaiser-Permanente multiphasic health examination data. *New Engl. J. Med.* **296**, 1194-200.

Klein, D. F., and Davis, J. M. (1969). *Diagnosis and Drug Treatment of Psychiatric Disorder*. Williams and Williams, Baltimore.

Kline, N. S., and Cooper, T. B. (1980). Monmoamine oxidase inhibitors as antidepressants. In *Psychotropic Agents Part I: Antipsychotics and Antidepressants*. (eds F. Hoffmeister, and G. Stille), pp. 369-97. Springer-Verlag, Berlin.

Klorman, R., and Ryan, R. M. (1980). Heart rate, contingent negative variation and evoked potentials during anticipation of affective stimulation. *Psychophysiology*, **17**, 513-23.

Knight, J. G. (1982). Dopamine receptor-stimulating autoantibodies; a possible cause of schizophrenia. *Lancet*, **ii**, 1073-6.

Knights, A., and Hirsch, S. R. (1981). Revealed depression and drug treatment for schizophrenia. *Arch. Gen. Psychiat.* **38**, 806-11.

Knorring, L., von., Almay, B. G. L., Johansson, F., and Terenius, L. (1978). Pain perception and endorphin levels in cerebrospinal fluid. *Pain*, **5**, 359-65.

Knorring, L., von., Perris, C., Eisemann, M., Eriksson, U., and Perris, H. (1983). Pain as a symptom in depressive disorders. I. Relationship to diagnostic subgroup and depressive symptomatology. *Pain*, **15**, 19-26.

Knott, V. J., and Venables, P. H. (1977). EEG alpha correlates of non-smokers, smokers, smoking and smoking deprivation. *Psychophysiology*, **14**, 150-6.

Knudsen. K., and Heath, A. (1984). Effects of self-poisoning with maprotiline. *Br. Med. J.* **288**, 601-2.

Koch, C., and Poggio, T. (1983). Electrical properties of dendritic spines. *Trends Neurosci.* **6**, 80-3.

Koch-Henriksen, N., and Nielsen. H. (1981). Vasopressin in post-traumatic amnesia. *Lancet*, **i**, 38-9.

Koe, B. K. (1983). A common mechanism of action for antidepressant drugs? *Trends Pharmac. Sci.* **6**, 110.

Koella, W. P. (1974). Serotonin—a hypnogenic transmitter and an anti-awaking agent. In *Serotonin—New Vistas, Adv. Biochem. Psychopharmacol. Vol. II*. (eds E. Costa, G. L. Gessa, and M. Sandler), pp.181-6. Raven Press, New York.

Koella, W. P. (1981a). Electroencephalographic signs of anxiety. *Prog. Neuropsychopharmacol.* **5**, 187-92.

Koella, W. P. (1981b). Neurotransmitters and sleep. In *Psychopharmacology of Sleep*. (ed D. Wheatly), pp.19-51. Raven Press, New York.

Koella, W. P. (1983). Polypeptides and sleep. *Trends Pharmac. Sci.* **4**, 210–11.

Koob, G. F., and Bloom, F. E. (1983). Behavioural effects of opioid peptides. *Br. Med. Bull.* **39**, 89–94.

Koolhas, J. M. (1984). The corticomedial amygdala and the behavioural change due to defeat. In *Modulation of Sensorimotor Activity During Alterations in Behavioural States.* (ed. R. Bandler), pp. 341–9. Alan R. Liss Inc., New York.

Kornetsky, C., Esposito, R. U., McLean, S., and Jacobson, O. (1979). Intracranial self-stimulation threshold. *Arch. Gen. Psychiat.* **36**, 289–92.

Kornmuller, A. E., Lux, H. D., Winkle, K., and Klee, M. (1961). Neurohumoral ausgeloste Schlafzustande an Tieren mit gekreuztem Kreislauf unter der kontrolle von EEG-Ableitungen. *Naturwissenschaften.* **48**, 503–5.

Korsgaard, S., Casey, D. E., Pedersen, N. E. D., Jorgensen, A., and Gerlach, J. (1981). Vasopressin in anergic schizophrenia; a cross-over study with lysine-8-vasopressin and placebo. *Psychopharmacology*, **74**, 379–82.

Koslow, S. H. (1974). 5-Methoxytryptamine: a possible central nervous system transmitter. In *Serotonin: New Vistas.* Adv. Biochem. Psychopharmacol. Vol. II. (eds E. Costa, G. L. Gessa, and M. Sandler), pp. 95–101. Raven Press, New York.

Kosterlitz, H. (1979). Endogenous peptides and the control of pain. *Psych. Med.* **9**, 1–4.

Kostowski, W. (1975). Brain serotonergic and catecholaminergic system: facts and hypothesis. In *Current Developments in Psychopharmacology.* (eds W. B. Essman, and L. Valzelli) Vol.I, pp. 39–64. Spectrum Publications, Inc. New York.

Kovacs, G. L., Bohus, B. E., Versteeg, D. H. G., Telegdy, G., and de Weid, D. (1982). Neurohypophyseal hormones and memory. In *Advances in Pharmacology and Therapeutics II, Vol. I, CNS Pharmacology-Neuropeptides.* (eds H. Yoshida, Y. Hagihara, and S. Ebashi), pp. 175–87. Pergamon Press, Oxford.

Kretschmer, E. (1936). *Physique and Character*, 2nd ed (translated by W. J. H. Sproff, and K. P. Trench). Trubner, New York.

Kruk, Z. L., and Pycock, C. J. (1979). *Neurotransmitters and Drugs.* Croom Helm, London.

Kupfer, D. J., and Bowers, M. B. (1972). REM sleep and central monoamine oxidase inhibition. *Psychopharmacologia*, **27**, 183–90.

Kupfer, D. J., and Foster, F. G. (1972). Interval between onset of sleep and rapid-eye-movement sleep as an indicator of depression. *Lancet*, **ii**, 684–6.

Kupferman, I. (1978). Learning. In *Principles of Neural Science.* (eds E. R. Kandel, and J. H. Schwartz), pp. 570–9. Edward Arnold Publishers Ltd., London.

Lader, M. H. (1967). Palmar skin conductance measures in anxiety and phobic states. *J. Psychosomatic Res.* **11**, 271–81.

Lader, M. (1978). Current psychophysiological theories of anxiety. In *Psychopharmacology: A Generation of Progress.* (eds M. A. Lipton, A. DiMascio, and K. F. Killam), pp. 1375–80. Raven Press, New York.

Lader, M. (1980). The psychophysiology of anxiety.. In *Handbook of Biological Psychiatry.* (ed H. M. van Praag) Part II, pp. 225–47. Marcel Dekker, Inc., New York.

Lader, M. (1981). The clinical assessment of depression. *Br. J. clin. Pharm.* **1**, 5–14.

Lader, M. (1982a). Summary and Commentary. In *Pharmacology of Benzodiazepines.* (eds E. Usdin, P. Skolnick, J. F. Tallman, D. Greenblatt, and S.M. Paul), pp. 53–60. Macmillan Co., London.

Lader, M. (1982b). Some newer antidepressants. *Hospital Update*, **8**, , pp. 895–902.

Lader, M., and Bhanji, S. (1980). Physiological and psychological effects of anti-depressants in man. In *Psychotropic Agents Part I: Antipsychotics and Anti-depressants*. (eds F.Hoffmeister, and G. Stille), pp. 573-82. Springer-Verlag, Berlin.

Lader, M. H., and Petursson, H. (1981). Benzodiazepine derivatives-side effects and dangers. *Biol. Psychiatry*. **16**, 1195-212.

Lader, M. H., Ron, M., and Petursson, H. (1984). Computed axial brain tomography in long-term benzodiazepine users. *Psychol. Med.* **14**, 203-6.

Lader, M. H., and Wing, L. (1964). Habituation of the psychogalvanic skin reflex in patients with anxiety states and in normal subjects. *J. Neurol. Neurosurg. Pscyhiat.* **27**, 210-8.

Lader, M. H., and Wing, L. (1966). *Physiological Measures, Sedative Drugs, and Morbid Anxiety*. Oxford University Press, Oxford.

Laduron, P. (1981). Dopamine receptor: from an in vivo concept towards a molecular characterisation. In *Towards Understanding Receptors*. (ed. J. W. Lamble), pp. 105-11. Elsevier/North-Holland Biochemical Press, Amsterdam.

Laduron, P. M. (1984). Lack of direct evidence for adrenergic and dopaminergic autoreceptors. *Trends Pharmac. Sci.* **5**, 459-61.

Lagergren, K., and Levander, S. (1974). A double blind study on the effects of Piracetam (l-acetamide-2-pyrrolidine) upon perceptual and psychomotor performance at varied heart rates in patients treated with artificial pacemakers. *J. Pharmacol. (Paris)* **,5,** (Suppl. 2) 55-6.

Lake, C. R., Sternberg, D. E., Kammen, D. P. van., Ballenger, J. C., Ziegler, M. G., Post, R. M., Kopin, I. J., and Bunney, W. E. (1980). Schizophrenia: elevated cerebrospinal fluid norepinephrine, *Science*, **207**, 331-3.

Lal, H., and Fielding, S. (1983). Clonidine in the treatment of narcotic addiction. *Trends Pharmac. Sci.* **4**, 70-1.

Lal, H., Miksic, S., Drawbaugh, R., Numan, R. and Smith, N. (1976). Alleviation of narcotic withdrawal syndrome by conditional stimuli. *Pavlovian J. Biol.Sci.* **11**, 251-62.

Lamberts. S. W. J., Quijada, M. de., Ree, J. M. van., and Wied, D. de. (1982). Non-opiate beta-endorphin fragments and dopamine: V gamma-type endorphin and prolactin secretion in rats. *Neuropharmacol.* **21**, 1129-36.

Lambiase, M., and Serra, C. (1957). Fume a sistema nervoso. I. modificazioni dell' attivita elettrica corticale da fumo. *Acta Neurologica (Napoli)*. **12**, 475-93.

Lance, J. W., and McLeod, J. G. (1981). *A Physiological Approach to Clinical Neurology*. Butterworth, London.

Lancet (1973). Beta-blockade for withdrawal symptoms? *Lancet*, **ii**, 650-1.

Lancet (1975). Narcolepsy and cataplexy. *Lancet*, **i**, 845.

Lancet (1979a). Sleep apnoea syndromes. *Lancet*, **i**, 25-6.

Lancet (1979b). What does prolactin do in man? *Lancet*, **ii**, 234-5.

Lancet (1980). Treatment of opiate-withdrawal symptoms. *Lancet*, **i**, 349-50.

Lancet (1982a). Naloxone for alcohol poisoning? *Lancet*, **ii**, 80.

Lancet (1982b). The CT Scan in schizophrenia. *Lancet*, **ii**, 968.

Lancet (1982c). Solvent abuse. *Lancet*, **ii**, 1139-40.

Lancet (1984a). Neuroleptic malignant syndrome, *Lancet*, **i**, 545-6.

Lancet (1984b). Management of trigeminal neuralgia. *Lancet*, **i**, 662-3.

Lancet (1984c). Psychotherapy: effective treatment or expensive placebo? *Lancet*, **i**, 83-4.

Lancet (1984d). The challenge of addiction. *Lancet*, **ii**, 1019-20.

Lancet (1985). Beta blockers in situational anxiety. *Lancet*, **ii**, 193.

Lands, A. M., Arnold, A., McAucliff, J. P., Luduena, F. P., and Brown, T. G. (1967). Differentiation of receptor systems activated by sympathomimetic amines. *Nature*, **214**, 597–8.

Lane, J. W., and McLeod, J. G. (1981). *A Physiological Approach to Clinical Neurology*. Butterworth, London.

Lanfumey, L., Dugovic, C., and Adrien, J. (1985). $Beta_1$ and $Beta_2$ adrenergic receptors: their role in the regulation of paradoxical sleep in the rat. *Electroenceph. clin. Neurophysiol.* **60**, 558–67.

Lang, P. J., Rice, D. G., and Sternbach, R. A. (1972). The psychophysiology of emotion. In *Handbook of Psychophysiology*. (eds N. S. Greenfield, and R. S. Sternbach), pp. 623–63. Holt, Rinehart and Winston, Inc., New York.

Langdon, N., Welsh, K. I., Dam, M. van., Vaughan, R. W., and Parkes, D. (1984). Genetic markers in narcolepsy. *Lancet*, **ii**, 1178–80.

Langer, G., and Karobath, M. (1980). Biochemical effects of antidepressants in man. In *Psychotropic Agents Part I: Antipsychotics and Antidepressants*. (eds F.Hoffmeister, and G. Stille), pp. 491–504. Springer-Verlag, Berlin.

Langer, G., and Sacher, E. J. (1977). Diet and growth-hormone response in affective illness. *Lancet*, **i**, 652.

Langer, S. Z. (1977). Presynaptic receptors and their role in the regulation of transmitter release. *Br. J. Pharmac.* **60**, 481–97.

Langer, S. Z. (1980). Presynaptic receptors and modulation of neurotransmission: pharmacological implications of therapeutic relevance. *Trends Neurosci.* **3**, 110–12.

Langer, S. Z. (1984). [^{3}H]Imipramine and [^{3}H]desipramine binding: non-specific displaceable sites or physiologically relevant sites associated with the uptake of serotonin and noradrenaline? *Trends Pharmac. Sci.* **5**, 51.

Langer, S. Z., and Arbilla, S. (1984). The amphetamine paradox in dopaminergic transmission. *Trends Pharmac. Sci.* **5**, 387–90.

Langer, S. Z., and Briley, M. (1981). High-affinity ^{3}H-imipramine binding: a new biological tool for studies in depression. *Trends Neurosci.* **4**, 28–31.

Langer, S. Z., Briley, M. S., and Raisman, M. (1980). Regulation of neurotransmission through presynaptic receptors and other mechanisms: possible clinical relevance and therapeutic potential. In *Receptors for Neurotransmitters and Peptides*. (eds G. Pepeu, and M.J. Kuhar), pp. 203–12. Raven Press, New York.

Langer, S. Z., and Dubocovich, M. L. (1977). Subsensitivity of presynaptic alpha-adrenoceptors after exposure to noradrenaline. *Eur. J. Pharmacol.* **41**, 87–8.

Larson, P. S., and Silvette, H. (1975). *Tobacco: Experimental and Clinical Studies*. Suppl. III. Williams and Wilkins, Baltimore.

Lashley, K. S. (1950). In search of the engram. *Symp. Soc. Exp. Biol.* **4**, 454–82.

Laurence, D. R. (1962). *Clinical Pharmacology*. J. A. Churchill Ltd., London.

LeBoeuf, A., Lodge, J., and Eames, P. G. (1978). Vasopressin and memory in Korsakoff's Syndrome. *Lancet*, **ii**, 1370.

Lecrubier, Y., Puech, A. J., Jouvent, R., Simon, P., and Widlocher, D. (1980). A beta adrenergic stimulant (salbutamol) versus clomipramine in depression: a controlled study. *Br. J. Psychiat.* **136**, 354–8.

Lee, K., Moller, L., Hardt, F., Haubek, A., and Jenson, E. (1979). Alcohol-induced brain damage and liver damage in young males. *Lancet*, **ii**, 759–61.

Lee, T., and Seeman, P. (1980a). Elevation of brain neuroleptic/dopamine receptors in schizophrenia. *Am. J. Psychiat.* **137**, 191–7.

Lee, T., and Seeman, P. (1980b). Abnormal neuroleptic/dopamine receptors in schizophrenia. In *Receptors for Neurotransmitters and Peptide Hormones*. (eds G. Pepeu, M.J. Kuhar, and S.J. Enna), pp. 435–41. Raven Press, New York.

Lees, A. J. (1985). Parkinson's disease and dementia. *Lancet*, **i**, 43–4.

Leff, J. P. (1978). Social and psychological causes of the acute attack. In *Schizophrenia: Towards a New Synthesis*. (ed. J. K. Wing), Academic Press, London.

Legros, J. J., Gilot, P., Seron, X., Claessens, J., Adam, A., Moeglin, J. M., Audibert, A., and Berchier, P. (1978). Influence of vasopressin on learning and memory. *Lancet*, **i**, 41–2.

Leith, N. J., and Barrett, R.J. (1981). Self-stimulation and amphetamine: tolerance to *d* and *l* isomers and cross tolerance to cocaine and methylphenidate. *Psychopharmacology*, **74**, 23–8.

LeMay, M. (1982). Morphological aspects of human brain asymmetry: an evolutionary perspective. *Trends Neurosci.* **5**, 273–5.

Lemberger, L., Fuller, R., Wong, D., and Stark, P. (1983). Fluoxetine: a clinically effective non-tricyclic antidepressant. In *Frontiers in Neuropsychiatric Research*. (eds E. Usdin, M. Goldstein, A. J. Friedhoff, and A. Georgatas), pp. 233–40. Macmillan Co., London.

Lenard, H. G., and Schulte, F. J. (1972). Polygraphic sleep study in craniophagus twins (where is the sleep transmitter?). *J. Neurol. Neurosurg. Psychiat.* **35**, 756–62.

Lenox, R. H., Ellis, J. E., van Riper, D. A., Ehrlich, Y. H., Peyser, J. M., Shipley, J. E., and Weaver, L. A. (1983). Platelet alpha₂ adrenergic receptor activity in clinical studies of depression. In *Frontiers in Neuropsychiatric Research*. (eds E. Usdin, M. Goldstein, A. J. Friedhoff, and A. Georgatas), pp. 331–56. Macmillam Co., London.

Leonard, B. E. (1985). New antidepressants and the biology of depression. *Stress Medicine*, **1**, 9–16.

Leppavuori, S. A., and Putkonen, P. T. S. (1980). Alpha-adrenoceptive influence on the control of the sleep waking cycle in the cat. *Brain Res.* **193**, 95–115.

Lerer, B., Ebstein, R. P., and Belmaker, R. H. (1981). Subsensitivity of human beta-adrenergic adenylate cyclase after salbutamol treatment of depression. *Psychopharmacology*, **75**, 169–72.

Leurs, J. W., and Liebeskind, J. C. (1983). Pain suppressive systems of the brain. *Trends Pharmac. Sci.* **4**, 73–5.

Levander, S., and Sachs, C. (1985). Vigilance performance and autonomic function in narcolepsy: effects of central stimulants. *Psychophysiology*, **22**, 24–31.

Levine, J. D., Gordon, N. C., Jones, R. T., and Fields, H. L. (1978). The nercotic antagonist naloxone enhances clinical pain. *Nature*, **272**, 826–7.

Levison, P. K. (1981). An analysis of commonalities in substance abuse and habitual behaviour. In *Behavioural Pharmacology of Human Drug Dependence*. (eds T. Thompson, and C. E. Johansson), N.I.D.A. Research Monograph 37. National Institute of Drug Abuse, Rochville, Maryland, U.S.A.

Levitt, R. A., and Goedel, G. D. (1975). Learning and memory. In *Psychopharmacology: A Biological Approach*. (ed. R. A. Levitt), pp. 299–326. Hemisphere Publishing Corporation, Washington D. C.

Levitt, R. A., and Lonowski, D. J. (1975). Adrenergic drugs. In *Psychopharmacology: A Biological Approach*. (ed. R. A. Levitt), pp. 51–91. Hemisphere Publishing Corporation, Washington D.C.

Levy, J. (1979). Human cognition and lateralisation of cerebral function. *Trends Neurosci.* **2**, 222–5.

Levy, R., Little, A., Chuaqui, P., Reith, M. (1983). Early results from double blind, placebo controlled trial of high doses phosphatidylcholine in Alzheimer's Disease. *Lancet*, **i**, 987–8.

Lewis, J. W., and Liebeskind, J. C. (1983). Pain suppressive systems of the brain. *Trends Pharmac. Sci.* **4**, 73–5.

Lewis, P. D. (1978). Neurohumoral influences on cell proliferation in brain development. *Trends Neurosci.* **1**, 158–60.

Lewis, S. A., Oswald, I., and Dunleavy, D. L. F. (1971). Chronic fenfluramine administration: some cerebral effects. *Br. Med. J.* **2**, 67–70.

Libiger, J., and Ban, T. (1981). Drug induced dementia. *Prog. Neuropsychopharmacol.* **4**, 561–7.

Lightman, S. L., Spokes, E. G., Sagnella, G. A., Gordon, D., and Bird. E.D. (1979). Distribution of beta-endorphin in normal and schizophrenic human brains. *Eur. J. Clin. Invest.* **9**, 377–9.

Liljequist, R., Linnoila, M., and Mattila, M. J. (1978). Effect of diazepam and chlorpromazine on memory functions in man. *Eur. J. clin. Pharmac.* **13**, 339–43.

Lindstrom, L. H., Widerlov, E., and Gunne, L. (1978). Endorphins in human cerebrospinal fluid: clinical correlations to some psychotic states. *Acta Psychiat. Scand.* **57**, 153–64.

Linnoila, M. (1974). Effect of drugs and alcohol on psychomotor skills related to driving. *Ann. Clin. Res.* **6**, 7–18.

Liskin, B., Roose, S. P., Walsh, B. T., and Jackson, W. K. (1985). Acute psychosis following phenelzine discontinuation. *J. Clin. Psychopharmacol.* **5**, 46–7.

List, S., and Seeman, P. (1980). Neuroleptic/dopamine receptors; elevation and reversal. In *Long-Term Effects of Neuroleptics.* Adv. Biochem. Psychopharmacol. Vol. 24. (ed F. Cattabeni), pp. 95–101. Raven Press, New York.

Listener, the. (1985). Britain's 50,000 heroin addicts. *Listener*, Jan 10, 10–14.

Littleton, J. M. (1983). Tolerance and physical dependence on alcohol at the level of synaptic membranes: a review. *J. Roy. Soc. Med.* **76**, 593–601.

Lloyd, K. J., Farley, I. J., Deck, J. H. N., and Hornykiewicz, O. (1974). Serotonin and 5-hydroxy-indoleacetic acid in discrete areas of the brainstem of suicide victims and control patients. *Adv. Biochem. Psychopharmacol.* **11**, 387–97.

Lorens, S. A. (1976). Comparison of the effects of morphine on hypothalamic and medial frontal cortex self-stimulation in the rat. *Psychopharmacology*, **48**, 217–24.

Lovick, T. A., and Wolstencroft, J. H. (1983). Actions of GABA, glycine, methionine-enkephalin and beta-endorphin compared with electrical stimulation of nucleus raphe magnus on responses evoked by tooth pulp stimulation in the medial reticular formation in the cat. *Pain*, **15**, 131–44.

Lowenstein, L. F.(1982). Glue sniffing: background features and treatment by aversion methods and group therapy. *Practitioner*, **226**, 1113–16.

Lukin, P. R., and Ray, A. B. (1982). Personality correlates of pain perception and tolerance. *J. clin. Psychol.* **38**, 317–20.

Lum, L. C. (1981). Hyperventilation and anxiety state. *J. Roy. Soc. Med.* **74**, 1–4.

Lundberg, J. M., and Hokfelt, T. (1985). Coexistence of peptides and classical neurotransmitters. In *Neurotransmitters in Action.* (ed. D. Bousfield), pp. 104–18. Elsevier Biomedical Press BV, Amsterdam.

Luttinger, D., Burgess, S. K., Nemeroff, C. B., and Prange, A. J. (1983). The effects of chronic morphine treatment on neurotensin-induced antinociception. *Psychopharmacology*, **81**, 10–13.

Lynch, G., and Baudry, M. (1984). The biochemistry of memory: a new and specific hypothesis. *Science*, **224**, 1057–63.

Lyon, L. J., and Anthony, J. (1982). Reversal of alcoholic coma by naloxone. *Ann. Int. Med.* **96**, 464–5.

Maas, J. W. (1979). Neurotransmitters in depression: too much, too little or too unstable? *Trends Neurosci.* **2**, 306–8.

Maas, J. W., Fawcett, J. A., and Dehirmenjian, H. (1972). Catecholamine metabolism, depressive illness and drug response. *Arch. Gen. Psychiat.* **26**, 252–62.

Macdonald, J. B., and Macdonald, E. T. (1977). Nocturnal femoral fracture and continuing widespread use of barbiturate hypnotics. *Br. Med. J.* **2**, 483–5.

MacKay, A. V. P. (1981). Endorphins and the psychiatrist. *Trends Neuorsci.* **4**, IX–XI.

MacKay, A. V. P. (1984). High dopamine in the left amygdala. *Trends Neurosci.* **7**, 107–8.

MacKay, A. V. P., Bird, E. D., Spokes, E. G., Rossor, M., Iversen, L. L., Creese, I., and Snyder, S. H. (1980). Dopamine receptors and schizophrenia: drug effect or illness? *Lancet*, **ii**, 915–16.

MacKenzie, A. I. (1979). Naloxone in alcohol intoxication. *Lancet*, **i**, 733–4.

MacLean, P. D. (1949). Psychosomatic disease and the 'visual brain'. *Psychosomatic Med.* **11**, 338–53.

MacLean, P. D. (1969). The hypothalamus and emotional behaviour. In *The Hypothalamus*. (eds E. Anderson, and W. J. H. Nauta), pp. 659–72. Charles C. Thomas, Springfield, Illinois.

MacLennan, J. A., Drugan, R. C., and Maier, S. F. (1983). Long-term stress analgesia blocked by scopolamine. *Psychopharmacology*, **80**, 267–8.

Macleod, A. G. (1973). *Cytology*, Upjohn Company, Kalamazoo, Michigan.

Madden, J. S. (1979). *Alcohol and Drug Dependence*. Wright, Bristol.

Madsen, J. A. (1974). Depressive illness and oral contraceptives. A study of urinary 5-hydroxyindoleactetic acid excretion. In *Serotonin—New Vistas*. (Adv. Biochem. Psychopharmacol. Vol. II. (eds E. Costa, G. L. Gessa, and M. Sandler), pp. 249–53. Raven Press, New York.

Mair, W. G. P., Warrington, E. K., and Weiskrantz, L. (1979). Memory disorder in Korsakoff's psychosis. *Brain*, **102**, 749–83.

Malmo, R. E. (1972). Overview. In *Handbook of Psychophysiology*. (eds N. S. Greenfield, and L. S. Sternbach), pp. 967–80. Holt, Rinehart, and Winston, Inc., New York.

Mamelak, M., Escriu, J. M., and Stokan, S. (1973). Sleep-inducing effects of gammahydroxybutyrate. *Lancet*, **ii**, 1973–4.

Manchanda, R., and Hirsch, R. (1981). (Des-Tyr-1)-gamma-endorphin in the treatment of schizophrenia. *Psychol. Med.* **11**, 401–4.

Mangan, G. L., and Golding, J. F. (1978). An 'enhancement' model of smoking maintenance. In *Smoking Behaviour: Physiological and Psychological Influences*. (ed R. E. Thornton), pp. 87–114. Churchill Livingstone, Edinburgh.

Mangan, G. L. and Golding, J. F. (1983). The effects of smoking on memory consolidation. *J. Psychol.* **115**, 65–77.

Manning, M. and Sawyer, W. H. (1984). Design and use of selective agonistic and antagonistic analogs of the neuropeptides oxytocin and vasopressin. *Trends Neurosci.* **7**, 6–9.

Marczynski, T. J., and Burns, L. L. (1976). Reward contingent positive variation

(RCPV) and post-reinforcement EEG synchronisation (PRS) in the cat: physiological aspects, the effect of morphine and LSD-25, and a new interpretation of cholinergic mechanisms. *Gen. Pharmacol.* **7**, 211–20.

Marczynski, T. J., and Hackett, J. T. (1976). Dose-dependent dual effect of morphine on electrophysiologic correlates of positive reinforcement (reward contingent positive variation: RCPV) in the cat. *Pharmacol. Biochem. Behav.* **5**, 95–105.

Mark, R. F. (1978). The developmental view of memory. In *Studies in Neurophysiology*. (ed. R. Porter), pp. 301–8. Cambridge University Press.

Marks, J. (1978). The Benzodiazepines: Use, Overuse, Misuse, Abuse. MTP Press, Lancaster.

Marks, J. (1983). The benzodiazepines: an international perspective. *J. Psychoactive Drugs*, **15**, 137–49.

Marks, J., and Nicholson, A. N. (1984). Drugs and insomnia. *Br. Med. J.* **288**, 261.

Marr, D., (1969). A theory of cerebellar cortex. *J. Physiol. (Lond.)*, **202**, 437–70.

Marsden, C. D. (1976). Cerebral atrophy and cognitive impairment in chronic schizophrenia. *Lancet*, **ii**, 1079.

Marshall, B. E., and Wollman, H. (1980). General Anaesthetics. In *The Pharmacological Basis of Therapeutics*. (eds A. G. Gilman, L. S. Goodman, and G. Gilman), pp. 276–98. Macmillan Co., New York.

Martin, W. R., Haertzen, C. A., and Hewett, B. B. (1978). Psychopathology and pathophysiology of narcotics addicts, alcoholics and drug abusers. In *Psychopharmacology: A Generation of Progress*. (eds M. A. Lipton, A. DiMascio, and K. I. Killam), pp. 1591–602. Raven Press, New York.

Martin, I. L. (1984). The benzodiazepine receptor: functional complexity. *Trends Neurosci.* **5**, 343–7.

Martin, W. R. (1982). Hypnotics. In *Psychotropic Agents Part III*. (eds F. Hoff meister, and G. Stille), pp. 305–29. Springer Verlag, Berlin.

Martindale. (1982). *The Extra Pharmacopoeia*, (ed. E. F. Reynolds), The Pharmaceutical Press, London.

Masek, K., and Kadlec, O. (1983). Sleep factor, muramyl peptides and the serotonergic system. *Lancet.* **i**, 1277.

Mason, J. W. (1972). Organisation of psychoendocrine mechanisms. In *Handbook of Psychophysiology*. (eds N. S. Greenfield, and R.S. Sternbach), pp.3–91. Holt, Rinehart and Winston, Inc., New York.

Mason, S. T. (1979). Noradrenaline and behaviour. *Trends Neurosci.* **2**, 82–4.

Mason, S. T. (1980). Noradrenaline and selective attention: a review of the model and the evidence. *Life Sci.* **27**, 617–31.

Mason, S. T. (1983). Designing a non-neuroleptic antischizophrenic drug: the noradrenergic strategy. *Trends Pharmac. Sci.* **4**, 353–5.

Mason, S. T., and Angel, A. (1983). Behavioural evidence that chronic treatment with the antidepressant desipramine causes reduced functioning of brain noradrenaline systems. *Psychopharmacology*, **81**, 73–7.

Mason, S. T., and Fibiger, H. C. (1979). Possible behavioural function for noradrenaline-acetycholine interaction in brain. *Nature*, **277**, 396–97.

Mathe, A. A., Sedvall, G., Wiesel, F. A., and Nyback, H. (1980). Increased content of immunoreactive prostaglandin E in cerebrospinal fluid of patients with schizophrenia. *Lancet*, **i**, 16–8.

Mathew, R. J., Meyer, J. S., Semchuk, K. M., Francis, D. M., Mortel, K., and Claghorn, J. L. (1980). Cerebral blood flow in depression. *Lancet*, **i**, 1308.

Mathies, H. (1980). Pharmacology of learning and memory. *Trends Pharmac. Sci.* **1**, 333-6.

Matsuzaki, M., and Dowling, K. C. (1985). Phencyclidine (PCP): effects of acute and chronic administration on EEG activities in the Rhesus monkey. *Electroenceph. clin. Neurophsyiol.* **60**, 356-66.

Matthew, H., and Lawson, A. A. H. (1979). *Treatment of Common Acute Poisonings.* Churchill Livingstone, Edinburgh.

Matus, A., Ackerman, M., Pehling, G., Byers, H. R., and Fujiwara, K. (1982). High actin concentrations in brain dendritic spines and postsynaptic densities. *Proc. Natl. Acad. Sci., U.S.A.* **79**, 7590-4.

Mayer-Gross, W., Slater, E., and Roth, M. (1954). *Clinical Psychiatry*, Cassell and Co. Ltd., London.

Mayer, J. M., Khauna, J. M., Kim, C., and Kalant, H. (1983). Differential pharmacological responses to ethanol, pentobarbital and morphine in rats selectively bred for ethanol sensitivity. *Psychopharmacology*, **18**, 6-9.

Mayes, A. (1983). The development and course of long-term memory. In *Memory in Animals and Humans*. (ed. A. Mayes), pp. 133-76. Van Nostrand Reinhold (UK) Co. Ltd.

Maykut, O. M. (1985). Health consequences of acute and chronic marihuana use. *Prog. Neuro-Psychopharmacol. Biol. Psychiat.* **9**, 209-238.

McCallum, W. C., and Walter, W. G. (1968). The effects of attention and distraction on the contingent negative variation in normal and neurotic subjects. *Electroenceph. clin. Neurophysiol.* **25**, 319-29.

McClelland, H. (1985). Psychiatric disorders. In *Textbook of Adverse Drug Reactions.* (ed D. M. Davies), pp. 549-77. Oxford University Press. Oxford.

McClelland, H. A. (1973a). Psychiatric complications of drug therapy Part I. *Adv. Drug Reaction Bull.* **40**, 128-31.

McClelland, H. A. (1973b). Psychiatric complications of drug therapy Part II. *Adv. Reaction Bull.* **41**, 132-5.

McClelland, H. A. (1986). Psychiatric reactions to psychotropic drugs. *Adv. Drug Reaction Bull.* **119**, 444-7

McDonald, R. J. (1982) Drug treatment of senile dementia. In *Psychopharmacology of Old Age*. (ed. D. Wheatley), pp. 113-38. Oxford University Press, Oxford.

McGeer, P. C., and Jakubovic, A. (1979). Ultrastructural and biochemical changes in CNS induced by marihuana. In *Marihuana: Biological Effects*. (eds G. G. Nahas, and W. D. M. Paton), pp. 519-31. Pergamon Press, Oxford.

McGinty, D. J., Harper, R. M., and Fairbanks, M.F. (1974). Neuronal unit activity and the control of sleep states. In *Advances in Sleep Research*. (ed. E. Weitzman), pp. 173-201. Spectrum Publications Inc., New York.

McGinty, D., and Harper, R. (1976). Dorsal raphe neurons: depression of firing during sleep in cats. *Brain Res.* **101**, 569-75.

McIsaac, W. M., Fritchie, G. E., Idanpaan-Heikkila, J. E., Ho, B. T., and Englert, L.F. (1971). Distribution of marihuana in monkey brain and concomitant behavioural effects. *Nature*, **230**, 593-5.

Mechoulam, R. (ed.) (1973). *Marijuana: Chemistry, Pharmacology, Metabolism and Clinical Effects.* Academic Press Inc., New York.

Mechoulam, R. (1982). Chemistry of cannabis. In *Psychotropic Agents Part III*. (eds F. Hoffmeister, and S. Stille), pp. 120-34. Springer-Verlag, Heidelberg.

Medical Research Council Brain Metabolism Unit (1972). Modified amine hypothesis for the aetiology of affective illness. *Lancet*, **ii**, 573-77.

Medical Research Council Drug Trials Subcommittee (1981). Continuation therapy with lithium and amitriptyline in unipolar depressive illness: a controlled clinical trial. *Psychol. Med.* **1**, 409–16.

Mednick, S. A., and Schulsinger, F. (1973). A learning theory of schizophrenia: thirteen years later. In *Psychopathology*. (eds M. Hammer, K. Salzinger, and S. Sutton), pp. 343–60. Wiley, New York.

Meier-Ruge, W., Enz, A., Gygax, P., Hunziker, O., Iwangoff, P., and Reichlmeier, K. (1975). Genesis and treatment of psychologic disorders in the elderly. In *Ageing*, (eds S. Gershon, and A. Rashin), pp. 55–126. Raven Press, New York.

Melgaard, B., Danielsen, U. T., Sorensen, H., and Ahlgren, P. (1986). The severity of alcoholism and its relation to intellectual impairment and cerebral atrophy. *Br. J. Addiction* **81**, 77–80.

Mellerup, E. T., and Rafaelson, O. J. (1979). Circadian rhythms in manic-melancholic disorders. In *Current Developments in Psychopharmacology*, (eds W. B. Essman, and W. B. Valzelli), Vol.5. pp. 51–66. Spectrum Publications, New York.

Mello, N. K. (1978). Alcoholism and the behavioural pharmacology of alcohol: 1967-1977. In *Psychopharmacology: A Generation of Progress*. (eds M. A. Lipton, A. DiMascio, and K. F. Killam), pp. 1619–37. Raven Press, New York.

Mellsop, G. W., Hutton, J. D., and Delahunt, J. W. (1985). Dexamethasone suppression test as a simple measure of stress? *Br. Med. J.* **290**, 1804–6.

Meltzer, H. Y. (1980). Relevance of dopamine autoreceptors for pscyhiatry: preclinical and clinical studies. *Schizophrenia Bull.* **6**, 456–74.

Meltzer, H. Y., and Fang, V. S. (1976). Serum prolactin levels in schizophrenia—effect of antipsychotic drugs: a preliminary report. In *Hormones, Behaviour and Psychopathology*. (ed. E. J. Sachar), pp. 178–91. Raven Press, New York.

Meltzer, H. Y., Goode, D. J., and Fang, V. S. (1978). The effect of psychotropic drugs on endocrine function I. Neuroleptics, precursors and agonists. In *Psychopharmacology: A Generation of Progress*. (eds M. A. Lipton, A. DiMascio, and K. F. Killam), pp. 509–29. Raven Press, New York.

Melzack, R. (1973). *The Puzzle of Pain*. Penguin Books Ltd., Harmondsworth, Middlesex.

Melzack, R., and Wall, P. D. (1965). Pain mechanisms: a new theory. *Science, N.Y.* **150**, 971–80.

Mendels, S., Secunda, S. K., and Dyson, P. (1972) A controlled study of the antidepressant effects of lithium carbonate. *Arch. Gen. Psychiat.* **26**, 154–7.

Mendlewicz, J., Linkowski, P., and Brauman, H. (1977). Growth hormone and prolactin response to laevodopa in affective illness. *Lancet*, **i**, 652.

Mendlewicz, J., Linkowski, P., and Rees, J. A. (1980). A double blind comparison of dothiepin and amitriptyline in patients with primary affective disorder: some levels and clinical response. *Br. J. Psychiat.* **136**, 154–60.

Mendlewicz, J., Canter, E. van., Linkowski, P., L'Hermitte, M., and Robyn, C. (1980). The 24-hour profile of prolactin in depression. *Life Sci.* **27**, 2015–24.

Menon, P., Evans, R., and Madden, J. S. (1986). Methadone withdrawal regime for heroin misusers: short-term outcome and effect of parental involvement. *Br. J. Addiction* **81**, 123–6.

Mered, B., Albrecht, P., Torrey, E. F., Weinberger, D. R., Potkin, S. G., and Winfrey, C. J. (1983). Failure to isolate viruses from CSF of schizophrenics. *Lancet*, **ii**, 919.

Mesulam, M-M. (1983). The functional anatomy and hemispheric specialisation for directed attention: the role of the parietal lobe and its connections. *Trends Neurosci.* **6**, 384–7.

Metz, A., Stump, K., Cowen, P.J., Elliott, J.M., Gelder, M.G., and Grahame-Smith, D.G. (1983). Changes in platelet alpha$_2$-adrenoceptor binding post-partum: possible relation to maternity blues. *Lancet*, **i**, 495-8.

Meyer, D. R., and Beattie, M.S. (1977). Some properties of substrates of memory. In *Neuropeptide Influences on the Brain and Behaviour*. (eds L. H. Miller, C. A. Sandman, and A. J. Kastin), pp. 145-62. Raven Press, New York.

Meyer, R. E. (1978). Behavioural pharmacology of marihuana. In *Psychopharmacology: A Generation of Progress*. (eds M. A. Lipton, A. DiMascio, and K. F. Killam), pp. 1639-52. Raven Press, New York.

Miles, J. (1977). Surgery for the relief of pain. . In *Persistent Pain*. (ed S. Lipton), Vol. 1, pp. 129-48. Academic Press, London, and Grune and Stratton, New York.

Millan, M. J., and Duka, Th. (1981) Anxiolytic properties of opiates and endogenous opioid peptides and their relationship to the actions of benzodiazepines. *Mod. Probl. Pharmacopsychiat.* **17**, 123-41.

Miller, L. L. (1979). Cannabis and the brain with special reference to the limbic system. In *Marihuana: Biological Effects*. (eds G. G. Nahas, and W. D. M. Paton), pp. 539-66. Pergamon Press, Oxford.

Miller, L., and Stern, W. (1983). Bupropion: an empirical pharmacological approach to drug development . In *Frontiers in Neurophyschiatric Research*. (eds E. Usdin, M. Goldstein, A.J. Friedhoff, and A. Georgatas), pp. 195-224. Macmillan Co., London.

Miller, R. (1984). How do opiates act? *Trends Neurosci.* **7**, 184-5.

Mills, I. H. (1977). Noradrenaline and the coping process in the brain. In *Depression—the Biochemical and Physiological Role of Ludiomil*. (ed. A. Jukes), pp. 53-8. Ciba Laboratories, Horsham, England.

Milner, B. (1970). Memory and the medial temporal lobes of the brain. In *Biology of Memory*. (eds K. H. Pribram, and D. E. Broadbent), pp. 29-50. Academic Press, New York.

Mindham, R. H. S. (1979). Tricyclic antidepressants and amine precursors. In *Psychopharmacology of Affective Disorders*. (eds E. S. Paykel, and A. Coppen), pp.123-58. Oxford University Press, Oxford.

Mindham, R. H. (1982). Tricyclic antidepressants. In *Drugs in Psychiatric Practice*. (ed. P. J. Tyrer), pp. 219-48. Butterworth, London.

Mishra, R., Gillespie, D. P., Youdem, M. B. H., and Sulser, F. (1983). Effect of selective monoamine oxidase inhibition by clorgyline and deprenyl on the norepinephrine receptor-coupled adenylate cyclase system in the rat cortex. *Psychopharmacology*, **81**, 220-3.

Mogenson, G. J. (1984). Limbic–motor integration—with emphasis on initiation of exploratory and goal–directed locomotion. In *Modulation of Sensorimotor Activity During Alterations in Behavioural States*. (ed R. Bandler), pp. 121-37. Alan R. Liss Inc., New York.

Mogenson, G. J., Jones, D. L., and Yim, C. Y. (1980). From motivation to action: functional interface between the limbic system and the motor system. In *Progress in Neurobiology*. (eds B. A. Kerkut, and J. W. Phillis), 14, pp. 69-97. Pergamon Press Ltd., Oxford.

Mohler, H. (1981). Benzodiazepine receptors: are there endogenous ligands in the brain? *Trends Pharmac. Sci.* **2**, 116-19.

Mohler, H., and Okada, T. (1977). Benzodiazepine receptor: demonstration in the central nervous system. *Science*, **198**, 849-51.

Mohler, H., and Okada, T. (1978). The benzodiazepine receptor in normal and pathological human brain. *Br. J. Psychiat.* **133**, B 261–8.

Mohler, H., Okada, T., and Enna, S. J. (1978). Benzodiazepine and neurotransmitter receptor binding in rat brain after chronic administration of diazepam and phenobarbitol. *Brain Res.* **156**, 391–5.

Moiseeva, N. I. (1979). Sleep as a regulator of brain electrical activity. *Human Physiology*, **4**, 283–8.

Moldofsky, H. (1982). Rheumatic pain modulation syndrome: the interrelationships between sleep, central nervous system serotonin, and pain. *Adv. Neurol.* **33**, 51–7.

Moller, S. E., Kirk, L., and Femming, K. H. (1976). Plasma amino acids as an index for subgroups in manic depressive psychosis: correlation with effect of tryptophan. *Psychopharmacology*, **49**, 205–13.

Mondadori, C. (1981). Pharmacological modulation of memory: trends and problems. *Acta Neurol. Scand.* Suppl. 89, **64**, 129–40.

Monnier, M., and Gaillard, J. M. (1981). Biochemical regulation of sleep. *Experimentia*, **36**, 21–4.

Monnier, M., and Hosli, L. (1965). Humoral regulation of sleep and wakefulness by hypnogenic and activating dialysable factors. In *Progress in Brain Research.* (eds K. Akert, C. Bally, and J. Schade), Vol. 18, pp. 118–23. Elsevier Publishing Co., New York.

Monnier, M., and Hosli, L. (1965). Humoral transmission of sleep and wakefulness. II. Hemodialysis of a sleep inducing humor during stimulation of the thalamic somnogenic area. *Pfluegers Arch.* **282**, 60–75.

Montgomery, S. A. (1980). Measurement of serum drug levels in the assessment of antidepressants. *Br. J. clin. Pharmac.* **10**, 411–6.

Montgomery, S. A. (1982). The non-selective effect of selective antidepressants. *Adv. Biochem. Psychopharmacol.* **31**, 49–56.

Monti, J. M. (1983). Noradrenergic modulation of REM sleep: pharmacological evidence. *Trends Pharmac. Sci.* **4**, 133–5.

Montigny, C. de., and Aghajanian, G. K. (1978). Tricyclic antidepressants: long-term treatment increases responsivity of rat forebrain neurons to serotonin. *Science*, **202**, 1303–6.

Montplaisir, J. Y. (1975). Cholinergic mechanisms involved in cortical activation during arousal. *Electroenceph. clin. Neurophysiol.* **38**, 263–72.

Morley, J. E., and Levine, A. S. (1983). The central control of appetite. *Lancet*, **i**, 398–401.

Morley, J. S. (1983). Chemistry of opioid peptides. *Br. Med. Bull.* **39**, 5–10.

Morrison, C. F., and Armitage, A. K. (1967). Effects of nicotine upon the free operant behaviour of rats and spontaneous motor activity of mice. *Ann. N.Y. Acad. Sci.* **142**, 268–76.

Morselli, P. L., Bianchetti, G., Tedeschi, G., and Braithwaite, R. (1981). Haloperidol: clinical pharmacokinetics and significance of therapeutic drug monitoring. In *Therapeutic Drug Monitoring.* (eds A. Richens, and V. Marks), pp. 296–306. Churchill Livingstone, Edinburgh.

Moruzzi, G., and Magoun, H. W. (1949). Brain stem reticular formation and evolution of the EEG. *Electroenceph. clin. Neurophysiol.* **1**, 455–73.

Moulin, M. A., Davy, J. P., Debruyne, D., Andersson, J. C., Bigot, M. C., Camsonne, R., and Poilpre, E. (1982). Serum level monitoring and therapeutic effects of haloperidol in schizophrenic patients. *Psychopharmacology*, **76**, 346–50.

Mountcastle, V. B. (1974). Sleep wakefulness and the conscious state: intrinsic regulatory mechanisms of the brain. In *Medical Physiology*. (ed V. B. Mountcastle), pp. 254–81. The C.V. Mosby Company. Saint Louis.

Mountcastle, V. B. (1978). An organising principle for cerebral function: the unit module and the distributed system. In *The Mindful Brain, Cortical Organisation and the Group-selective Theory of Higher Brain Function*. (eds G. M. Edelman, and V. B. Mountcastle), pp. 7–50. MIT Press, Cambridge. Mass.

Mountjoy, C. Q., Price, J. S., Weller, M., Hunter, P., Hall, R., and Dewar J.H. (1974). A double-blind crossover sequential trial of oral thyrotrophin-releasing hormone in depression. *Lancet*, **i**, 958–60.

Muhlethaler, M., Dreifuss, J. J., and Gohwiler, B. H. (1982). Vasopressin excites hippocampal neurones. *Nature*, **296**, 749–51.

Mullaney, D. J., Kripke, D. F., Fleck, P. A., and Johnson, L.C. (1983). Sleep loss and nap effects on sustained continuous performance. *Psychphysiol.* **20**, 643–51.

Mullen, A., and Wilson, C. W. M. (1974). Fenfluramine and dreaming. *Lancet*, **ii**, 594.

Muller-Oerlinghausen, B. (1980). Clinical pharmacology (pharmacokinetics). In *Psychotropic Agents Part I: Antipsychotics and Antidepressants*. (eds F. Hoffmeister, and G. Stille), pp. 267–85. Springer-Verlag, Berlin.

Mullin, M. J., and Ferko, A. P. (1983). Alterations in dopaminergic function after subacute ethanol administration. *J. Pharmac. Exp. Therap.* **225**, 694–98.

Murphree, H. B., Pfeiffer, C. C., and Price, L. M. (1967). Electroencephalographic changes in man following smoking. *Ann.N.Y. Acad. Sci.* **142**, 245–60.

Murphy, D. L., Campbell, I., and Costa, J. L. (1978). Current status of indole amine hypothesis of affective disorders. In *Psychopharmacology: A Generation of Progress*. (eds M. A. Lipton, A. DiMascio, and K. F.Killam), pp. 1235–49. Raven Press, New York.

Murphy, D. L., Goodwin, F. K., Miller, H., Kotin, J., and Bunney, W. E. (1974). L-tryptophan in affective disorders: indoleamine changes and differential clinical effects. *Psychopharmacology*, **34**, 11–13.

Murphy, P., Hindmarch, I., and Hyland, C. M. (1982). Aspects of short-term use of two benzodiazepine hypnotics in the elderly. *Age and Ageing*, **11**, 222–8.

Murphy, S. M., Owen, R. T., and Tyrer, P. J. (1984). Withdrawal symptoms after six week's treatment with diazepam. *Lancet*, **ii**, 1389.

Murray, C. L., and Fibiger, H. C. (1986). The effect of pramizacetam (CI–879) on the acquisition of a radial arm maze task. *Psychopharmacology*. **89**, 378–81.

Murray, J. B. (1986). Marihuana's effects on human cognitive functions, psychomotor functions, and personality. *J. Gen. Psychol.* **113**, 23–55.

Murray, R. M., Lewis, S. W., and Reveley, A. M. (1985). Towards an aetiological classification of schizophrenia. *Lancet*, **i**, 1023–6.

Murray, R. M., and Oon, C. H. (1976). The excretion of dimethyltryptamine in psychiatric patients. *Proc. Roy. Soc. Med.* **69**, 831–2.

Murray, R. M., and Reveley, A. M. (1983). Schizophrenia as an infection. *Lancet*, **i**, 583.

Myers, D. H. (1978). Prognosis of schizophrenia. *Br. J. Hosp. Med.* 516–22.

Myers, R. D. (1978). Psychopharmacology of alcohol. *Ann. Rev. Pharmac. Toxicol.* **18**, 125–44.

Nagasaki, H., Iriki, M., Indue, S., and Uchizona, K. (1974). The presence of a sleep promoting material in the brain of sleep-deprived rats. *Proc. Jap. Acad.* **50**, 241–6.

Nagasaki, H., Iriki, M., and Uchizona, K. (1976). Inhibitory effect of the brain extract of sleep-deprived rats (BE-SDR) on the spontaneous discharges of crayfish abdominal ganglion. *Physiol. Behav.* **5**, 243–6.

Nahas, G. G., and Paton, W. D. M. (1979). *Marihuana: Biological Effects*. (eds) pp. Pergamon Press, Oxford.

Nakahama, H., Shima, K., Aya, K., Kisara, K., and Sakarada, S. (1981). Anti-nociceptive action of morphine and pentacozine on unit activity in the nucleus centralis lateralis, nucleus ventralis lateralis and nearby structures of the cat. *Pain*, **10**, 47–56.

Nathan, R. S., and van Kammon, D. P. (1985). Neuroendocrine effects of antipsychotic drugs. In *Drugs in Psychiatry*. Vol. 3. Antipsychotics (eds G. D. Burrows, T. R. Norman, and B. Davies), pp. 11–26. Elsevier, Amsterdam.

Nelsen, J. M. (1978). Psychological consequences of chronic nicotinisation: a focus on arousal. In *Behavioural Effects of Nicotine*. (ed K. Battig), pp. 1–17. S. Karger, Basel.

Nelson, W. T., Steiner, S. S., Brutus, M., Farrell, R., and Ellman, S. J. (1981). Brain site variation in effects of morphine on electrical self-stimulation. *Psychopharmacology*, **74**, 58–65.

Nestoros, J. N. (1980). Ethanol selectively potentiates GABA-mediated inhibition of single feline cortical neurons. *Life Sci.* **26**, 519–23.

Newlin, D. B. (1986). Conditional compensatory response to alcohol placebo in humans. *Psychopharmacology*, **88**, 247–51.

Newnham, J. P., Tomlin, S., Ratter, S. J., Bourne, G. L., and Rees, L. H. (1983). Endogenous opioids in pregnancy. *Br. J. Obstet. Gynaecol.* **90**, 535–8.

Nicholson, A. N. (1980a). Hypnotics: rebound insomnia and residual sequelae. *Br. J. clin. Pharmac.* **9**, 223–5.

Nicholson, A. N. (1980b). The use of short and long-acting hypnotics in clinical medicine. *Br. J. clin. Pharmac.* **11**, *Suppl. 1*, 61–9.

Nicholson, A. N., and Stone, B. (1980). Activity of the hypnotics flunitrazepam and triazolam, in man. *Br. J. clin. Pharmac.* **9**, 187–94.

Nicoll, R. (1978). Selective actions of barbiturates on synaptic transmission. In: *Psychopharmacology: A Generation of Progress*. (eds M. A. Lipton, A. DiMascio, and K. F. Killam), pp. 1337–48. Raven Press, New York.

Nicoll, R. A. (1975). Presynaptic action of barbiturates in the frog spinal cord. *Proc. Natl. Acad. Sci. USA*, **72**, 1460–3.

Nielsen, I. M. (1980). Tricyclic antidepressants: general pharmacology. In *Psychotropic Agents Part I: Antipsychotics and Antidepressants*. (eds F.Hoffmeister, and G. Stille), pp. 399–414. Springer-Verlag, Berlin.

Nielsen, M., Braestrup, C. and Squires, R. F. (1978). Evidence for a late evolutionary appearance of brain-specific benzodiazepine receptors: an investigation of 18 vertebrate and 5 invertebrate species. *Brain Res.* **141**, 342–6.

Nilsson, J. L., and Carlsson, A. (1982). Dopamine-receptor agonist with apparent selectivity for autoreceptors: a new principle for antipsychotic action? *Trends Pharmac. Sci.* **3**, 322–5.

Nishikawa, T., Tsuda, A., Tanaka, M., Koga, I., and Uchida, Y. (1982). Prophylactic effect of neuroleptics in symptom free schizophrenics. *Psychopharmacology*, **77**, 301–4.

Nistri, A. (1975). Are benzodiazepines antipsychotic agents? *Lancet*, **ii**, 1040.

Norman, T. R., and Burrows, G. D. (1983). Plasma concentrations of antidepressant drugs and clinical responses. In *Antidepressants*. (eds G. D. Burrows, T. R. Norman, and R. Davies), pp. 111–20. Elsevier Science Publishers, Amsterdam.

North, R. A. and Williams, J. T. (1983). How do opiates inhibit neurotransmitter release? *Trends Neurosci.* **6**, 337–9.

Norton, A. (1981). Old men forget. *Br. Med. J.* **283**, 1201–2.

Noyes, R., Dempsey, G. M., Blum, A., and Cavanaugh, G. L. (1974). Lithium treatment of depression. *Comp. Psychiat.* **15**, 187–93.

Nuotto, E., Palva, E. S., and Lahdenranta, U. (1983). Naloxone fails to counteract heavy alcohol intoxication. *Lancet*, **ii**, 167.

Oakley, D. A. (1979). Neocortex and learning. *Trends Neurosci.* **2**, 149–52.

Oakley, D. A. (1981). Brain mechanisms of mammalian memory. *Br. Med. Bull.* **37**, 175–80.

Oblowitz, H., and Robins, A. H. (1983). The effect of clobazam and lorazepam on the psychomotor performance of anxious patients. *Br. J. clin. Pharmac.* **16**, 95–9.

O'Boyle, C. A., Harris, D., Barry, H., and Cullen, J. H. (1986). Differential effects of benzodiazepine sedation in high and low anxious patients in 'real life' stress setting. *Psychopharmacology*, **88**, 266–9.

O'Connor, D. (1982). The use of suggestion techniques with adolescents in the treatment of glue sniffing and solvent abuse. *Human Toxicol.* **1**, 313–20.

O'Connor, D. (1984). *Glue Sniffing and Volatile Substance Abuse*. Gower Publishing Co. Ltd., Aldershot.

Oehme, P., and Krivoy, W. A. (1983). Substance P: a peptide with unusual features. *Trends Pharmac. Sci.* **4**, 521–3.

Offermeier, J., and Rooyen, J. H. van. (1982). Is it possible to integrate dopamine receptor terminology? In *More About Receptors*. (ed. J. W. Lamble), pp. 93–97. Elsevier Biomed. Press, Amsterdam.

Ogren, S-O. (1981). Studies on the role of serotonin in avoidance learning. *Psychopharmacol. Bull.* **17**, 17–19.

Ogren, S-O., Fuxe, K., Berge, O. G., and Agnati, L. F. (1983). Effects of chronic administration of antidepressant drugs on central serotonergic receptor mechanisms.. In *Frontiers in Neuropscyhiatric Research*. (eds E. Usdin, M. Goldstein, A. J. Friedhoff, and A. Georgatas), pp. 93–108. Macmillan Co., London.

Ogunremi, O. O., Adamson, L., Brezinova, V., Hunter, W. M., Maclean, A. W., Oswald, I., and Percy-Robb, I. W. (1973). Two antianxiety drugs: a psychoendocrine study. *Br. Med. J.* **2**, 202–7.

Ohman, A., Erikson, A., Fredriksson, M., Hugdahl, K., and Olofsson, C. (1974). Habituation of the electrodermal orienting reaction to potentially phobic and supposedly neutral stimuli in normal human subjects. *Biol. Psychol.* **2**, 85–93.

Ojemann, G. A. (1983). The intrahemispheric organisation of human language, derived with electrical stimulation techniques. *Trends Neurosci.* **6**, 184–9.

Okamoto, M. (1978). Barbiturates and alcohol: Comparative overviews on neurophysiology and neurochemistry. In *Psychopharmacology: A Generation of Progress*. (eds M. A. Lipton, A. DiMascio, and K. F. Killam), pp. 1575–90. Raven Press, New York.

O'Keefe, J. and Nadel, L. (1978). *The Hippocampus as a Cognitive Map*. Clarendon Press, Oxford.

Okuma, T., Koga, I., and Uchida, Y. (1976). Sensitivity to chlorpromazine effects on brain function in schizophrenics and normals. *Psychopharmacology*, **51**, 101–5.

Olds, J. (1956). Pleasure centres in the brain. *Scientific Am.* **195**, 105–17.

Olds, J. (1962). Hypothalamic substances of reward. *Physiol. Rev.* **42**, 554–604.

Olds, J. (1975). In *Brain-stimulation Reward.* (ed A. Wauguier, and E. T. Rolls), pp. 1–27. North Holland, Amsterdam.

Olds, J. (1977). *Drives and Reinforcements: behavioural studies of hypothalamic functions.* Raven Press, New York.

Olds, J., and Milner, P. (1954). Positive reinforcement produced by electrical stimulation of septal area and other regions of rat brain. *J. Comp. Physiol. Psychol.* **47**, 419–27.

Olds, J., and Travis, R. P. (1960). Effects of chlorpromazine, meprobamate, pentobarbital and morphine on self-stimulation. *J. Pharmac. Exp. Therap.* **128**, 397–404.

Olds, M. E., and Olds, J. (1963). Approach avoidance analysis of the rat diencephalon. *J. Comp. Neurol.* **120**, 259–62.

Oliver, J. S., and Watson, J. M. (1977). Abuse of solvents 'for kicks': a review of 50 cases. *Lancet,* **i,** 84–6.

Oliveros, J. C., Jandali, M. K., Timsit-Berthier, M., Remy, R., Benghezal, A., Audibert, P., and Moeglen, P. (1978). Vasopressin in amnesia. *Lancet,* **i,** 42.

Oomura, Y., and Aou, S. (1984). Catecholaminergic and cholinergic involvement in reward related responses in monkey orbitofrontal cortex. In *Modulation of Sensorimotor Activity During Alterations in Behavioural States.* (ed R. Bandler), pp. 269–90. Alan R Liss Inc., New York.

Oppenheimer, S. J. (1985). Oncogenes in scrapie and Creutzfeld-Jacob diseases. *Proc. Roy. Soc. Med.* **78**, 347.

Ostergaard, G. Z., and Pedersen, S. E. (1982). Neonatal convulsions caused by withdrawal from maternal clomipramine. *Pediat.* **69**, 233–4.

Oswald, I. (1976). The function of sleep. *Postgrad. Med. J.* **52**, 15–18.

Oswald, I. (1980). *Sleep.* Penguin Books, Ltd., Harmondsworth, Middlesex.

Oswald, I., Adam, K., and Spiegel, R. (1982). Human EEG slow-wave sleep increased by a serotonin antagonist. *Electroenceph. clin. Neurophysiol.* **54**, 583–6.

Oswald, I., Brezinova, V., and Dunleavy, D. L. F. (1972). On the slowness of action of tricyclic antidepressant drugs. *Br. J. Psychiat.* **120**, 673–7.

Oswald, I., French, C., Adam, K. and Gilham, J. (1982) Benzodiazepine hypnotics remain effective for 24 weeks. *Br. Med. J.* **284**, 860–3.

Oswald, I., Lewis, S. A., Dunleavy, D. L. F., Brezinova, V., and Briggs, M. (1971). Drugs of dependence though not of abuse: fenfluramine and imipramine. *Br. Med. J.* **2,** 70–3.

Otsuka, M. and Konishi, S. (1983) Substance P—the first peptide neurotransmitter? *Trends Neurosci.* **6**, 317–320.

Owen, F., Cross, A. J., Crow, T. J., Deakin, J. F. W., Ferrier, N., Lofthouse, R., and Poulter, M. (1983). Brain 5-HT2 receptors and suicide. *Lancet,* **ii,** 1256.

Owen, F., Cross, A. J., Crow, T. J., Lofthouse, R., and Poulter, M. (1981). Neurotransmitter receptors in brain in schizophrenia. *Acta. Psychiat. Scand.* **63,** *Suppl. 289*, 20–6.

Owen, F., Cross, A. J., Crow, T. J., Longden, A., Poulter, M., and Riley, G. J. (1978). Increased dopamine-receptor sensitivity in schizophrenia. *Lancet,* **ii,** 223–6.

Owen, R. T., and Tyrer, P. (1983). Benzodiazepine dependence: a review of the evidence. *Drugs,* **25**, 385–98.

Oxaprotaline Study Group (1983). A double-blind comparative trial of oxapprotaline with amitriptyline and placebo in outpatients with moderate depression: relationship of urinary MHPG levels. In *Frontiers in Neuropsychiatric Research*. (eds E. Usdin, M. Goldstein, A. J. Friedhoff, and A. Georgatas), pp. 319-30. Macmillan Co., London.

Oyama, T., Jin, T., Yamaya, R., Ling, N., and Guillemin, R. (1980). Profound analgesic effects of beta-endorphin in man. *Lancet*, **i**, 122-4.

Oyama, T., Jin, T., Yamaya, R., Matsuki, A., Ling, N., and Guillemin, R. (1982). Intrathecal use of beta-endorphin as a powerful analgesic agent in man. In *Advances in Pharmacology & Therapeutics II. Vol. 1. CNS Pharmacology—Neuropeptides*. (eds H. Yoshida, Y. Hagihara, and S. Ebashi), pp. 39-43. Pergamon Press, Oxford.

Palfai, T., Brown, O. M., and Walsh, T. J. (1978). Catecholamine levels in whole brain and the probability of memory formation are not related. *Pharmacol. Biochem. Behav.* **8**, 717-21.

Pandya, D. N., and Seltzer, B. (1982). Association areas of the cerebral cortex. *Trends Neurosci.* **5**, 386-90.

Panksepp, J. (1981). Brain opioids—a neurochemical substrate for narcotic and social dependence. In *Theory in Psychopharmacology. Vol.1* (ed. S. J. Cooper), pp. 149-76. Academic Press, London.

Papez, J. (1937). A proposed mechanism of emotion. *Arch. Neurol. Psychiat.* **38**, 725-43.

Pappenheimer, J. R., Miller, T. B., and Goodrich, C. A. (1967). Sleep-promoting effects of cerebrospinal fluid from sleep-deprived goats. *Proc. Natl. Acad. Sci.* **58**, 513-17.

Pare, C. M., Yeung, D. P., Price, K., and Stacey, R. S. (1969). 5-hydroxytryptophan, noradrenaline, and dopamine in brainstem, hypothalamus and caudate nucleus of controls and of patients committing suicide by gas poisoning. *Lancet*, **ii**, 133-5.

Parker, E. S., Morihina, J. M., Wyatt, R. J., Schwartz, B. L., Weingartner, H., and Stillman, C. (1981). The alcohol facilitation effect on memory: a dose-response study. *Psychopharmacology*, **74**, 88-92.

Parkes, J. D. (1977). The sleepy patient. *Lancet*, **i**, 990-3.

Parkes, J. D. (1981). Day-time drowsiness. *Lancet*, **ii**, 1213-17.

Parkes, J. D., Langdon, N., and Lock, C. (1986). Narcolepsy and immunity. *Br. Med. J.* **292**, 359-60.

Parrott, A. C., and Davies, S. (1983). Effects of a 1-5 benzodiazepine derivative upon performance in an experimental stress situation. *Psychopharmacology*, **79**, 367-9.

Parrott, A. C., and Kentridge, R. (1982). Personal constructs of anxiety under the 1,5 benzodiazepine derivative clobazam related to trait-anxiety levels of the personality. *Psychopharmacology*, **75**, 353-7.

Paterson, S. J., Robson, L. E., and Kosterlitz, H. W. (1983). Classification of opioid receptors. *Br. Med. Bull.* **39**, 31-6.

Paton, A. (1985) The politics of alcohol. *Br. Med. J.* **290**, 1-2.

Paton, J. A., and Nottebohm, F. N. (1984). Neurons generated in the adult brain are recruited into functional circuits. *Science*, **225**, 1046-8.

Paton, W. D. M. (1979). Concluding summary. In *Marihuana: Biological Effects*. (eds G. G. Nahas, and W. D. M. Paton), pp. 735-8. Pergamon Press, Oxford.

Paton, W. D. M., and Crown J. (eds) (1972). *Cannabis and its Derivatives. Pharmacology and Experimental Psychology*. Oxford University Press, Oxford.

Paton W. D. M., Pertwee, R. G., and Tylden, E. (1983). Clinical aspects of cannabis action. In *Marihuana: Biological Effects*. (eds G. G. Nahas, and W. D. M. Paton), pp. 335–65. Pergamon Press, Oxford.

Paul, G. J., and Whitehouse, L. W. (1977). Metabolic basis for the supra-additive effect of the combination of the ethanol-diazepam combination in mice. *Br. J. Pharmac.* **60**, 83–90.

Paulson, G. W. (1975). Tardive dyskinesia. *Ann. Rev. Med.* **25**, 75–81.

Pavlov, I. P. (1927). *Conditioned Reflexes: An Investigation of the Physiological Activity of the Cerebral Cortex*. Oxford University Press, Oxford.

Paykel, E. S. (1974) Recent life events and clinical depression.. In *Life Stress and Illness*. (eds E. G. Gunderson, and R. H. Rahe), pp. 134–63. Thomas Springfield, Illinois.

Paykel, E. S. (1979a). Predictors of treatment response. In *Psychopharmacology of Affective Disorders*. (eds E. S. Paykel, and A. Coppen), pp. 193–220. Oxford University Press, Oxford.

Paykel, E. S. (1979b). Management of acute depression. In *Psychopharmacology of Affective Disorders*. (eds E. S. Paykel, and A. Coppen), pp. 235–47. Oxford University Press, Oxford.

Paykel, E. S. (1983). The classification of depression. *Br. J. clin. Pharmac.* **15**, 155– 9.

Paykel, E. S., West, P. S., Rowan, P. R., and Parker, R. R. (1982). Influence of acetylator phenotype on antidepressant effects of phenelzine. *Br. J. Psychiat.* **141**, 243–8.

Pearce, J. M. S. (1984a). Migraine: a cerebral disorder. *Lancet*, **ii**, 86–9.

Pearce, J. M. S. (1984b). Boxer's brains. *Br. Med. J.* **288**, 933–4.

Pearce, J. M. S. (1985). Is migraine explained by Leao's spreading depression? *Lancet*, **ii**, 763–6.

Peet, M. (1981). Is propranolol antischizophrenic? *Neuropharmacol.* **20**, 1303–7.

Peet, M., and Coppen, A. (1979). The pharmacokinetics of antidepressant drugs: relevance to their therapeutic effect. In *Psychopharmacology of Affective Disorders*. (eds E. S. Paykel, and A. Coppen), pp. 9–107. Oxford University Press, Oxford.

Pellow, S., and File, S. E. (1984). Multiple sites of action for anxiogenic drugs. *Psychopharmacology*, **83**, 304–15.

Penfield, W., and Jasper, H. (1954). *Epilepsy and the Functional Anatomy of the Human Brain*. Little, Brown & Co., Boston.

Penfield, W., and Perot, P. (1963). The brain's record of auditory and visual experience. *Brain*, **86**, 595–9.

Perkins, J. P. (1982). Catecholamine-induced modification of the functional state of beta-adrenergic receptors. In *More About Receptors*. (ed J. W. Lamble), pp. 48–53. Elsevier Biomedical Press, Amsterdam.

Peroutka, S. J., Lebkovitz, R. M., and Snyder, S. H. (1981). Two distinct central serotonin receptors with different physiological function. *Science*, **212**, 827–9.

Peroutka, S. J., and Snyder, S. H. (1980). Long-term antidepressant treatment decreases spiroperidol-labelled serotonin receptor binding. *Science*, **210**, 88–90.

Perris, C. (1980). Central measures of depression. In *Handbook of Biological Psychiatry Part II Brain Mechanisms and Abnormal Behaviour — Psychophysiology*. (ed H. M. van Praag), pp. 183–224. Marcel Dekker Inc., New York and Basel.

Perry, E. K., and Perry, R. H. (1985). New insights into the nature of senile (Alzheimer-type) plaques. *Trends Neurosci.* **8**, 301–3.

Perry, T. L., Kish, S. J., Buchanan, J., and Hanson, S. (1979). Gamma-aminobutyric acid deficiency in brain of schizophrenic patients. *Lancet*, **i**, 237–9.

Pert, A., and Hulsebus, R. (1975). Effect of morphine on intracranial self-stimulation behaviour following brain amine depletion. *Life Sci.* **17**, 19-20.

Pert, C. B., and Quirion, R. (1983). The phencyclidine receptor. *Trends Pharmac. Sci.* **4**, 12.

Peters, A., Palay, S. L., and Webster, H. deF. (1976). *The Fine Structure of the Nervous System.* W. B. Saunders Company, Philadelphia.

Peters, T. J. (1983). Aldehyde dehydrogenase and alcoholism. *Lancet*, **i**, 364.

Pettigrew, J. D. (1978). The locus coeruleus and cortical plasticity. *Trends Neurosci.* **1**, 73-4.

Pettit, H-O., Ettenberg, A., Bloom, F. E., and Koob, G. F. (1984). Destruction of dopamine in the nucleus accumbens selectively attenuates cocaine but not heroin self-administration in rats. *Psychopharmacology*, **84**, 167-73.

Petursson, H., and Lader, M. H. (1981a). Withdrawal from long-term benzodiazepine treatment. *Br. Med. J.* **283**, 643-5.

Petursson, H., and Lader, M. H. (1981b). Benzodiazepine dependence. *Br. J. Addiction*, **76**, 133-45.

Petursson, H., and Lader, M. H. (1984). *Dependence on Tranquillisers.* Oxford University Press, Oxford.

Petursson, H., Shur, E., Checkley, S., Slade, A., and Lader, M. H. (1981). A neuroendocrine approach to benzodiazepine tolerance and dependence. *Br. J. clin. Pharmac.* **11**, 526-8.

Pfeiffer, C. C., Goldstein, L., Murphree, H. B., and Jenney, E. H. (1964). Electroencephalographic assay of anti-anxiety drugs. *Arch. Gen. Psychiat.* **10**, 446-53.

Phillis, J. W., and Jhamandas, K. (1971). The effects of chlorpromazine and ethanol on in vivo release of acteylcholine from the cerebral cortex. *Comp. Gen. Pharmac.* **2**, 306-10.

Piaget, J., and Inhelder, B. (1969). *The Psychology of the Child.* Basic Books, New York.

Pickar, D. (1983). Naloxone in schizophrenia. *Lancet*, **i**, 819.

Pickar, D., Cutler, N. R., Naber, D., Post, R. M., Pert, C. B., and Bunney, W. E. (1980). Plasma opioid activity in manic-depressive illness. *Lancet*, **i**, 937.

Piercy, M. F. (1977). Experimental studies of the organic amnesic syndrome. In *Amnesia.* (eds C. W. M. Whitty, and O. L. Zangwill), pp. 1-51. Butterworth, London.

Pilotto, R., Singer, G., and Overstreet, D. (1984). Self-injection of diazepam in naive rats: effects of dose, schedule and blockade of different receptors. *Psychopharmacology*, **84**, 174-7.

Poling, A. D., and Appel, J. B. (1982). Dependence-producing liability of LSD and similar psychotomimetics. In *Psychotropic Agents Part III.* (eds F. Hoffmeister and S. Stille), pp. 111-6. Springer-Verlag, Heidelberg.

Polkey, C. E. (1983). Effects of anterior temporal lobectomy apart from the relief of seizures: a study of 40 patients. *J. Roy. Soc. Med.* **76**, 354-8.

Pollitt, J. (1982). Moodiness: a heavenly problem? *J. Roy. Soc. Med.* **75**, 7-16.

Pomara, N., and Stanley, M. (1982). Cholinergic precursors in Alzheimer's disease. *Lancet*, **ii**, 1049.

Pomerleau, O. F., Fertig, J. B., Seyler, L. E., and Jaffe, J. (1983). Neuroendocrine reactivity to nicotine in smokers. *Psychopharmacology*, **81**, 61-7.

Pomerleau, O. F., Turk, D. C., and Fertig, J. B. (1984). The effects of smoking on pain and anxiety. *Addictive Behaviours*, **9**, 265-71.

Pompeiano, O. (1967). The neurophysiological mechanisms of postural and motor events during desynchronised sleep. *Res. Publ. Assoc. Res. Nerv. Ment. Dis.* **45**, 351–423.

Post, R. M. (1978). Frontiers in affective disorder research: new pharmacological agents and new methodologies. In *Psychopharmacology: A Generation of Progress.* (eds M. A. Lipton, A. DiMascio, and K. F. Killam), pp. 1323–36. Raven Press, New York.

Post, R. M., Rubinow, D. R., Uhde, T. W., Ballenger, J. C., Lake, C. R., Linnoila, M. Jimerson, D. C., and Reus, V. (1985). Effects of carbamazepine on noradrenergic mechanisms in affectively ill patients. *Psychopharmacology*, **87**, 59–63.

Post, R. M., and Uhde, T. W. (1983). Biochemical and physiological mechanisms of action of carbamazepine in affective illness. In *Frontiers in Neuropsychiatric Research.* (eds E. Usdin, M. Goldstein, A. J. Friedhoff, and A. Georgatas), pp. 175–91. Macmillan Co., London.

Praag, H. M. van., (1980a). Central monoamine metabolism in depression. I Serotonin and related compounds. *Comp. Psychiat.* **21**, 30–43.

Praag, H. M. van., (1980b). Central monoamine metabolism in depression. II Catecholamines and related compounds. *Comp. Psychiat.* **21**, 44–54.

Praag, H. M. van., (1982). Neurotransmitters and CNS disease. *Lancet*, **ii**, 1259–63.

Praag, H. M. van., and Verhoeven, W. M. A. (1981). Endorphin research in schizophrenic psychoses. *Comp. Psychiat.* **22**, 135–46.

Prange, A. J., Nemeroff, C. B., and Lipton, M. A. (1978). Behavioural effects of peptides: basic and clinical studies. In *Psychopharmacology: A Generation of Progress.* (eds M. A. Lipton, A. DiMascio, and K. F. Killam), pp. 441–58. Raven Press, New York.

Prange, A. J., Wilson, I. C., Lara, P. P., Alltop, L. B., and Breese, G. R. (1972). Effects of thyrotropin-releasing hormone in depression. *Lancet*, **ii**, 999–1002.

Prichard, D. C. U., Perry, B. D., Wang, C. M., Mitrius, J. C., and Kahn, D. J. (1983). Molecular aspects of regulation of alpha$_2$-adrenergic receptors. In *Frontiers in Neuropsychiatric Research.* (eds E Usdin, M. Goldstein, A. J. Friedhoff, and A. Goergatas), pp. 65–82. Macmillan Co., London.

Prien, R. F., Caffey, E. M., and Klett, C. J. (1972). Comparison of lithium carbonate and chlorpromazine in the treatment of mania. *Arch. Gen. Psychiat.* **26**, 146–53.

Proudfoot, A. (1982). *Diagnosis and Management of Acute Poisoning.* Blackwell Scientific Publications, Oxford.

Putkonen, P. T. S. (1979). Alpha and beta adrenergic mechanisms in the control of sleep stages. In *Sleep Research.* (eds R. G. Priest, A. Pletscher, and J. Ward), pp. 19–34. MTP Press, Ltd., Lancaster.

Quarantotti, B. P., Carolis, A. S., de, and Longo, V. G. (1975). Behavioural effects of intracerebrally administered catecholamines in mice and their modifications by some adrenergic blocking agents. *Psychopharmacologia (Berl.)* **45**, 83–6.

Quintero, S., Henney, S., Lawson, P., Mellanby, J. and Gray, J. A. (1985). The effects of compounds related to gamma-aminobutyrate and benzodiazepine receptors on behavioural responses to anxiogenic stimuli in the rat: punished barpressing. *Psychopharmacology*, **85**, 244–51.

Quitkin, F., Rifkin, A., and Klein, D. F. (1976). Neurologic soft signs in schizophrenia and character disorders. *Arch. Gen. Psychiat.* **33**, 845–53.

Racagni, G., and Brunello, N. (1984). Transynaptic mechanisms in the action of antidepressant drugs. *Trends Pharmac. Sci.* **5**, 527–31.

Rago, L. K., Allikonets, L. H., and Zarkovsky, A. M. (1981). Effects of piracetam on the central dopaminergic transmission. *Naunyn-Schmiedeberg's Arch. Pharmacol.* **318**, 36-7.

Raisman, G. (1969). Neuronal plasticity in the septal nuclei of the adult rat. *Brain Res.* **14**, 25-48.

Rall, T. W. (1980). Central nervous system stimulants. In *The Pharmacological Basis of Therapeutics.* (eds A. G. Gilman, L. S. Goodman, and A. Gilman), pp. 592-607. Macmillan Co., New York.

Rall, T. W., and Schleifer, S. (1980). Drugs effective in the therapy of the epilepsies. In *The Pharmacological Basis of Therapeutics.* (eds A. G. Gilman, L. S. Goodman, and A. Gilman), 6th edn, pp. 448-74. Macmillan Co., New York.

Rance, M. J. (1983). The antagonist analgesics: actions at multiple opiate receptors. In *Persistent Pain.* (eds S. Lipton, and J. Miles), Vol.4, pp. 21-40. Grune and Stratton, London.

Rao, V. A. R., and Norris, J. R. (1972). A double-blind investigation of Hydergine in the treatment of cerebrovascular insufficiency in the elderly. *Johns Hopkins Med. J.* **130**, 317-24.

Raw, M. (1978). The treatment of cigarette dependence. In *Research Advances in Alcohol and Drug Problems.* (ed Y. Israels, F. B. Glaser, H. Kalant, R. C. Pophan, W. Schmidt, and R. G. Smart), Plenum Press, New York.

Rawlins, J. N. P. (1984). Some neurophysiological properties of the septo-hippocampal system.. In *Psychopharmacology of the Limbic System.* (eds M. R. Trimble, and E. Zarifian), pp. 17-50. Oxford University Press, Oxford.

Rebert, C. S. (1973). Elements of a general cerebral system related to CNV genesis. *Electroenceph. clin. Neurophysiol.* Suppl. 33, 63-7.

Redgrave, P., and Dean, P. (1981). Intracranial self-stimulation. *Br. Med. Bull.* **37**, 141-6.

Redmond, D. E. (1982). Does clonidine alter anxiety in humans? *Trends Pharmac. Sci.* **3**, 477-80.

Ree, J. M. van. (1982). Non opiate beta-endorphin 2-9 enhances apomorphine-induced stereotypy following subcutaneous and intrastriatal injection. *Neuropharmacol.* **21**, 1103-10.

Ree, J. M. van., Caffe, A. R., and Wolterink, G. (1982a). Non-opiate beta-endorphin fragments and dopamine-III. Gamma-type endorphins and various neuroleptics counteract the hyperactivity elicited by injection of apomorphine into the nucleus accumbens. *Neuropharmacol.* **21**, 1111-18.

Ree, J. M. van., Innemce, H., Louwerens, J. W., Kahn, R. S., and Wied, D. de. (1982b). Non-opiate beta-endorphin fragments and dopamine-I. The nueroleptic-like gamma-endorhin fragments interfere with the behavioural effects elicited by small doses of apomorphine. *Neuropharmacol.* **21**, 1095-102.

Ree, J. M. van., and Wied, D. de. (1981). Endorphins in schizophrenia. *Neuropharmacol.* **20**, 1271-7.

Ree, J. M. van., and Wied, D. de. (1982). Neuroleptic-like profile of gamma-type endorphins as related to schizophrenia. *Trends Pharmac. Sci.* **3**, 358-61.

Ree, J. M. van., Verhoeven, W. M. A., Praag, H. M. van., and Wied, D. de. (1981). Neuroleptic-like and antipsychotic effects of gamma-type endorphins. *Mod. Probl. Pharmacopsychiat.* **17**, 266-78.

Ree, J. M. van., Wolterink, G., Fekete, M., and Wied, D. de. (1982c). Non-opiate beta-endorphin fragments and dopamine-IV. Gamma-type endorphins may control dopaminergic systems in the nucleus accumbens. *Neuropharmacol.* **21**, 1119-28.

Reggiani, A., Barbaccia, M. L., Spano, P. F., and Trabucchi, M. (1980). Dopamine metabolism and receptor function after acute and chronic ethanol. *J. Neurochem.* **35**, 34–7.

Reich, W. (1975). The spectrum concept of schizophrenia; problems for diagnostic practice. *Arch. Gen. Psychiat.* **32**, 489–98.

Reisberg, B., Ferris, S. H., Anand, R., Mir, P., Geibel, V., DeLeon, M. J., and Roberts, E. (1983). Effects of naloxone in senile dementia: a double blind trial. *New Engl. J. Med.* **308**, 721–2.

Reisberg, B., Ferris, S. H., and Gershon, S. (1981). An overview of pharmacologic treatment of cognitive decline. *Am. J. Psychiat.* **138**, 593–600.

Reisine, T. D., Rossor, M., Spokes, E., Iverson, L. L., and Yamamura, H. I. (1980). Opiate and neuroleptic receptor alterations in human schizophrenic brain tissue. In *Receptors for Neurotransmitters and Peptide Hormones.* (eds G. Pepeu, M. J. Kuhar, and S. J. Enna), pp. 443–50. Raven Press, New York.

Revely, A. M., Revely, M. A., and Murray, R. M. (1983). Enlargement of cerebral ventricles in schizophrenics is confined to those without genetic prodisposition. *Lancet*, **ii**, 525.

Reynolds, E. H. (1983). Interictal behaviour in temporal lobe epilepsy. *Br. Med. J.* **286**, 918–9.

Reynolds, E. H., Carney, M. W. P., and Toone, B. K. (1984) Methylation and mood. *Lancet*, **ii**, 196–8.

Reynolds, G. P. (1983). Increased concentrations and lateral asymmetry of amygdala dopamine in schizophrenia. *Nature*, **305**, 527–9.

Reynolds, G. P. (1984). Noradrenaline and schizophrenia. *Trends Pharmac. Sci.* **5**, 138.

Reynolds, G. P., Reynolds, L. M., Reiderer, P., Jellinger, K., and Gabriel, E. (1980). Dopamine receptors and schizophrenia; drug effect or illness. *Lancet*, **ii**, 1251.

Reynolds, G. P., Riederer, P., Jellinger, K., and Gabriel, E. (1981). Dopamine receptors and schizophrenia: the neuroleptic drug problem. *Neuropharmacol.* **20**, 1319–20.

Richards, C. D. (1972). On the mechanism of barbiturate anaesthesia. *J. Physiol.* **227**, 749–67.

Richards, C. D. (1980). In search of the mechanisms of anaesthesia. *Trends Neurosci.* **3**, 9–13.

Richards, C. D., and Smaje, J. O. (1976). Anaesthetics depress the sensitivity of cortical neurones to L-glutamate. *Br. J. Pharmac.* **58**, 347–57.

Richardson, A. E., and Bereeny, F. J. (1977). Effect of piracetam on level of consciousness after neurosurgery. *Lancet*, **ii**, 1110–11.

Richelson, E. (1981). Pharmacology and clinical considerations of the neuroleptics. In *Neuropharmacology of Central Nervous System and Behavioural disorders.* (ed G. C. Palmer), pp. 125–46. Academic Press, New York.

Richter, D. (1978). Clues to the causation of schizophrenia. In *The Biological Basis of Schizophrenia.* (eds G. Hemmings, and W. A. Hemmings), pp. 55–61. MTP Press Ltd., Lancaster.

Rickels, K. (1978). Use of antianxiety agents in anxious out patients. *Psychopharmacology*, **58**, 1–17.

Rifkin, A., and Siris, S. (1984). Sodium lactate response as a model for panic disorders. *Trends Neurosci.* **7**, 188–9.

Rigter, H., and Riezen, H. van. (1978). Hormones and Memory. In *Psy-*

chopharmacology: A Generation of Progress . (eds M. A. Lipton, A. DiMascio, and K. F. Killam), pp. 677–89. Raven Press, New York.

Rimon, R., Terenius, L., and Kampman, R. (1980). Cerebrospinal fluid endorphins in schizophrenia. *Acta. Psychiat. Scand.* **61**, 375-403.

Ritchie, J. M. (1980). The aliphatic alcohols. In *The Pharmacological Basis of Therapeutics*. (eds A. G. Gilman, L. S. Goodman, and A. Gilman), pp. 376-90. Macmillan Co., New York.

Ritchie, J. M., and Greene, N. B. (1981). Local anaesthetics. In *The Pharmacological Basis of Therapeutics*. (eds A. G. Gilman, L. S. Goodman, and A. Gilman), pp. 300-20. Macmillan Co., New York.

Roberts, J. K. A. (1984). Frontal lobe hypofunction in schizophrenia. *Lancet*, **i**, 969-70.

Robertson, M. N., and Trimble, M. R. (1981). Neuroleptics as antidepressants. *Neuropharmacol.* **20**, 1355-6.

Robinson, D. S., Cooper, T. B., Ravaris, C. L., Ives, J. O., Nies, A., Bartlett, D., and Lamborn, K. R. (1979a). Plasma tricyclic drug levels in amitriptyline-treated depressed patients. *Psychopharmacology*, **63**, 223-31.

Robinson, J. H., and Wang, S. C. (1979). Unit activity of limbic system neurones: effects of morphine, diazepam and neuroleptic agents. *Brain Res.* **166**, 149-59.

Robinson, S. E., Berney, S., Mishra, R., and Sulser, F. (1979b). The relative role of dopamine and norepinephrine receptor blockade in the action of antipsychotic drugs: metoclopramide, triethylperazine, and molindone as pharmacological tools. *Psychopharmacology*, **64**, 141-7.

Rogers, H. J., Spector, R. G., and Trounce, J. R. (1981). *A Textbook of Clinical Pharmacology*. Hodder and Stoughton Ltd., Kent.

Rolls, E. T., and Cooper, S. J. (1973). Activation of neurones in prefrontal cortex by brain stimulation reward in the rat. *Brain Res.* **60**, 351-68.

Rolls, E. T., and Cooper, S. J. (1974). Anesthetization and stimulation of the sulcal prefrontal cortex and brain stimulation reward. *Physiol. Behav.* **12**, 563-71.

Rolls, T., Caan, A. W., Perrett, D. I., and Wilson, F. A. W. (1981). Neuronal activity related to long term memory. *Acta neurol. Scand.* Suppl.89, **64**, 121-4.

Root-Bernstein, R. S., and Westall, F. E. (1983). Sleep factors: do muramyl peptides activate serotonin binding sites? *Lancet*, **i**, 653.

Rosenbaum, A. H., and de le Fuenta, J. R. (1979). Benzodiazepines and tardive dyskinesia. *Lancet*, **ii**, 900.

Rosenbaum, A. H., Schatzberg, A. F., Maruta, T., Orsulak, P. J., Cole, J. O., Grab, E. L., and Schildkraut, J. J. (1980). MHPG as a predictor of antidepressant response to imipramine and maprotiline. *Am. J. Psychiat.* **137**, 1090-2.

Rosenthal, R., and Bigelow, L. B. (1972). Quantitative brain measurements in chronic schizophrenia. *Br. J. Psychiat.* **121**, 259-64.

Ross, E. D. (1982). Disorders of recent memory in humans. *Trends Neurosci.* **5**, 170-3.

Ross, E. D. (1984). Right hemisphere's role in language, affective behaviour and emotion. *Trends Neurosci.* **7**, 342-6.

Rossor, M. N. (1982). Neurotransmitters and CNS disease: dementia. *Lancet*, **ii**, 1200-4.

Rossor, M. N., Iverson, L. L., Mountjoy, C. W., Roth, M., Hawthorn, J., Aug, V. Y., and Jenkins, J. S. (1980). Arginine vasopressin and choline acetyltransferase in brains of patients with Alzheimer type senile dementia. *Lancet*, **ii**, 1367-8.

Rossor, M. N., Iverson, L. L., Reynolds, G. P., Mountjoy, C. Q., and Roth, M. (1984). Neurochemical characteristics of early and late onset types of Alzheimer's disease. *Br. Med. J.* **288**, 961-4.

Roth, M. (1984). Agoraphobia, panic disorder and generalised anxiety disorder: some implications of recent advances. *Psychiat. Devel.* **2**, 31-52.

Roth, M., and Barnes, T. R. E. (1981). The classification of affective disorders: a synthesis of old and new concepts. *Comp. Psychiat.* **22**, 54-77.

Roth, R. (1979). Dopamine autoreceptors; pharmacology, function and comparison with postsynaptic dopamine receptors. Communications in *Psychopharmacology*, **3**, 429-45.

Rottanburg, D., Robins, A. H., Ben-Arie, O., Teggin, A., and Esk, R. (1982). Cannabis-associated psychosis with hypomanic features. *Lancet*, **ii**, 1364-6.

Roubicek, J. (1980). Antipsychotics: neuropsychological properties (in man). In *Psychotropic Agents Part I: Antipsychotics and Antidepressants.* (eds F. Hoffmeister, and G. Stille), pp. 177-92. Springer-Verlag, Berlin.

Routtenberg, A. (1968). The two arousal hypothesis: reticular formation and limbic system. *Psychol. Rev.* **75**, 51-80.

Routtenberg, A. (1978). Reward systems of the brain. *Scientific Am.* **239**, 125-31.

Routtenberg, A., and Santos-Anderson, R. (1977). The role of prefrontal cortex in intracranial self-stimulation. In *Handbook of Psychopharmacology.* (eds L. L. Iversen, S. D. Iversen, S. H. Snyder) pp. 1-24. Plenum Press, New York.

Royal College of Psychiatrists (1979). *Alcohol and Alcoholism.* Tavistock Publications, London.

Royall, D. R., and Klemm, W. R. (1981). Dopaminergic mediation of reward: evidence gained using a natural reinforcer in a behavioural contrast paradigm. *Neurosci. Lett.* **21**, 223-9.

Rubenstein, G., and Norman, T. R. (1984). Newer antianxiety agents. In *Antianxiety Agents.* (eds G. D. Burrows, T. R. Norman, and B. Davies), pp. 1-11 Elsevier Science Publishers BV, Amsterdam

Rudeberg, C. (1983). Effects of single and multiple doses of antidepressant drugs on the 3H-spiperone-labelled serotonin receptors in the frontal cortex of the rat. In *Frontiers in Neuropsychiatric Research.* (eds E. Usdin, M. Goldstein, A. S. Friedhoff, and A. Georgatas), pp. 135-43. Macmillan Co., London.

Rupniak, N. M. J., Kilpatrick, G., Hall, M. D., Jenner, P., and Marsden, C. D., (1984a). Differential alterations in striatal dopamine receptor sensitivity induced by repeated administration of clinically equivalent doses of haloperidol, sulpiride or clozapine in rats. *Psychopharmacology*, **84**, 512-9.

Rupniak, N. M. J., Mann, S., Hall, M. D., Fleminger, S., Kilpatrick, G., Jenner, P., and Marsden, C. D. (1984b). Differential effects of continuous administration of haloperidol or sulpiride on striatal dopamine function in the rat. *Psychopharmacology*, **84**, 503-11.

Russell, M. A. H. (1978a). Cigarette smoking: a dependence on high nicotine boli. *Drug Metabolism Reviews.* **8**, 29-57.

Russell, M. A. H. (1978b). Smoking Addiction. In *Progress in Smoking Cessation.* (ed J. L. Schwartz), American Cancer Soc., WHO, New York.

Russell, M. A. H., Raw, M., and Jarvis, M. J. (1980). Clinical use of nicotine chewing gum. *Br. Med. J.* **280**, 1599.

Ruthrich, H. L., Wetzel, W., and Matthies, H. (1983). Memory retention in old rats: improvement by orotic acid. *Psychopharmacology*, **79**, 348-51.

Sachar, E. J. (1982). Endocrine abnormalities in depression. In *Handbook of Affective Disorders*. (ed E. S. Paykel), pp. 191–201. Churchill Livingstone, Edinburgh.

Sachar, E. J., Gruen, P. H., Altman, N., Halpern, F. S., and Frantz, A. G. (1976). Use of neuroendocrine techniques in psychopharmacological research. In *Hormones, Behaviour and Psychopathology*. (ed E. J. Sachar), pp. 161–76. Raven Press, New York.

Salamy, J. G. (1976). Sleep: some concepts and constructs. In *Pharmacology of Sleep*. (eds R. L. Williams, and I. Karacan), pp. 53–82. John Wiley & Sons Inc., New York.

Saletu, B. (1980). Central measures in schizophrenia. In *Biological Psychiatry Part II. Brain Mechanisms and Abnormal Behaviour — Psychophysiology*. (eds M. H. van Praag, M. H. Lader, O. J. Rafaelson, and E. J. Sachar), pp. 97–144. Marcel Dekker Inc., New York.

Saletu, B., Saletu, M., and Itil, T. (1972). Effect of minor and major tranquillisers on somatosensory evoked potentials. *Psychopharmacologia*, **24**, 347–58.

Salkind, M. (1982). *Topics in Drug Therapy*, Module 2. Open University Press, Milton Keynes.

Sandler, M. (1982). The emergence of tribulin. *Trends Neurosci.* **5**, 471–2.

Sandler, M., and Reynolds, G. P. (1976). Does phenylethylamine cause schizophrenia? *Lancet*, **i**, 70–1.

Sandoz (1977). *Hydergine*. Sandoz Information Service, Sandoz Products, Ltd., Middlesex.

Sara, S. J. (1980). Memory retrieval deficits: alleviation by etiracetam, a nootropic drug. *Psychopharmacology*, **68**, 235–41.

Sara, S. J., David-Remacle, M., Weyers, M., and Giurgea, C. (1979). Piracetam facilitates retrieval but does not impair extinction of bar-pressing in rats. *Psychopharmacology*, **61**, 71–5.

Savage, D. D., Mendels, J., and Frazer, A. (1980). Decrease in [3-H]-serotonin binding in rat brain produced by the repeated administration of either monoamine oxidase inhibitors or centrally acting serotonin agonists. *Neuropharmac.* **19**, 1063–70.

Scanlon, M. F., Weightman, D. R., Mora, B., Heath, M., Shale, D. J., Snow, M. H., and Hall, R. (1977). Evidence for dopaminergic control of thyrotrophin secretion in man. *Lancet*, **ii**, 421–3.

Scatton, B., Loo, H., Dennis, T., Benkelfat, C., Gay, C., and Poirer-Littre, M-F. (1986). Decreases in plasma levels of 3,4-dihydroxyphenylethyleneglycol in major depression. *Psychopharmacology*, **88**, 220–5.

Schachter, S. (1971). *Emotion, Obesity and Crime*. Academic Press, New York.

Schaffer, C. E., Pandey, G. N., Noll, K. M., Killian, G. A., and Davis, J. M. (1981). Introduction and theories of affective disorders. In *Neuropharmacology of Central Nervous System and Behavioural Disorders*. (ed G. C. Palmer), pp. 1–36. Academic Press, New York.

Schardein, J. L. (1976). *Drugs as Teratogens*. CRC Press, Cleveland, Ohio.

Schatzberg, A. F., Rosenbaum, A. H., Orsulak, P. J., Rhode, W. A., Maruta, T., Kruger, E. R., Cole, M. D. and Schildkraut, J. J. (1981). Towards a biochemical classification of depressive disorders III: Pretreatment urinary MHPG levels as predictors of response to treatment with maprotiline. *Psychopharmacology*, **75**, 34–8.

Schiff, A. A. (1977). Propranolol in schizophrenia. *Lancet*, **ii**, 761–2.

Schildkraut, J. J. (1965). The catecholamine hypothesis of affective disorders: a review of supporting evidence. *Am. J. Psychiat.* **122**, 509–22.

Schildkraut, J. J. (1973a). Pharmacology—the effects of lithium on biogenic amines. In *Lithium: Its Role in Psychiatric Research and Medical Treatment.* (eds S. Gershon, and B. Shopsin), pp. 51–73. Plenum Press, New York.

Schildkraut, J. J. (1973b). Norepinephrine metabolites as biochemical criteria for classifying depressive disorders and predicting responses to treatment—preliminary findings. *M. J. Psychiat.* **130**, 695–9.

Schildkraut, J. J. (1978). Current status of the catecholamine hypothesis of affective disorders. In *Psychopharmacology: A Generation of Progress.* (eds M. A. Lipton, A. DiMascio, and K. F. Killam), pp. 1223–34. Raven Press, New York.

Schmiterlow, C. G., Hansson, E., Andersson, G., Applegren, L. E., and Hoffman, P.C. (1967). Distribution of nicotine in the central nervous system. *Am. N.Y. Acad. Sci.* **142**, 2–14.

Schmitt, P., Di Scala, G., Jenck, F., and Sander, G. (1984). Periventricular structures, elaboration of aversive effects and processing of sensory information.. In *Modulation of Sensorimotor Activity During Alterations in Behavioural States.* (ed R. Bandler), pp. 393–414. Alan R Liss Inc., New York.

Schmutz, J., and Picard, C. W. (1980). Tricyclic neuroleptics; structure-activity relationships. In *Psychotropic Agents Part I: Antipsychotics and Antidepressants.* (eds F. Hoffmeister, and G. Stille), pp. 3–26. Springer-Verlag, Berlin.

Schneider-Helmert, D. and Spinweber, C. L. (1986). Evaluation of L-tryptophan for treatment of insomnia: a review. *Psychopharmacology* **89**, 1-7.

Schneider-Helmert, D., Graf, M., and Schoenenberger, G. A. (1981). Synthetic delta-sleep-inducing peptide improves sleep in insomniacs. *Lancet*, **i**, 1256.

Schoenenberger, G. A., and Schneider-Helmert, D. (1983). Psychophysiological functions of DSIP. *Trends Neurosci.* **4**, 307–10.

Schopf, J., Laurian, S, and Gaillard, Le, J-M. (1984). Intrinsic activity of the benzodiazepine antagonist RO 15-1788 in man: and electrophysiological investigation. *Pharmacopsychiatry*, **17**, 79–83.

Schulsinger, F. (1985). Schizophrenia: genetics and environment. In *Psychopharmacology. Recent Advances and Future Prospects.* (ed S. D. Iverson), pp. 185–95. Oxford University Press, Oxford.

Schultz, H., Lund, R., and Doerr, P. (1978). The measurement of change in sleep during depression and remission. *Arch. Psychiat. Nervenkr.* **225**, 233–41.

Schultz, R., Wuster. M., Duka, T., and Herz, A. (1980). Acute and chronic ethanol treatment changes endorphin levels in brain and pituitary. *Psychopharmacology*, **68**, 221–7.

Schulz, S. C., Koller, M. M., Kishore, P. R., Hamer, R. M., Gehl, J. J., and Friedel, R.O. (1983). Ventricular enlargement in teenage patients with schizophrenic spectrum disorder. *Am. J. Psychiat.* **140**, 1592–5.

Schwartz, G. E., Davidson, R. J., and Maer, F. (1975). Right-hemisphere lateralisation for emotion in the human brain: interactions with cognition. *Science*, **190**, 286–90.

Scott, D. F. (1981). Other sleep disorders and their treatments. In *Psychopharmacology of Sleep.* (ed D. Wheatley), pp. 214–31. Raven Press, New York.

Scott, F. L. (1979). A review of some current drugs used in the pharmacotherapy of organic brain syndromes. In *Physiology of Cell Biology of Ageing*, Ageing volumn

8 (eds A. Cherkin, C. E. Finch, N. Kharasch, T. Makinodam, F. L. Scott, and B. Strehler), pp. 151–84. Raven Press, New York.

Scoville, W. B., and Milner, B. (1957). Loss of recent memory after bilateral hippocampal lesions. *J. Neurol. Neurosurg.Psychiat.* **20**, 11–21.

Seligman, M. E. P. (1975). *Helplessness: on Depression, Development and Death.* Freeman, San Francisco.

Selkoe, D. J. (1982). Molecular pathology of the aging human brain. *Trends Neurosci.* **5**, 332–6.

Selye, H. (1956). *The Stress of Life.* McGraw Hill, New York.

Senn, H-J., Jungi, W. F., Kunz, H., and Poldinger, W. (1977). Clozepine and agranulocytosis. *Lancet*, **i**, 547.

Sepinwall, J., and Cook, L. (1979). Mechanism of action of the benzodiazepines: behavioural aspect. *Fed. Proc.* **39**, 3024–31.

Serafetinides, E. A., Coger, R. W., Martin, J., and Dymond, A. M. (1981). Schizophrenic symptomatology and cerebral dominance patterns: a comparison of EEG, AER and BPRS measures. *Comp. Psychiat.* **22**, 218–25.

Shader, R. I., Goodman, M., and Gever, J. (1982). Panic disorders: current perspectives. *J. Clin. Psychopharmacol.* **2**, *Suppl. 6*, 2–10.

Shagass, C. (1977). Twisted thoughts, twisted brainwaves? In *Psychopathology and Brain Dysfunction.* (eds C. Shagass, S. Gershon, and A. J. Friedhoff), pp. 353–78. Raven Press, New York.

Shagass, C., Ornitz, E. M., Sutton, S., and Tueting, P. (1978). Event related potentials and psychopathology. In *Event-related Brain Potentials in Man.* (eds E. Callaway, P. Tueting, and S. H. Koslow), pp. 443–95. Academic Press, New York.

Shagass, C., and Straumenis, J. J. (1978). Drugs and human sensory evoked potentials. In *Psychopharmacology: A Generation of Progress.* (eds M. A. Lipton, A. DiMascio, and K. F. Killam), pp. 699–709. Raven Press, New York.

Shapiro, A. P., and Nathan, P. E. (1986). Human tolerance to alcohol: the role of Pavlovian conditioning processes. *Psychopharmcology*, **88**, 90–5.

Sharpless, S. K. (1970). Hypnotics and sedatives. I. The barbiturates. In *The Pharmacological Basis of Therapeutics.* (ed L. S. Goodman, and A. Gilman), 4th edn. pp. 98–120. Macmillan Co., London.

Shaw, D. (1979). Lithium and antimanic drugs: clinical usage and efficacy. In *Psychopharmacology of Affective Disorders.* (eds E. S. Paykel, and A. Coppen), pp. 179–92. Oxford University Press, Oxford.

Shaw, D. M., Kellam,. A. M. P., and Mottram, R. F. (1982). *Brain Sciences in Psychiatry.* Butterworth, London.

Shea, V. T. (1982). State-dependent learning in children receiving methyl phenidate. *Psychopharmacology*, **78**, 266–70.

Shearman, G. T., and Herz, A. (1983). Ethanol and tetrahydroquinoline alkaloids do not produce discriminative stimulus effects. *Psychopharmacology*, **81**, 224–7.

Sheehan, D. V., Ballinger, J., and Jacobson, G. (1980). Treatment of endogenous anxiety with phobic, hysterical and hypochondriacal symptoms. *Arch. Gen. Psychiat.* **37**, 51–9.

Sheppard, G. P., Gruzelier, J., Manchanda, R., Hirsch, S. R., Wise, R., Frackowiak, R., and Jones, R. (1983). [15]-O positron emission tomographic scanning in predominantly never-treated acute schizophrenic patients. *Lancet*, **ii**, 1448–52.

Sheppard, G. P., Jutai, J., Manchanda, R., Gruzelier, J., Hirsch, S. R., Wise, R., Frackowiak, R., and Jones, T. (1984). Frontal lobe hypofunction in schizophrenia. *Lancet*, **i,** 970–1.

Frackowiak, R., and Jones, T. (1984). Frontal lobe hypofunction in schizophrenia. *Lancet*, **i,** 970–1.

Sherlock, S. (ed) (1982). Alcohol and disease. *Br. Med. Bull.* **38.**

Sherman, G. F., Galaburda, A. M., and Geschwind, N. (1982). Neuroanatomical asymmetries in non-human species. *Trends Neurosci.* **5,** 429–31.

Shore, D. (1979). Psychobiological interactions and schizophrenia. In *Current Developments in Psychopharmacology.* (eds W. B. Essman, and L. Valzelli), Vol. 5. pp. 263–91. Spectrum Publications, New York.

Sicuteri, F. (1981). Persistent non-organic central pain: headache and central panalgesia. In *Persistent Pain.* (eds S. Lipton and J. Miles) Vol. 3. pp. 119–40. Academic Press, London, and Grune and Stratton, New York.

Siegel, A. (1984). Anatomical and functional differentiation within the amygdala-behavioural state modulation. In *Modulation of Sensorimotor Activity During Alterations in Behavioural States.* (ed R. Bandler), pp. 299–303. Alan R. Liss Inc., New York.

Siegel, S. (1975). Evidence from rats that morphine tolerance is a learned response. *J. Comp. Physiol. Psychol.* **89,** 498–506.

Siegel, S. (1978). A Pavlovian conditioning analysis of morphine tolerance. *Natl. Inst. Drug Abuse (MDA) Res. Monograph*, **18,** pp. 27–53.

Siegel, S. (1983). Classical conditioning, drug tolerance and drug dependence. In *Research Advances in Alcohol and Drug Problems.* (eds Y. Israel, F. B. Glaser, H. Kalant, R. E. Popham, W. Schmidt, and R. G. Smart), Vol. 7, pp. 207–46. Plenum Press, New York.

Siever, L. J., Pickar, D., Lake, C. R., Cohen, R. M., Uhde, T. W., and Murphy, D. L. (1983). Extreme elevations in plasma norepinephrine associated with decreased alpha-adrenergic responsivity in major depressive disorders; two case reports. *J. Clin. Psychopharm.* **3,** 39–41.

Siman, R., Baudry, M., and Lynch, G. (1985). Regulation of glutamate receptor binding by the cytoskeletal protein fodrin. *Nature*, **313,** 225–8.

Simon, E. J. (1981). Opiate receptors: some recent developments. In *Towards Understanding Receptors.* (ed J. W. Lamble), pp. 159–65. Elsevier/North Holland Biomedical Press, Amsterdam.

Simon, P., Lecrubier, Y., Jouvent, R., Puech, A. J., Allilaire, J. F., and Widlocher, D. (1978). Experimental and clinical evidence of the antidepressant effect of a beta-adrenergic stimulant. *Psychol. Med.* **8,** 335–8.

Singh, S., and Mirkin, B. L. (1973). Drug effects on the foetus. *New Ethicals.* **10,** 150–66.

Sjoquist, B., Eriksson, A., and Winblad, B. (1982). Brain salsolinol levels in alcoholism. *Lancet*, **i,** 675–6.

Skegg, D. C. G., Richards, S. M., and Doll, R. (1979). Minor tranquillisers and road accidents. *Br. Med. J.* **1,** 917–19.

Skjelbred, P., and Lokken, P. (1980). Effects of naloxone on post-operative pain and steroid-induced analgesia. *Br. J. clin. Pharmac.* **1,** 221–6.

Skolnick, P., Hommer, D., and Paul, S. M. (1982). Benzodiazepine antagonists. In *Pharmacology of Benzodiazepines.* (eds E. Usdin, P. Skolnick, J. F. Tallman, D. Greenblatt, and S. M. Paul), pp. 441–54. Macmillam Co., London.

Small, G., and Jarvik, L. F. (1982). The dementia syndrome. *Lancet*, **ii,** 1443–5.

Small, J. G., and Small, I. F. (1973). Pharmacology and neurophysiology of lithium. In *Lithium. Its Role in Psychiatric Research and Medical Treatment.* (eds S. Gershon, and B. Shopsin), pp. 83-106. Plenum Press, New York.

Smith, C. B., Garcia-Savilla, J. A., and Hollingworth, P. J. (1981). Alpha$_2$-adrenoceptors in rat brain are decreased after long-term tricycline antidepressant drug treatment. *Brain Res.* **210,** 413-8.

Smith, D. E., and Wesson, D. R. (1983). Benzodiazepine dependency syndromes. *J. Psychoactive Drugs,* **15,** 85-95.

Smith, G. C., and Copolov, D. (1979). Brain amines and peptides—their relevance to psychiatry. *Aust. N.Z. J. Psychiat.* **13,** 283-91.

Smith, S. E., and Rawlins, M. D. (1973). *Variability in Human Drug Response.* Butterworth, London.

Smythies, J. R. (1984). the transmethylation hypotheses of schizophrenia re-evaluated. *Trends Neurosci.* **7,** 45-7.

Snyder, S. H. (1981a). Opiate and benzodiazepine receptors. *Psychosomatics,* **22,** 986-9.

Snyder, S. H. (1981b). Dopamine receptors, neuroleptics and schizophrenia. *Am. J. Psychiat.* **138,** 460-4.

Snyder, S. H. (1981c). Adenosine receptors and the actions of methylxanthines. *Trends Neurosci.* **4,** 242-4.

Snyder, S. H. (1982) Schizophrenia. *Lancet,* **ii,** 970-3.

Sovner, R. and DiMascio, A. (1978). Extrapyramidal syndromes and other neurological side effects of psychotropic drugs. In *Psychopharmacology: A Generation of Progress.* (eds M. A. Lipton, A. DiMascio, and K. F. Killam), pp. 1021-32. Raven Press, New York.

Spealman, R. D., and Goldberg, S. R. (1982). Maintenance of schedule-controlled behaviour by intravenous injection of nicotine in quirrel monkeys. *J. Pharm. Exp. Therap.* **223,** 402-8.

Sperry, R. W. (1973). Lateral specialisation of cerebral function in the surgically separated hemispheres. In *The Psychophysiology of Thinking.* (eds F. J. McGuigan, and R. A. Schoonover), Academic Press, New York.

Sperry, R. W. (1974). Lateral specialisation in surgically separated hemispheres. In *The Neurosciences; Third Study Program.* (eds F. O. Schmitt, and F. G. Worden), MIT Press, Cambridge, Mass.

Sperry, R. W. (1976). Mental phenomenona as causal determinants in brain function. In *Consciousness and the Brain: A Scientific and Philosophic Enquiry.* (eds G. G. Globus, G. Maxwell, and I. Savodnik), Plenum Press, New York.

Speth, R. C., Guidotti, A., and Yamamura, H. (1980). The pharmacology of the benzodiazepines. In *Neuropharmacology of Central Nervous System and Behavioural Disorders.* (ed G. C. Palmer), pp. 243-83. Academic Press, New York.

Spinweber, C. L., Ursin, R., Hilbert, R. P., and Hilderbrand, R. L. (1983). L-tryptophan: effects on daytime sleep latency and the waking EEG. *Electroenceph. clin. Neurophysiol.* **55,** 652-61.

Spitzer, R. L., Endicott, J., and Gibbon, M. (1979). Crossing the border into borderline personality and borderline schizophrenia; the development criteria. *Arch. Gen. Psychiat.* **39,** 17-24.

Spitzer, R. L., Endicott, J., and Robins, E. (1975). Clinical criteria for psychiatric diagnosis and DSM III. *Am. J. Psychiat.* **132,** 1187-92.

Spokes, E. G. S. (1981). The neurochemistry of Huntingdon's chorea. *Trends Neurosci.* **4,** 115-18.

Spohn, H. E., and Patterson, T. (1979). Recent studies of psychophysiology in schizophrenia. *Schizophrenia Bull.* **5,** 581–611.

Squire, L. R. (1980). The anatomy of amnesia. *Trends Neurosci.* **3,** 52–4.

Squire, L. R., and Davis, H. P. (1981). The pharmacology of memory: a neurobiological perspective. *Ann. Rev. Pharmac. Toxicol.* **21,** 323–56.

Squires, R. F. (1983). Benzodiazepine receptor multiplicity. *Neuropharmacol.* **22,** 1443–50.

Squires, R. F., and Braestrup, C. (1977). Benzodiazepine receptors in the rat brain. *Nature,* **266,** 732–4.

Stanes, M. D., Brown, C. P., and Singer, G. (1976). Effect of physostigmine on Y-maze discrimination retention in the rat. *Psychopharmacologia,* (*Berl.*) **46,** 269–76.

Stanley, M., and Mann, J. J. (1983). Increased serotonin-2 binding sites in frontal cortex of suicide victims. *Lancet,* **i,** 214–16.

Stanley, M., and Mann, J. J. (1984). Suicide and serotonin receptors. *Lancet,* **i,** 349.

Stanley, M., Virgilio, J. and Gershon, S. (1982). Tritiated imipramine binding sites are decreased in the frontal cortex of suicide victims. *Science,* **216,** 1337–9.

Stein, G. S., Milton, F., Bebbington, P., Wood, K., and Coppen, A. (1976). A relationship between mood disturbance and free and total plasma tryptophan in postpartum women. *Br. Med. J.* **2,** 457.

Stein, J. F. (1982). *An Introduction to Neurophysiology.* Blackwell Scientific Publications, Oxford.

Stein, J. F. (1985). The control of movement. *In Functions of the Brain* (ed. C. W. Coen) pp. 67–97. Clarendon Press, Oxford.

Stein, L. (1968). Chemistry of reward and punishment. In *Psychopharmacology—A Review of Progress 1957–1967.* (ed D. H. Efron), Publ. No. 1836, pp. 105–23. U.S. Government Printing Office, Washington D.C.

Stein, L. (1971). Neurochemistry of reward and punishment. Some implications for the etiology of schizophrenia. *J. Psychiat. Res.* **8,** 345–61.

Stein, L. (1978). Reward transmitters: catecholamines and opioid peptides. In *Psychopharmacology: A Generation of Progress.* (eds M. A. Lipton, A. DiMascio, and K. F. Killam), pp. 569–81. Raven Press, New York.

Stein, L., and Wise, C. D. (1969). Release of norepinephrine from hypothalamus and amygdala by rewarding median forebrain bundle stimulation and amphetamine. *J. Comp. Physiol. Psychol.* **67,** 189–98.

Stein, L., and Wise, C. D. (1974). Serotonin and behavioural inhibition. *Adv. Biochem. Psychopharmacol.* **11,** 281–91.

Stein, L., Wise, C. D., and Belluzzi, J. D. (1977). Neuropharmacology of reward and punishment. In *Handbook of Psychopharmacology.* 8 (eds L. L. Iverson, S. D. Iverson, S. H. Snyder), pp. 23–53. Plenum Press, New York.

Steinert, J., and Pugh, C. R. (1979). Two patients with schizophrenic-like psychosis after treatment with beta-adrenergic blockers. *Br. Med. J.* **1,** 790.

Stern, W. C., and Morgane, P.J. (1977). Sleep and memory: effects of growth hormone on sleep, brain neurochemistry and behaviour. In *Neurobiology of Sleep and Memory.* (eds R. R. Drucker-Colin, and J. L. McGaugh), pp. 373–401. Academic Press, New York.

Sternbach, R. A. (1981). Chronic pain as a disease entity. *Triangle* (*Sandoz*), **20,** 27–32.

Stevens, J. R. (1979a). Schizophrenia and dopamine regulation in the mesolimbic system. *Trends Neurosci.* **2**, 102–5.

Stevens, J. R. (1979b). Rapid eye movements of paradoxical sleep—photic modulation of central monoamine activity. *Trends Neurosci.* **2**, 163–6.

Stewart, M. (1976). MAOIs and food-fact and fiction. *Adv. Drug. Reaction Bull.* **58**, 200–3.

Stiglick, A., Llewellyn, M. E., and Kalant, H. (1984). Residual effects of prolonged cannabis treatment on shuttle-box avoidance in the rat. *Psychopharmacology*, **84**, 476–9.

Stinus, L., Kelley, A. E., and Winnock, M. (1984). Neuropeptides and limbic system function.. In *Psychopharmacology of the Limbic System*. (eds M. R. Trimble, and E. Zarifian), pp. 209–25. Oxford University Press, Oxford.

Stirrat, G. M., and Beard, R. W. (1973). Drugs to be avoided or given with caution in the second and third trimesters of pregnancy. *Prescrib. J.* **13**, 135–9.

Stokes, P. E., Stoll, P. M., Shamoian, C. A., and Patton, M. J. (1971). Efficacy of lithium as acute treatment of manic-depressive illness. *Lancet*, **i**, 1319–25.

Strang, J. (1984). Intravenous benzodiazepine abuse. *Br. Med. J.* **289**, 964.

Sugrue, M. F. (1980). Effects of acutely and chronically administered antidepressants on the clonidine-induced decrease in rat brain of 3-methoxy-4-hydroxy phenethyleneglycol sulphate. *Life Sci.* **28**, 377–84.

Sugrue, M. F. (1981) Effect of chronic antidepressant administration on rat frontal cortex alpha$_2$ and beta-adrenoceptor binding. *Br. J. Pharmac.* **74**, 760P.

Sullivan, C. E., Issa, F. G., Berthon-Jones, M., and Eves, L. (1981). Reversal of obstructive sleep apnoea by continuous positive airway pressure applied through the nares. *Lancet*, **i**, 862–5.

Sulman, F. G., and Givant, Y. (1986). Endocrine effects of neuroleptics. In *Psychotropic Agents Part I: Antipsychotics and Antidepressants*. (eds F. Hoffmeister, and G. Stille), pp. 337–48. Springer-Verlag, Berlin.

Sulser, F., (1981). Perspectives on the mode of action of antidepressant drugs. In *Towards Understanding Receptors*. (ed J. W.Lamble), pp. 99–104. Elsevier/North Holland Biomedical Press, Amsterdam.

Sulser, F., and Mobley, P. L. (1980). Biochemical effects of antidepressants in animals. In *Psychotropic Agents Part I: Antipsychotics and Antidepressants*. (eds F. Hoffmeister, and G. Stille), pp. 471–90. Springer-Verlag, Berlin.

Sulser, F., Vetulani, J., and Mobley. P. L. (1978). Mode of action of antidepressant drugs. *Biochem. Pharmac.* **27**, 257–61.

Sulser, S., Okada, F., Manier, D. H., Gillespie, D. D., Janowsky, A., and Mishra, R. (1983). Noradreneragic signal transfer as a target of antidepressant therapy. In *Frontiers in Neuropsychiatric Research*. (eds E. Usdin, M. Goldstein A. J. Friedhoff, and A. Georgatas), pp. 3–17. Macmillan Co., London.

Sutherland, R. J., Wishaw, I. Q., and Kolb, B. (1981). A ghost in a different guise. *Behav. Brain Sci.* **4**, 492.

Svensson, T. H. (1980). Effect of chronic treatment with tricyclic antidepressant drugs on indentified brain noradrenergic and serotonergic neurons. *Acta Psychiat. Scand.* **61**, Suppl. 280, pp. 121–31.

Svensson, T. H., Dahlhof, C., Engberg. G., and Hallberg, H. (1981). Central pre- and postsynaptic monoamine receptors in antidepressant therapy. *Acta. Psychiat. Scand.* **63**, *Suppl. 289*, pp. 67–78.

Svensson, T. H., and Usdin, T. (1978). Feedback inhibition of brain noradrenaline neurones by tricyclics: alpha-receptor mediation after acute and chronic treatment. *Science*, **202**, 1081–91.

Sweet, W. H. (1980). Neuropeptides and nonoaminergic neuro-transmitters: their relation to pain. *J. Roy. Soc. Med.* **73**, 482–91.

Swerdlow, M. (1984). Anticonvulsant drugs and chronic pain. *Clin. neuropharmacol.*, **7**, 51–82.

Swett, J. E., and Bourassa, C. M. (1981). Electrical stimulation of peripheral nerve. In *Electrical Stimulation Research Techniques*. (eds M. M. Patterson, and R. P. Kesner), pp. 243–95. Academic Press, New York.

Swyer, G. I. M. (1985). Postpartum mental disturbance and hormone changes. *Br. Med. J.* **290**, 1232–3.

Taggart, P., Carruthers, M., and Somerville, W. (1973). Electrocardiogram, plasma catecholamines and lipids, and their modification by oxprenolol when speaking before an audience. *Lancet*, **ii**, 341–5.

Tagliavini, F., and Pilleri, G. (1983). Neuronal counts in basal nucleus of Meynert in Alzheimer Disease and in simple senile dementia. *Lancet*, **i**, 469–70.

Taha, A., and Ball, K. (1980). Smoking and Africa; the coming epidemic. *Br. Med. J.* **280**, 991–3.

Takemori, A. E., Vaught, J. L., and Contreras, P. C. (1982). Neuropeptides and morphine tolerance. In *CNS Pharmacology: Neuropeptides*. (eds H. Yoshida, Y. Hagira, and S. Ebashi), pp. 189–98. Pergamon Press, Oxford.

Tamminga, C. A., Crayton, J. W., and Chase, T. N. (1979). Improvement in tardive dyskinesia after muscimol therapy. *Arch. Gen. Psychiat.* **36**, 595–8.

Tarriere, C., and Hartemann, F. (1964). Investigation into the effects of tobacco smoke on a visual vigilance task. In *Proceedings of the Second International Congress of Ergonomics* (suppl. 1 to *Ergonomics*) Dortmund. 525–30.

Taylor, P. (1980). Ganglion stimulating and blocking agents. In *The Pharmacological Basis of Therapeutics*. (eds A. G. Gilman, L. S. Goodman, and A. Gilman), pp. 211–9. Macmillan Co., New York.

Taylor, S. H., and Meeran, M. K. (1973). Different effects of adrenergic beta-receptor blockade on heart rate response to mental stress, catecholamines and exercise. *Br. Med. J.* **4**, 257–9.

Tecce, J. J., and Cole, J. O. (1974). Amphetamine effects in man: paradoxical drowsiness and lowered electrical brain activity (CNV). *Science*, **185**, 451–3.

Tecce, J. J., Cole, J. O., and Savignano-Bowman, J. (1975). Chlorpromazine effects on brain activity (contingent negative variation) and reaction time in normal women. *Psychopharmacologia (Berl.)* **43**, 293–5.

Tecce, J. J., Friedman, S. B., and Mason, J. W. (1965). Anxiety, defensiveness and 17-hydroxycorticosteroid excretion. *J. Nerv. Ment. Dis.* **141**, 549–54.

Tecce, J. J., Savignano-Bowman, J., and Cole, J. O. (1978). Drugs effects on contingent negative variation and eyeblinks: the distraction-arousal hypothesis. In *Psychopharmacology: A Generation of Progress*. (eds M. A. Lipton, A. DiMascio, and K. F. Killam), pp. 745–58. Raven Press, New York.

Tepper, J. M., Groves, P. M., and Young, S. J. (1985) The neuropharmacology of the autoinhibition of monoamine release. *Trends Pharmac. Sci.* **6**, 251–6.

Terenius, L. (1977). *Physiological and clinical relevance of endorphins*. Communication to symposium on Centrally Acting Peptides. Biological Council, April 4/5 1977, Middlesex Hospital Medical School. London

Terenius, L. (1980). Opiates and their receptors. In *Brain and Pituitary Peptides*. Ferring Symposium, Munich 1979. pp. 27-34. Karger, Basel.

Terenius, L. (1981). Biochemical mediators of pain. *Triangle (Sandoz)*. **20**, 19-26.

Terenius, L. (1982). Endorhphins—clinical relevance in neurology. In *Advances in Pharmacology and Therapeutics II Vol. 1. CNS Pharmacology—Neuropeptides*. (eds H. Yoshida, Y.Hagihara, and S. Ebashi), pp. 57-65. Pergamon Press, Oxford.

Theories of Drug Abuse (1980). (eds D. J. Lettieri, M. Sayers, and H. W. Pearson), Dept. of Health and Human Services, National Institute of Drug Abuse. Rockville, Md., U.S.A.

Thibault, A. (1974). A double blind evaluation of 'Hydergine' and placebo in the treatment of patients with organic brain syndrome and cerebral arteriosclerosis in a nursing home. *Curr. Med. Res. and Opinion*, **2**, 482-7.

Thomas, C. B. (1973). The relationship of smoking and habits of nervous tension. In *Smoking Behaviour: Motives and Incentives*. (ed W. L. Dunn), pp. 157-70. Winston and Sons, Washington D.C.

Thomas. M., Halsall, S., and Peters, T. J. (1982). Role of hepatic aldehyde dehydrogenase in alcoholism: demonstration of persistent reduction of cytosolic activity in abstaining patients. *Lancet*, **ii**, 1057-9.

Thompson, C., Checkley, S. A., Corn, T., Franey, C., and Arendt, J. (1983a). Downregulation at pineal beta-adrenoceptors in depressed patients treated with desipramine? *Lancet*, **i**, 1101.

Thompson, C., Checkley, S. A., Corn, T., Franey, C., and Arendt, J. (1983b). Downregulation at pineal beta-adrenoceptors in depressed patients treated with desipramine? *Lancet*, **ii**, 735.

Thompson, J. W. (1984a). Pain: mechanisms and principles of management. In *Advanced Geriatric Medicine*. (eds J. Grimley Evans, and F. I. Caird), Vol.4, pp. 3-16 Pitman Publishing Ltd.

Thompson, J. W. (1984b). Opioid peptides. *Br. Med. J.* **288**, 259-61.

Thompson, J. W., Newton, P., Pocock, P. V., Cooper, R., Crow, H., McCallum, W. C., and Papakostopoulos, D. (1978). Preliminary study of pharmacology of contingent negative variation in man. In *Multidisciplinary Perspective in Event-Related Brain Potential Research*. (ed D. A. Otto), Epic IV, pp. 51-5. N. Carolina, Hendersonville, U.S.A.

Thompson, J., and Oswald, I. (1977). Effect of oestrogen on the sleep, mood and anxiety of menopausal women. *Br Med. J.* **2**, 1317-19.

Thorndike, E. L. (1911). *Animal Intelligence*. Macmillan Co., New York.

Ticku, M. K. (1983). Benzodiazepine-GABA receptor -ionophore complex: current concepts. *Neuropharmacol.* **22**, 1459-70.

Timsit-Berthier, M. (1973). CNV, slow potentials and motor potential studies in normal subjects and psychiatric patients. In *Human Neurophysiology, Psychology, Psychiatry: Averaged evoked responses and their conditioning in normal subjects and psychiatric patients*. (eds A. Fessard, and G. Lelord), pp. 327-66. Inserm, Paris.

Timsit-Berthier, M. (1981). A propos de l'interpretation de la variation contingente negative en psychiatrie. *Rev. EEG Neurophysiol.* **11**, 236-44.

Tiwary, C. M. (1974). Testoserone, L.H.R.H., and behaviour. *Lancet*, **i**, 993.

Toffano, G., Leon, A., Massotti, M., Guidotti, A., and Costa, E. (1980). GABA-modulin; a regulatory protein for GABA receptors. In *Receptors for Neurotransmitters and Peptide Hormones*. (eds G. Pepeu, M. J. Kuhar, and S. J. Enna), pp. 133-42. Raven Press, New York.

Torrey, E. F., and Peterson, M. R. (1974). Schizophrenia and the limbic system. *Lancet*, **ii**, 942–6.

Towell, J. F., Cho, J-K., Byung, L. R., and Wang, R. I. H. (1983). Aldehyde dehydrogenase and alcoholism. *Lancet*, **i**, 364–5.

Trabucchi, M., and Ba, G. (1975). Are benzodiazepines antipsychotic agents? *Lancet*, **ii**, 868.

Tranel, D. T. (1983). The effects of monetary incentive and frustrative non-reward on heart rate and electrodermal activity. *Psychophysiology*, **20**, 652–7.

Traskman, L., Asberg, M., Bartilsson, L., and Sjostrand, L. (1981). Monoamine metabolites in CSF and suicidal behaviour. *Arch. Gen. Psychiat.* **38**, 631–6.

Trethowan, W. H. (1975). Pills for personal problems. *Br. Med. J.* **2**, 749–51.

Triggle, D. J. (1981). Desensitization. In *Towards Understanding Receptors*. (ed J. W. Lamble), pp. 28–33. Elsevier/North Holland Biomedical Press, Amsterdam.

Trimble, M. R. (1981). Visual and auditory hallucinations. *Trends Neurosci.* **4**, I–IV.

Trimble, M. R., Meldrum, B. S., and Anglezark, G. (1977). Effect of nomifensine on brain amines and epilepsy in photosensitive baboons. *Br. J. clin. Pharmac.* **4**, 101–7.

Trimble, M. R., and Thompson, P. J. (1981). Memory, anticonvulsant drugs and seizures. *Acta Neurol. Scand.* **64**, *Suppl. 89*, 31–41.

Tsuang, M. T. (1982). Long-term outcome in schizophrenia. *Trends Neurosci.* **5**, 203–5.

Tsuchiya, T., and Kitagawa, S. (1976). Effects of benzodiazepines and pentobarbital on the evoked potentials in the cat brain. *Japan. J. Pharmacol.* **26**, 411–8.

Tsukahara, N. (1981). Sprouting and the neuronal basis of learning. *Trends Neurosci.* **4**, 234–7.

Tucker, D. M., Antes, J. R., Stenslie, C. E., and Barnhardt, T. M. (1978). Anxiety and lateral cerebral function. *J. Abn. Psychol.* **87**, 380–3.

Tucker, D. M., Roth, R. S., Arneson, B. A., and Buckingham, V. (1977). Right hemisphere activation during stress. *Neuropsychologia*, **15**, 697–700.

Tucker, D. M. (1981). Lateral brain function, emotion and conceptualisation. *Psychol. Bull.* **89**, 19–46.

Tuomisto, J., Tukiainen, E., and Ahlfors, U. G. (1979). Decreased uptake of 5-hydroxytryptamine in blood platelets in patients with endogenous depression. *Psychopharmacology*, **65**, 141–7.

Turner, P. (1976). Beta-adrenoceptor blockade in hyperthyroidism and anxiety. *Proc. Roy. Soc. Med.* **69**, 375–7.

Twycross, R. G., and Lack, S. A. (1983). *Symptom Control in Far Advanced Cancer: Pain Relief*. Pitman Publishing Ltd., London.

Tyrer, P. J. (1977). Propranolol in schizophrenia. *Lancet*, **ii**, 761.

Tyrer, P. J. (1981). Drug-induced depression. *Prescribers J.* **21**, 237–42.

Tyrer, P. J. (1982). Monoamine oxidase inhibitors and amine precursors. In *Drugs in Psychiatric Practice*. (ed P. J. Tyrer), pp. 249–79. Butterworth, London.

Tyrer, P. J. (1983). In *The Benzodiazepines: from Molecular Biology to Clinical Practice*. (ed E. Costa), pp. 400–6. Raven Press, New York.

Tyrer, P. J. (1984). Clinical effects of abrupt withdrawal from tricyclic antidepressants and monoamine oxidase inhibitors after long-term treatment. *J. Affect. Dis.* B6, 1–7.

Tyrer, P. J. (1985). Neurosis divisible? *Lancet*, **i**, 685–8.

Tyrer, P. J., and Lader, M. H. (1974). Response to propranolol and diazepam in somatic and psychic anxiety. *Br. Med. J.* **2**, 14-6.

Tyrer, P. J., and Lader, M. H. (1976). Central and peripheral correlates of anxiety: a comparative study. *J. Nerv. Ment. Dis.* **162**, 99-104.

Tyrer, P., Owen, R. and Dawling, S. (1983). Gradual withdrawal of diazepam after long-term therapy. *Lancet*, **i**, 1402-6.

Tyrer. S. P., Capon, M. N., Peterson, D. M., Charlton, J. E., and Thompson, J. W. (1986). The identification, nature and extent of psychiatric and psychological handicaps in a British pain clinic population. *Pain*, (in the press).

Tyrer, S., and Shaw, D. M. (1982). Lithium carbonate. In *Drugs in Psychiatric Practice* . (ed P. J. Tyrer), pp. 280-312. Butterworth, London.

Tyrer, S., and Shopsin, B. (1980). Neural and Neuromuscular side-effects of lithium. In *Handbook of Lithium Therapy*. (ed F. N. Johnson), pp. 289-309. MTP Press Ltd., Lancaster.

Tyrrell, D. A. J., Parry, R. P., Crow, T. J., Johnstone, E., and Ferrier, I. N. (1979). Possible virus in schizophrenia and some neurological disorders. *Lancet*, **i**, 839-41.

Vandel, B., Vandel, S., Allers, G., Bechtel, P., and Volmat, R. (1979). Interaction between amitriptyline and phenothiazine in man: effects on plasma concentration of amitriptyline and its metabolite nortriptyline and the correlation between clinical response. *Psychopharmacology*, **65**, 187-90.

Vanderwolf, C. H., and Robinson, T. E. (1981). Reticulo-cortical activity and behaviour: a critique of the arousal theory and a new synthesis. *Behav. Brain Sci.* **4**, 459-514.

Vaughan, C. E., and Leff, J. P. (1976). The influence of family and social factors on the course of psychiatric illness. *Br. J. Psychiat.* **129**, 125-37.

Veith, R. C., Bielski, R. J., Bloom, V., Fawcett, J., Narasimhachari, N., and Friedel, R.O. (1983). Urinary MHPG excretion and treatment with desipramine or amitriptyline: prediction of response, effect of treatment and methodological hazards. *J. Clin. Psychopharmacol.* **3**, 18-27.

Venables, P. H. (1980). Peripheral measures of schizophrenia. In *Handbook of Biological Psychiatry Part II. Brain Mechanisms and Abnormal Behaviour—Psychophysiology*. (eds H. M. van Praag, M. A. Lader, O. J. Rafaelson, and E. J. Sachar), pp. 79-96. Marcel Dekker Inc., New York.

Venables, P.H. (1981). Psychophysiology of abnormal behaviour. *Br. Med. Bull.* **37**, 199-203.

Venables, P. M. (1973). Input regulation and psychopathology. In *Psychopathology: contributions from the social, behavioural and biological sciences*. (eds M. Hammer, K. Salzinger, and S. Sutton), pp. 261-284. J. Wiley & Sons, New York.

Venables, P. M. (1977). The electrodermal physiology of schizophrenia and children at risk for schizophrenia. *Schizophrenia Bull.* **3**, 28-48.

Verhoeven, W. M. A., van Praag, H. M., Botter, P. A., Sunier, A., van Ree, J. M., and de Wied, D. (1978). [Des-Tyr-1]-gamma-endorphin in schizophrenia. *Lancet*, **i**, 1046-7.

Verhoeven, W. M. A., van Praag, H. M., van Ree, J. M., and de Wied, D. (1979). Improvement of schizophrenic patients treated with [Des-Tyr-1]-gamma-endorphin (DT-gamma-E). *Arch. Gen. Psychiat.* **36**, 294-8.

Vestergaard, P., Amdisen, A., and Schou, M. (1980). Clinically significant side effects of lithium treatment. A survey of 237 patients in long-term treatment. *Acta Psychiat. Scand.* **62**, 193-200.

Vetulani, J., and Sulser, F. (1975). Action of various antidepressant treatments reduces reactivity of noradrenergic cyclic AMP- generating system in limbic fore-brain. *Nature*, **257**, 495–6.

Villarreal, J. E., and Salazar, L. A. (1981). The dependence-producing properties of psychomotor stimulants. In *Psychotropic Agents Part II.* (eds F. Hoffmeister, and S. Stille), pp. 607–35. Springer-Verlag, Heidelberg.

Vogel, G. W. (1975). A review of REM sleep deprivation. *Arch. Gen. Psychiat.* **32**, 749–61.

Vogel, G. W. (1978). An alternative view of the neurobiology of dreaming. *Am. J. Psychiat.* **135**, 1531–5.

Volavka, J., Dorubush, R., Mallya, A., and Cho, D. (1979). Naloxone fails to affect short term memory in man. *Psychiat. Res.* **1**, 89–92.

Volicer, L., and Biagioni, T. M. (1982). Effect of ethanol administration and with-drawal on benzodiazepine receptor binding in the rat brain. *Neuropharmacol.* **21**, 223–6.

Waddington, J. L. (1985). Further anomalies in the dopamine receptor super-sensitivity hypothesis of tardive dyskinesia. *Trends Neurosci.* **8**, 200.

Wahlstrom, A., and Terenius, L. (1981). Endorphin hypothesis of schizophrenia. *Mod. Probl. Pharmacopsychiat.* **17**, 181–91.

Wakelin, J. S. (1983). A review of the properties of a new specific 5-HT reuptake inhibitor—fluvoxamine moleate. In *Frontiers in Neuropsychiatric Research.* (eds E. Usdin, M. Goldstein, A. J. Friedhoff, and A. Georgatas), pp. 159–73. Macmillan Co., London.

Waldron, H.A. (1981). Effects of organic solvents. *Br.J. Hosp. Med.* **26**, 645–9.

Wall, P. D. (1978). The gate control theory of pain mechanisms: a re-examination and re-statement. *Brain*, **101**, 1–18.

Wall, R., Linford, S. M. J., and Akhter, M. (1980). Addiction to Distalgesic (dextro-propoxyphene). *Br. Med. J.* **280**, 1213–4.

Walter, W. G. (1964). Slow potential waves in the human brain associated with expectancy, attention and decision. *Arch. Psychiat. Nervenkr.* **206**, 309–22.

Walter, W. G., Cooper, R., Aldridge, V. J., McCallum, W.C., and Winter, A. L. (1964). Contingent negative variation: an electric sign of sensorimotor assocation and expectancy in the human brain. *Nature*, **203**, 380–4.

Walton, J. M. (1977). *Brain's Diseases of the Nervous System.* 8th edn, revised by J.M. Walton. Oxford University Press, Oxford.

Warrington, E. K. (1981). Neuropsychological evidence for multiple memory systems. *Acta Neurol. Scand.* **64**, *Suppl. 89*, 13–19.

Warrington, E. K., and Weiskrantz, L. (1970). Amnesic syndrome: consolidation or retrieval? *Nature (Lond.)* **228**, 628–30.

Watson, S. J. (1977). Hallucinogens and other psychotomimetics; biological mech-anisms. In *Psychopharmacology: from Theory to Practice..* (eds J. P. Barchas, P. A. Berger, R. D. Ciaranello, and G. R. Elliott), pp. 341–54. Oxford University Press, New York.

Watson, S. J., Akil, H., Berger, P. A., and Barchas, J. D. (1979). Some observations on the opiate peptides and schizophrenia. *Arch. Gen. Psychiat.* **36**, 35–41.

Way, E. L. (1978). Basic mechanisms in narcotic tolerance and physical dependence. *Ann. N.Y. Acad. Sci.* **75**, 61–8.

Way, E. L. (1983). Brain neurohormones in morphine tolerance and dependence. In *Pharmacology and the the Future of Man. Proceedings of the Fifth International Congress in Pharmacology.* (ed J. Cochin), pp. 77–94. Karger, Basel.

Way, E. L., and Glasgow, C. (1978). Recent developments in morphine analgesia: tolerance and dependence. In *Psychopharmacology: A Generation of Progress*. (eds M. A. Lipton, A. DiMascio, and K. F. Killam), pp. 1535–56. Raven Press, New York.

Way, E. L., Loh, H. H., and Shen, F. H. (1969). Simultaneous quantitative assessment of morphine tolerance and physical dependence. *J. Pharmac. Exp. Therap.* **167**, 1–8.

Webberly, M. S., and Cuschieri, A. (1982). Response of patients to upper gastro-intestinal endoscopy: effect of inherent personality traits and premedication with diazepam. *Br. Med. J.* **285**, 251–2.

Webster, K. E. (1978). The brainstem reticular formation. In *The Biological Basis of Schizophrenia*. (eds G. Hemmings, and W. A. Hemmings), pp. 3–27. MTP Press Ltd., Lancaster.

Webster, P. A. C. (1973). Withdrawal symptoms in neonates associated with maternal antidepressant therapy. *Lancet*, **ii**, 318.

Weckowicz, T. E., Tam, C-N, I., Mason, J., and Bay, K. S. (1978). Speed test performance in depressed patients. *J. Abnormal Psychol.* **87**, 578–82.

Weinberger, D. R., Torrey, E. F., Neophytides, A. N., and Wyatt, R. J. (1979a). Lateral cerebral ventricular enlargement in chronic schizophrenia. *Arch. Gen. Psychiat.* **36**, 735–9.

Weinberger, D. R., Torrey, E. F., Neophytides, A. N., and Wyatt, R. J. (1979b). Structural abnormalities in the cerebral cortex of schizophrenic patients. *Arch. Gen. Psychiat.* **36**, 935–9.

Weinberger, D. R., Torrey, E. F., and Wyatt, R. J. (1979c). Cerebellar atrophy in chronic schizophrenia. *Lancet*, **i**, 718–19.

Weinberger, D. R., and Wyatt, R. J. (1980). Schizophrenia and cerebral atrophy. *Lancet*, **i**, 1130.

Weiner, N. (1980a). Atropine, scopolamine and related antimuscarinic drugs. In *The Pharmacological Basis of Therapeutics*. (eds A. G. Gilman, L. S. Goodman, and A. Gilman), pp. 120–37. Macmillan Co., New York.

Weiner, N. (1980b). Norepinephrine, epinephrine and the sympathomimetic amines. In *The Pharmacological Basis of Therapeutics*. (eds A. G. Gilman, L. S. Goodman, and A. Gilman), pp. 138–75. Macmillan Co., New York.

Weingartner, H., Gold, P., Ballenger, J. C., Smallberg, S. A., Summers, R., Rubinow, D. R., Post, R. M., and Goodwin, F. K. (1981). Effects of vasopressin on human memory functions. *Science*, **211**, 601–3.

Weinstein, M. R. (1980). Lithium treatment of women during pregnancy and in the post-delivery period. In *Handbook of Lithium Therapy* . (ed F. N. Johnson), pp. 421–31. MTP Press, Ltd., Lancaster.

Weiskrantz, L. (1977). Trying to bridge some neurophysiological gaps between monkey and man. *Br. J. Psychol.* **66**, 431–45.

Wen, H. L., and Cheung, S. Y. C. (1973). Treatment of drug addiction by acupuncture and electrical stimulation. *Asian J. Med.* **9**, 138–41.

Wesnes, K., and Warburton, D. M. (1978). The effects of cigarette smoking and nicotine tablets upon human attention. In *Smoking Behaviour: Physiological and Psychological Influences*. (ed R. E. Thornton), pp. 131–47. Churchill Livingstone, Edinburgh.

West, E. D. (1981). Electric convulsive therapy in depression: a double-blind controlled trial. *Br. Med. J.* **1**, 355–7.

West, R. E., and Miller, R. J. (1983). Opiates, second messengers and cell response. *Br. Med. Bull.* **39**, 53–8.

Wexler, B. E. (1980). Cerebral laterality and psychiatry: a review of the literature. *Am. J. Psychiat.* **137**, 279–91.

Wexler, B. E., and Heminger, G. R. (1979). Alterations in cerebral laterality during acute psychotic illness. *Arch. Gen. Psychiat.* **36**, 278–84.

Whalley, L. J., Christie, J. E., Bennie, J., Dick, H., Blackburn, I. M., Blackwood, D., Sanchez Watts, G., and Fink, G. (1985). Selective increase in plasma luteinising hormone in drug free young men with mania. *Br. Med. J.* **290**, 99–102.

Whalley, L. J., Rosie, R., Heinz, D., Levy, G., Watt, A. G., Sheward, W. J., Christie, J. E., and Fink, G. (1982). Immediate increases in plasma prolactin and neurophysin but not other hormones after electroconvulsive therapy. *Lancet*, **ii**, 1064–7.

Wheatley, D. (1981). Effects of drugs on sleep. In *Psychopharmacology of Sleep.* (ed D. Wheatley), pp. 153–76. Raven Press, New York.

Whitaker, P. M., Crow, T. J., and Ferrier, N. (1981). Tritiated LSD binding in frontal cortex in schizophrenia. *Arch. Gen. Psychiat.* **38**, 278–80.

White, F. J., Wang, R. Y. (1983). Differential effects of classical and atypical antipsychotic drugs on A_9 and A_{10} dopamine neurones. *Science*, **221**, 1054–7.

Whitehouse, P. J., Price, D. L., Struble, R. G., Clark, A. W., Coyle, J. T., and DeLong, M.R. (1982). Alzheimer's disease and senile dementia: loss of neurones in the basal forebrain. *Science*, **215**, 1237–9.

Whitty, C. W. M., Stores, G., and Lishman, W. A. (1977). Amnesia in cerebral disease. In *Amnesia.* (eds C. W. M. Whitty, and O. L. Zangwill), pp. 52–92. Butterworth, London.

Whitty, C. W. M., and Zangwill, O. L. (1977). Traumatic amnesia. In *Amnesia.* (eds C. W. M.Whitty, and O. L. Zangwill), pp. 118–35. Butterworth, London.

Widlocher, D. Lecrubier, Y, Jouvent, R., Puech, A. J., and Simmon, P. (1977). Antidepressant effect of salbutamol. *Lancet*, **ii**, 767–8.

Wied, D., de., (1969). Effects of peptide hormones on behaviour. In *Frontiers of Neuroendocrinology.* (eds. W. F. Ganong, and L. Martini), pp. 97–140. Oxford University Press, New York.

Wied, D., de., (1974). Pituitary-adrenal system hormones and behaviour. In *The Neurosciences.* Third Study Program (eds. F. O. Schmidt, and F. G. Warden), pp. 653–66. MIT Press, Cambridge, Mass.

Wied, D., de., (1984a). The importance of vasopressin in memory. *Trends Neurosci.* **7**, 63–4.

Wied, D., de., (1984b). The importance of vasopressin in memory. *Trends Neurosci.* **7**, 109.

Wied, D., de., and Gispen, W. H. (1977). Behavioural effects of peptides. In *Peptides in Neurobiology.* (ed. H. Gainer), pp. 397–448. Plenum Press, New York.

Wiesel, T. N., and Hubel, D. H. (1963). Single cell response in striate cortex of kittens deprived of vision in one eye. *J. Neurophysiol.* **26**, 1003–17.

Wiesnieski, H. M., and Iqbal, K. (1980). Ageing of the brain and dementia. *Trends Neurosci.* **3**, 226–8.

Wilbur, R., and Kulik, F. A. (1981). Gray's cybernetic theory of anxiety. *Lancet*, **ii**, 803.

Wilbur, R., and Kulik, A. V. (1983). Propranolol for akathisia. *Lancet*, **ii**, 917.

Wilcock, G. K., and Esiri, M. M. (1983). Age and Alzheimer's disease. *Lancet*, **ii**, 346.

Wilkins, A. J., Jenkins, W. J., and Steiner, J. A. (1983). Efficacy of clonidine in treatment of alcohol withdrawal state. *Psychopharmacology*, **81**, 78-80.

Wilkinson, R. T. (1965). Sleep deprivation. In *The Physiology of Human Survival*. (eds O. G. Edholm, and A. L. Bacharach), pp. 399-430. Academic Press, London.

Williams, D. G. (1980). Effects of cigarette smoking on immediate memory and performance in different kinds of smoker. *Br. J. Psychol*. **71**, 83-90.

Williams, M. (1977). Memory disorders associated with electroconvulsive therapy. In *Amnesia*. (eds C. W. M. Whitty, and O. L. Zangwill), pp. 183-98. Butterworth, London.

Williams, M. (1984). Adenosine—a selective neuromodulator in mammalian CNS? *Trends Neurosci*. **7**, 164-8.

Willner, P. (1984). The validity of animal models of depression. *Psychopharmacology*, **83**, 1-16.

Willner, P., and Montgomery, T. (1980). Neurotransmitters and depression: too much, too little, too unstable—or not unstable enough? *Trends Neurosci*. **3**, 201.

Wilson, P. R., and Yaksh, T. L. (1980). Pharmacology of pain and analgesia. *Anaesth. Intens. Care*. **8**, 248-56.

Wise, R. A. (1980). The dopamine synapse and the notion of 'pleasure centres' in the brain. *Trends Neurosci*. **3**, 91-5.

Wodak, A. D., Saunders, J. B., Ewusi-Mensah, I., Davis, M., and Williams, R. (1983). Severity of alcohol dependence in patients with alcoholic liver disease. *Br. Med. J*. **287**, 1420-2.

Wolfe, B. B., Harden, T. K., Sporn, J. R., and Molinoff, M. (1978). Presynaptic modulation of beta adrenergic receptors in rat cerebral cortex after treatment with antidepressants. *J. Pharmac. Exp. Therap*. **207**, 446-57.

Wood, P. L., and Stotland, L. M. (1980). Actions of enkephalin, mu and partial agonist analgesics on acetylcholine turnover in the rat brain. *Neuropharmacol*. **19**, 975-82.

Woods, B. T. (1983). Is the left hemisphere specialised for language at birth? *Trends Neurosci*. **6**, 115-17.

Woods, B. T., and Wolf, J. (1983). A reconsideration of the relation of ventricular enlargement to duration of schizophrenic illness in schizophrenia. *Am. J. Psychiat*. **140**, 1564-70.

Woods, J. H. (1978). Behavioural pharmacology of drug self-administration. In *Psychopharmacology: A Generation of Progress*. (eds M. A. Lipton, A. DiMascio, and K. F. Killam), pp. 595-607. Raven Press, New York.

World Health Organisation (1979). *Schizophrenia: an International Follow-up Study*. J. Wiley & Sons, Chichester.

Worrall, E. P., Moody, J. P., Peet, M., Dick, P., Smith, A., Chambers, C., Adams, M., and Naylor, G. J. (1979). Controlled studies of the acute antidepressant effects of lithium. *Br. J. Psychiat*. **135**, 255-62.

Wouters, W., and Bercken, J. van den.(1980). Effects of met-enkephalin on slow synaptic inhibition in frog sympathetic ganglion. *Neuropharmacol*. **19**, 237-43.

Wyatt, R. J., Fram, D. H., Buchbinder, R., and Snyder, F. (1971a). Treatment of intractible narcolepsy with a monoamine oxidase inhibitor. *New Engl. J. Med*. **285**, 987-91.

Wyatt, R. J., and Gillin, J. C. (1976). Biochemistry and human sleep. In *Pharmacology of Sleep*. (eds R. L.Williams, I. Karacan, and J. H. Masserman), pp. 239–74. John Wiley & Sons Inc., New York.

Wyatt, R. J., Neff, N. H., Vaughan, T., Franz, J., and Ommaya, A. (1974). Ventricular fluid 5-hydroxyindoleacetic acid concentrations during human sleep. In *Serotonin—New Vistas*, Adv. Biochem. Psychopharmacol. Vol. II. (eds E. Costa, G. L. Gessa, and M. Sandler), pp. 193–7. Raven Press, New York.

Wyatt, R. J., Portnoy, B., Kupfer, D. J., Snyder, F., and Engleman, K. (1971b). Resting plasma catecholamine concentrations in patients with depression and anxiety. *Arch. Gen. Psychiat.* **24**, 65–70.

Yaksh, T. L. (1982). Opioid peptides and analgesics: sites of action. In *Advances in Pharmacology and Therapeutics II Vol.1. CNS Pharmacology—Neuropeptides.* (eds H. Yoshida, Y. Hagihara, and S. Ebashi), pp. 29–38. Pergamon Press, Oxford.

Yaksh, T. L., and Hammond, D. L. (1982). Peripheral and central substrates involved in the rostral transmission of nociceptive information. *Pain*, **13**, 1–85.

Yaksh, T. L., and Rudy, T. A. (1978). Narcotic analgetics: CNS sites and mechanisms of action as revealed by intracerebral injection techniques. *Pain*, **4**, 299–359.

Yamminga, C. A., Crayton, J. W., and Chase, T. N. (1979). Improvement in tardive dyskinesia after muscimol therapy. *Arch. Gen. Psychiat.* **36**, 595–8.

Yanagida, H. (1978). Congenital insensitivity and naloxone. *Lancet*, **ii**, 520–1.

Yanagita, T. (1981). Dependence-producing effects of anxiolytics. In *Handbook of Experimental Pharmacology*, (eds H. Hoffmeister, and G. Stille), Vol. 55. pp. 395–408. Springer-Verlag, Berlin.

Yorkston, N. J., Gruzelier, J. H., Zaki, S. A., Hollander, D., Pitcher, D. R., and Sergeant, H. G. S. (1977a). Propranolol as an adjunct to the treatment of schizophrenia. *Lancet*, **ii**, 575–8.

Yorkston, N. J., Gruzelier, J. H., Zaki, S. A., Hollander, D. Pitcher, D. R., and Sergeant, H. G. S. (1977b). Propranolol in chronic schizophrenia. *Lancet*, **ii**, 1082–3.

Yorkston, N. J., Zaki, S. A., Malik, M. K. W., Morrison, R. C., and Havard, C. W. H. (1974). Propranolol in the control of schizophrenic symptoms. *Br. Med. J.* **4**, 633–5.

Yorkston, N. J., Zaki, S. A., Weller, M. P., Gruzelier, J. H., and Hirsch, S. R. (1981). L-propranolol and chlorpromazine following admission for schizophrenia. *Acta. Psychiat. Scand.* **63**, 13–27.

Young, B. G. (1974). A phenomenological comparison of LSD and schizophrenic states. *Br. J. Psychiat.* **124**, 64–74.

Young, J. P. R., Hughes, W. C., and Lader, M. H. (1976). A controlled comparison of flupenthixol and amitriptyline in depressed outpatients. *Br. Med. J.* **1**, 1116–18.

Young, J. Z. (1966). *The Memory System of the Brain.* Oxford University Press, Oxford.

Young, J. Z. (1979). Learning as a process of selection and amplification. *J. Roy. Soc. Med.* **72**, 801–14.

Zacur, H. A., Foster, G. V., and Tyson, J. E. (1976). Multifactorial regulation of prolactin secretion. *Lancet*, **i**, 410–12.

Zander, K. J., Fischer, B., Zimmer, R., and Ackenheil, M. (1981). Long-term treatment of chronic schizophrenic patients: clinical and biochemical effects of withdrawal. *Psychopharmacology*, **73**, 43–7.

Zangwill, O. L. (1977). The Amnesic Syndrome. In *Amnesia*. (eds C. W. M. Whitty, and O. L. Zangwill), pp. 104–35. Butterworth, London, Boston.

Zebrowska-Lupina, I. (1980). Presynaptic alpha-adrenoceptors and the action of tricyclic antidepressant drugs in behavioural despair in rats. *Psychopharmacology*, **71**, 169–72.

Zeelen, F. J. (1980). Chemistry (Structure and Activity). In *Frontiers in Neuropsychiatric Research*. (eds E. Usdin, M. Goldstein, A. J. Friedhoff, and A. Georgatas), pp. 352–68. Macmillan Co., London.

Zeisel, S. H., Reinstein, D. K., Wurtman, R. J., Corkin, S., and Growdon, J. H. (1981). Memory disorders associated with ageing. *Trends Neurosci.* **4**, viii–ix.

Zelsen, C., Lee, S. J., and Casalino, M. (1973). Comparative effects of maternal intake of heroin and methadone. *New Engl. J. Med.* **289**, 1216–19.

Ziegler, W. H., and Schalch, E. (1982). Antagonism of benzodiazepine-induced sedation in man. In *6th European Congress of sleep research abstracts*. Zurich: Pharmakologisches Institut der Universitat Zurich. (ed. A. Borbely), p. 128.

Zimmerman, M. (1981). Physiological mechanisms of pain and pain therapy. *Triangle (Sandoz)*. **20**, 7–17.

Zornetzer, S. F. (1978). Neurotransmitter Modulation and Memory: A New Neuropharmacological phrenology. In *Psychopharmacology: A Generation of Progress*. (eds M. A. Lipton, A. DiMascio, and K. F. Killam), pp. 637–49. Raven Press, New York.

Index